Ergonomics

for Therapists

Ergonomics
for Therapists

KAREN JACOBS
EdD, OTR/L, CPE, FAOTA

Clinical Professor
Department of Occupational Therapy and Rehabilitation Counseling
Sargent College of Health and Rehabilitation Sciences
Boston University
Boston, Massachusetts

third edition

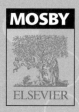

MOSBY

ELSEVIER

MOSBY
ELSEVIER

11830 Westline Industrial Drive
St. Louis, Missouri 63146

ERGONOMICS FOR THERAPISTS   978-0-323-04853-8

Notice

Neither the Publisher nor the Author assumes any responsibility for any loss or injury and/or damage to persons or property arising out of or related to any use of the material contained in this book. It is the responsibility of the treating practitioner, relying on independent expertise and knowledge of the patient, to determine the best treatment and method of application for the patient.

The Publisher

Library of Congress Control Number 2007928087

ISBN: 978-0-323-04853-8

Publishing Director: Linda Duncan
Acquisitions Editor: Kathy Falk
Senior Developmental Editor: Melissa Kuster Deutsch
Publishing Services Manager: Patricia Tannian
Senior Project Manager: Sarah Wunderly
Design Direction: Julia Dummitt

Printed in the United States

Last digit is the print number: 9 8 7 6 5 4 3

This book is dedicated to my dear friend
and outstanding occupational therapist
Diana Aja

Love is the bond between heaven and earth

Contributors

Naomi Abrams, MOT, OTR/L
Occupational Therapist, Ergonomic Consultant
NRH Regional Rehab
Bethesda, Maryland

Nancy A. Baker, ScD, OTR/L
Assistant Professor
School of Health and Rehabilitation Sciences
University of Pittsburgh
Pittsburgh, Pennsylvania

Mary Frances Baxter, PhD, OT
Associate Professor
Texas Woman's University
Denton, Texas
Research Coordinator
Rehabilitation Services
The University of Texas MD Anderson Cancer
    Center
Houston, Texas

Valerie J. Berg Rice, PhD, CPE, OTR/L
Human Factors Engineer/Ergonomist, Occupational
    Therapist
US Army
Universal City, Texas

Chetwyn Che Hin Chan, PhD, OT(C)
Professor
Department of Rehabilitation Sciences
The Hong Kong Polytechnic University
Hung Hom, Kowloon
Hong Kong

Susan A. Domanski, BScOT, OT Reg (Ont)
Occupational Therapist
Waterloo, Ontario

Asnat Bar-Haim Erez, PhD
Occupational Therapist
The School of Occupational Therapy
Hadassah and the Hebrew University
Jerusalem, Israel

Daniel Focht, MA, OTR
Therapy Services Coordinator
Tri-State Occupational Health
Medical Associates/Mercy Health Center
Dubuque, Iowa

Robin Mary Gillespie, PhD, MPH
Director
Whole Ergonomics
New York, New York

E. Kent Gillin, MSc
Professor of Ergonomics
Department of Kinesiology
The University of Western Ontario
London, Ontario

Nancy J. Gowan, BHSc(OT), OT Reg(Ont), CDMP
Occupational Therapist, President
Gowan Health Consultants
Wallacetown, Ontario

Ev Innes, BAppSc(OT), MHPEd, PhD, AccOT, MHFESA
Senior Lecturer
School of Occupation and Leisure Sciences
Faculty of Health Sciences
University of Sydney
Lidcombe, New South Wales
Australia

Karen Jacobs, EdD, OTR/L, CPE, FAOTA
Clinical Professor
Department of Occupational Therapy and Rehabilitation Counseling
Sargent College of Health and Rehabilitation Counseling
Boston University
Boston, Massachusetts

Paul C.W. Lam, PhD
Occupational Therapist
Elderly Resources Centre
Hong Kong Housing Society
Hong Kong

Tatia M.C. Lee, PhD
Professor
Laboratory of Neuropsychology
The University of Hong Kong
Pok Fu Lam Road
Hong Kong

Jenny Legge, BPhty, Merg
Founder/Managing Director/CEO
JobFit Systems International
Mt. Pleasant, Queensland
Australia

Rhysa Tagen Leyshon, MSc(OT), CHT, OT(c)
Graduate Student
Department of Health and Rehabilitation Sciences
The University of Western Ontario
London, Ontario

Cecilia W.P. Li-Tsang, PhD, MPhil, PDOT, OT(C), HKROT
Associate Head and Associate Professor
Department of Rehabilitation Sciences
The Hong Kong Polytechnic University
Hung Hom, Kowloon
Hong Kong

Rosemary Lysaght, PhD, OT
Assistant Professor
School of Rehabilitation Therapy
Queen's University
Kingston, Ontario

Denise M. Miller, MBA, OTR/L
Outpatient Supervisor
Glendale Adventist Therapy and Wellness Center
Los Angeles, California

Jill J. Page, OTR/L
Industrial Rehabilitation Consultant
Ergoscience, Inc.
Birmingham, Alabama

Alan Salmoni, PhD
Professor
School of Kinesiology
The University of Western Ontario
London, Ontario

Charissa C. Shaw, MA, OTR
President
Elysian Integrated Health Solutions
Long Beach, California

Lynn Shaw, PhD
Assistant Professor
School of Occupational Therapy
Faculty of Health Sciences
The University of Western Ontario
London, Ontario

Orit Shenkar, MSc, PhD
Occupational Therapist
The School of Occupational Therapy
Hadassah and the Hebrew University
Jerusalem, Israel

Ellen Rader Smith, MA, OTR, CPE
Principal Ergonomist
Ergo & Rehab Services
Towaco, New Jersey

Sandi J. Spaulding, PhD, OTR, OT(C)
Associate Professor
School of Occupational Therapy
Faculty of Health Sciences
The University of Western Ontario
London, Ontario

Susan Strong, BScOT Reg (ON), MSc(DME)
Associate Clinical Professor
School of Rehabilitation Science
McMaster University
Coordinator of Program Evaluation/Research
Schizophrenia Service
St. Joseph's Healthcare
Hamilton, Ontario

Connie Y.Y. Sung, MPhil
Graduate Student
Department of Rehabilitation Services
The Hong Kong Polytechnic University
Hung Hom, Kowloon
Hong Kong

Patrice L. (Tamar) Weiss, PhD
Professor
Department of Occupational Therapy
University of Haifa
Haifa, Israel

Melanie Weller, BHScOT, OT Reg. (Ont.)
Occupational Therapist
Gowan Health Consultants
Wallacetown, Ontario

Foreword

The fields of ergonomics, occupational therapy, and physical therapy have grown increasingly intertwined as professional knowledge and skills are blended to advance applications that optimize human well-being and performance. Practice applications cover many different populations, from able-bodied individuals to those with disabilities, and from infants to senior citizens. Societal trends play a major role in influencing the focus and expansion of practice. An aging population and the proliferation of technologies into seemingly all facets of life are examples of trends having a profound impact on populations, environments, and occupations.

The impact these trends have on human performance continues to challenge ergonomics and therapy practices. Interactions between people, environment, and occupations are often complex. As workforce demographics, work methods, schedules, and environments become increasingly nontraditional, the need for analysis of human capabilities, limitations, and characteristics to design for efficiency, effectiveness, and safety will continue to be paramount.

Not only do societal trends shape ergonomics and therapy practice, but practice applications can influence societal trends. The future is rich with opportunities for collaboration between the fields to create more sophisticated and comprehensive analyses of conditions that present risks to health and safety and inform decision making to promote health and productivity. Advancements in practice have the potential to revolutionize our world of work, home life, and leisure activities. Practice skills, coupled with creativity and ingenuity, have the power to spark innovations in the design of new products, technologies, and services. This text serves as a valuable resource to those with a passion to make a difference.

Phyllis M. King, PhD, OT, FAOTA
Professor
Director, Occupational Therapy Program
Associate Director, Center for
Ergonomics
University of Wisconsin-Milwaukee

Preface

Ergonomics—a science that continues to evolve and grow and a field that provides almost limitless opportunities for occupational and physical therapists with expertise in this area.

I am delighted that you have selected *Ergonomics for Therapists* to help guide your best practice. It is a tool to help you develop expertise in ergonomics as well as a resource for those of you already practicing in ergonomics. The contributors and I feel great satisfaction in providing you with cutting-edge chapters on important aspects of ergonomics.

Organization

This third edition of *Ergonomics for Therapists*, like its predecessor, is a user-friendly text divided into six parts:
1. Overview and Conceptual Framework
2. Knowledge, Tools, and Techniques
3. Special Considerations
4. Application Process
5. Resources
6. Appendixes

New to This Edition

All the chapters included in the last edition have been thoroughly revised or rewritten for this edition to include the current evidence-based science by 31 experts from five countries who contributed to this text. The following new chapters that broaden the scope of this book are included:
- Macroergonomics
- Ergonomics and work assessments
- Ergonomics of children and youths
- Ergonomics of aging
- Ergonomics of play and leisure
- Entrepreneurship

Distinctive Features of This Book

To facilitate your using *Ergonomics for Therapists* as a training tool, each chapter has the following features:
- *Learning objectives*
- *Glossary boxes* containing key words and definitions

- *Case studies* that are threaded throughout the chapter
- *Learning exercises,* which engage the reader to apply the chapter information to real-life situations and help the reader perform assessments
- *Multiple choice review questions*

Another feature is the *Appendixes* that contain additional case studies, ergonomic information sheets for consumers that can be photocopied to give to clients, and measurement conversions commonly used in ergonomics.

Acknowledgments

"The quality of life is determined by its activities."

Aristotle

My appreciation and gratitude are extended to all of the authors who have shared their expertise within the pages of this book. I offer appreciation to Kathy Falk, Melissa Kuster, and Sarah Wunderly at Elsevier for using their creative skills to make this edition of *Ergonomics for Therapists* even better than its predecessor.

To my family and friends, you are always the "wind beneath my wings." Thank you for always being there for me.

Karen Jacobs
kjacobs@bu.edu

Contents

Ergonomics

for Therapists

1

Ergonomics and Therapy: An Introduction

Valerie J. Berg Rice

Learning Objectives

After reading this chapter and completing the exercises, the reader should be able to do the following:

1. Understand the unique contributions of occupational therapy, physical therapy, and ergonomics (human factors engineering) professionals to the study, analysis, and improvement of work and work conditions; returning individuals with disabilities to work; and designing products specifically for human use.
2. Describe the historical beginnings of the professions of occupational therapy, physical therapy, and ergonomics.
3. List some basic principles of ergonomics.
4. List professional terms that have been considered synonymous with *ergonomics.*
5. Understand and discuss the need for and limitations of the current state of the art of research and design efforts for populations with disabilities.

Ergonomics. The study of work performance with an emphasis on worker safety and productivity.
Occupational therapy. Skilled treatment that helps individuals achieve independence in all facets of their lives (www.aota.org).

Physical therapy. The assessment, prevention, and treatment of movement dysfunction and physical disability, with the overall goal of enhancing human movement and function.

CASE STUDY

A large health care company just heard about ergonomics. They own a number of full-service hospitals, rehabilitation centers, and even day-care centers for children with disabilities. They want to improve their services and heard that occupational therapy and physical therapy often deal with ergonomics, so they have called your group and asked for "full ergonomic consultation services" for all of their facilities. Your group could certainly use the income and reputation in the field. What do you tell them? Do you accept immediately? How will you discover what they really need and what you can comfortably offer within your areas of expertise?

This chapter defines *ergonomics* and provides brief histories of the fields of occupational therapy (OT), physical therapy, and ergonomics. It also describes the relationships between therapists and ergonomists in three areas of practice: (1) workplace analysis, (2) environment and product design and redesign, and (3) research. Principles of therapy and ergonomics are considered in relation to persons with permanent disabilities; persons with temporary injuries, such as work-related musculoskeletal disorders; and persons without disabilities. This chapter also profiles considerations for joint ventures between therapists and ergonomists.

HISTORICAL BACKGROUND

Occupational Therapy

OT is predicated on the belief that eradication of disease alone is insufficient for complete recovery. Before the advent of OT, individuals who had been injured or ill were hospitalized, treated, and discharged, only to find themselves unable to function sufficiently because of physical and mental exhaustion. George Barton, an originator of OT, spent extensive time as a client in a tuberculosis hospital and recognized the need for additional therapy. Trained as an architect, he formed his own rehabilitation program after leaving the hospital by working with the tools of his profession to strengthen himself physically and mentally. In 1914 he opened Consolation House to provide similar services for others. Other founders of the field of OT held similar beliefs that occupying one's time and doing something of purpose serve both as evaluative tests and as tools for "strength, reserve force, nerve and mental poise, and of the several elements that we take together as character."[7]

What was important for the founders of OT was that the individual have pursuits that were important to him or her. The purposeful involvement helped reduce weaknesses caused by illness or injury by building on personal strengths, allowing people to return as productive members of their families and society. Dr. Adolph Meyer, another of the founders of OT, asked his colleagues at the Chicago Pathological Society in 1893 for their opinions on the types of occupations that could best be used during patient treatment. Gardening, ward, and shop work were mentioned, including raffia and basket work, weaving, bookbinding, carpentry, and metal and leather working.[55] These crafts were not considered leisure activities as they are today; instead, the practice of a craft was an assignment that provided rehabilitation for the client and could be used as full-time employment to support the client and client's family after discharge. Thus, the OT rehabilitation process focused on improving physical and mental functioning, as well as returning the patient to a functional status in society. Indeed, these activities were often used to train patients for specific jobs, and it was with great alarm that therapists first realized their patients did not always enter the craft field for which they had been trained. Questions arose regarding whether time, effort, and funds had been wasted in training if the clients did not enter the field for which they had been trained. It was noted, however, that with just a few carefully chosen, occupationally based crafts, the habits and skills needed for rehabilitation and employment could be learned and transferred to numerous jobs.[62] Crafts were categorized according to the physical movements (upper and lower extremity, torso, head and neck), balance, and coordination required, as well as according to complexity, pace, stimulation level provided (monotonous or stimulating), the level of problem-solving skills required, initial cost, final product use, level of concentration needed, initiative required, noise created, amount of mental capacity required, and type of client for which it might be appropriate.[5] Thus, the need for simulating the job each client wanted to return to, or undergoing specific new training for a particular occupation, was eliminated.

The question of whether using a few well-chosen activities for rehabilitation is more effective than individual job simulation has still not been clearly answered through outcome research. Work hardening, or the simulation of the work environment as a means for recovery of ability, has revived the idea that each job and its commensurate job tasks need to be recreated to provide the best possible rehabilitation and return-to-work programs for the industrial worker, but no proof for either argument exists, except anecdotally. The intent is clear, however, that actively engaging the patient in carefully guided physical and mental activities enhances the chances for a more successful return to work.

The fundamental goal of OT is to enhance "the capacity [of the client] throughout the life span, to perform with satisfaction to self and others those tasks and roles essential to productive living and to the mastery of self and the environment."[33] OT should also help clients obtain their highest functional performance in all areas of life, including work, recreational activities, and life at home. Clearly, though, the main focus of OT is working with clients (as opposed to the global workforce population). That is, OT focuses on those individuals who need assistance in order to achieve independent and satisfying lives. According to the American Occupational Therapy Association's website (www.aota.org), OT is skilled treatment that helps individuals achieve independence in all facets of their lives. OT assists people in developing the "skills for the job of living" necessary for independent and satisfying lives. Services typically include the following:

- Customized treatment programs to improve one's ability to perform daily activities
- Comprehensive home and job site evaluations with adaptation recommendations
- Performance skills assessments and treatment
- Adaptive equipment recommendations and usage training
- Guidance for family members and caregivers

Both occupational therapists and ergonomists are trained to be aware of normal human abilities. Therapists must be aware of clients' current physical, cognitive, and psychologic limitations and capabilities; their potential abilities and disabilities; and the physiologic and psychologic demands of the clients' activities (including work). Therapists must also be aware of the performance competencies and limitations of people without injuries to be able to assess whether a client is functioning within normal range. Maximal functional performance has been the goal of OT since the inception of the profession in 1917 (beginning with the founding of the National Society for the Promotion of Occupational Therapy). The use of purposeful activities (e.g., work simulation) as treatment modalities was integral to the development of the profession, as suggested by its name: *occupational* therapy. It must be noted, however, that work or activity used in a therapeutic manner is not ergonomics, nor is work hardening necessarily a part of ergonomics.

The first articles appearing in OT literature to use ergonomic principles were published by Haas in the late 1920s and early 1930s. The first article involved what has been termed *ergonomics-for–special populations*.[64] Haas designed and constructed a weaving frame that could be used for those who were bedridden.[30] The second article described the combination of the principles of OT (therapeutic activity) with the needs of the hospital (increasing work efficiency): the clients were assigned to build a folding conveying chair for the hospital.[28] As described in a subsequent article, the building of an adjustable stool that encouraged "good" posture helped hasten recovery, maintain health, and increase productivity through the principles of anatomy.[29] None of the early articles applied to the general population; instead, the articles were designs for special client populations.

Physical Therapy

The American Women's Physical Therapeutic Association was founded in 1921, becoming the American Physiotherapy Association in the 1930s, and the American Physical Therapy Association in the 1940s. The early fundamental intention of physical therapy (PT) was "to assess, prevent, and treat movement dysfunction and physical disability, with the overall goal of enhancing human movement and function."[59]

In terms of injury prevention, the overall goal conforms to the objectives delineated by ergonomic engineers, particularly those who design workplaces and equipment for physical safety and effective work performance. That is, the goal of ergonomics, in terms of injury prevention, is to design products, processes, and places to enhance human performance while simultaneously keeping the environment safe. In turn, as industrial consultants, physical therapists often use knowledge of human motion to evaluate safe and effective working postures. Physical and occupational therapists who work in industrial environments also evaluate the limitations and capabilities of workers with injuries (functional capacity assessment) and the demands of the work role (workplace analysis) to establish treatment regimens for those individuals. Assessment and treatment roles are sometimes targeted toward specialty areas, such as back care, strength training, or work hardening. The benefit to companies of having an occupational or physical therapist on an ergonomic team is the increased likelihood of the employee's returning to work earlier, matching worker capabilities with work demands, and preventing injuries. Each of these benefits can translate into increased revenues for a company.[37] A therapist can often provide information about the prognosis of an injury or illness, along with knowledge of the Americans with Disabilities Act (ADA).

The American Physical Therapy Association has established guidelines for "Occupational Health Physical Therapy," which focuses on work conditioning and work hardening programs (available at www.apta.org). Although physical therapists participate in team approaches to solving ergonomic issues, their focus appears to be on the worker with an injury and preventive education.

Ergonomics

Although the concept of ergonomics (also called *human factors*) existed during the Stone Age (humans constructed tools to fit their own hands for hunting and gathering needs), the first documented mention of the field came in 1857, when Wojciech Jastrzebowski published *An Outline of Ergonomics, or The Science of Work Based upon the Truths Drawn from the Science of Nature*[34]:

> "Hail, Thou great unbounded idea of work! God, Who, as the Bible teaches us, cursed mankind and subjected him to work, cursed him with a father's heart; for the punishment was also a consolation. He who complains against his work knoweth not life; work is an uplifting force by which all things may be moved. Repose is death, and work is life!"

Jastrzebowski felt the ideas of work should be studied and preached with the same rigor applied to the more philosophical studies of his time, for he believed that "affections (i.e., beliefs, emotions) are nothing else, but accessories to deeds."[34] According to Jastrzebowski, the study of work, or ergonomics, should involve all aspects of useful work, the four main components of which are physical, aesthetic, rational, and moral (Table 1-1). Jastrzebowski taught that applying each of the four components of work to whatever endeavors one is involved with increases the benefits of those activities exponentially. For example, whereas pure physical work applied to planting might yield a two-for-one harvest, applying aesthetic or sensory forces would increase the yield fourfold. Additional application of intellectual forces would then yield an eightfold gain at harvest time, and so on.[34] His treatise is more complex than this chapter shows; he further subdivided all areas of work. He also sought to identify further areas of study including (1) the animals with which we share work categories, (2) the periods of our lives that are particularly suited to various types of work, (3) the manner of work, and (4) the benefits drawn from work for both the individual and the common good of society. His views are remarkably similar to those of the founders of OT, although the latter applied the theories to

TABLE 1-1	Jastrzebowski's Divisions of Useful Work			
Physical	**Aesthetic**	**Rational**	**Moral**	
Kinetic or motor	Emotional or sensory	Intellectual or rational	Spiritual	
Labor or toil	Entertainment or pastime	Thinking or reasoning	Devotion or dedication	
Breaking stones	Playing with stones	Investigation of a stone's natural properties	Removing stones from the road to remove untidiness and possible suffering for other persons and animals	

Adapted from Jastrzebowski W: *An outline of ergonomics, or the science of work based upon the truths drawn from the science of nature,* Warsaw, 1997, Central Institute for Labor Protection (translated by T Baluk-Ulewiczowa).

individuals who were injured or ill, whereas Jastrzebowski primarily applied his theories to able-bodied persons, with the ultimate objective of bettering humankind.

Ergonomics as a specialty made gains as technologic developments emerged during the industrial revolution. Time and motion studies, considered predecessors of our present day ergonomic discipline, focused on evaluation of work methods, workstation design, and equipment design. They were conducted by numerous investigators, including the Gilbreths, Taylor, Muensterberg, and Binet.[17]

The field of ergonomics received particular attention during World War II, when the complexity of military equipment frequently surpassed the abilities of human operators[18]: "Man had become the weak link."[19] As during World War I, the primary focus was selection and training of personnel; however, even with extensive training, personnel could not always perform as needed.[66] Because selection and training were not providing an acceptable solution, the focus changed to fitting the task or equipment to the person by using human dimensions, capabilities, and limitations as factors in the design process.

After World War II, the Ergonomics Research Society (the current Ergonomics Society) was founded in England, and the first ergonomics text, *Applied Experimental Psychology: Human Factors in Engineering Design* by Chapanis, Garner, and Morgan, was published.[16] In 1957, the Human Factors Society was formed in the United States,

and *Ergonomics,* the journal of the Ergonomics Research Society, began publication. The International Ergonomics Association was formed in 1959 to join ergonomics societies from several countries. Since that time, the field of ergonomics has had tremendous growth, and many areas of specialization have been developed. The interface between humans and computers has given rise to new specializations in ergonomics, and the incident at Three Mile Island accelerated the study of the role of ergonomics in the nuclear power industry. In addition, more attention to product liability has increased the number of ergonomics experts needed in forensics to address design deficiencies, instructions, and warning labels.[66] Other areas that are experiencing considerable growth in awareness of ergonomic issues involve designing for special populations including children (Figure 1-1),[14,50] older adults,[56] and persons with disabilities.[45]

Ergonomics developed from the common interests of a number of professions, particularly engineering, psychology, and medicine. It has remained a multidisciplinary field of study. Ergonomists include professionals with degrees in psychology, engineering, ergonomics, industrial design, education, physiology, medicine, health and rehabilitation sciences, business administration, computer science, and industrial hygiene. However, as the discipline evolved, specific areas of knowledge and practice have been identified, giving rise to bachelor's, master's, and doctoral degree programs, specifically in ergonomics or human

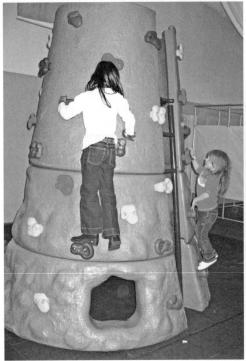

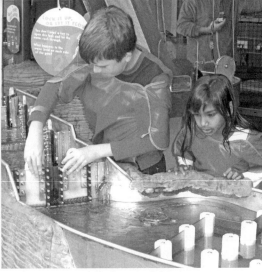

FIGURE 1-1 Ergonomic design for children is challenging. Designs must meet the current physical and cognitive development of the users while simultaneously challenging users to attempt activities at a slightly higher level. Designs must also be appropriate for a relatively wide age range, such as these activities shown at the children's museum in Chattanooga, Tennessee.

factors. The Human Factors and Ergonomics Society (www.hfes.org) offers an accreditation process for these programs. Individual certification is also offered through the Board of Certification in Professional Ergonomics (P.O. Box 2811, Bellingham, WA 98227-2811; www.bcpe.org) (see Chapter 19).

ERGONOMICS DEFINED

Ergonomics (Greek *ergon* [work] + *nomos* [law]) focuses on the study of work performance with an emphasis on worker safety and productivity. Although several definitions have been proposed, one of the best was provided by Chapanis, who used the terms *ergonomics* and *human factors* interchangeably: "Human factors (ergonomics) is a body of knowledge about human abilities, human limitations, and other human characteristics that

are relevant to design. *Human factors engineering* (ergonomics implementation) is the application of human factors information to the design of tools, machines, systems, tasks, jobs, and environments for safe, comfortable, and effective human use."[15] According to the International Ergonomics Association (www.iea.cc), ergonomics (or human factors) is the scientific discipline concerned with the understanding of interactions among humans and other elements of a system, and the profession that applies theory, principles, data, and other methods to design in order to optimize human well-being and overall system performance. Ergonomists contribute to the design and evaluation of tasks, jobs, products, environments, and systems in order to make them compatible with the needs, abilities, and limitations of people.

Considerable debate on the definitions of *ergonomics* and *human factors* has persisted. The controversy has been especially fervent regarding the differentiation of the terms. Proponents of differentiation argue that the term *human factors* was first used in psychology and refers primarily to the interface of humans with technology, whereas *ergonomics* originated in human physiology and biomechanics and therefore refers primarily to physically demanding work.[21] The differentiation is capricious at best, and both the classic and newer human factors and ergonomics texts encourage use of the two terms interchangeably.* In their introduction, Sanders and McCormick state that "some people have tried to distinguish between the two, but we believe that any distinctions are arbitrary and that, for all practical purposes, the terms are synonymous."[66]

In this chapter, as well as throughout this book, the two terms are used interchangeably. It is true that originally *ergonomics* was not as widely used in the United States and Canada as in other parts of the world. In the United States, the terms *human factors engineering, human engineering, engineering psychology,* and *human factors* have all been used, although the current term of choice is *human factors.* As noted by Chapanis, "whether we call ourselves human factors engineers or ergonomists is mostly an accident of where we happen to live and where we were trained."[15] *Ergonomics* is the more recognized term among the general public, even in the United States.

Part I of this text establishes the context in which a therapist chooses to specialize in dealing with work-related issues such as occupational health and ergonomics. It includes both a client-centered approach, as well as a broader macroergonomic perspective.

Ergonomics focuses on humans and their interactions with the environment. It involves interactions with tools, equipment, consumer products, work methods, jobs, instruction books, facilities, and organizations. Kantowitz and Sorkin noted that "the first commandment of human factors is 'Honor Thy User'."[36] Ergonomists design environments and products according to the physical (visual, auditory, tactile, strength, anthropometric), cognitive (learning, information processing, retention), and psychosocial (cultural influences,

behavior, background) characteristics of humans. Accordingly, ergonomics is not solely confined to the workplace. Products and environments should match the abilities, needs, and perceptions of the people who use them. In self-care, ergonomically designed toothbrushes and spigots are found. These spigots conform to users' expectations (e.g., water should emerge when the spigot is turned counterclockwise, and cold water should be controlled by the spigot on the user's right). Bicycles and snow skis are designed with riders and skiers of differing abilities in mind and are designed differently for men and women. Numerous examples of proper and improper designs can be found throughout homes and offices. The concept of making the devices and systems "user-friendly" extends beyond the workplace.[60]

To attain the goal of designing user-friendly devices and systems, ergonomists conduct scientific investigations to identify the limitations, capabilities, and responses of humans in a variety of climates and circumstances. This information is used to produce designs that match human characteristics. Part II of this book, Knowledge, Tools, and Techniques, provides some necessary basic information, as well as examples of how physical and cognitive information can be applied in the workplace.

Part III, Special Considerations, demonstrates how human characteristics are applied to specific situations. Ergonomists evaluate equipment, jobs, work methods, and environments to ensure they meet their intended objectives. This section is more specific, using a microergonomic approach.

Ergonomics can be considered a design philosophy that focuses on supplying a product that ensures safety, ease of use, comfort, and efficiency. However, many distinguished human factors practitioners and ergonomists contend that ergonomics is a unitary, scholarly discipline with unique characteristics, just as OT and PT are unique disciplines.[52-54]

WHY USE ERGONOMICS?

For the lay person, ergonomics is most noted when absent. This is because the focus is to optimize the relationship between the environment and the person.[12,36] When an appropriate ergo-

---

*References 21, 26, 32, 38, 46, 54, 72.

nomic design is in use, the user should be unaware of environmental design deficiencies and should be able to concentrate on the task at hand. For example, in a well-designed office workstation, a worker should not have to hold his or her neck in an awkward posture to use a visual display terminal and should not experience neck and shoulder discomfort. According to Osborne, good ergonomic design in the workplace offers a means to "victory over the oppressive forces that continue to make work less productive, less pleasant, less comfortable, and less safe."[58]

In the past, industry focused on product outcome, and the needs of workers took second place. Humanistic and economic concerns and litigation, however, have convinced industry that consideration of the worker is good business. The use of sound ergonomic principles has generated many examples of increased worker productivity and safety. One older example demonstrated that less training is required if workers' abilities are considered in the design of equipment. In this example, the detection efficiency of machine parts inspectors was evaluated after either a 4-hour training program or the use of a set of visual aids and displays that assisted with the detection of defects. A 32% increase in detected defects was found with the training, a 42% increase was found with the use of appropriate visual aids, and a 71% increase was found when training and visual aids were combined.[13] Although training was useful, a properly designed environment was needed for superior results.

In terms of the case study mentioned at the beginning of the chapter, asking to have ergonomic consultation for all of their facilities and services is a huge endeavor! Ergonomists could start by evaluating the following:

- Safety practices, procedures, and records, including deaths, injuries, and near-miss occurrences in terms of patient safety
- Injuries, illnesses, turnover, and workers' compensation cases among the employees
- The health care practitioners' perceptions regarding the products they use and environments they work in to determine if the designs are as complementary to their work as they should be
- Costs and revenues to see where they might have the most impact on a redesign effort
- Information flow throughout the facilities, including client care, team interactions, and data management

Any of these initial approaches would be within the purview of ergonomics as they seek to design products and places to improve efficiency, effectiveness, and safety. However, it is doubtful that most therapists would be comfortable handling any of these approaches based solely on their entry-level education. With advanced education in the area of work, perhaps they would be most comfortable handling the second approach, especially if the target subset of injuries involved musculoskeletal overuse injuries.

THE INTERRELATIONSHIP BETWEEN THERAPISTS AND ERGONOMISTS

The interrelationship between rehabilitation and ergonomics has received a great deal of attention.[2-4,63,64] More recent efforts by ergonomists are focusing on design issues.[47,48] In fact, ergonomic practice within the field of health care is burgeoning, with research being conducted in areas as varied as teamwork,[6,51] client safety,[9,70] information transfer,[27] cognitive strategies used by clinicians,[8] and the design of equipment,[35] client care areas,[23] and protocol workflow.[1]

Therapists and ergonomists share some common interests, and therapists can contribute their unique strengths to the practice of ergonomics in five principal areas: ergonomics-for-one (individuals who have a disability); ergonomics for special populations; prevention of musculoskeletal injuries; equipment design; and the application of the ADA.[64] These five areas can be simplified into three major practice application arenas, in addition to integrating ergonomic principles into therapeutic clinical practice: (1) workplace analysis aimed at prevention of work-related musculoskeletal trauma; (2) workplace and tool design for individuals with disabilities; and (3) research through the development and use of databases.

Work-Site Analysis

Therapists should be familiar with the field of ergonomics as a whole to understand terminology being used, know how to best describe their own expertise, and recognize when an ergonomist with specialized training should be consulted.[61,68] A review of introductory ergonomics texts (as well as university accreditation requirements for OTs, PTs, and ergonomics) produced the following observations about the knowledge base of therapists compared with that of ergonomists.*

Some areas of ergonomics with which therapists are familiar are sensory nervous system considerations, anthropometry, kinesiology, human development, anatomy and physiology, work capability analysis, and basic research. Areas familiar to occupational therapists (less so to physical therapists, based on their required training) include communication, learning, motivation, normal and abnormal psychology (including the effects of stress), job and task analysis, and measures of job satisfaction. Workplace design, seating and posture, and safety may or may not be included in the knowledge of entry-level therapists. Topics in ergonomics with which entry-level therapists may be unfamiliar include person-machine communication (displays and controls), workstation design, vibration, noise, temperature, illumination, training, inspection and maintenance, error and reliability, signal detection theory, visual displays, legal aspects of product liability, physics as applied to machinery as well as human motion, and advanced statistical research methods. Although therapists may consider themselves educated in safety, they may be unfamiliar with safety as it is taught in ergonomics curricula. In these classes, safety includes accident losses; the Occupational Safety and Health Act; standards, codes, and safety documents; designing, planning, and production errors; hazards; acceleration, falls, and other impacts; pressure and electrical hazards; explosions and explosives; toxic materials; radiation; vibration and noise; slip, trip, and fall (traction and physical materials, as well as biomechanics and physiology); and methods of safety analysis.[22,31]

Therapists are well educated in the procedures of problem identification, interviewing, observation, and record review. Their considerable knowledge of anatomy and physiology, neuroanatomy and neurophysiology, kinesiology, and the mechanism and treatment of injuries makes therapists excellent allies for ergonomists. Knowledge of ergonomics allows therapists to apply their expertise by specializing in the field of work-related musculoskeletal ergonomics and injury prevention.

The application of ergonomics for therapists primarily implies workplace consultation directed at preventing musculoskeletal injuries. Therefore, in the case study presented at the beginning of the chapter, therapists' goals would be to promote safety and to decrease the financial costs associated with lost work time, medical treatment, and retraining of hospital employees. Consultative services could be combined with direct services (client treatment) or offered alone. When providing consultative services in addition to direct services, therapists could offer functional capacity testing, work hardening, and graded return-to-work placements along with workplace evaluations. They could also conduct ergonomics workplace evaluations specifically to identify situations that might contribute to musculoskeletal injuries such as task analysis, videotaping, measurement and analysis of equipment and workstations, and workspace analysis (see Lopez[49] and Sanders[65] for technique suggestions in addition to this text). The consultations may be primarily based on physical considerations or may involve psychosocial factors.[10,42] The last part of this book addresses the ergonomics intervention process from the beginning (program development and marketing) through problem identification, analysis, and implementation to the final product (evaluation and report of results).

Design for Individuals with Disabilities

More than 51 million Americans have a physical or mental disability, and 32.5 million have a severe disability.[69] This means that between 11.5% and 18.1% of the total population in the United States has a disability. Individuals who have a disability are less likely to finish high school or to attend college and are more likely to live in poverty.[69] Many of these individuals either do not work or have difficulty finding a job (Figure

---

*References 25, 36, 38, 46, 66, 68.

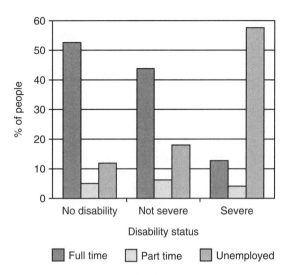

FIGURE 1-2 Percentage of individuals 21 to 64 years of age employed year round in the previous 12 months by disability status in 2002. (Data from U.S. Census Bureau, Survey of Income and Program Participation, June-Sept 2002.)

1-2). Ergonomic intervention could do much to enhance quality of life, at work and home, for these people.

Cannon, an ergonomics consultant in Colorado who has designed equipment for persons with visual impairments, stated, "No segment of the population suffers more from neglect of human factors requirements in product design than the severely handicapped."[26] Unfortunately, that statement remains true 20 years later. Opportunities abound within the areas of overlap between ergonomics and health care. For example, modifications and design features of buildings, vehicles, and appliances could improve independent living prospects for those with physical, cognitive, and emotional disabilities. In the hospital case study running throughout this chapter, therapists might also contribute by evaluating hiring and placement practices with special consideration for those who have disabilities and how the company is meeting ADA compliance. Yet much remains to be done.

Many factors contribute to the lapse of information: seeming unavailability of appropriate resources, lack of data, scarcity of ergonomic concept application in health care and rehabilitation, financial expense, lack of public support for funding, and insufficient databases on which to base designs for special populations. Although the enactment of the ADA in 1990 encouraged both public and private entities to consider individuals with disabilities in the initial designs of workplaces, accommodations, transportation systems, and communication services, the achievements have not been as great as some hoped. Databases are available on hardware and software for persons with disabilities who use computers,[11] and the increase in the geriatric population has increased spending and research on the needs of older Americans. By designing specifically for the older population, their independence and ability to be active and engaged in life improves. Many even learn advanced technologies.[57,67]

Few data exist, however, on the anthropometric characteristics, capabilities, and limitations of individuals with disabilities and elderly populations in varying climates and conditions. The argument that has prevented the collection of such information is that the capabilities and limitations differ with each disease process and each person. This argument contends that all of the individual differences that exist within an able-bodied population also exist within a population of persons with disabilities; however, the differences are compounded because of the additional contrasts in residual capabilities of individuals with disabilities. Until the abilities and restrictions of individuals with disabilities and elderly populations are identified, however, suitable products for their use will not be developed on a consistent basis. As noted, the expansion of the older population has resulted in an increased interest and generation of research in geriatrics.[45,67] A commensurate increase in research for individuals with disabilities has not occurred, however. The resistance, location, and shape of hand and foot controls; workplace design for people who must sit; and seat pan depth and width requirements differ for people with disabilities and vary according to the disabling condition. Therapists have the skills and are in the settings to gather information for a database on various populations with disabilities. Cases of good research exist, however, and one notable exception to the paucity of information is the research conducted by Das[20] on paraplegic workers. Das has carefully researched anthropometric information used in design guidelines for paraplegics, annotated measurements of his own, and developed isometric strength profiles for male and female paraplegics.[20,43,44] Another noteworthy epidemiologic research project identified injuries of wheelchair users and design and selection criteria to assist in injury prevention.[24]

Technologic aids for individuals with disabilities are expensive because small-scale production is not cost-effective. Although this situation may continue for high-level technologic equipment, the concept that assistive equipment designed for individuals with disabilities could also be attractive and useful for the able-bodied population could be further examined.[71] This would entail greater attention to *universal design*—that is, design that is useful for all persons, regardless of age or functional capability. For example, use of large numerals on telephones; large, well-marked keys on television remote controls; and door levers rather than knobs may be equally desirable for people with and without disabilities. Curb cuts outside supermarkets are a fairly simple example of universal design; they make entering and exiting easier for shoppers pushing grocery carts, elderly persons with mobility difficulties, small children, and wheelchair users (Figure 1-3). Another excellent resource is the TRACE Center, which focuses on universal design and accessibility of advanced technologies (information is available at http://trace.wisc.edu).

The development and design of products and places for individuals with disabilities include a need for developmental and operational testing of those products during the prototyping and final design processes. Although therapists and medical practitioners may not typically be involved in product development and user testing, this is another area ripe for collaboration between ergonomists and therapists. Medical and rehabilitation equipment must be designed with the users (medical practitioners, clients, and clients' family members and caregivers) in mind. Thus, iterative testing, including usability testing, is essential to achieve an ergonomic product—one that truly fits

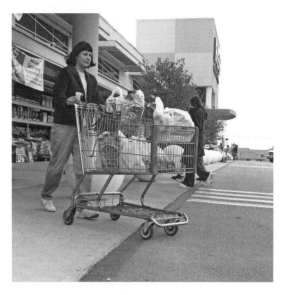

FIGURE **1-3** Curb cuts are an example of universal design. Although they help those in wheelchairs or using walkers, they also benefit children, elderly, and those pushing grocery carts.

the user. Such products can increase user acceptance, decrease errors, increase productivity, and improve quality of life (see Chapter 10).

Therapists can provide ergonomists and design engineers with valuable information on the functional capabilities and limitations of, environmental effects on, and overall prognosis of individual clients and diagnostic groups. The information is essential to development of products for those with disabilities, as well as for identifying needed accommodations for workers with disabilities. These issues are particularly important in accordance with the ADA[39-41] and as our population ages.[45]

Ergonomics applies equally to the interaction of humans and the tools and environments involved in pursuits other than work. Both therapists and ergonomists consult about human performance with regard to recreation, transportation, the hospitality industry, city planning, and the layout and design of home construction. Typically therapists consult regarding those with disabilities, ergonomists consult regarding the healthy population, and both consult regarding musculo-skeletal injury prevention.

Research Interests

Therapists and ergonomists often need the same information on human performance. Therapists can and do use ergonomics data in clinical treatment and prevention programs. For example, when treating hospitalized clients, a therapist should be aware of the effects of diurnal variation on muscle strength during muscle strength testing. Therapists should also be aware of the effects of sleep deprivation on cognition, perceptual-motor performance, and learning. Much of this information is found in ergonomics research among the populations without disabilities.

Therapists use ergonomic data from both able-bodied persons and individuals with disabilities during the evaluation of, goal-setting with, and treatment of clients. It is easy to envision therapists, perhaps primarily those serving in academia, contributing to the body of knowledge in areas such as human performance, neurosensory function, and strength testing, especially as they reflect the functionality of those with disabling conditions.

Certainly, national research goals could be established that would cover the common areas between ergonomics and health care and rehabilitation. Some of these goals might include anthropometric and strength (capabilities and limitations) databases to assist with design for special populations, technology use by and design for special populations, epidemiologic investigations of injuries and illnesses common to people with disabilities with suggestions for prevention, and compilations of ergonomics-for-one success stories.[64]

CONCLUSION

Common interests and areas of practice can allow ergonomists and therapists to blend their knowledge to benefit both populations of individuals with and without disabilities. Three broad practice areas of common interest are workplace evaluation for the prevention of musculoskeletal injuries; environment, workspace, and product design; and research.

Learning Exercises

Overview
These learning exercises are designed to help you use recently acquired information within a professional therapeutic context.

Purpose
These exercises will guide you to an understanding of the interactions between professionals to solve ergonomic challenges in a work setting, as well as encouraging them to think in terms of research and design.

Exercises
1. Have colleagues role-play as an employer, corporate safety officer, and a facilities or plant floor manager experiencing concerns about injuries and ergonomics in a workplace. Have others role-play healthcare and ergonomic team members to include several professionals (minimum: an OT, PT, and an ergonomist). Role play their initial meeting to discover what the healthcare and ergonomic team may have to offer.
   a. Have the employer and the healthcare and ergonomic teams work together to define pertinent issues and areas that need further exploration.
   b. For each issue or area of further exploration, identify what each healthcare and ergonomic team member's role will be, according to their professional expertise. Identify any additional professionals who might assist the team effort.
   c. Write a sequential plan of action, including when reports on progress and findings will be given to the employer team.
   d. Identify questions associated with each issue that might benefit from additional research.
2. Pick an environment, an associated job or task, and an injury or disability (you could even write several on slips of paper and draw them from a hat). Conduct a mental "walk-through" of a person with the injury or disability in that environment. Identify functional issues that could arise, along with some potential design solutions.

Ergonomics, in its broadest sense, is the design of products, environments, and processes to make the world user-friendly for humans by creating items and places that enhance productivity, are pleasant to use and view, and do not injure the user. Although a more specific definition of *ergonomics* has been identified, it is equally important to recognize what ergonomics is not. Ergonomics is not simply "(1) applying checklists and guidelines, (2) using oneself (or non-target populations) as the model(s) for designing objects, or (3) common sense."[66] A "cookbook" approach to ergonomics (checklists) is an embarrassment to the therapist or ergonomist who uses it and is inherently dangerous. Ergonomics also applies to much more than the prevention of work-related musculoskeletal disorders, although it is in this realm that therapists are most adept.

Ergonomics can be a satisfying area of specialization for therapists. It provides therapists with a growth area of specialization in injury prevention. It also is an area that presents considerable challenge for designing better equipment and environments for the clients that therapists serve. Clients, and all persons, deserve to be considered in the design of their equipment and environments. Therapists have the skills, knowledge, and abilities to contribute to the field of ergonomics, and this book provides information and tools to enhance that process.

Multiple Choice Review Questions

1. Which of the following is (are) *not* true regarding the occupational therapy profession? (More than one may be selected.)
   A. Rehabilitation should improve physical and mental functioning.
   B. Rehabilitation should assist with returning an individual to a functional status in society.
   C. Each job a person returns to should be replicated in a therapeutic setting in order to ensure the person can return to his or her job.
   D. Transfer of training occurs easily; therefore work skills in a craft will transfer to a work environment.
   E. Actively engaging a person in carefully guided physical and mental activities enhances the chances for a more successful return to work.

2. Ergonomics began as a multidisciplinary field and developed from the common interests of a number of professions, particularly which of the following? (More than one may be selected.)
   A. Engineering, sociology, and health care
   B. Physical aspects of therapy, industrial psychology, and occupational medicine
   C. Engineering, psychology, and medicine
   D. Anatomy, disability, and work methods (such as those introduced by the Gilbreths)

3. The first commandment of human factors is "Honor thy user."
   A. True
   B. False

4. The primary focus of occupational and physical therapy is to improve the physical and cognitive function of the individual person who has suffered an injury or disability.
   A. True
   B. False

5. The primary focus of ergonomics is design.
   A. True
   B. False

6. Which term has *not* historically been used interchangeably with *ergonomics?* (More than one may be selected.)
   A. Occupational medicine
   B. Human factors engineering
   C. Human engineering
   D. Engineering psychology
   E. Industrial and organizational psychology

7. What percentage of the U.S. population has a disability?
   A. Between 5% and 10%
   B. Between 11% and 18%
   C. Between 19% and 30%
   D. No one really knows, as the research has not been done.

8. Which of the following statements regarding individuals with disabilities is *not* true? (More than one may be selected.)
   A. Those with disabilities have more difficulty locating a job.
   B. Those with disabilities have the same likelihood of finding a job but are less likely to keep a job throughout their lifetime.
   C. Those with disabilities are as likely to finish high school as those who do not have a disability.
   D. Those with disabilities are less likely to attend college.
   E. Those with disabilities are more likely to live in poverty.

9. Some unique contributions of therapists to ergonomic teams include which of the following (*unique* meaning that ergonomists would not also have this knowledge from their basic professional education)? (More than one may be selected.)
   A. Knowledge of disability and disease processes
   B. Knowledge of design
   C. Knowledge of work processes, such as work and communication flow
   D. Knowledge of task analysis, such as the breakdown of tasks into their smallest component parts (sometimes known as "therbligs")
   E. An understanding of the "big picture" of one's work life, such as corporate culture and systems interactions
   F. An understanding of all the aspects of an individual and the impact they can have on his or her functionality, such as family dynamics, personal motivation, and the assumption of the "worker role"

10. Universal design is the design of equipment and products for use by individuals with disabling conditions.
    A. True
    B. False

REFERENCES

1. Alper SJ, Karsh B, Holden RJ et al: Protocol violations during medication administration in pediatrics. In *Proceedings of the Human Factors and Ergonomics Society 50th Annual Meeting*, San Francisco, Calif, 2006, Human Factors and Ergonomics Society.
2. Bogner MS: *Human error in medicine: a frontier for change*, Hillsdale, NJ, 1994, Lawrence Erlbaum.
3. Bogner MS: Medical human factors. In *Proceedings of the Human Factors and Ergonomics Society 40th Annual Meeting*, Santa Monica, Calif, 1996, Human Factors and Ergonomics Society.
4. Bogner MS: Special section preface, *Hum Factors* 38:551, 1996.
5. Bowman M: Report of the round table on crafts for the physically disabled, *Arch Occup Ther* 2:467, 1928.
6. Brown J, Dominguez C, Stahl G: Multidisciplinary perspectives on collaborative care. In *Proceedings of the Human Factors and Ergonomics Society 50th Annual Meeting*, San Francisco, Calif, 2006, Human Factors and Ergonomics Society.
7. Brush F: Occupational therapy for men in the convalescent period, *Arch Occup Ther* 2:87, 1923.
8. Burns C, Momtahan K, Enomoto Y: Supporting the strategies of cardiac nurse coordinators using cognitive work analysis. In *Proceedings of the Human Factors and Ergonomics Society 50th Annual Meeting*, San Francisco, Calif, 2006, Human Factors and Ergonomics Society.
9. Carayon P: *Handbook of human factors and ergonomics in health care and patient safety*, Hillsdale, NJ, 2006, Lawrence Erlbaum.
10. Carayon P, Haims MC: Balanced work system and participation: applications in the community, *Artif Intell Soc* 17(2), 2003.
11. Casali SP, Williges RC: Data bases of accommodative aids for computer users with disabilities, *Hum Factors* 32:407, 1990.

12. Casey S: *The atomic chef,* Santa Barbara, California, 2006, Aegean.

13. Chaney FB, Teel KS: Improving inspector performance through training and visual aids, *J Appl Psychol* 51:311, 1967.

14. Chang HY, Jacobs K, Orsmond G: Gender-age environmental associates of middle school students' low back pain, *Work* 26(1):19, 2006.

15. Chapanis A: To communicate the human factors message, you have to know what the message is and how to communicate it, *Hum Factors Soc Bull* 34:1, 1991.

16. Chapanis A, Garner WR, Morgan CT: *Appl Exp Psychol,* New York, 1949, Wiley.

17. Christensen JM: The human factors profession. In Salvendy G, editor: *Handbook of human factors,* New York, 1987, Wiley.

18. Damon A, Randall FE: Physical anthropology in the Army Air Forces, *Am J Phys Anthropol* 2:293, 1944.

19. Damon A, Stoudt HW, McFarland RA: *The human body in equipment design,* Cambridge, Mass, 1966, Harvard University Press.

20. Das B: Physical disability case study: an ergonomics approach to workstation design for paraplegics. In Rice VJB, editor: *Ergonomics in health care and rehabilitation,* Boston, 1998, Butterworth-Heinemann.

21. Fraser TM: *The worker at work: a textbook concerned with men and women in the workplace,* New York, 1989, Taylor and Francis.

22. Friend MA, Kohn JP: *Fundamentals of occupational safety and health,* 2006, Lunham, Md, Government Institutes.

23. Funk KH, Doolen T, Nicolalde J, et al: A methodology to identify systemic vulnerabilities to human error in the operating room. In *Proceedings of the Human Factors and Ergonomics Society 50th Annual Meeting,* San Francisco, Calif, 2006, Human Factors and Ergonomics Society.

24. Gaal RP, Rebholtz N, Hotchkiss RD, et al: Wheelchair rider injuries: causes and consequences for wheelchair design and selection, *J Rehabil Res Dev* 34(1):58, 1997.

25. Gamache G: *Essentials in human factors,* 2004, Bloomington, Ind, Authorhouse.

26. Gay K: *Ergonomics: making products and places fit people,* Hillside, NJ, 1986, Enslow.

27. Gurses A, Xiao Y, Gorman P et al: A distributed cognition approach to understanding information transfer in mission critical domains. In *Proceedings of the Human Factors and Ergonomics Society 50th Annual Meeting,* San Francisco, Calif, 2006, Human Factors and Ergonomics Society.

28. Haas LJ: A folding conveying chair, *Arch Occup Ther* 7:21, 1928.

29. Haas LJ: An adjustable stool chair, *Arch Occup Ther* 8:367, 1930.

30. Haas LJ: Weaving frame for bedside occupational therapy, *Arch Occup Ther* 4:135, 1925.

31. Hammer W, Price D: *Occupational safety management and engineering,* Englewood Cliffs, NJ, 2000, Prentice-Hall.

32. Helander M: *A guide to human factors and ergonomics,* ed 2, New York, 2005, Taylor and Francis.

33. Hopkins HL: Current basis for theory and philosophy of occupational therapy. In Willard HS, Spackman CS, editors: *Occupational theory,* Philadelphia, 1978, Lippincott.

34. Jastrzebowski W: *An outline of ergonomics, or the science of work based upon the truths drawn from the science of nature,* Warsaw, 1997, Central Institute for Labor Protection [translated by T Baluk-Ulewiczowa].

35. Jessa M, Cafazzo J, Chagpar A et al: Human factors evaluation of automatic external defibrillators in a hospital setting. In *Proceedings of the Human Factors and Ergonomics Society 50th Annual Meeting,* San Francisco, Calif, 2006, Human Factors and Ergonomics Society.

36. Kantowitz BH, Sorkin RD: *Human factors: understanding people-system relationships,* New York, 1983, Wiley.

37. Key GL: Work capacity analysis. In Scully RM, Barnes MR, editors: *Physical therapy,* New York, 1989, Lippincott.

38. Konz S, Johnson S: *Work design: occupational ergonomics,* Scottsdale, Ariz, 2004, Holcomb Hathaway.

39. Kornblau BL: Americans with Disabilities Act and related laws that promote participation in work, leisure, and activities of daily living. In Pendleton J, Schultz-Krohn W, editors: *Pedretti's occupational therapy: practice skills for physical dysfunction,* ed 6, St Louis, 2006, Mosby.

40. Kornblau BL, Hines M: Advocating for clients and legal issues. In Bachner S, Ross M, editors: *Adults with developmental disabilities,* ed 2, Bethesda, Md, 2004, American Occupational Therapy Association.

41. Kornblau BL, Shamberg S, Klein R: Occupational therapy and the Americans with Disabilities Act. Official position paper of the American Occupational Therapy Association, replacing the 1993 position paper, Bethesda, Md, 2000, American Occupational Therapy Association.

42. Korunka C, Scharitzer D, Sainfort F et al: Employee strain and job satisfaction related to an implementation of quality in a public service organization: a longitudinal study, *Work Stress* 17(1):52, 2003.

43. Kozey J, Das B: An evaluation of existing anthropometric measurements of wheelchair mobile individuals. In *Proceedings of the Annual Human Factors Association of Canada Meeting,* Hamilton, Ontario, 1992, Human Factors Association of Canada.

44. Kozey JW, Das B: Determination of the normal and maximum reach measures of adult wheelchair users, *Int J Ind Ergon* 33(3):205, 2004.

45. Kroemer KHE: "Extra-ordinary" ergonomics: how to accommodate small and big persons, the disabled and elderly, expectant mothers, and children, Santa Monica, Calif, 2005, HFES.

46. Kroemer K, Kroemer H, Kroemer-Elbert K: *Ergonomics: how to design for ease and efficiency,* Englewood Cliffs, NJ, 2000, Prentice-Hall.

47. Lin J, Drury CG, Paquet V: A quantitative methodology for assessment of wheelchair controllability. In *Proceedings of the Human Factors and Ergonomics Society 50th Annual Meeting,* San Francisco, Calif, 2006, Human Factors and Ergonomics Society.

48. Loewenhardt RAK: Analysis of bread bag closures for individuals with rheumatoid arthritis. In *Proceedings of the Human Factors and Ergonomics Society 50th Annual Meeting,* San Francisco, Calif, 2006, Human Factors and Ergonomics Society.

49. Lopez MS: Musculoskeletal ergonomics: an introduction. In Rice VJB, editor: *Ergonomics in health care and rehabilitation,* Boston, 1998, Butterworth-Heinemann.

50. Lueder R, Rice V: *Ergonomics for children: designing products and places for toddlers to teens*, New York, Taylor and Francis. In press.

51. McHugh A, Crandall B, Miller T: Barriers and facilitators of common ground in critical care teams. In *Proceedings of the Human Factors and Ergonomics Society 50th Annual Meeting,* San Francisco, Calif, 2006, Human Factors and Ergonomics Society.

52. Meister D: *Conceptual aspects of human factors,* Baltimore, 1989, Johns Hopkins University Press.

53. Meister D: *The practice of ergonomics: reflections on a profession,* Bellingham, Wash, 1997, Board of Certification in Professional Ergonomics.

54. Meister D: *Conceptual foundations of human factors measurement,* Hillsdale, NJ, 2003, Lawrence Erlbaum.

55. Meyer A: The philosophy of occupational therapy, *Arch Occup Ther* 1:1, 1921.

56. Mouloua M, Hancock PA: Preface: the importance of technological solutions to the asymmetric pattern of global aging, *Hum Factors* 47(2):217, 2005.

57. Murata A, Hrokazu I: Usability of touch-panel interfaces for older adults, *Hum Factors* 47(4):767, 2005.

58. Osborne DJ: *Ergonomics at work,* New York, 1982, Wiley.

59. Pinkston D: Evolution of the practice of physical therapy in the United States. In Scully RM, Barnes MR, editors: *Physical therapy,* New York, 1989, Lippincott.

60. Pruitt J, Adlin T: *The persona lifecycle: keeping people in mind throughout product design,* Boston, 2006, Elsevier.

61. Rader Smith E: Evolution of health care and rehabilitation ergonomics. In Rice VJB, editor: *Ergonomics in health care and rehabilitation,* Boston, 1998, Butterworth-Heinemann.

62. Report of the Committee on Installations and Advice: Analysis of crafts, *Arch Occup Ther* 6:417, 1928.

63. Rice VJB: Defining common ground: human factors engineering and rehabilitation, *Rehabil Manage* 5:30, 1992.

64. Rice VJB: *Ergonomics in health care and rehabilitation,* Boston, 1998, Butterworth-Heinemann.

65. Sanders MJ: *Management of cumulative trauma disorders,* Boston, 1997, Butterworth-Heineman.

66. Sanders MS, McCormick EJ: *Human factors in engineering and design,* New York, 1987, McGraw-Hill.

67. Sharit J, Rogers W, Charness N et al: *Designing for older adults: principles and creative human factors approaches,* New York, 2004, Taylor and Francis.

68. Stanton N, Hedge A, Brookhuis K et al: *Handbook of human factors and ergonomics methods,* Boca Raton, 2004, CRC Press.

69. Steinmetz E: Current population reports. In *Americans with Disabilities: 2002,* Washington DC, 2006, U.S. Department of Commerce, Economics and Statistics Administration, U.S. Census Bureau.

70. Tartaglia R: *Healthcare systems ergonomics and patient safety,* Boca Raton, 2005, CRC Press.

71. Wilkoff WL, Abed LW: *Practicing universal design: an interpretation of the ADA,* New York, 1994, Van Nostrand Reinhold.

72. Wilson JR, Corlett EN, editors: *Evaluation of human work: a practical ergonomics methodology,* New York, 1990, Taylor and Francis.

A Client-Centered Framework for Therapists in Ergonomics

Lynn Shaw, Susan Strong

Learning Objectives

After reading this chapter and completing the exercises, the reader should be able to do the following:

1. Understand why a client-centered approach is an integral part of therapists' ergonomic practice.
2. Understand the theory and concepts of a client-centered approach.
3. Understand and apply client-centered practice concepts in return to work and occupational ergonomics to address worker and organizational concerns.
4. Use tools that will help address barriers and support implementation of client-centered principles in practice with a focus on the Person-Environment-Occupation model.

Client-centered ergonomic approach. This approach emphasizes participation of the worker and organization in return to work and occupational ergonomic processes. It is characterized by the equitable involvement, partnership, and clearly understood responsibilities of all key stakeholders such as the worker, the employer, the union or worker representative, health and safety representatives, allied health professionals, ergonomists, engineers, and, where appropriate, vendors or manufacturers.

Occupational ergonomics. The strategies and processes that aim to prevent injury and to promote optimal human performance and functioning at work through workplace systems design, equipment, and tool design.

Return to work. The collaborative processes among the worker, employer and health professional involved in establishing, implementing, progressing, and evaluating a work reintegration plan for enabling a worker with an injury to resume a preinjury job or start a new one.

Person-Environment-Occupation model. This model elaborates an understanding of occupational performance that is characterized by the complex interaction of factors and relationships among the person, the environment, and the occupation. In ergonomics, the person refers to the worker with the ergonomic concern, the environment refers to the workplace, and the occupation refers to the work demands.

For therapists who work in ergonomics, the need to engage the participation of workers and workplaces in the ergonomic process is essential for improving health and productivity outcomes.[26] However, therapists continue to experience many challenges that make it difficult to integrate client-centered values and principles into practice.* Historically, ergonomics has examined the person-machine interface through time and motion studies and anthropometric, biomechanical, and kinesiologic measurements. In these traditional ergonomic applications, ergonomists, therapists, engineers, and kinesiologists provided an expert approach to improving work demands. The current client-centered practice emphasizes participation of the worker and organizations in the process of fitting work to the worker according to the conditions of a particular workplace. The ability of an individual to safely, efficiently, and consistently produce a high-quality product is now viewed as a collection of complex relationships among the worker, his or her occupation, and his or her work environment. Therapists are beginning to examine ergonomic issues in terms of these relationships.[1,26] The concept of *client* in a client-centered ergonomic practice is broadened to refer to the individual worker, but also workplace groups such as unions or work units composed of workers, and the organization such as the employer or supervisors. This broader focus on all of the clients involved in ergonomics builds capacity in the workplace to achieve improved health, safety, and productivity. For instance, attending to worker needs helps enable individuals to proactively manage and apply ergonomic principles in the midst of performing job tasks. Including workgroups or units in ergonomics encourages involvement of worker teams in generating solutions to common problems. Engaging organizations helps to foster a workplace culture that supports the mobilization of resources and implementation of best practices in ergonomics.

A number of factors have shaped this transition toward involvement of workers in the ergonomic process and the needs of the workplace. One factor is the economic climate of restricted costs

and increasing accountability in rehabilitation practice. This trend has encouraged therapists to focus efforts on effectively achieving clients' goals. An underlying premise of client-centered practice is that time and resources are effectively used by concentrating on the issues that are most important to the client (workers and organizations) and by involving the client or clients throughout the process. Furthermore, the evidence suggests that worker involvement leads to positive outcomes. The client-centered approach and increased client participation are associated with better health outcomes,[22,29,34,41] improved practice outcomes such as adherence to goals,[15,19,27] and increased client satisfaction.[24] Involving clients also supports greater client control through ownership of responsibilities and participation in care processes.[37] All of these elements support quality management. Organizations now recognize that happy and satisfied workers perform better.[20,48] It follows that a client-centered practice is consistent with good business practices.

Another factor supporting client-centered approaches is the growing disconnect between providers and employers in the health, return-to-work, and rehabilitation systems in returning workers with injuries to work.[21] Loisel and colleagues[26] recognize the need for greater collaboration in ergonomics through participatory ergonomics not only to prevent injury reoccurrence, but also to reduce chronic disability arising from unsafe and inadequate ergonomic practices. Collaboration underscores the behavior of all persons involved in a client-centered approach. Collaboration assists workers, health providers, insurers, and workplace parties to focus their efforts on shared goals for the client in the return-to-work process.

The other influencing factor for adopting a client-centered approach is the growing endorsement and legitimization of a client-centered approach as a standard of practice through documents and texts (e.g., policies, acts, professional position papers). From the early 1980s to the 1990s, a number of regulations, acts, accreditation criteria, and guiding principles of care within professional associations began to incorporate language in support of more client involvement in

*References 8, 9, 31, 32, 39, 43, 44.

care processes. There are many examples of documents that, in principle, support the adoption of client-centered ideologies within health care. In 1992 the United States introduced amendments to the Rehabilitation Act to include persons with disabilities in making choices and decisions in both rehabilitation and education. Canada followed suit, albeit not at the regulatory level, but through a position paper in 1996 mandating inclusionary practices for the delivery of health and social services for persons with disabilities. This document, entitled *In Unison,*[16] was a step toward participatory health practices in Canada. As early as the 1980s, guidelines for occupational therapy (OT) practice introduced the term *client-centered.*[4-6] Rehabilitation professionals similarly adopted consumer empowerment and involvement as central tenets of practice in United States[35] and Canada.[28] Acceptance of consumers' rights to self-determination by rehabilitation professionals[28] also served to advance the adoption of participatory approaches in North America and Europe.[10,12,25,46]

Such supporting texts have helped to shape and legitimize the implementation of practice models that are more inclusive of health care clients in the delivery of health and rehabilitation services. It follows then that service delivery systems and professional values have evolved to be more client-focused, and that collaborative approaches are becoming central to ergonomic practice in workplaces.

PARTICIPATION AND ERGONOMIC APPROACHES

Many different theoretic approaches are used in ergonomics. The approaches presented are used by therapists within the context of therapeutic practice (enabling return to safe work after injury) or occupational ergonomics (preventing injury and promoting optimal human performance and functioning at work through workplace systems design, equipment, and tool design). Some have roots in other ergonomic applications, and others draw on theories from other disciplines. The seven ergonomic approaches discussed in the following sections are occupational biomechanics,[7] the functional approach,[17] the systems approach,[47] the Ergonomic Tool Kit approach,[3] the multidisciplinary approach,[18] the Person-Process-Environment model approach,[45] and participatory ergonomics.[26]

Theoretically these approaches offer therapists a guide or conceptual framework for applying ergonomic applications in workplaces or in client-therapist interactions. All of these approaches require information about human performance to establish just the right interface with equipment, tools, and work processes. However, the extent of participation and involvement of key stakeholders in the ergonomic process varies depending on the theoretic concepts that underpin the approach and how the therapist applies these concepts in practice. For instance, occupational biomechanics[7] and the systems approach[47] involve information gathering and analysis that leads to including organizations in the design and change process to improve the worker-workplace interface, product design, and/or workplace productivity. The functional approach,[17] the Ergonomic Tool Kit approach,[3] the multidisciplinary approach,[18] and participatory ergonomics[26] may involve the worker and other stakeholders in evaluation and/or change processes to prevent injury or disability as well as supporting return to function and return to work. Incorporating a client-centered approach to ergonomics can provide therapists with a means to achieve greater consistency for quality management by including workers and organizations throughout interactions, assessments, planning, interventions, and monitoring. In addition, the principles underlying a client-centered approach can be used by therapists to foster the necessary positive working relationships needed to improve workplace safety and performance with workers and employers.

CLIENT-CENTERED PRACTICE IN ERGONOMICS

Routinely client-centered practice is a collaborative alliance between client and therapist designed to use their combined skills, strengths, and resources to work toward the client's occupational performance goals. "Occupational therapists demonstrate respect for clients, involve clients in decision making, advocate with and for clients in meeting clients' needs, and otherwise recognize clients' experience and knowledge" (p. 49).[6] The clients may be individuals, groups, agencies, governments, or systems such as families, businesses, organizations, and communities. "Occupational performance refers to the ability to choose, organize, and satisfactorily perform meaningful occupations that are culturally defined and age appropriate for looking after one's self, enjoying life, and contributing to the social and economic fabric of community life" (p. 30).[6] The goal of client-centered practice is to enhance occupational performance, health, and well-being.

When therapists work in the field of occupational ergonomics, they may work with businesses or other organizations that are not directly experiencing occupational performance problems; rather, they may be attempting to promote safety and prevent injury. For instance, a new concern of many workplaces is addressing the needs of aging workers (see Chapter 15). Organizations are seeking consultation with therapists in purchasing equipment or in renovating work sites to proactively redesign workspaces that will optimize occupational performance as workers age. In occupational ergonomics, client-centered practice fosters partnerships and encourages collaborative identification of obstacles and options for intervention that are not only people focused, but also system related. Organizations may have individuals with occupational performance problems (e.g., workers with persistent complaints of inability to perform specific work tasks because of back pain). In addition, various sectors of the organizations may experience occupational performance problems such as decreased productivity owing to a very hot or a very cold work environment, high absenteeism rates, lack of computerization for manual work, or ineffective communication and conflict resolution strategies. Depending on the contractual arrangement, the therapist's consultation may also be with the organization, or with the organization and an external agency (e.g., an insurance agency). This assists the overall process of managing the changes necessary for individuals or groups of workers to perform safely, efficiently, and effectively while maintaining the organization's goals.

A review of client-centered texts such as *Client-Centered Occupational Therapy*[24] and *Client-Centered Practice in Occupational Therapy*[43] and the current literature on involving clients in practice[13,36-38,40] revealed nine principles for consideration in creating a context for participation and partnership in ergonomic practice. These principles represent the concepts and actions common across client-centered approaches and frameworks and are relevant for therapists in return to work and occupational ergonomics. In addition, these principles can guide therapists in enacting a client-centered approach in the worker-therapist dyad, in workgroup interactions as well as in expanded collaborations with workplace stakeholders such as employers, insurers, and health or safety personnel in addressing workplace needs. Each principle is elaborated in the following pages for use in either workplace practice or in occupational ergonomics and then applied to the case study of the Centralized Booking Company. Questions are then posed for students to further explore and integrate concepts and actions required to enact a client-centered practice. Box 2-1 lists the nine principles of client-centered practice in ergonomics.

Box 2-1   *Principles of Client-Centered Practice*

1. Enacting participation and partnering throughout the process
2. Respecting and enabling worker and organization choices, needs, and knowledge
3. Focusing on person-environment-occupation (PEO) relationships in the practice context
4. Addressing physical comfort and emotional support needs of clients
5. Fostering open and transparent communications and knowledge exchange
6. Establishing a shared vision for ergonomic management
7. Establishing shared and realistic goals among work parties
8. Creating opportunities that engage workplace parties in problem solving and decision making
9. Ensuring a flexible and individualized occupational therapy approach

CASE STUDY

An occupational therapist received a request from the manager-owner of a company called the Centralized Booking Company (CBC) to conduct a work site visit and make recommendations to assist in managing ongoing problems with musculoskeletal injuries. The manager of CBC shared his concerns about the growing costs of injuries and the negative impact on profitability. He employs 100 workers to provide a 24-hour booking service for medical, dental, community care, and hospital appointments for national and international clients. At CBC all office workers are required to rotate office duties on a 12-hour basis: 3 days on, 3 days off, 3 nights on, and 3 nights off. Duties include computerized scheduling and booking of appointments for thousands of companies and organizations via a national and international network, invoicing and billing clients, and managing telephone inquiries and customer service relations.

During the initial work site visit the therapist discovered the following:

1. The company purchased and installed new office equipment to improve worker comfort, reduce time lost because of injuries associated with musculoskeletal strain, and improve productivity. Six months after the office redesign, productivity is unchanged and lost-time injury rates and levels of absenteeism remain high. During the work site visit, workers consistently complained of dissatisfaction with the new workstations.

2. The manager requested specific assistance with how to manage a return-to-work for Jean, an employee requesting an accommodation of no shift work. Jean was an office worker who was well liked by her co-workers, and before her injury engaged in social activities with co-workers. Jean was in a car accident and sustained multiple crush injuries to the dominant right hand and a head injury. Her current limitations include decreased sensation and coordination in the hand and fingers as well as figure-ground and visual-perceptual problems.

3. The manager also revealed that he has received complaints from workers regarding fairness of workload in light of the workers who are on limited duties. Up to this point the employer has tried to follow the recommendations from insurance companies and medical professionals; however, he now recognizes that assistance is needed to find better ways to manage disability and workload issues.

Enacting Participation and Partnering Throughout the Process

Enacting a client-centered approach requires a collaborative partnership between workers, workplace parties, employers, external agencies such as insurers, and therapists. These partnerships require a power shift in the expertise and knowledge from the therapist to clients. It goes beyond the conventional involvement of these clients to include a shared responsibility for the identification of ergonomic risks, implementation of goals, and a shared accountability for partnering in administrative activities such as identifying the need to meet, setting meeting agendas, communicating among workers, and giving and receiving feedback about commitment to roles and responsibilities.[32,37] This may involve therapists helping workers and workplace groups develop partnering expertise, for instance, by improving confidence and skills in giving and receiving feedback in groups or as it pertains to occupational performance problems. The therapist can also take a leadership role in educating workers, workgroups, and organizations about the appropriateness and effectiveness of collaboration in facilitating the best approach to solving complex ergonomic issues in the workplace. At this time the therapist can share with organizations and workgroups the growing evidence on collaboration, importance of worker engagement, and the need for multiple perspectives in the management of ergonomics.[1,14,26,37] These actions are required for the worker and workgroups to develop capacity for collaboration in the implementation and evaluation of ergonomic activities at work.

At CBC the therapist recognized the need to evaluate the extent of the workers' and the manager's knowledge about the importance of a collaborative approach in solving ergonomic problems in the workplace. The therapist recommended that an initial meeting with a group of worker representatives and the manager take place to focus on information exchange. To promote engagement and a sense of partnering, each worker and the manager were asked to bring one rule or suggestion for how to make the group meeting successful and to identify how he or she might contribute to the group.

As a therapist you may need to become more aware of your own partnering skills and approach to collaborative care. What are the skills you feel are essential to partnering and collaboration? What skills are you confident in performing? Reflect on and consider an example of how you have practiced or used this skill. Identify the additional skills you need and how you might learn or acquire this expertise.

Respecting and Enabling Clients' Choices, Needs, and Knowledge

Understanding worker, workgroups, and employer preferences, needs, and knowledge is important when enacting a client-centered approach. Respect is demonstrated through listening, actively learning, and understanding. At the worker level, therapists need to consider workers' diverse life experiences, coping styles, and unique backgrounds. Inviting workers to express their preferences, needs, and perceptions about their capacities for work opens the door for workers to feel that their views are valued.

Insight into the workplace culture will also help the therapist gain an appreciation of and demonstrate respect for the past choices, purchases, and knowledge of workers and organizations. This understanding can be achieved through gathering information about the nature and history of ergonomic experiences, responsibilities for ergonomics, and decisions made among workers, unions, and management, as well as the values and attitudes toward safety. Meeting with organizational representatives from management, human resources, and/or occupational health and safety and taking a plant or work site tour will assist the therapist in finding information about safety culture and practices. While on a tour, the therapist can find out how organizational changes are made to improve worker and workplace productivity. Therapists can further reflect on this information to identify potential gaps and new opportunities for organizations to improve programs and involve workers in the ergonomic process.

The therapist respected CBC's recent purchase of workstations and reinforced with the employer that the workstations offered workers the ergonomic flexibility to support safe work practices.

However, during the work site visit the therapist discovered that the workers were not involved in the purchasing decision. This insight provided information on one area where worker choice had been overlooked and the need to emphasize opportunities to include workers and support their input in future in ergonomic processes.

How would you find out about the choices that workers have in managing their health safety at work? What questions would you ask? How would you as a therapist explore the preferences of workers and workplace parties? What kinds of documents would you need? Who would you talk to about workplace culture?

Focusing on Person-Environment-Occupation Relationships in the Practice Context

One of the opportunities in using a client-centered approach is that it supports a holistic approach in the management of ergonomic concerns. At the core of this process is the examination of relationships among the capacities, skills, and resources of workers (person), the multidimensional factors of the work environment (environment), and work demands and processes (occupation) that may contribute to occupational performance issues and their resolution. Occupational performance difficulties of workers and those commonly experienced by groups of workers are closely interwoven with their environments and occupations. Environments are multidimensional and vary from one organization to another (e.g., with respect to policies, norms of behavior, methods of communication, approaches to dispute resolution). Similarly, workers vary in the skills and capacities to meet the physical, emotional, and cognitive demands of work. The person-environment-occupation (PEO) perspective provides therapists with an approach that considers the worker's ergonomic needs in the workplace context while recognizing that the worker's issues are also embedded in the realities and complexities of his or her workplace culture. Implementing an exploration of ergonomic problems using a PEO approach can help all workplace parties stay focused on the problem and solutions and avoid pitfalls such as blaming individuals and/or inadvertently creating tensions and feelings of guilt.

In the following section the full application of using a PEO perspective is elaborated for the case study example.

Addressing Physical Comfort and Emotional Support Needs of Clients

To make informed and effective decisions, clients need to feel comfortable and receive adequate information about occupational performance issues. Frameworks emphasize that therapists need to have an open, caring manner and need to carefully listen to workers' or employer descriptions of problems and needs. The issue of comfort arises when workers are placed in unfamiliar settings or situations such as in planning a return to work after illness or injury. For instance, a worker's comfort may involve the presence of a union representative in the evaluation. No matter the setting, the relationship that the therapist has with the worker or organization ultimately enables success. Recent evidence strongly supports that early and caring supervisor contact with the worker influences return to work. Supervisors who demonstrate concern for the worker's early and safe return to work have positive outcomes.[2,11,33]

The therapist must also pay particular attention to the development and maintenance of relationships with different members of the organization (e.g., union representatives, management, workers, human resources personnel, and health and safety representatives). Information needs to be provided in an understandable format, and the use of language becomes a focus to address potential tensions that may arise from different workplace parties. Most workplaces have previous negative experiences and histories with accommodations or return to work that lead to stereotyping and negative attitudes about workers in co-workers and supervisors. The therapist must emphasize that these attitudes and beliefs need to be bracketed; understood, but also put aside, when interacting with each new worker and each new situation. Likewise, the therapist must also bracket his or her assumptions. Each situation must be addressed anew with an openness to possibilities. The workplace parties must work jointly with the therapist to create an individualized and humanistic context when addressing worker's needs.

Jean and the therapist decided that the best way to conduct an assessment of Jean's workstation needs was to do this at the work site. However, Jean raised concerns about doing this evaluation when many of the other staff may be present. Jean was concerned that she might be perceived as disruptive to others if they went during peak hours and as receiving more attention than other workers. To minimize Jean's anxieties and concerns the therapist and Jean identified opportunities when the work site visit might be conducted. Together they decided to do the workstation evaluation at the beginning of the evening shift when fewer work stations were in use.

What other suggestions would you make to Jean in preparation for this work site visit? What tools and resources does Jean need? What tools and resources do you need?

Fostering Open and Transparent Communications and Knowledge Exchange

To foster open and transparent communications the therapist must identify barriers and challenges that can hinder communications at the individual level when interacting with workers as well as with other workplace parties. At the worker level, workers may fear disclosing information for fear of reprisals in the workplace from employers and co-workers. It is imperative that the therapist be sensitive to the worker's relationship with the employer and that an environment of trust that encourages knowledge sharing and exchange be created. Likewise, at the organizational level the therapist must respect the confidentiality of proprietary information. The therapist must be aware of his or her responsibilities and roles within a client-centered ergonomic approach that will also support knowledge exchange and application by the workers and the organization. Building a foundation of trust involves the therapist, worker, and workplace parties establishing ground rules for what information will be shared with co-workers, employers, and insurers and the information that will remain confidential. In addition, efforts are needed to establish a location and space for requesting information (all questions and concerns are worthy of consideration) and providing opportunities for feedback. In the return-to-work process, the therapist can take the lead in initiating a discussion about disclosure of information as part of the planning process. The therapist can elicit concerns the worker may have and offer potential options for the worker to consider. A proactive approach to help workers identify and resolve communication issues is to rehearse or role-play how the worker will share information with the employer and co-workers. With the worker's consent, the therapist can also meet with co-workers and provide information about co-worker concerns, the return-to-work process, and how co-workers might offer support and encouragement to workers on modified duties.

In consultations about occupational ergonomic concerns, being client-centered requires therapists to engage in sharing knowledge and expertise about ergonomics with all workplace parties rather than withholding information and maintaining a power differential. The aim of this process is to provide the workplace with tools needed to help workplace parties understand and apply ergonomic principles and concepts in the identification and management of ergonomic risks. Educating workers, supervisors, and employers about ergonomics will help them build capacity to evaluate and address workplace concerns.

In discussing a return-to-work plan Jean conveyed her anxieties about how to respond to questions or negative attitudes of co-workers concerning her illness and when she will be back to full duties. To help Jean prepare for these questions the therapist suggested that Jean write out a list of potential questions other people might ask her, then together they would role-play and rehearse appropriate and comfortable responses to these questions before her return to work.

What types of questions and negative attitudes might Jean encounter in returning to work? Generate a list of comments or concerns that other co-workers might express. Create a response to each concern that would assist Jean in maintaining a positive relationship with co-workers and at the same time allow Jean to maintain confidentiality. What information tools or brochures are available in your region that might help you explore with Jean responses about disclosure and her rights in the workplace?

Establishing a Shared Vision for Ergonomic Management

In the workplace, different parties may have different views on how ergonomic outcomes are achieved. Thus, the therapist needs to elicit an understanding of workers', unions', and management beliefs about responsibilities for safe work behaviors. Some parties perceive that safety and ergonomics are an employer's responsibility, or a health and safety department's responsibility, or the therapist's responsibility. In the absence of a shared vision about ergonomic management, therapists need to work with workers and employers to generate a common understanding about ergonomic principles and the types of actions and efforts required at the individual and workplace levels to create opportunities for safe and optimal work performance. A common vision for ergonomic management should outline responsibilities and actions for the identification of risks, the generation of solutions, and a process for evaluation of outcomes. The acceptance of a shared vision for managing ergonomic concerns will lend support for collaboration of all stakeholders as well as provide stakeholders with specific accountabilities. For instance, establishing and implementing a shared vision would allow workers to contribute their knowledge and help them realize their obligations as workers to work safely. Similarly, development of a shared vision on how ergonomic concerns will be managed will support the employer as well as the workers to implement a proactive approach to injury prevention that includes shared responsibilities for addressing problems and supporting safe and optimal occupational performance of workers. In turn, this vision will support workers, supervisors, and management to become partners in the ergonomic process.

CBC does not have a procedure or policy for managing ergonomics. In this workplace, the workers felt left out of previous decision-making processes about the purchase of new workstations and subsequently devalued. This led to negative worker concerns that the employer views safety as something that can be purchased in terms of equipment. On the other hand, the employer is feeling as though he has exhausted all ideas and resources on how to address ergonomic problems and reduce costs associated with injuries. To address these workplace tensions, the therapist recommended that the employer and worker representatives at CBC define and establish a common vision and components of an ergonomic program.

Work in a group and write a vision for ergonomic management at CBC. Include the actions, activities, and responsibilities of workers and management and identify potential outcomes.

Establishing Shared and Realistic Goals

Therapists work in partnership with workers, workgroups, and employers to set goals for outcomes. As mentioned previously, the therapist seeks to understand the knowledge and preferences of workers and managers as well as the resources within the workplace context. This information is also valuable in establishing shared and feasible goals to address ergonomic and return-to-work concerns and to improve outcomes in the workplace. In a collaborative approach, responsibility for goals and outcomes is shared, and thus the success is dependent on the commitment of workers and organizations. This type of process can also support setting goals and a shared action plan for how the interventions will proceed with a clear ownership for worker and employer responsibilities in the plan. In this process workplace parties need to identify what they view as a successful ergonomic program so that their standards are built into the goals and objectives, and their expectations are in line with the shared goals.

Workers will require resources and support to monitor ergonomic needs and forward input needed to generate shared goals. For instance, engaging workers in setting shared goals with management for ergonomics requires that workers engage in the process of evaluating and monitoring ergonomic needs at work. Introducing a form to capture information about common ergonomic problems that cannot be solved at the worker level will support collaboration.

Organizations need objectives not only to help them commit to ergonomics, but also to plan for and mobilize resources needed to ensure the implementation of safe ergonomic practices at work. Resources can include strategic financing of new equipment, workstations, and tools, and it can also include time. Providing the time for people to meet and address ergonomic issues as well as generate solutions is vital to the proactive management of concerns. Shared goals and explicit objectives will ultimately assist organizations in using evidence and knowledge as well as building internal capacity and accountability for addressing ongoing and future ergonomic concerns.

At CBC, the therapist gained worker and management support to set a shared vision for ergonomic management with specific objectives for improving ergonomic outcomes. A committee was set up to meet quarterly to address ergonomic concerns. At the initial meeting the committee decided to establish priorities and goals for immediate, long-term, and ongoing solutions. The committee asked for information from workers, supervisors, and the therapist to identify common and unique problems. For each problem the committee set an action plan, a target date for implementation, and a plan for evaluation of the outcomes. This was then shared with workers.

What type of information could the workers provide to help the committee evaluate worker commitment to ergonomics? Likewise, what type of information could the manager-owner provide to demonstrate commitment to and success in achieving goals?

Creating Opportunities That Engage Clients in Decision Making and Problem Solving

Involving workers and workplaces in decision making to solve and manage ergonomic problems is key to developing a sense of ownership and accountability for implementing safe practices. Therapists can support this through recognizing that workers and employers are the experts when it comes to knowing their problems, how they solve problems, and how these problems affect their lives, especially at work. The workers and supervisors have access to invaluable information and often can make practical, relevant suggestions about how to address concerns.

It is important that the therapist contributes to and facilitates a culture of self-management and self-monitoring of ergonomic concerns. The therapist can achieve this through translating policy, health and safety legislation, procedural information, and research evidence on ergonomics and return to work into an understandable format for the end-users. Workers and workplace parties can then reframe this information and apply it to the workplace. The therapist can offer strategies to support the actions and efforts of workplace parties in self-management through identifying and sharing credible sources of information located on the Internet or through tools and resources for workers to manage their ongoing ergonomic needs. In addition, the therapist would encourage the active solicitation of suggestions and solutions from various levels of the organization and that information collected across workgroups be incorporated into an ongoing process to support informed and collaborative decision making.

Involvement and participation of the workers in developing confidence and capacity to make decisions and apply ergonomic information is key to enabling and sustaining a proactive ergonomic program. Workers need a process and tools to support effective decision making and changes in work behavior to perform work safely. The therapist can offer education, training, and opportunities for reflection to support workers enacting ergonomic responsibilities. For instance, the ergonomic action form (Figure 2-1) is designed to engage workers in gathering information, evaluating potential problem areas, making adjustments, and documenting outcomes. This form can support the ongoing reflection and self-monitoring by workers and help them in taking proactive steps in managing their health and safety at work and in forwarding unresolved issues for further input and action.

At CBC, the workers did not receive education on how to adjust or alter workstations to specific needs. Some workers accessed information on the Internet; however, many did not know how to apply ergonomic information about their chairs, placement of telephones, lighting, and computer posture, nor did they understand its application to personal characteristics. The therapist encouraged workers to review a credible online video on workstation design for office workers and provided them with a tool for recording and analyzing problems. The form also provided them with a place to document the actions taken to adjust or alter equipment, processes, or work behaviors. Workers were asked to identify concerns that were not answered through the video. A session was held with workers to review this experience and to share information with one another on corrective strategies and to identify additional information they felt they needed to self-monitor ergonomic issues.

How would you go about ensuring that workers have the information they need about ergonomics? Would you provide it or would you help them find it? How might you assist the workers apply information to personal factors such as height, age, weight, and gender? What ergonomic approaches will inform the information you provide? What strategies will you use to ensure that workers can use this information to self-manage and to solve ergonomic problems in their daily work lives?

Ensuring a Flexible and Individualized Occupational Therapy Approach

Ensuring a flexible and individualized OT approach in ergonomics requires therapists to attend to the structures of health care systems, return-to-work systems, and workplace demands. For instance, when working in industry, the therapist needs to clearly communicate what he or she has to offer employers or managers and explain how services may or may not help resolve the ergonomic issues under discussion. To be effective, the therapist must be flexible in meeting client needs, respecting the resources and services available uniquely to each organization.

Therapists also need to be reflective—to become more aware of their actions and the efforts needed to remain within the scope of practice and to gain a deeper appreciation of the influence of their actions on others. This is especially important in client-centered practice. It is often easier to tell workers and employers what they need to do to improve safety than it is to help them assume

Ergonomic Action Form

Job Title:	Job Code:	Location:
Job Demand/Duty:	**Date Initiated:**	

Type of Ergonomic Concern: Physical/Psychological/Sensory/Cognitive/Behavioral

Physical Demands or Task (describe the demand or processes/procedures)

Mobility
Strength
Time performing demand
Effort required
Speed
Frequency # of repetitions
Body posture (neutral or awkward)
Equipment

Summary of Concern:

Sensory/Cognitive/Behavioral (describe the demand or processes/procedures)

Person resources or skills
Effort
Speed
Interactions with others

Summary of Concern:

Work Environment Factors (weather, hot, cold, tools, workstation design or structures, and work location)

Summary of Factors and Concern:

Actions: (include date and steps taken to address, change, or modify concern, and plans for further action)
1. **Date**
   Action
   Follow-up plan

2. **Date**
   Action
   Follow-up plan

FIGURE **2-1** Ergonomic action form.

shared responsibilities and enact accountabilities in the workplace. Taking time for active reflection is essential in helping therapists become aware of how to communicate and act as team members as well as understand how a therapist's efforts influence or motivate others to engage in partnering. Therapists must also become aware of personal biases from previous interactions with other employers and learn how to bracket perceptions to maintain a consistently open and responsive approach with each new client. Therapists can be reflexive and learn about themselves in a number of ways—keeping a reflective log of assumptions, debriefing with peers about challenges and experiences, and inviting feedback from clients.

After working with the workers at CBC for a number of months the therapist wanted feedback on her performance and what things she did that kept workers interested and committed to ergonomics at work. To do this, she invited workers to share this information anonymously by responding to three questions: What, if at all, does the therapist do to help the workers and managers function as a team? How does the therapist contribute to the team? What, if at all, does the therapist do to help you feel part of the team? The therapist reflected on the responses to gain insights into the impact of her actions on empowering others to work collaboratively.

Based on your previous work experiences, write down your current attitudes and assumptions about workers on modified duty programs and your views about an employer's commitment to health and safety. Hypothesize on how these views might influence your actions in dealing with returning workers with injuries to work. How might you prepare for your next interaction with an employer and worker in planning a return to work? What can you do before the meeting and during the meeting to maintain a client-centered approach in discussing return-to-work plans?

THE PERSON-ENVIRONMENT-OCCUPATION MODEL

Derived from environment behavior studies and principles of client-centered practice, the PEO model[23] is suitable for planning client-centered interventions on both personal and environmental levels. The *environment* is defined broadly to include cultural, socioeconomic, institutional or structural, and social elements. The model has been used by therapists in various roles in a variety of settings. It has been shown to be a practical tool to conceptualize, communicate, plan, and evaluate occupational performance interventions.[42]

The model (Figure 2-2) has three components: the person, the environment, and the occupation, imagined as interrelated spheres that move with respect to one another over time. The spheres represent how a person continuously engages in occupations and interacts with environments. Environments, occupations, and people have enabling or constraining effects on one another; the components shape one another. A cross-section taken at any discrete point in time would reveal different interactions.

The greater the degree of overlap between the three components represents increased congruence, or PEO match, resulting in improved occupational performance and improved job experience or satisfaction. Occupational performance is the product of PEO transactions. The aim of interventions is to improve occupational performance and increase the PEO congruence by removing obstacles or providing supports for more harmonious PEO relationships.

The PEO model can be used as a tool in client-therapist alliances to systematically examine complex occupational performance issues. The model focuses on the relationships among the worker, the work environment, and the work itself to create a structure for problem-solving strategies. This approach can assist therapists to address not only worker issues, but also the impact of organizational relationships, systems, and attitudes. Ultimately the PEO model is designed to help facilitate communication with all members of the workplace.

Application of the Person-Environment-Occupation Model to Ergonomics Practice

To illustrate the PEO model as a practical tool for therapists in ergonomics, the model has been applied to the same three ergonomic problems

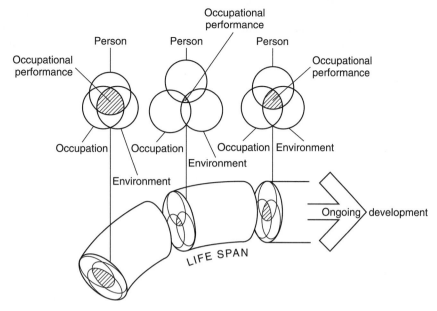

FIGURE **2-2** The person-environment-occupation model. (From Law M, Cooper B, Strong S et al: The Person-Environment-Occupation model: a transactive approach to occupational performance, *Can J Occup Ther* 63:9, 1996.)

identified earlier in the case example of the Centralized Booking Company. This model is particularly of value to the therapist for identifying and clarifying barriers to the resolution of ergonomic problems such as worker attitudes, systems issues, organizational issues (e.g., policy, leadership style), and interpersonal relationships within an organization.

Ergonomic Problem 1

A worker who sustained injuries in a car accident wants to return to work on temporarily modified duties, day shift only. Barriers include the resistance of co-workers and the need to identify the work tasks that will enable the worker to return to work on modified duties.

Analysis and Assessment

The therapist gathers information from the worker regarding his or her current abilities (e.g., physical, cognitive, affective, emotional). In addition, the therapist works in partnership with clients to gather data on the actual demands and processes involved in managing customer accounts and the

service desk. Information is gathered from the worker, the supervisor, and the employer. Analysis of person-occupation, person-environment, and environment-occupation relationships reveals a number of issues.

Person-Occupation Issues
- The worker's physical abilities and physical restrictions do not match the physical demands of the job (e.g., pain in hand with prolonged repetitive posture of right hand, visual-perceptual problems working with standard computer screen, right hand coordination and sensory impairment make it difficult to manipulate paper and writing utensils, which reduces the speed of performing tasks). Jean likes her job and receives a great deal of satisfaction in helping customers get the information and assistance they need in a timely fashion. Currently, Jean has reduced confidence in her capacity to effectively perform job tasks and resume her preinjury level of performance. Primarily, she is concerned about the increased time it takes to handle and manipulate paperwork and the multitasking demands such as

talking on the phone to customers, searching for information on the computer and in manuals, and recording information.

Person-Environment Issues

- Poor match of physical abilities with work expectations (e.g., temporary inability to perform all shifts because of fatigue related to sleep disturbance problems).
- The employer anticipates a lack of cooperation from co-workers based on co-workers' previous responses when other workers returned to work. Jean is also worried about how she will handle any negative attitudes. In the past, Jean perceived her co-workers as liking her and viewing her as friendly, and Jean often socialized with them outside of work.

Environment-Occupation Issues

- A lack of formal policy for rehabilitation of workers with injuries, in particular no formalized modified duty program
- Workload during modified duty programs perceived as inequitable by co-workers
- Management wishes to reduce occurences of lost time injuries
- Management identified issues with workplace safety practices and desires a program to eliminate workplace injuries
- Management identified issues with team functioning and wants to improve human relations of staff

Person-Environment-Occupation Interventions

The therapist works in consultation with all parties, including the workers, co-workers, and management, to develop a modified duty program. The PEO model is used to help workers, supervisors, and employers understand the impact of relationships among the workers and the organization *(person),* the work *(occupation),* and the workplace *(environment)* that influences human performance and workplace productivity. Next, the model is used to highlight the barriers to and facilitators of return to work. This information, along with legislation, can inform the development of a modified duty program and supporting guidelines.

The modified duty program guidelines provide a focus for discussions on issues surrounding the particular worker with an injury, and the opportu-

nity to negotiate a return to work plan. The guidelines also help other co-workers gain awareness needed to accept co-workers on modified duties beginning with initial rotations into the day shift, and a gradual return to all shifts (afternoons followed by night shifts). Subsequently a plan is developed to match the worker's current abilities with work demands. The development of this plan involves dialogue with the supervisor and the worker and negotiation of duties that match the worker's abilities and under what circumstances they are performed (i.e., the parties work together to explore ways to improve the PEO congruence). The supervisor, the worker, and the therapist create a plan to gradually increase the worker's duties as endurance and pain control improves. For instance, to address Jean's difficulties with decreased coordination, she is assigned a group of customer accounts for which all the information she needs to source is on one computer. It is anticipated that this type of collaborative planning using a PEO perspective will help Jean achieve success and gain confidence in transitioning back to work.

The therapist in this case also teaches Jean to adjust the sensitivity of keys on the keypad and her computer mouse and helps Jean to use a process to self-monitor her performance during the return-to-work process. This process entails documenting problems, successes, and strategies she uses to address problems and evaluate her progress over time in terms of endurance, effort, and speed. The process of self-monitoring provides Jean with an active role in the return-to-work process by giving her responsibilities for managing her needs in the midst of performing her work and helps her prepare for and participate in feedback of her progress with the therapist and employer.

Ergonomic Problem 2

After the corporation-wide installation of new ergonomically designed office equipment, office workers continued to complain of musculoskeletal pain in their necks, shoulders, backs, and wrists.

Analysis and Assessment

The therapist began her assessment of this problem by conducting interviews with the staff to ask about the factors they perceive to be contributing to musculoskeletal pain. In addition, the therapist reviews the office equipment and gathers information associated with the purchase and installation of the new ergonomic office workstations. The following issues were identified.

Person-Occupation Issues

- Pain while performing duties, fears of increasing incapacitation, and reluctance to engage in some duties
- Stress believed to be associated with some work duties in the rotation
- Not all employees were trained in all work duties within the rotation

Person-Environment Issues

- People were not consulted concerning the identification of solutions or factors that potentially contributed to original problems.
- Workers perceived that the manager was somewhat interested in health and safety; however, they were aware that the employer was very busy in the day-to-day running of an expanding business, generating new accounts, and ensuring that customers were satisfied. Thus, the proactive leadership in managing health and safety was compromised.

Environment-Occupation Issues

- Increased workload demands for each employee
- Rotation of work limited because of absenteeism (i.e., staff experiencing prolonged periods of high-stress duties)
- New equipment installed, but workers received no training on how to manage and adjust it

Person-Environment-Occupation Interventions

The therapist's recommendations include training of staff on basic ergonomic principles to promote the application of this knowledge in identifying and self-managing problems with their workstations. Training recommendations include adjustment and mechanical management of workstations (to be provided to employees by the vendor) and workplace training on basic principles of ergonomics such as methods to evaluate, modify, and prevent workplace risks (to be provided to employees and management by the therapist). Stretching and exercise programs are also included as part of the training package. Part of the recommenda-

tions include implementing a new process to engage employees in providing input and generation of solutions. The therapist recommends a tool be used by employees to self-monitor and correct ergonomic issues in performing daily work tasks and a process be adopted to forward more complex problems to an ergonomics committee for consideration and resolution.

Ergonomic Problem 3

The Centralized Booking Company identified that the continuation of lost-time claims, absenteeism, and worker dissatisfaction and discomfort contributed to lost productivity, decreased efficiency, difficulty with staffing, and overall poor staff relations.

Analysis and Assessment

To address this problem the therapist gathers information on claims experience, types of injuries, work flow processes, and so forth to understand and evaluate the workplace injury management program. In addition, the therapist considers the ergonomic problems within the greater legislative and organizational systems, such as the workplace collective agreements, workplace policy, and health and safety legislation.

Person-Occupation Issues

- Lack of management experience and training in health and safety in office settings
- Lack of understanding of joint or shared responsibilities and processes for enacting safety obligations and accountabilities
- Lack of successful outcomes in previous situations, despite the fact that management was motivated to return employees to work
- Lack of employee satisfaction with workload and duties

Person-Environment Issues

- Lack of systems monitoring and opportunities for input, feedback, and collaboration

Environment-Occupation Issues

- Time and manpower constraints have limited implementation of work rotation and limited accommodation of workers.
- Purchase of ergonomic equipment did not reduce lost-time injuries.
- Workplace injury management strategy lacked direction.

Person-Environment-Occupation Interventions

A collaborative approach to identifying a rotation strategy and efficient sequencing of tasks per rotation is recommended by the therapist. This requires involvement of the therapist, worker representative, and management to design a suitable rotation. An additional complementary recommendation is the training of office staff on all accounts and the development of skill requirements to enable rotation through all tasks, minimizing the length of time on stressful work and allowing recovery time after the most demanding duties. To test the applicability and feasibility of the rotation a trial of the new job rotation with self-monitoring is recommended. Then a worker-to-worker training program will be implemented to ensure all staff receive cross-training in all work tasks.

ETHICS AND CHALLENGES IN IMPLEMENTING A CLIENT-CENTERED APPROACH

Ethical dilemmas can arise when using a client-centered approach in the ergonomics field. For example, the priorities of key parties may conflict. The workers may believe that the most urgent ergonomic issues relate to poor equipment, whereas the employer may identify the worker's unsatisfactory performance and compliance with proper techniques as the priorities. The therapist is confronted with the question of which of these clients' issues and priorities take precedence. Being client-centered does not mean that the therapist must agree with the client or "take sides." Rather, the therapist focuses on the issues as directed by the client and enters the client's world in a collaborative partnership. The therapist may reclarify and ascertain the priorities and needs of both parties and with them may negotiate which issues will be addressed and at what time. For the scenario described, an objective evaluation of the views of all participants is necessary to identify the extent of all problems. The therapist ensures that all issues are addressed from all perspectives. The goal is to encourage each party to see all points of view. With the introduction of the PEO model, the parties have a more objective focus and develop a shared understanding of the impact of PEO relationships on occupational performance

from which to collaboratively move forward. In turn, this shared understanding helps to build trust from the outset among the therapist, workers, employers, and external agencies.

The therapist may encounter attitudinal barriers that have a negative impact on relationships between supervisors and workers. With the client-centered approach, these issues need to be addressed in an objective and respectful manner. Negative attitudes can be identified as barriers to effective solutions. For example, a supervisor may label a worker "unmotivated" or "lazy." Thus, when the worker returns to work on modified duties because of injury, the supervisor may attribute all concerns raised by the worker to laziness. Niemeyer describes how labeling and stereotyping can bias observers' (i.e., supervisors') beliefs and can delay recovery if the individual accepts the label.[30] The early identification of destructive attitudes allows the therapist to take steps before plans are undermined. The importance of offering a caring and supportive return-to-work experience must not be overlooked. For example, current evidence suggests that a humanistic approach can have a positive influence on return-to-work outcomes.[2,11] This approach translates to simple steps such as early supervisor contact with the employee with an illness or injury and a sincere expression of concern for the employee. Therapists can work with employers to translate research evidence on effective return-to-work programs that in turn help employers create workplace environments that support return to work.

Problems with negative attitudes also extend to co-workers. For example, the therapist can provide informed information to co-workers that helps to counter misinformation and stereotypes. This can be achieved through information sessions with co-workers about the difficulties and anxieties that workers face when they are alienated from work and attempting to return to work. Positive moral peer support can help ease the transition of workers returning to work and help them regain their sense of belonging.

Funding issues may also pose ethical dilemmas for the therapist. The employer or insurance company may not be able to fund what the worker and therapist identify as necessary to resolve the ergonomic problems. The therapist needs to work with workers and organizations to identify options for funding and other methods for arriving at an appropriate solution. It is important that the therapist address funding proactively to maintain trust throughout the process.

Lack of compliance of the worker or employer in carrying out the agreed-on changes also presents the therapist with a dilemma. The client-centered approach is intended to foster partnerships and actively engage key parties in meaningful plans from the beginning. In this way, the situation of noncompliance can often be avoided. An effective client-centered approach to ergonomics includes the establishment of target dates and identifies an individual responsible for monitoring and re-evaluating changes (e.g., therapist, supervisor, employee). The responsible individual(s) notifies the group if issues are not resolved efficiently and completely. However, it is recognized that the best intentions to implement ergonomic changes may be impeded by competing priorities in running a business or in managing customer needs. Thus, it is truly essential that a client-centered approach in ergonomics also aims to help organizations establish an accountability process for linking ergonomics with organizational outcomes of productivity and safety. Linking ergonomics to strategic priorities will support organizations in refocusing on and targeting ergonomic risks and solutions as a natural, routine part of doing business.

CONCLUSION

Organizations are challenged with complying with changes in legislation concerning health and safety, human rights, and disability to ensure healthy work environments. A highly competitive marketplace has contributed to the incorporation of ergonomics to maximize productivity and redesign for efficiency. The practice of ergonomics must continue to develop to meet the changing, complex needs of clients through evidence-based evaluations (see Chapter 18). A client-centered approach can be instrumental to workers and organizations in building capacity to assume control and management of ergonomics in the workplace. In this process, not only are workers viewed as a valuable resource, but they are ac-

tively involved with employers in the identification, assessment, and resolution of ergonomic concerns. Using a client-centered approach that embraces the PEO model can help therapists and clients think critically about ergonomic issues, create innovative solutions, and further develop the practice of ergonomics.

Learning Exercises

Overview

The learning exercise is designed to help you identify, deconstruct, and articulate the components of the PEO model as it applies to a worker with an injury.

Purpose

The purpose of these exercises is to encourage you to analyze the barriers and challenges to occupational performance using a PEO ap-proach and to consider client-centered strategies to address ergonomic concerns.

Exercises

1. Use a PEO approach to evaluate the problems in a workplace setting. Invite colleagues to share their experiences where they have encountered a workplace ergonomic problem. Choose one example in which a colleague developed a strain or injury.
2. Use a role-play that involves the colleague role-playing the worker with the ergonomic concern and the remaining members of the class role-playing the therapist.
3. The "therapists" will conduct a group interview with the "worker" to identify and create a list of P-E, E-O, and P-O concerns or issues that limit optimal performance.
4. For each PEO issue, identify two potential interventions for each performance problem.
5. Evaluate each intervention to ensure that the processes and steps in the interventions are consistent with a client-centered approach. Consider the involvement, accountability, and responsibilities of all of the people involved in the intervention process.

Multiple Choice Review Questions

1. To be client-centered, therapists must:
   A. Always agree with the client.
   B. Create a collaborative partnership and enter the client's world from the client's perspective.
   C. Avoid dealing with ethical issues.
   D. Rely solely on the client's skills and resources to the exclusion of the therapist's skills and resources.

2. Concepts central to client-centered practice include:
   A. Facilitation of client participation in all aspects of service.
   B. Flexible, individualized service.
   C. Respect for clients and the choices they make.
   D. All of the above

3. Why does a therapist use an ergonomic framework?
   A. A framework allows the therapist to understand ergonomic problems.
   B. A framework directs the therapist's observations, data collection, and interpretation of findings.
   C. A framework lends comprehensiveness to assessments and intervention plans.
   D. All of the above

4. The PEO model is:
   A. A tool for therapists' use to facilitate client-centered practice.
   B. An intervention model applicable to ergonomics.
   C. Flexible and a guide rather than something that dictates practice.
   D. All of the above

5. Why does a therapist encourage worker involvement in self-monitoring responsibilities?
   A. To give a worker more things to do while on modified duties
   B. To give a worker control over work tasks
   C. To help a worker work with co-workers
   D. To help a worker document productivity

6. In the case of the CBC, the problem of a lack of time and manpower constraints limiting the implementation of a work rotation schedule is an example of what PEO component?
   A. A person-environment issue
   B. A person-occupation issue
   C. An environment-occupation issue
   D. A person-environment-occupation issue

7. In the case of the CBC, the problem of a worker experiencing pain while performing duties is an example of what PEO component?
   A. A person-environment issue
   B. A person-occupation issue
   C. A person-environment-occupation issue
   D. An environment-occupation issue

8. In the case of the CBC, the problem of workers not being consulted concerning the identification of solutions or identification of potential factors that contributed to original problems is an example of what PEO component?
   A. A person-environment-occupation issue
   B. A person-occupation issue
   C. An environment-occupation issue
   D. A person-environment issue

9. Therapists who adopt a client-centered approach to address occupational ergonomic problems will:
   A. Develop a partnership with workers and managers to establish a return-to-work plan.
   B. Develop a partnership with workers and management to prevent injuries.
   C. Develop an educational session for employers and workers on attitudes toward injured workers.
   D. Develop a relationship with the union.

10. A therapist who brackets his or her assumptions and biases in working with workers with injuries and employers is enacting which client-centered principle?
    A. Ensuring a flexible and individualized approach
    B. Establishing shared or realistic goals
    C. Fostering open and transparent communications
    D. Enacting participation and partnering throughout the process

REFERENCES

1. Anema JR, Steenstra IA, Urlings IJM et al: Participatory ergonomics as return-to-work intervention: a future challenge? *Am J Ind Med* 44:273, 2003.
2. Baril R, Clarke J, Friesen M et al: Management of return-to-work programs for workers with musculoskeletal disorders: a qualitative study in three Canadian provinces, *Soc Sci Med* 57:2101, 2003.
3. Burke M: *Ergonomics tool kit: practical applications,* Gaithersburg, Md, 1998, Aspen.
4. Canadian Association of Occupational Therapists, Health Services Directorate, and Health Services and Promotion Branch: *Guidelines for the client-centred practice of occupational therapy,* Ottawa, 1983, Minister of National Health and Welfare.
5. Canadian Association of Occupational Therapists: *Occupational therapy guidelines for client-centered practice,* Toronto, 1991, CAOT Publications ACE.
6. Canadian Association of Occupational Therapists: *Enabling occupation: an occupational therapy perspective,* Ottawa, 1997, CAOT Publications ACE.
7. Chaffin DB, Anderson G: *Occupational biomechanics,* ed 2, New York, 1991, Wiley & Sons.
8. Christiansen C, Baum C: *Occupational therapy: overcoming human performance deficits,* Thorofare, NJ, 1991, Slack.
9. Christiansen C, Baum C: Person-environment occupational performance: a conceptual model for practice. In Christiansen C, Baum C, editors: *Occupational therapy: enabling function and well-being,* ed 2, Thorofare, NJ, 1997, Slack.
10. England S, Evans J: Patients' choices and perceptions after an invitation to participate in treatment, *Soc Sci Med* 34:1217, 1992.
11. Friesen M, Yassi A, Cooper J: Return-to-work: the importance of human interactions and organizational structures, *Work* 17:11, 2001.
12. Gage M, Polatajko HJ: Naming practice: the case for the term client-driven, *Can J Occup Ther* 62:115, 1995.
13. Gerteis M, Edgman-Levitan S, Daley J et al: *Through the patient's eyes,* San Francisco, 1993, Jossey-Bass.
14. Hignett S, Wilson JR, Morris W: Finding ergonomics solutions: participatory approaches, *Occup Med* 55:200, 2005.
15. Horvath A: Research on the alliance. In Horvath A, Greenberg L, editors: *The working alliance: theory, research and practice,* New York, 1994, Wiley.
16. Human Resources Development Canada: *In unison: a Canadian approach to disability issue,* 1996, Government of Canada.
17. Isernhagen SJ: *The comprehensive guide to work injury management,* Gaithersburg, Md, 1995, Aspen.
18. Jequier JC, Gauthier JM, Lapointe C et al: Model for a multidisciplinary approach. In Poirier F, editor: *Rehabilitation and ergonomics,* Mississauga, Ontario, 1989, Human Factors Association of Canada.
19. Kivlighan D, Shaughnessy P: Patterns of working alliance development: a typology of client's working alliance ratings, *J Couns Psychol* 47:362, 2000.
20. Koehoorn M, Lowe G, Rondeau K et al: *Creating high quality health care workplaces,* CPRN Discussion Paper No. W/14, 2002.
21. Korzycki M, Korzycki M, Shaw L: Tug of war between health and return to work: consumer experiences with system tensions. In *Proceedings of the University of Western Ontario Occupational Therapy Conference on Evidence-Based Practice* 6:87, 2006, London, Ontario.
22. Law M: Participation in the occupations of everyday life, *Am J Occup Ther* 56:640, 2002.
23. Law M, Cooper B, Strong S et al: The person-environment-occupation model: a transactive approach to occupational performance, *Can J Occup Ther* 63:9, 1996.

24. Law M, Mills J: Client-centered occupational therapy. In Law M, editor: *Client-centered occupational therapy,* Thorofare, NJ, 1998, Slack.

25. Levine S, Greenlick M: Removing barriers to the empowerment of the elderly in health programs, *Gerontologist* 3:581, 1991.

26. Loisel P, Durand M, Berthelette D et al: Disability prevention: a new paradigm for the management of occupational back pain, *Dis Manage Health Outcomes* 9:351, 2001.

27. Lustig DC, Strauser DR, Rice ND et al: The relationship between working alliance and rehabilitation outcomes, *Rehabil Couns Bull* 46:25, 2002.

28. MacDonald JW, Crozier C: Organizations in transition series. Rehabilitation in the 90s and beyond: the challenge for the British Columbia rehabilitation society, *Can J Rehabil* 5:237, 1992.

29. McWilliam CL, Stewart M, Brown JB et al: Home-based health promotion for chronically ill older persons: results of a randomized controlled trial of a critical reflection approach, *Health Promot Int* 14:27, 1999.

30. Niemeyer LO: Social labeling, stereotyping, and observer bias in worker's compensation: the impact of provider-patient interaction on outcome, *J Occup Rehabil* 1:251, 1991.

31. Rebeiro K: Client perspectives on occupational therapy practice: are we truly client-centered? *Can J Occup Ther* 67(1):7, 2000.

32. Rebeiro K: Partnerships for participation in occupation, *Ment Health Spec Interest Sect Q* 25(3):1, 2002.

33. Roberts-Yates C: The concerns and issues of injured workers in relation to claims/injury management and rehabilitation: the need for new operational frameworks, *Disabil Rehabil* 25:898, 2003.

34. Roter D: The enduring and evolving nature of the patient-physician relationship, *Patient Educ Couns* 39:5, 2000.

35. Rumrill PD, Koch LC, Harris EJ: Future trends in assessment and planning: priorities for vocational rehabilitation in the 21st century, *Work* 10:271, 1998.

36. Shaw L, MacKinnon J, McWilliam C et al: Consumer participation in the work rehabilitation process: contextual factors and implications for practice, *Work* 23:182, 2004.

37. Shaw L, McWilliam C, Sumsion T et al: Optimizing environments for consumer participation and self-direction in finding employment, *OTJR: Occupation, Participation Health,* in press.

38. Shaw L, Sumsion T, McWilliam C et al: Service provider challenges in implementing participatory approaches in employment rehabilitation, *J Vocat Rehabil* 21:123, 2004.

39. Soever L, Cott CA, Boyle J: Client-centered rehabilitation II: health care professionals' perspectives, Toronto, 2003, Arthritis Community Research Evaluation Unit (ACREU).

40. Stevenson FE: Launching the Tidal Model in an adult mental health programme, *Art Sci Res* 15:33, 2001.

41. Stewart M, Belle Brown J, Donner A et al: The impact of patient-centered care on outcomes, *J Fam Med* 49:796, 2000.

42. Strong S, Rigby P, Stewart D et al: Application of the person-environment-occupation model: a practical tool, *Can J Occup Ther* 66:122, 1999.

43. Sumsion T: *Client-centered practice in occupational therapy: a guide to implementation,* ed 2, Philadelphia, 2006, Elsevier.

44. Townsend E: *Good intentions overruled: a critique of empowerment in the routine organization of mental health services,* Toronto, 1998, University of Toronto Press.

45. Webb RDC: Rehabilitation of the injured worker. In Poirier F, editor: *Rehabilitation and ergonomics,* Mississauga, Ontario, 1989, Human Factors Association of Canada.

46. Wehmeyer M: Self-determination and the education of students with mental retardation, *Educ Train Ment Retard* 27:302, 1992.

47. Woodson WE, Tillman B, Tillman P: *Human factors design handbook: information and guidelines for the design of systems, facilities, equipment, and products for human use,* New York, 1992, McGraw-Hill.

48. Yardley JK: *Healthy employment relationships: the heart of hospitals.* A discussion paper prepared and circulated at the Second Annual OHA Healthy Hospitals Innovative Practices Symposium, Toronto, Sept. 30–Oct. 1, 2004.

Macroergonomics

Valerie J. Berg Rice

Learning Objectives

After reading this chapter and completing the exercises, the reader should be able to do the following:

1. Understand the definition, principles, and use of macroergonomics.
2. Describe the role of therapists in assisting in macroergonomic interventions or research efforts.
3. List the ways in which macroergonomics may differ from as well as interface with other disciplines, such as industrial engineering, organizational psychology, physical therapy, and occupational therapy.
4. List some basic principles of macroergonomics and how they may contribute to long-term, lasting change within an organization.
5. Select, understand, and discuss a macroergonomic versus a microergonomic approach, when to use each, and their pros and cons.

Participatory ergonomics. The process by which workers of all levels help identify ergonomic problems and solutions.

Macroergonomics. A subdiscipline of human factors or ergonomics that emphasizes a broad system view of design and fitting the organization to the person or persons within that organization.

Microergonomics. An approach to ergonomics that emphasizes the examination of the interface between person and the product, as opposed to other factors.

CASE STUDY

An example may help the reader understand macroergonomics, as well as why a macroergonomic approach is more likely to lead to large scale, long-lasting results. In this case, the Army Medical Department Center and School commander asked ergonomists (also known as *human factors engineers)* to assist with reducing musculoskeletal injuries among soldiers attending advanced individual training (AIT) to become U.S. Army Health Care Specialists (Figure 3-1). Soldiers attend this rigorous training program at Fort Sam Houston in San Antonio, Texas, after completing basic training.[5,7] At the time of the intervention the training program was 10 weeks in length. The hope was that the intervention program developed at this training site, if successful, might also be duplicated at other training sites. The ergonomic team quickly recognized that the most effective method of evaluation and intervention would involve a macroergonomic approach.

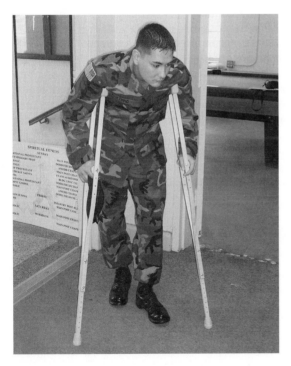

FIGURE **3-1** Musculoskeletal injuries are high among soldiers attending basic combat training as well as advanced individual training programs.

This chapter defines macroergonomics and provides a brief introduction to macroergonomics as a subdiscipline of human factors or ergonomics and as a problem-solving approach. The chapter also investigates the potential role of occupational and physical therapists in using macroergonomics, lists governing principles of macroergonomics, and demonstrates with a case study example. Finally, guidance is given for helping therapists decide when to use a micro versus a macro approach.

MACROERGONOMIC ORIGINS AND MOVEMENT

In 1978 the Select Committee on Human Factors Futures (1980-2000) was initiated to study societal trends and their impact on human factors and ergonomics.[1] The sixth item identified was the "failure of traditional (micro-) ergonomics." The point was that a specific solution to a known ergonomic issue, regardless of how well it was conceived or implemented, did not always result in the expected positive results. Paying attention to specific components of the system, such as a workstation, might mean the bigger picture of the work environment was lost. Therefore, although an ergonomist might evaluate and redesign a single workstation to fit an individual, overall work effectiveness, including productivity, safety, and the overall work environment, might not change at all. For more on the history of the development of macroergonomics, consult Hendrick and Kleiner,[1] Kleiner,[4] and Robertson.[10]

More recently, organizational design and management (ODAM) has been integrated into the human factors or ergonomics field, with venues including the Macroergonomics Technical Group within the Human Factors and Ergonomics Society and other countries' societies. The Human Factors in ODAM symposium occurs every 2 to 4 years. Macroergonomics has also been a major topic at the International Ergonomics Association triennial conferences since 1985.

MACROERGONOMICS DEFINED

Depending on whom you speak with, macroergonomics can be defined as a perspective, an approach, a specific discipline, or a subdiscipline of human factors or ergonomics. Basically, rather than a "fitting the task to the man," macroergonomics proposes to "fit the organization to the person or persons within that organization." Yet it is more than even that. In fitting the organization to the people, the ergonomist assesses each element of an organization with the thought that each element has the potential for redesign. In addition, the ergonomist must also consider systems outside the organization that affect the organization. From the highest level of the organizational hierarchy to the entry-level worker and from the most intricate technology to the simple interactions by the water fountain, all elements are interconnected with one another. All have an impact on the achievement of an organization's objectives.

Because of the nature of organizations (as systems of systems), the design process is neither linear nor singular, the way the design of a coffee cup or a computer wrist rest might be. Instead, the process is complex, iterative, and ever-changing as people, societies, technologies, goals, missions, and knowledge change. Although humans are apt to stay with what is familiar to them, metamorphosis is a constant; perhaps it is the only constant. Metamorphosis can occur by chance or it can be managed according to evidence-based facts, but it will continue nonetheless.

According to Hendrick and Kleiner,[1] organizational psychology and macroergonomics differ in their focus and approach; organization psychologists are more inclined to use selection, incentives, climate, and leadership to achieve objectives, whereas ergonomists redesign to ensure optimal human interactions with "jobs, machines, and systems." It is my opinion that any separation of the two is arbitrary—that is, the examination and design (or redesign) of a work system will potentially include personnel systems, selection processes, and climate (described as part of organizational psychology). Only by examining the whole can an ergonomist know which portions need redesign. To leave out a part because it is psychology or industrial engineering rather than macroergonomics defeats the broader approach that macroergonomics brings. Instead, an initial wide-ranging analysis will identify existing elements of the organization, along with the links and the gaps. It will demonstrate work flow, information flow, decision points, and the need for decision aids. In short, when designing an organization, the ergonomist needs to understand each of the systems within that organization, the inside and outside pressures, and the overarching mission and goals, as well as the intricacies of the culture and subcultures. Only by knowing these things, as well as knowing the research literature on organizational effectiveness, hierarchic structures, teamwork and so on, can the ergonomist assist with designing a thoroughly harmonized organization.

Macroergonomics evaluates and optimizes the interface among human, machine, organization, technology, and environment by examining the personnel subsystem, the technologic subsystem, and the internal and external environments. At the same time, the assessment includes looking at the organization's *complexity*—that is, both the segmentation of the organization, known as *differentiation,* and the integration of the organization, known as *integration, formalization* (degree of standardization), and *centralization.*[1,4,10] The bottom line is that in a true macroergonomic project, the goal is to design (or redesign) any and all parts of the organization in order for the entire organization to operate in a harmonized fashion. A harmonized fashion means that because of the design the organization (or work system) operates as smoothly, efficiently, and safely as possible and everyone working there experiences a sense of value, satisfaction, and commitment.

Although this sounds like workplace nirvana, it is close to the goal of all ergonomic design: to create products, places, and procedures that are simultaneously efficient, effective, easy-to-use, and sufficiently challenging enough to be interesting, as well as safe and comfortable. The difference between "regular" ergonomics, also known as *microergonomics,* and macroergonomics lies primarily in the complexity, both in terms of effort and time.

THE MACROERGONOMIC PROCESS

Initial Evaluation

As seen by this explanation of ergonomics, the first step in the process is to examine all systems that influence the issue in question. In the case study mentioned previously, all systems and subsystems that might affect soldier fitness and musculoskeletal injury status were examined. This included external factors such as level of fitness before enlisting on active duty, previous dietary habits, history of exercise and injury during and before basic training, and recommendations by various organizations such as the Centers for Disease Control and Prevention (CDC) and the American College of Sports Medicine. Internal factors included the military structure and schedule, the physical training regimen, current marching requirements, dietary habits, methods of seeking medical care, attitudes of the trainers, intramural sports and accessible exercise facilities, doctrine and standard operating procedures, and so on. In this way, what existed before the assessment was annotated and what existed at the time of the assessment was plainly delineated.

In addition, each system and each level within a system, including the organizational structure, resources, agencies, personnel, policies, surveillance systems, and communication systems, were examined using a broad-to-focused approach. Meetings, interviews, and focus groups were conducted with local supervisors and managers to ascertain attitudes, as well as noting who would assist with change and who would resist change.

Participatory Ergonomics

Orchestrating organizational change takes time. Introducing changes systematically and gradually using a participatory process throughout each level of the organization will vastly improve the probability of success. The participatory process is one of the primary methods used during a macroergonomic project. During this process, workers and managers participate in identifying problems, methods to investigate those problems, and the development of solutions. They are actively en-

gaged in the decision-making process concerning the work practices and activities that directly affect their work lives. Because of this, knowledge and power spread to each organizational level. Although some individuals refer to this as "buy-in," there is more to it. It is a means and process to steadily introduce change into the everyday business practices of an organization. During this progression, workers at all levels discover how to investigate and understand their own organization, as well as how to introduce lasting change. In fact, at the end of a successful macroergonomic program, workers and managers may wonder what the researchers did, because they "did all the work themselves."

It is important to understand the perspectives of the workers and supervisors at the start, as they may have preconceived ideas that conflict with either the process or the research results. For example, in this case, not all of the supervisors believed that musculoskeletal injuries were a problem during AIT (Figure 3-2, *A*) or later at a soldier's permanent duty station or in a deployed war-time situation. Yet, there were sufficient data to show that all three are true. In fact, supervisors were not at all sure they could effect changes by the way they trained (and worked with) their soldiers, which was the basis for the intervention (Figure 3-2, *B*).

In investigating and reducing musculoskeletal injuries during the case study, careful attention was paid to building communication systems between researchers, workers, and supervisors on a regular basis.[8] In fact, weekly meetings were held between ergonomists and stakeholders (Table 3-1). The best team member was identified for each interaction. For example, commanders reacted more positively when dealing directly with the research team leader, whereas our civilian researchers or our physical therapy assistant, who was an active duty sergeant, achieved better results with drill sergeants and instructors. When initially developing unit-led injury prevention teams, the research team leader, who was also an occupational therapist with considerable experience running groups (as well as being a human factors engineer), worked with the team leaders to help them understand the important role of

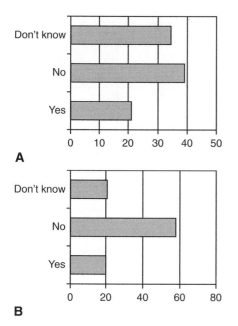

FIGURE 3-2 **A,** Supervisors' responses to the question, "Are there too many overuse injuries occurring in your unit?" **B,** Supervisors' responses to the question, "Can injuries be decreased by changing the way you train your soldiers?"

TABLE 3-1	Weekly Meetings Between Ergonomists and Stakeholders

Month of Macroergonomic Project	Number of Meetings per Week
1-6	4
7-12	3.5
13-18	2

Data from Rice VJ, Pekarek D, Connolly V et al: Participatory ergonomics: determining injury control "buy-in" of U.S. Army cadre, *Work* 18(2):191-204, 2002.

Note: Numerous participatory meetings are required to involve all levels of workers in the process. These are the average number of meetings per week during the macroergonomic injury prevention program at Fort Sam Houston, Texas.

facilitating interaction among group members. This was particularly important, as many soldiers do not learn how to facilitate open communication among soldiers, but merely expect that it will happen. They are trained in leadership but not in group process, group dynamics, motivation, and methods of recognizing and recording issues for later resolution. The soldiers often know many of the involved issues, but they must feel free to disclose them and often need subtle, yet pointed questions or suggestions to help them recall and share pertinent information.

Using a Team Approach to Identify and Fill the Gaps

The immediate team included personnel with backgrounds in research, ergonomics, physical and occupational therapy, and athletic training. In addition, a team of consultants was developed from the initiation of the project. These individuals received updates and could voice their opinions and provide feedback throughout the process. The consultants included personnel with backgrounds in preventive medicine, kinesiology, exercise physiology, epidemiology, physical and occupational therapy, and ergonomics. They worked all over the country and were from organizations that included the CDC, the Department of Defense Injury Prevention Integrated Processing Team, the U.S. Army Physical Fitness School, the U.S. Army Center for Health Promotion and Physical Fitness, and the U.S. Army Research Institute for Environmental Medicine.

The existing structure, procedures, and processes were evaluated by trainee supervisors and subject matter experts (SMEs) from the immediate ergonomic team. This information was compared with research findings and recommendations for preventing musculoskeletal injuries, as well as being used to examine alternate methods of injury identification and early treatment. Consequently the gaps between what existed and what should exist (according to the literature, supervisors, and SMEs) were used to develop best practice scenarios for physical training of the soldiers.[9] This included educational programs as well as changes in standard operating procedures and exercise regimens. These solutions were broad-based, as opposed to being targeted toward a specific causality or type of injury. However, by carefully documenting the number and types of injuries throughout the investigation process, we could track how our implemented solutions influenced injury rates. In this case, musculoskeletal injury rates were measured in terms of medical clinic visits. This overarching set of changes resulted in a decrease in medical clinic visits of approximately 11% for musculoskeletal injuries.[5,9]

A Research-Based and Community Process

By tracking clinic visits as well as the reasons for the visits, we were able to identify the type and severity of each injury (as measured by time of limited duty per injury). We also gathered information from a soldier with an injury and the health care practitioner who treated the soldier. With this information, we could begin to identify potential contributing factors in order to target interventions. Clear outcome data should drive decision making and intervention strategies. Macroergonomic evaluations and interventions can be costly. It is up to the ergonomic team to assure the funding is well spent by demonstrating results through evidence-based outcomes.

Simultaneously with the above system, process, and procedural evaluations, as well as clinical tracking, we administered surveys. Surveys were gathered from all new health care specialist trainees and all graduating health care trainees, including those experiencing a musculoskeletal injury and the health care practitioners who treated their injuries. This information allowed us to identify soldiers at greatest risk of injury, as well as the primary contributing factors. Based on this information, a targeted program of intervention was put into place. The primary contributor to injuries during AIT was the running portion of the Army physical fitness program.

Significant organizational changes were required to put such a targeted intervention program into place. Enacting these changes was possible only because of the rapport, processes, regular injury prevention and fitness council meetings, and cultural changes that had begun to take place over the previous 18 months. Although the previous changes had resulted in decreased injuries

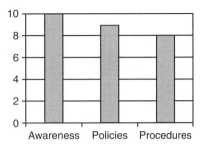

FIGURE 3-3 Number of clinic visits for musculoskeletal injuries per 100 soldiers in training.

after initial interventions such as increasing awareness, changing policies, and changing procedures (Figure 3-3), the targeted interventions achieved even greater results. The targeted interventions resulted in a 36.5% reduction in medical clinic visit rates for musculoskeletal injuries and a 48.6% reduction in limited duty assignments for musculoskeletal injuries.[5,7] All findings were also described in terms of dollars expended and troops readily deployable, both of which are important in a military environment.

THE ROLE OF OCCUPATIONAL AND PHYSICAL THERAPISTS

Most occupational or physical therapists will not take an assignment or consultation job that requires true macroergonomics. Therapists are not trained to evaluate and design organizations or the interactions between humans and technologies from a systems perspective. Therapists spend years studying and understanding normal and abnormal human development, interruptions to normal functioning, and therapeutic interventions to help their clients return to their roles as spouses, parents, workers, students, and children. Well-trained therapists should understand the individual. They should recognize how that individual can potentially fit into various environments during and after treatment, and they provide the guidance to help the individual get back to the "job" of life. Most therapists have been involved in task analysis, especially on a physical and biomechanical level. Yet few therapists have studied organizational effectiveness, work behavior, criterion characteristics of performance, judgmental measures of performance, or the psychosocial context of work performance from a systems perspective. Most know little about human systems integration, just as few ergonomists know when and how to construct an ulnar splint or what type of movement patterns might be most efficient for a person with cerebral palsy; each profession has its own unique set of knowledge and skills.

However, therapists can apply a macroergonomic approach to a specific problem or participate on an ergonomic team. For example, individuals in a work setting might be experiencing a large number of work-related musculoskeletal disorders (WRMD). A typical microergonomic approach would be to examine and redesign the workstations of all individuals who have sought health care for a WRMD. A more comprehensive approach might be to examine all workstations and have employees complete a survey on their symptoms or identify the tasks associated with their job, in order to help determine physical risk factors. An even larger perspective might involve addressing other contributing factors, such as the physical and psychosocial considerations associated with an impending plant closing, the aging workforce, a predominance of workers who no longer fit the physical profile to easily use the equipment (being overweight or underweight, too short or too tall, or under strength), or an influx of workers from a different culture with differing values associated with work. Without a broader approach, a simple workstation change may influence very little.

A FEW PRINCIPLES

Ergonomics involves the applied study of humans and their capabilities and limitations across a broad spectrum of performance in order to design products, places, and procedures to match those capabilities and limitations. Thus all ergonomic design is human-centered, including designs as diverse as a particular medical tool and a road system to produce a more fluid traffic flow. This does not mean that all design is individual-centered, as organizational design must also ac-

count for collective groups of individuals who can work and behave quite differently under diverse conditions and situations. Some basic principles of macroergonomics follow.

- *All relationships within an organization are reflected throughout the organization.* In using a macroergonomic perspective, ergonomists recognize the impact of all relationships within an organization. For example, a hierarchic structure will work well for certain types of organizations and people, whereas a flat system will work better for others. The balanced scorecard approach,[2,3] which helps each person and each section know their role and how they contribute to the good of the whole, is based on this principle.
- *Each potential solution, and each decision about design, depends on the results of assessments of the organization.* Assessment results drive the design. These assessments can be formal or informal and can consist of observations, interviews, focus groups, surveys, or record reviews. If the goal is to conduct an analysis and redesign of an organization, then a 10-step process described as macroergonomic analysis and design (MEAD) might be used.[1,4]

LARGE-SCALE AND LASTING CHANGE

Ergonomists often choose a macroergonomic approach to achieve large-scale and lasting change (LSLC). The following additional principles apply:

- Any change must clearly support the mission and goals of the organization.
- Any change must clearly reflect the culture and values of the organization.
- LSLC is unlikely to occur unless all relevant aspects of a system are involved.
- LSLC is unlikely unless workers of all levels understand and agree with the need for change. Dictated changes do not last; attitude and belief changes do last.
- LSLC is more likely when workers of all levels help identify the problems and solutions (participatory ergonomics).

- LSLC occurs when each individual recognizes his or her role.
- LSLC occurs more readily when participatory ergonomic methods are conducted from the top down, bottom up, and sideways in.
- LSLC tends to occur when carefully and methodically introduced, not when introduced quickly and dictatorially.
- Although evidence-based design can persuade others that change is necessary, both the evidence and the display of the evidence must be relevant to the viewer.
- Overall system change sets the stage, so that targeted change can occur in a climate of acceptance, yielding the greatest results.
- Top-level support is essential.

When the macroergonomic effort involves injury prevention, it must also be recognized that health care practitioners are consultants only. The workers and supervisors bear the primary responsibility for maintaining their fitness and health.

Although it is not always possible to examine the same facility years later, in this case study a follow-up evaluation occurred 2 years later. Data revealed that injuries and limited duty assignments had been reduced even further, with no additional assistance from researchers or health care providers.[6] In the opinion of the researchers, this was because the knowledge and the tools were given to the soldiers and supervisors during the macroergonomic intervention. They had numerous classes on the most recent literature on injury prevention, given on arrival at their assignment, annually during recertification as drill sergeants, and during other regularly scheduled training times. They were taught how to track injuries and look for variations and possible causes of those variations. Most importantly, this information was permanently included in their standard operating procedures. They owned it. It became part of their normal, everyday job.

WHEN SHOULD A PRACTITIONER USE A MICROERGONOMIC APPROACH?

A microergonomic approach is appropriate when the identified problem is *limited in scope*. An example would be conducting an evaluation and finding a solution for a single individual with a history of back pain and/or back surgery who could benefit from a supportive chair and a better workstation design. Another example would be if a rash of injuries occurred after the introduction of a new process or tool. If that tool or process is undoubtedly the culprit, then large-scale evaluations and interventions are unwarranted. Basically, a microergonomic approach is best when there is no indication that a larger scale approach will yield greater results.

Limitations in resources can also dictate a microergonomic approach. A macroergonomic approach is impossible without sufficient funds, personnel, time, or interest on the part of the client. Sometimes, when resources are limited, a linear, stepwise approach can be used for problem solving, prioritizing those issues that are most important and implementing solutions as resources become available. An alternative would be to investigate with a macro approach but to implement changes or interventions in a linear, one-at-a-time fashion. A third option with low-level funding is to make changes but incur the charges over time.

Many ergonomists move from micro to macro approaches, using the "low-hanging fruit"—that is, quick achievement of lesser goals—to fuel their future work to make bigger, lasting changes. This technique works well in situations where costs and benefits of ergonomics are relatively unknown, or held suspect, by managers. As managers see improvements and cost savings, they are more willing to invest in additional ventures to improve conditions.

CONCLUSION

Therapists are unlikely to perform MEAD unless they obtain substantial additional training, such as attending a degree program or a series of college courses. These are not skills that can be gained in a short course. However, therapists can play a significant role in helping individuals and managers see the value of ergonomics through microergonomic applications. Subsequently they can suggest a supplementation of their efforts, and a

Although the occupational therapy department in your educational institution is a microcosm of the overall university, it is a good place to start thinking about the use of a macroergonomic approach. Imagine you are a consultant and your job is to evaluate the department regarding overuse injuries for both students and staff. The following are some questions and exercises to help you think about the issues.

1. List all the systems that might affect musculoskeletal injuries among students and staff.
2. List all the issues that might also affect musculoskeletal injuries among students and staff.
3. Identify information you would like to have from students, staff, and the college or university.
   a. Develop structured interviews for each group.
   b. Develop survey questions for both students and staff for which you can quantify the answers (or identify existing surveys you could use).
4. Discuss the evidenced-based outcome measures that might be of interest to the students, staff, department head, and college president. Consider the ethics of such a question. Which interests are more important? Which one is your "client"?
5. What other colleagues might you want on your team, and how do you think they contribute to the project?
6. Imagine you find other issues outside the realm of musculoskeletal injuries. One involves an instructor with partial blindness who does not seem to have the appropriate tools and assistance to do the best job possible. How would you handle that situation, being that you were hired for a different purpose? Role-play talking with this instructor. Role-play talking with the department head about the issue.

team approach, in order to attain large-scale, long-lasting organizational changes through macroergonomics. Having an understanding of the power of system-wide evaluations and interventions can help therapists explain why certain levels of achievement may, or may not, be met using a specific technique or technology.

Based on the case study provided in this chapter, what actions might an ergonomic team take during the initial evaluation phase of a macroergonomic project? What actions did the ergonomic team evaluating musculoskeletal injuries take? Which principles of macroergonomics did the ergonomic team evaluating musculoskeletal injuries seem to consider? How would you have done things differently? What evidence-based outcome measures did the ergonomics team use? What other measures do you assume they used (but that may not be mentioned in this chapter)?

Multiple Choice Review Questions

1. Macroergonomics is:
   A. fitting a task to the individuals who do the task.
   B. designing physical items so they fit the person using them and can be used by other employees also.
   C. fitting the organization to the people in the organization.
   D. harmonizing the operation of an organization by designing or redesigning any and all parts of the organization.

2. A macroergonomic project may involve which of the following evaluations? (Select all that apply.)
   A. Work flow
   B. Decision points
   C. Periods of high-volume or high-stress work
   D. Mission and goals of the organization
   E. Functional work capacities of the workers

3. Differentiation, when speaking of macroergonomics, refers to:
   A. the integration of the organization.
   B. the degree of standardization in the organization.
   C. the segmentation of the organization.
   D. the centralization of the organization.

4. Participatory ergonomics refers to:
   A. involving the members of the work force in the ergonomic evaluation and solution process.
   B. the communication and integration among the ergonomic team members.
   C. the interactions among the workers that may affect ergonomics in the workplace.
   D. considering the hierarchy and communication systems as part of the ergonomic evaluation process.

5. A macroergonomic evaluation process looking at musculoskeletal injuries in the workplace would include:
   A. identifying the gaps between what currently exists within an organization and the best practices within the research literature.
   B. evaluating all systems that affect the workforce.
   C. evaluating hiring, firing, and prehire practices.
   D. evaluating the workforce population, including demographics such as gender and race.
   E. all of the above

6. Evidenced-based outcomes, when considering macroergonomics, include which of the following? (Select the best single answer.)
   A. Consideration of the basic mission of the organization
   B. The individual characteristics of the employees (such as strength and endurance)
   C. Alignment with traditional clinic-based outcomes in occupational therapy practices, such as functional lifting and carrying abilities of workers
   D. Are not important; we cannot measure everything anyway

7. Research, data collection, and data comparison after a design intervention are part of the ergonomic process.
   A. True
   B. False

8. Which of the following should drive design decisions within an organization? (Select the single best answer.)
   A. Interview results
   B. The top decision maker for the organization
   C. Ergonomic assessments results
   D. Subject matter expert opinions
   E. Open-literature research results

9. Principles that apply to using macroergonomics to achieve large-scale and lasting changes (LSLC) within an organization include which of the following? (Select all that apply.)
   A. Dictated changes can result in LSLC, while attitudes and beliefs change.
   B. LSLC is more likely when workers of all levels help identify the problems and solutions (participatory ergonomics).
   C. Typically the culture and values of an organization, although important, do not affect issues of an ergonomic nature, such as musculoskeletal injuries.

D. If workers of all levels understand and agree with the need for change, LSLC is more likely.

10. A macroergonomic approach is used when which of the following are true? (Select all that apply.)
   A. The ergonomic consultant is an academic researcher.
   B. The complexity of the situation demands that a larger scale evaluation and set of solutions be developed.
   C. The ergonomic consultant wants a long, involved project, so they will have a greater income for a longer period of time.
   D. A company wants long-term, lasting organizational change.
   E. When there are sufficient subject matter experts available to put together a good, strong ergonomic team approach.

REFERENCES

1. Hendrick H, Kleiner B: *Macroergonomics: an introduction to work system design,* Santa Monica, Calif, 2000, Human Factors and Ergonomics Society.
2. Kaplan RS, Norton DP: *Alignment: using the balanced scorecard to create corporate synergies,* Cambridge, 2006, Harvard Business School Press.
3. Kaplan RS, Norton DP: *Translating strategy into action: the balanced scorecard,* Cambridge, 1996, Harvard Business School Press.
4. Kleiner BM: Macroergonomics: analysis and design of work systems, *Appl Ergon* 37:81, 2006.
5. Rice VJ, Bergeron A, Connolly V et al: *A macroergonomic and public health approach to injury control,* San Antonio, 2002, presented to the Association of the United States Army.
6. Rice VJ, Gable C: A combined macroergonomics & public health approach to injury prevention: two years later. In *Proceedings of the Human Factors Society 46th Annual Meeting,* Santa Monica, Calif, 2004, Human Factors Society.
7. Rice VJ, Mays MZ: Combining models to solve the problem: macroergonomics and public health. In *Proceedings of the Human Factors Society 46th Annual Meeting,* Santa Monica, Calif, 2002, Human Factors Society.
8. Rice VJ, Pekarek D, Connolly V et al: Participatory ergonomics: determining injury control "buy-in" of U.S. Army cadre, *Work* 18(2):191, 2002.
9. Rice VJB, Connolly V, Bergeron A et al: *Evaluation of a progressive unit-based running program during advanced individual training,* Technical Report No. Aegis T02-1, Fort Sam Houston, Tex, 2002, U.S. Army Medical Department Center and School.
10. Robertson MM: Macroergonomics: a work system design perspective. In *Proceedings of the SELF-ACE 2001 Conference—Ergonomics for Changing Work, Montreal,* 2001.

SUGGESTED READING

Brown O: Participatory ergonomics: from participation research to high involvement ergonomics. In Brown O, Hendrick H, editors: *Human factors in organizational design and management,* Amsterdam, 1996, North-Holland.

Dray SM, Eason K, Gower J, Henderson DA: Macroergonomics in organizations. In Brown ID, Goldsmith R, Coombes K, Sinclair MA, editors: *Ergonomics International (Proceedings of the 9th Congress of the International Ergonomics Association, Bournemouth, England, September, 1985),* Philadelphia, 1985, Taylor & Francis.

Haines H, Wilson JR, Vink P and others: Validating a framework for participatory ergonomics (the PEF), *Ergonomics* 45(4):309, 2002.

Heacox NJ, Holly AH: Separate sides of the same coin: organizational design and (good) design of a decision support tool. In *Proceedings of the Human Factors and Ergonomics Society 49th Annual Meeting,* Orlando, Fla, 2005.

Hendrick HW: Macroergonomics: a conceptual model for integrating human factors with organizational design. In Brown O, Hendrick H, editors: *Human factors in organizational design and management,* Amsterdam, 1996, North-Holland.

Hendrick HW: Organizational design and macroergonomics. In Salvendy G, editor: *Handbook of human factors and ergonomics,* New York, 1997, Wiley.

4

Ergonomics and Work Assessments

Ev Innes

Learning Objectives

After reading this chapter and completing the exercises, the reader will be able to do the following:

1. Identify when to use various types of work-related assessments for individuals and job requirements.
2. Identify a range of work-related assessments that have acceptable reliability and validity for use in clinical practice.
3. Describe a range of assessments used in workplace assessment and job analysis, including ManTRA, OWAS, REBA, RULA, and the Strain Index.

Functional capacity evaluation (no job) (FCENJ). Assessments of this type are "focused on an individual worker performing physical demands related to work in general, rather than to a specific job or duties. Results [are] considered generalisable to general work demands or occupational categories, but not to specific jobs. . . . [FCENJs are] performed to determine the worker's ability to safely perform general physical demands and skills related to work, rather than a specific job. . . . [FCENJs are] also used to identify further rehabilitation, training and/or education options for the worker." (pp. 56-67) [52]

Functional capacity evaluation (job) (FCEJ). Assessments of this type are "focused on an individual worker performing specific tasks within a specific work-place with an identified employer. Results [are] considered not generalisable to other tasks or workplaces. . . . [FCEJs are] primarily conducted to determine the worker's suitability to return to work and develop an appropriate rehabilitation plan, either in the form of a Return to Work (RTW) plan or a clinic-based work conditioning/hardening program" (p. 57) [52]

Physical ergonomic assessment. Assessments that examine and measure the physical aspects of a job, task, and/or environment. This may include measurement and observation of workers' posture, movements, strength, and range of motion; weight handled; force exerted; distances traveled; working heights; exposure times; and light, sound, and temperature levels.

CASE STUDY

Kim is a therapist employed by a vocational and occupational rehabilitation provider. The company provides injury prevention and ergonomic assessment services to industry and case management and occupational rehabilitation services for workers with injuries. The referred workers with injuries have varying types of predominantly musculoskeletal injuries; although the aim is to return them to their preinjury jobs and employers, this is not always possible. Kim has a number of new referrals, including the following:

- Trevor, a 33-year-old crane chaser. A crane chaser fixes slings to loads for cranes and winches and directs the movement of loads, ensuring they do not exceed lifting capacities. Trevor sustained a severe crush injury to his left lower leg 8 months ago when a sling slipped on a load and a large (1-tonne [1.1-ton]) coil of steel fell on his leg. Trevor's left ankle is fused; he has reduced lower limb strength and reduced tolerance for standing and walking. He is unable to return to his previous job and has been referred to determine what work he is capable of doing.
- Lucy, a 38-year-old office administrator. She has developed an overuse injury affecting her nondominant right upper limb after a significant increase in keyboard work (numeric data entry and word processing) related to producing end-of-financial-year reports. She has had 2 weeks off work and has been referred for a return-to-work program.
- The "Women's Health at Work" program, run by an area health service, is concerned about the musculoskeletal risks for female workers on small family-run market gardens in the area. They want the risks identified and assessed and recommendations for risk control provided.
- A manufacturing company with some sections reporting a large number of injuries affecting workers' upper limbs and backs. The company has requested an assessment of these areas to identify potential hazards and develop interventions to control these risks.

T his chapter will introduce a range of work-related assessments used by therapists to assess workers' abilities to perform general phys-ical work demands, and also tools to determine a range of physical hazards associated with work. The case study of Kim is used to explore the range of assessments therapists may consider using and the clinical decision making associated with the scenarios presented.

SELECTION OF WORK-RELATED ASSESSMENTS

As the first step in all these new referrals, Kim must decide what information is needed and the best way to obtain it. The most common methods of data collection therapists use are observation, interview, and measurement.[52] We will look at the range of assessment options Kim will consider for each of these referrals.

In order to select appropriate work-related assessments to use, Kim must consider the purpose of the assessment, the level of assessment (ensuring consistency between the purpose and level), and then the attributes of the assessment, including utility and dependability (Figure 4-1).[47] Work-related assessments[48] purposes are as follows:

To determine the need for intervention

To assess an individual's ability to perform the roles, duties, tasks, task elements, and physical demands of work

To determine effort during work tasks

To measure and document outcomes of work-related interventions

To evaluate programs and engage in research

The level of the assessment is determined by ensuring consistency between the worker's level of function being assessed (role, activity, tasks, skill, and/or body system function) and the job level (job position, duties, tasks, task elements, and/or elemental motions) (Table 4-1; Figure 4-2).[49,93]

FUNCTIONAL CAPACITY EVALUATION (NO JOB)

Functional capacity evaluations (FCEs) conducted when there is no specifically identified job or employer to return to are referred to here as *functional capacity evaluation (no job)*, or FCENJ.

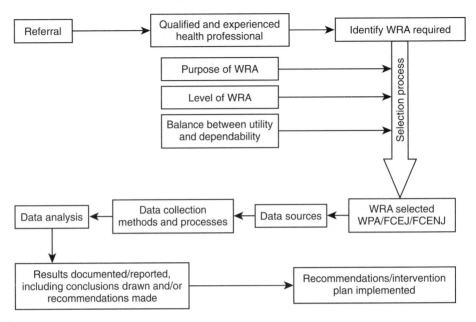

FIGURE 4-1 Model process of excellence in work-related assessments (WRA). (From Innes E: Factors influencing the excellence of work-related assessments in Australia, Unpublished PhD thesis, Perth, Western Australia, 2001, Curtin University of Technology.)

TABLE 4-1   **Definitions of Individual Performance and Work Levels**

Individual	Work
Lifetime role—career developed over lifetime; not context dependent	Career—general course of action or progress through life; may be linear, expert, spiral or transitory, or a combination
Current role—worker; dependent on context	Job position—complex of tasks and duties for any individual
Activities—complex collection of tasks that result in an identifiable whole (e.g., making a table)	Job duties—major activities involved in the job, consisting of several related tasks
Task—discrete identifiable component that contributes to a whole activity (e.g., hammering a nail)	Task—a discrete unit of work performed by an individual; logical and necessary step of a duty; typically has identifiable beginning and end
Skill—ability to perform specific physical tasks (e.g., manual dexterity)	Task elements—smallest step into which it is practical to subdivide any work activity without analyzing separate motions, and so on
Body system—physical, cognitive, and psychologic aspects of function (e.g., strength, balance, color discrimination)	Elemental components—very specific separate motions or movements (biomechanical aspects); may also include cognitive and psychologic variables

From O'Halloran D, Innes E: Understanding work in society. In Whiteford G, Wright-St Clair V, editors: *Occupation and practice in context*, London, 2005, Churchill Livingstone.

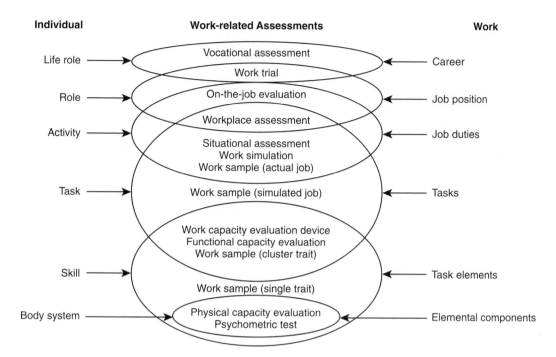

FIGURE 4-2 Work-related assessments relevant to individual performance and work levels. (From O'Halloran D, Innes E: Understanding work in society. In Whiteford G, Wright-St Clair V, editors: *Occupation and practice in context,* London, 2005, Churchill Livingstone.)

They are "performed to determine the worker's ability to safely perform general physical demands and skills related to work, rather than a specific job" (p. 57)[52] or job duties. These types of assessments are considered generalizable to general work demands but not to specific jobs and can be used to identify further rehabilitation, training, and/or education options for workers.[52]

Therapists may use a range of commercially available or published FCEs. The assessments commonly used vary from country to country. In Australia the most popular systems are WorkHab FCE, Isernhagen Work Systems (IWS) FCE, Ergoscience Physical Work Performance Evaluation (PWPE), Blankenship FCE, Key Functional Capacity Assessment, Workability Mk III, EPIC Lift Capacity (ELC) Test, WEST Standard Evaluation, Progressive Isoinertial Lifting Evaluation (PILE), and Valpar Component Work Samples (VCWSs).[18,55,122] In the United States, the IWS FCE, PWPE, Blankenship FCE, WorkSTEPS, and ERGOS Work Simulator are more commonly used,[72] and

in Hong Kong, VCWS and Baltimore Therapeutic Equipment Technologies (BTE) equipment are popular (Figure 4-3).[70] In Europe the IWS FCE, ERGOS, Ergo-Kit FCE, Blankenship FCE, and VCWS are used.[34,57,104,110]

Kim needs to decide which FCENJ will be appropriate to use to determine Trevor's physical abilities for work in general *(purpose of assessment).* As the specific job or position has not been identified, the assessment will focus on the general tasks and task elements associated with work that Trevor can do *(level of assessment).* The *utility* and *dependability* of the FCENJ also need to be considered. Kim will consider which work capacity evaluation devices, FCE systems, and/or lifting assessments will be used (Figure 4-4).

WORK CAPACITY EVALUATION DEVICES

Work capacity evaluation devices are computer-linked and capture assessment information. They can also be programmed for work conditioning

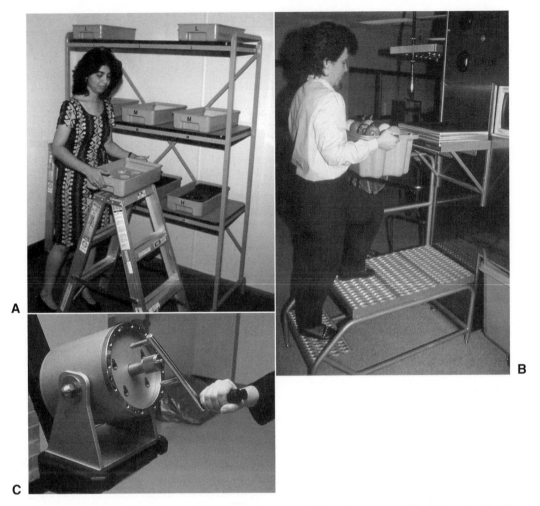

FIGURE 4-3 Examples of popular work-related assessments. **A,** Valpar Component Work Sample 19—Dynamic Physical Capacities. **B,** ERGOS Work Simulator—Panel 3 Work Endurance Component. **C,** Baltimore Therapeutic Equipment Technologies Work Simulator II.

or hardening programs. Work capacity evaluation devices tend to assess at the task and task element levels.

Baltimore Therapeutic Equipment Technologies

BTE has three work capacity evaluation devices: the BTE Work Simulator II (BTE WS), the BTE Primus, and the BTE Evaluation Rehabilitation (ER).

Baltimore Therapeutic Equipment Technologies Work Simulator II

The BTE WS was the first developed and has static and dynamic modes. With its various attachments, a wide range of movements associated with various functional tasks can be simulated. It is used primarily for upper limb assessment and intervention. Test-retest reliability for a range of attachments is considered good to excellent, with the static mode more reliable and accurate than

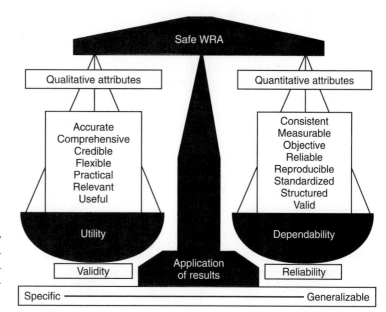

FIGURE **4-4** Utility and dependability constructs of work-related assessments. (From Innes E, Straker L: Attributes of excellence in work-related assessments, *Work* 20[1]:63, 2003.)

the dynamic mode.* Studies examining aspects of validity have also been conducted, with varying results.†

Baltimore Therapeutic Equipment Technologies Primus

The BTE Primus is also able to simulate a range of movements associated with functional tasks. It has isotonic, isometric, and isokinetic modes and has applications for the upper and lower limbs and trunk. As for the BTE WS, the static testing mode of the BTE Primus has better test-retest reliability than the dynamic mode.[65,108] Fewer attachments have been examined for reliability and validity than for the BTE WS, possibly because it was developed more recently.

Baltimore Therapeutic Equipment Technologies Evaluation Rehabilitation

The BTE ER Functional Testing System was formerly known as the *Hanoun Medical Functional Occupational Capacity Unbiased System (FOCUS).*

It incorporates a computerized version of the ELC Test and the Functional Range of Motion (FROM) Assembly Test as part of its overall FCE. Test-retest reliability of the FROM Assembly Test is good to excellent,[79] but no other studies using other parts of this system have been published. The research on the ELC Test also applies, as it is included in the BTE ER.

ERGOS Work Simulator

The ERGOS Work Simulator consists of five test panels that use simulated work tasks to assess strength, body mechanics, cardiovascular endurance, movement speed, and accuracy. Results are criterion-referenced and use Methods-Time-Measurement (MTM) industrial standards to interpret a person's performance.

Published reliability studies have examined only Panel 1 (lifting—static and dynamic) (reliability of computer versus human instructions)[75] and Panel 5 (seated work tolerances and upper limb/hand function).[8] Concurrent validity of the ERGOS with other FCE approaches was not demonstrated,[25,102] indicating that the various systems measure different aspects.

---

*References 14, 15, 28, 29, 50, 60, 87, 115, 116.
†References 4, 5, 7, 27, 30, 32, 51, 60, 101, 121.

FUNCTIONAL CAPACITY EVALUATION

Almost all the FCE systems in use are based on the U.S. Department of Labor's physical demands for work[118] or include similar aspects. Each system has protocols and subtests for determining the following:

Working positions—sitting, standing

Manual handling/exertion—lifting, carrying, pushing, pulling

Mobility—walking, climbing, crawling

Other work postures and nonmaterials handling—stooping or bending, crouching, kneeling, balancing

Upper limb and hand function and manipulation—reaching, handling, fingering, feeling (most systems incorporate pre-existing and established upper limb and hand function tests, such as the Crawford Small Parts Dexterity Test, Hand Tool Test, Minnesota Rate of Manipulation Test/Minnesota Dexterity Test, O'Connor Finger Dexterity Test, O'Connor Tweezer Dexterity Test, Purdue Pegboard, and/or Jamar Grip Strength Dynamometer [Figure 4-5])

Other demands, such as seeing, hearing, and speaking, are usually not formally tested but are commented on if there are difficulties evident during testing.

Although many of the FCEs assess similar items (e.g., lifting, carrying), they determine these in

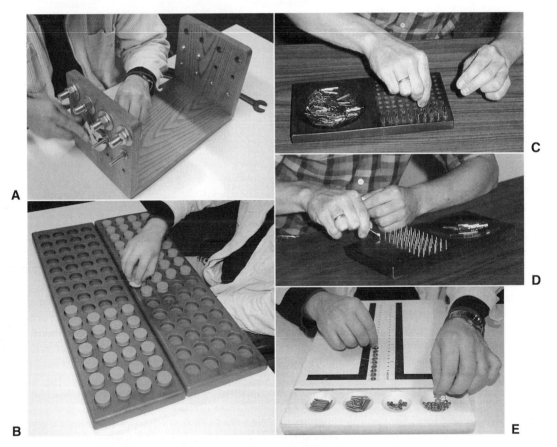

FIGURE 4-5 Examples of various hand function assessments. **A,** Hand-Tool Dexterity Test. **B,** Minnesota Rate of Manipulation Test. **C,** O'Connor Finger Dexterity Test. **D,** O'Connor Tweezer Dexterity Test. **E,** Purdue Pegboard.

different ways, and so results cannot be used interchangeably or compared. This has been demonstrated by poor correlations among several FCEs measuring apparently the same physical demands.[46,102,103]

Ergo-Kit Functional Capacity Evaluation

The Ergo-Kit FCE (Figure 4-6) is a relatively recently developed FCE that incorporates 55 standardized work-related tasks. It includes the Physical Agility Tester (PAT), which is used to test work postures and movements, handling and dexterity, lifting and carrying, and simulation of work-related tasks. Commercial information about the Ergo-Kit is currently available only in Dutch, although a number of research publications are available in English.[33,46,63,102]

Test-retest reliability ranges from moderate to good for lifting tests, and poor for manipulation tests.[33] Inter-rater reliability was moderate to good for the same subtests. Construct and concurrent validity have also been examined for the Ergo-Kit.[46,63,102] Findings indicate that results are not interchangeable between different FCEs, and self-reports of lifting capacity should not replace actual testing of lifting capacity.

Ergoscience Physical Work Performance Evaluation

The PWPE consists of 36 standardized tasks covering six areas: dynamic strength, position tolerance, mobility, balance, endurance, and coordination and fine motor skills.[24] It has substantial test-retest reliability for the dynamic strength

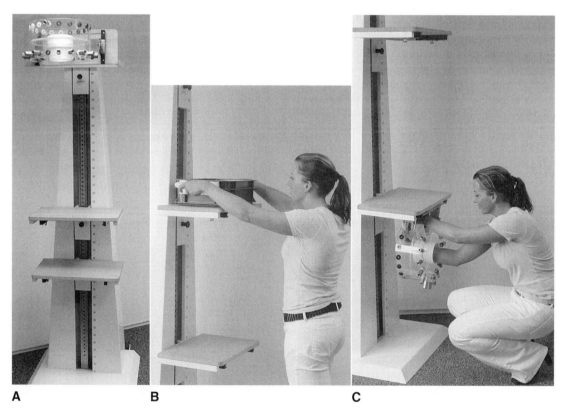

A   **B**   **C**

FIGURE 4-6 Ergo-Kit Functional Capacity Evaluation. **A,** Ergo-Kit FCE. **B,** Lifting a weighted crate. **C,** Physical Agility Tester (PAT), set for low-level task. (Courtesy of Ergo Control.)

tests, fair to substantial for position tolerance tests, and poor to moderate for mobility tests.[117] Inter-rater reliability is also substantial for most tests, with the mobility tests having only fair to moderate reliability.[24] The PWPE has been examined for some aspects of concurrent validity, with moderate correlation between the overall work level recommended and the level of work currently performed.[64]

Isernhagen Work Systems Functional Capacity Evaluation

The IWS FCE consists of 20 work-related tests covering weighted tasks, flexibility and positional tasks, static work, ambulation and mobility tasks, and upper limb coordination.[54] End-points of the assessment are primarily based on therapists' ratings of physiologic and biomechanical signs of effort to determine safe, maximum performance levels (kinesiophysical approach).[36,53]

The IWS FCE is the most extensively researched FCE available (in 2007). It has well-established test-retest reliability for those with and without back pain, especially the lifting subtests.[10,96,97] Although the IWS FCE was originally developed as a 2-day assessment, recent research has indicated that 1 day is adequate, without losing reliability.[98] Intra-rater reliability is also good.[31,35,99,100]

Validity has also been extensively studied and found to be weakly linked to a greater likelihood and speedier return to work[38,39,76]; however, it did not predict recurrence of back injury.[37,38] Comparison with other FCEs indicated that results were not interchangeable.[46,103] This was also the case when self-reported lifting capacity and clinical examination by a physician were compared with IWS FCE results,[9,63] indicating that assessing actual physical abilities through an FCE is necessary to gain an accurate picture of a worker's performance.

Other Functional Capacity Evaluation Systems

Other FCE systems commonly in use have limited peer-reviewed publications regarding their reliability and validity. The Blankenship FCE, Key FCA, WorkHab FCE, and WorkSTEPS have no peer-reviewed studies published on reliability or validity,[34,50,51] although some papers have been published in conference proceedings.[6,67,107] Workability Mk III has moderate content validity,[51,109] but no recent studies have been published.

LIFTING ASSESSMENTS

EPIC Lift Capacity Test

The ELC Test[77,78] has superseded the WEST Standard Evaluation[74,92] as a test of lifting (Figure 4-7). It tests occasional and frequent lifting over three

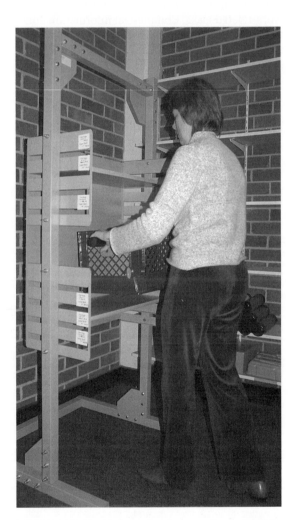

FIGURE 4-7 EPIC Lift Capacity Test—waist to shoulder lift.

ranges (waist-to-shoulder, floor-to-waist, floor-to-shoulder), and uses multiple measures to determine safe end-points for the lifts (biomechanical, psychophysical, and aerobic). Normative data are available. It has good to excellent test-retest and inter-rater reliability[1,50,77] and is able to determine change after treatment.[78]

Progressive Isoinertial Lifting Evaluation

The PILE[81-83] is a lifting assessment using two ranges; the lumbar test from floor to waist (0 to 76 cm [30 inches]) and the cervical test from waist to shoulder (76 cm [30 inches] to 137 cm [54 inches]). The PILE uses endpoints based on psychophysical, aerobic, and safety criteria. Normative data are available.

The PILE has good to excellent test-retest and inter-rater reliability for both people without injuries and those with back and neck pain.[41,45,69,71,81] Construct validity to determine change in lifting ability after intervention has been demonstrated in a number of studies.[20,40,68,84,123]

WORK SAMPLES

Valpar Component Work Samples

There are over 20 Work Samples that use generalized worklike tasks administered in a standardized manner. Results are compared with industrial standards (MTMs). The work samples can also be used as part of a work hardening program. The work samples cited most frequently in the literature are VCWSs 4 (upper extremity range of motion), 8 (simulated assembly), 9 (whole body range of motion), 11 (eye-hand-foot coordination), 19 (dynamic physical capacities) and 204 (fine finger dexterity) (Figure 4-8).

Other than information reported by Valpar on its website regarding data used to establish learning curves for the work samples,[119] no peer-reviewed studies on reliability for these work samples have been published. Good test-retest (VCWSs 4, 9, and 19) and inter-rater reliability (VCWS 19) have been reported in conference proceedings and research theses.[2,3,114] Construct validity for the ability to differentiate between groups (those who are sick-listed and those who are not; formwork carpenters and office workers) has also been demonstrated (VCWSs 8, 19, and 204).[66,104,105,110]

FUNCTIONAL CAPACITY EVALUATION (JOB)

Functional capacity evaluations (job) (FCEJ) are "primarily conducted to determine the worker's suitability to return to work and develop an appropriate rehabilitation plan, either in the form of a return-to-work program or a clinic-based work conditioning/hardening program" (p. 57).[52] In Australia FCEJs are often conducted in conjunction with a workplace assessment (WPA) in which the therapist does an on-site assessment of the worker's preinjury duties and potential suitable duties that may be included in a return-to-work plan. The WPA also includes assessment of the work environment, including any equipment or tools that may be used. In New South Wales, Australia, a return-to-work plan cannot be approved unless a WPA has been conducted by an occupational therapist or physiotherapist.

Therapists often design their own FCEs, especially if assessing a worker's ability to return to a specific job.[18,55,72] The preferred type of FCEJ for many therapists is a battery of tests of the therapist's own design that may use elements of established FCEs, when the subtests are appropriate and relevant to the specific job to which the worker is returning.[18,52,72] Many also use work simulation, such as setting up a keyboard task for a worker returning to computer-based duties.

Kim will use an FCEJ to determine Lucy's current abilities and how these relate to her specific work requirements in order to develop an appropriate return-to-work plan. Some components of standardized FCEs will be used, such as upper limb reaching components. Kim will also simulate some of Lucy's job demands by setting up a data-entry task on a computer workstation similar to that used by Lucy at work. Kim will make modifications and adjustments to the workstation to determine what is optimal for Lucy. Kim may use computer workstation checklists as well as observing and measuring Lucy's performance.

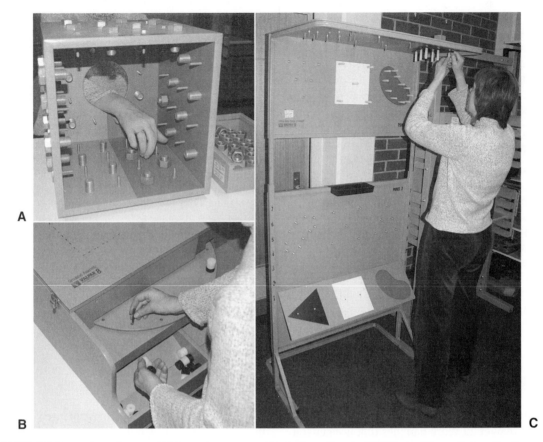

FIGURE 4-8 Examples of several Valpar Component Work Samples. **A,** VCWS 4—Upper Extremity Range of Motion. **B,** VCWS 8—Simulated Assembly. **C,** VCWS 9—Whole Body Range of Motion.

ASSESSMENT OF PHYSICAL ERGONOMICS OF JOBS

In a survey of certified professional ergonomists,[22] the most common tools used by more than 80% of respondents were tape measures, video and digital cameras, stopwatches, and laptop computers. More than half also used spring gauges, scales (load cells), goniometers, light meters, sound pressure meters, and thermometers. The most common direct measurement techniques were the use of grip and pinch dynamometers and push-pull force sensors. The most popular observational techniques included the National Institute for Occupational Safety and Health (NIOSH) lifting equation, psychophysical material handling data,

body discomfort maps, and Rapid Upper Limb Assessment (RULA). More than 70% also used ergonomic checklists.

Other observational techniques frequently referred to in the literature are whole body postural assessments—Ovako Working Posture Analysis System (OWAS)[58,59] and Rapid Entire Body Assessment (REBA)[44]—and upper limb posture and hand use assessments—RULA[85] and the Strain Index.[89,90] A recently developed observational technique for whole body assessment also in use is Manual Tasks Risk Assessment (ManTRA).[13]

Kim considers the various options regarding assessing the musculoskeletal hazards and risks for the "Women's Health at Work" program in family-run market gardens and the manufacturing company.

GENERAL ERGONOMIC ASSESSMENT AND JOB ANALYSIS CHECKLISTS

There are almost as many ergonomic and job analysis checklists as there are therapists who conduct assessments of work. Each therapist has his or her preferred checklist or has developed one based on components from others. As with FCEs, the ergonomic and job analysis checklists most commonly used are custom-made (by self or company).[22] Two main types of checklists have been identified: analysis and action checklists.[62] Analysis checklists present a list of items that are analyzed and evaluated by the user. They are useful for inventory purposes to ensure that important aspects of a job or workplace are considered, to identify problem areas and compare different jobs or workplaces.[62] Action checklists present a list of actions that can be taken to improve the existing designs or conditions and are useful for prioritizing improvement options and training needs.[62]

Checklists rely on the observation skills of the people using them and are often based on subjective assessment, which may lack precision.[62] The role of checklists is "as one of a range of practical evaluation tools for conducting social dialogue between employers, workers, users, and others concerned" (p. 1750).[62] Many occupational health and safety authorities in various countries have a range of checklists available. There are also many published in various ergonomics texts, such as *Kodak's Ergonomic Design for People at Work.*[26]

An example of job analysis based on observation of physical demands that Kim conducted for the "Women's Health at Work" program is Figure 4-9.

WHOLE BODY POSTURAL ASSESSMENT

Manual Tasks Risk Assessment

ManTRA was developed to assist health and safety inspectors audit workplaces for compliance with the Queensland Manual Tasks Advisory Standard and to make an assessment of exposure to musculoskeletal risk factors.[13] When used in the workplace it is used by a team, including workers who perform the tasks assessed and staff responsible for manual task risk management.[13] ManTRA has been used in a variety of workplaces such as mining, food production, construction, and health.[11-13,113]

A task is assessed as a whole, rather than as task elements, and the assessment is based on a specific person's performance of the task, not people generally. The tool "combines information about the total time for which a person performs the task in a typical day (exposure) and the typical time for which the task is performed without break (duration)" (p. 2).[13] Four body regions (lower limbs, back, neck/shoulder, and arm/wrist/hand) are all considered for five characteristics of the task (cycle time, force, speed, awkwardness, and vibration).[13] Scores are calculated, and intervention may be indicated if certain critical values are exceeded (Figure 4-10).

Ovako Working Posture Analysing System

The Ovako Working Posture Analysing System (OWAS) was developed as a "practical method for identifying and evaluating poor working postures" (p. 199).[59] It requires observation of work tasks every 30 or 60 seconds, and the postures of the back, upper limbs, and lower limbs are rated.[80] The various posture combinations are classified into four action categories to determine whether intervention is required and how quickly the problem should be addressed. The length of time spent in various postures is also considered.[80] Figure 4-11 demonstrates OWAS postures. OWAS is considered easy to use and is focused on assessing posture, not risk of manual handling.[94] Therefore, if you wish to determine the risk of manual handling operations, other tools should be used,[94] such as ManTRA, the NIOSH lifting equation (see Chapter 11), or Manual Handling Assessment Charts.[42]

The OWAS method was originally developed for use in the Finnish steel industry, but it has also been used in a wide range of other areas, including in the mining industry,[43] with cleaners, with mechanics, with construction workers, with

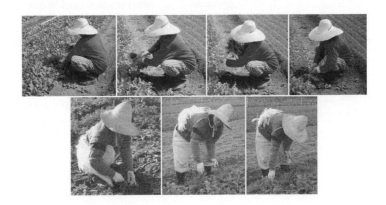

Description:
1. Squat (with or without stool) or stand and bend at hips
2. Reach forward bilaterally
3. Using dominant hand, push knife beneath surface to cut roots
4. Pull plant from the soil with nondominant hand
5. Tap roots with knife to remove soil
6. Place to the side to be bundled
7. Repeat steps 2-6 with nondominant hand
8. Gather a bundle (2-3 plants)
9. Tie using a plastic tie (bilateral movement)
10. Place bundle to the side

Environment: Outdoors during daylight hours
Duration: Task performed for up to 3 hours at a time
Equipment: Plastic ties, blunt curved knife, gloves, hat, sunglasses, boots, sleeve protectors

Physical demand	Frequency	Comments
Squatting	Constant	Without stool
Kneeling/crawling	Infrequent	Moving while squatting
Reaching: a) Forward b) Sideways	 Constant Frequently	 Mostly bilateral; repetitive over whole task and sustained for short periods Predominantly with nondominant hand; repetitive
Neck postures: a) Flexion b) Rotation	 Constant Infrequent	 Sustained
Side flexion	Infrequent	Sometimes work for short instances in this position
Shoulder postures a) Abduction b) Flexion	 Constant Constant	 Sustained/repetitive–bilateral Sustained/repetitive–bilateral
Wrist postures: a) Flexion b) Extension c) Pronation d) Supination	 Occasional Frequent Constant Occasional	 Ulnar deviation (occasional) To push knife into soil, repetitive, dominant hand Main position–bilateral Bilateral
Fine hand coord.	Occasional	Tying and picking roots
Gripping/grasping	Constant	Constantly grasping knife and/or vegetables while cutting and tying
Lifting: a) Floor-to-knee transfer	 Infrequent	 Transferring vegetables from one side to the other–v. light
Pulling	Occasional	Pull plant out; pull roots off
Exposure to extreme temps	Constant	Work outdoors
Exposure to chemicals	Constant	Fertilizer and pesticides; low-level exposure

FIGURE **4-9** Example of Task Analysis based on observation: cutting and bunching English spinach. (From Crowther A, Fonti F, Quayle L: *Musculoskeletal pain and injury experienced by Chinese women working on market gardens: workplace assessment report,* Sydney, New South Wales, 2005, Sydney West Area Health Service Women's Health at Work Program and The University of Sydney.)

Manual Tasks Risk Assessment Tool (ManTRA) V 2.0 Scoring Matrix

Body region	Total time	Duration	Cycle time	Repetition risk	Speed	Force	Exertion risk	Awkwardness	Vibration	Cumulative risk
Lower limbs										
Back										
Neck										
Shoulder/arm										
Wrist/hand										

Cumulative risk is the sum of unshaded cells.

Task codes

Total time

1	2	3	4	5
0-2 hours/day	2-4 hours/day	4-6 hours/day	6-8 hours/day	>8 hours/day

Duration of continuous performance

1	2	3	4	5
<10 minutes	10 min-30 min	30 min-1 hr	1 hr-2 hr	>2 hr

Cycle time

1	2	3	4	5
>5 minutes	1-5 minute	30 s-1 min	10 s-30 s	<10 s

Force

1	2	3	4	5
Minimal force		Moderate force		Maximal force

Speed

1	2	3	4	5
Slow movements	Moderately paced	Little or no movement– static posture	Fast and smooth movements	Fast, jerky movements

Awkwardness

1	2	3	4	5
All postures close to neutral	Moderate deviations from neutral in one direction	Moderate deviations in more than one direction	Near end range of motion posture in one direction	Near end range of motion in more than one direction

Vibration (whole body or peripheral)

1	2	3	4	5
None	Minimal	Moderate	Large amplitude	Severe amplitude

Scoring keys for repetition and exertion

Scoring key for repetition

Cycle time	1	2		Duration		
			3	4	5
1	1	1	3	4	5
2	1	2	3	4	4
3	2	3	4	4	5
4	2	3	4	5	5
5	3	4	5	5	5

Scoring key for exertion

Speed	1	2		Force		
			3	4	5
1	1	1	3	4	5
2	1	2	2	3	4
3	2	3	3	4	4
4	2	3	4	4	5
5	3	4	5	5	5

Action may be indicated if, for any region, the exertion risk factor is 5, the sum of exertion and awkwardness is 8 or greater, or the cumulative risk is 15 or greater.

FIGURE **4-10** ManTRA. (From Straker L, Burgess-Limerick R, Pollock C, Egeskov R et al: A randomized and controlled trial of a participative ergonomics intervention to reduce injuries associated with manual tasks: physical risk and legislative compliance, *Ergonomics* 47[2]:166, 2004.)

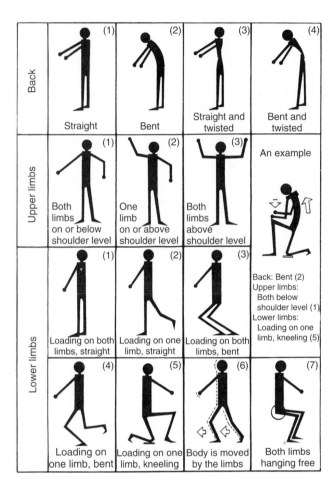

FIGURE 4-11 OWAS postures. (From Karhu O, Kansi P, Kuorinka I: Correcting working postures in industry: a practical method for analysis, *Appl Ergon* 8(4):199, 1977.)

dairy farmers, with nurses,[80] in the building industry,[88] in the fishing industry,[106] and in the seafood retail industry.[120] OWAS has also been suggested for use in occupational rehabilitation.[95] Inter-rater and test-retest (intra-rater) reliability of OWAS is considered good.[21]

Rapid Entire Body Assessment

REBA was developed as a postural analysis tool sensitive to the type of unpredictable working postures found in health care and other service industries.[44] It has been used to assess jobs in health care and hospitals,[44,56] supermarkets,[19] and dental professions.[91] REBA's approach and scoring system are based on RULA.[85] Scoring is based on trunk, neck, and leg postures and load or force (Score A), upper and lower arms, wrist and coupling (Score B), and an activity rating.[44] The score is then converted into a recommendation for action.[44,94]

As with OWAS, REBA is focused on assessment of posture rather than manual handling risk.[94] It is sensitive to detecting changes or improvements after ergonomic intervention; however, its focus is biomechanical, and workplace changes based on task repetition, length of shifts, and other factors that affect worker performance are not reflected in REBA scores.[19] Initial studies indicate that REBA has acceptable inter-rater reliability; however, more detailed examination of reliability and validity is recommended by REBA's developers.[44]

UPPER LIMB POSTURAL ASSESSMENT

Rapid Upper Limb Assessment

RULA was developed "to investigate the exposure of individual workers to risk factors associated with work-related upper limb disorders" (p. 91).[85] It is intended to be used as a screening tool and as part of a broader ergonomic survey covering epidemiologic, physical, mental, environmental and organizational factors.[85,86] RULA assesses biomechanical and postural loading of the whole body, with particular focus on the neck, trunk, and upper limbs.

Deciding at what point of the work cycle to perform a RULA assessment is important. It can be based on the posture held for the longest time or the "worst" posture adopted or taken at regular intervals over the working period.[86] The postures for the upper arm, lower arm, wrist, and forearm ("wrist twist") are scored (Posture Score A). Static loading or repetition, and force/load scores are then estimated. This is repeated for the neck, trunk, and legs (Posture Score B). Combining these scores produces a grand score that is used to determine an action level indicating whether the posture is acceptable or requires investigation and change.[17,85] Right and left upper limbs can be scored separately if necessary (Figure 4-12).

RULA was originally developed using workers in the garment-making industry, with computer operators, and with workers performing a variety of manufacturing tasks.[85,86] It has also been used with formwork carpenters,[66] with truck drivers,[73] in the retail seafood industry,[120] in automotive assembly plants,[23] and to assess the impact of different mouse positions when doing a computer task.[16]

Construct validity of the RULA method has been established with significant associations between RULA scores and reported pain.[73,85] Inter-rater reliability indicated "high consistency of scoring" (p. 98).[85]

Strain Index

The Strain Index is a semi-quantitative job analysis method used to identify jobs that expose workers to increased risk of developing distal upper extremity (elbow, forearm, wrist, hand) disorders.[89,90] The Strain Index produces a score representing the product of six task variables: intensity of exertion, duration of exertion, exertions per minute, hand and wrist posture, speed of work, and duration of task per day.[89,90] It was originally developed for use in a pork processing plant and has also been used in turkey processing[61] and automotive assembly.[23]

The Strain Index has good test-retest and inter-rater reliability[111,112] and has demonstrated predictive validity.[61,89] When compared with RULA, however, results had very little correlation, indicating that results were not interchangeable and the instruments measured different constructs.[23] It was recommended that if the job involved high hand intensity the Strain Index could be used, whereas if there were awkward upper limb postures adopted, then RULA could be used.[23]

Following a walk-through survey of the manufacturing company, discussion with supervisors and workers and examination of injury records, Kim has identified the areas with high incidences of back and upper limb injuries and also those at increased risk. For areas with manual handling tasks, ManTRA will be used, whereas in areas that require a range of postures (static and dynamic) OWAS or REBA will be used. To address upper limb injury concerns, RULA will be used for tasks involving awkward upper limb postures, and the Strain Index will be used when tasks require high hand force and intensity.

CONCLUSION

This chapter has presented work-related assessments that can be used to assess individuals' work abilities when there is a specific job available or more generally to consider the physical demands of work. Although there are many commercial and home-grown systems available, those that have been included here are in more common use around the world, and evidence for their reli-

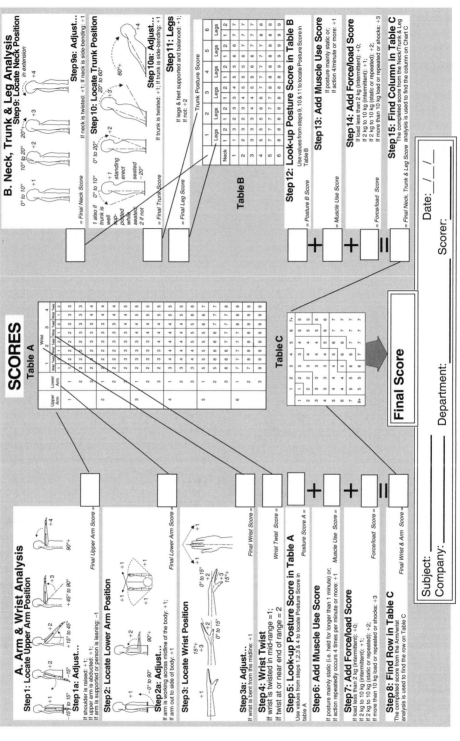

FIGURE 4-12 RULA worksheet. (Reprinted with permission from Professor Alan Hedge, http://ergo.human.cornell.edu/ahRULA.html.)

Overview

The learning exercises provided are designed to increase your practical understanding of some basic issues associated with work-related assessments for individuals and job requirements.

Purpose

The purpose of these learning exercises is to consider the referrals Kim has received and examine the types of work-related assessments for individuals and job requirements that may be most appropriate to use.

Exercises

1. Consider Kim's referral for Trevor. Kim needs to decide which FCENJ will be appropriate to use to determine Trevor's physical abilities for work in general *(purpose of assessment)*. As the specific job or position has not been identified, the assessment will focus on the general tasks and task elements associated with work that Trevor can do *(level of assessment)*. The *utility* and *dependability* of the FCENJ also need to be considered. Considering all these aspects, make recommendations regarding which work capacity evaluation devices, FCE systems, and/or lifting assessments would be most appropriate for Kim to use.

2. Identify two workplaces you are familiar with that are from different industry sectors and engage in different activities (e.g., a supermarket and a dental surgery office). Consider the types of work-related injuries that people in these workplaces may experience. Select ergonomic assessment tools that would be appropriate to use in these workplaces. Justify your selection and explain why the tools you selected are the same or different for the two workplaces.

ability and validity has been published. This enables therapists such as Kim to select the assessments to use based on a model that presents a process of excellence in work-related assessments (see Figure 4-1).

Therapists also use job analysis techniques to assess the physical requirements and demands of jobs, identifying potential risks to which workers may be exposed. This enables therapists to make recommendations regarding the prevention of musculoskeletal injuries in the workplace. Various approaches have been presented, including observation, checklists, and more quantitative instruments. Tools addressing manual handling risks (ManTRA), postural concerns (OWAS, REBA, and RULA) and high-intensity hand use (Strain Index) have been included. Therapists are encouraged to investigate these tools further and develop expertise in their use.

Multiple Choice Review Questions

1. When Kim received the referral for Trevor, what was the first thing that needed to be determined?
   A. Identify whether to do an FCE (No Job) or FCE (Job)
   B. Identify which Valpar Component Work Samples would be most appropriate
   C. Determine the purpose of the work-related assessment
   D. Determine how the data will be collected and from what sources

2. What type of work-related assessment is focused on an individual worker performing physical demands related to work in general, rather than to a specific job or duties?
   A. Physical ergonomic assessment
   B. Workplace assessment
   C. Functional capacity evaluation (job)
   D. Functional capacity evaluation (no job)

3. Which of the following hand function assessments (see Figure 4-5) is the most suitable to assess gross grasp and placement?
   A. Minnesota Rate of Manipulation Test
   B. Purdue Pegboard
   C. O'Connor Finger Dexterity Test
   D. O'Connor Tweezer Dexterity Test

4. The EPIC Lift Capacity Test and the PILE (Progressive Isoinertial Lifting Evaluation) both assess a person's lifting ability. At what individual or job level (see Figure 4-2) would these assessments be?
   A. Role/Activity (individual) or Job Position/Job Duties (job)
   B. Task/Skill (individual) or Tasks/Task Elements (job)
   C. Skill/Body System (individual) or Task Elements/Elemental Motions (job)
   D. Activity/Task (individual) or Job Duties/Tasks (job)

5. Kim needs to determine Lucy's ability to perform her usual duties, such as data entry and word processing. What would be the most appropriate way to do this?
   A. Interview Lucy about her perceived capacity to return to performing these duties.
   B. Check with Lucy's supervisor or manager to determine her capacity to return to performing these duties.
   C. Perform a range of standardized hand function assessments, such as the Minnesota Rate of Manipulation Test, Purdue Pegboard, and O'Connor Finger Dexterity Test.

   D. Simulate Lucy's job demands using a computer workstation that can be adjusted to suit Lucy.

6. Which of the following would be most suitable to assess the musculoskeletal risk factors associated with manual handling?
   A. OWAS
   B. RULA
   C. REBA
   D. ManTRA

7. Which of the following would be most suitable to assess unpredictable working postures, such as those found in the health care industry?
   A. OWAS
   B. RULA
   C. REBA
   D. ManTRA

8. Using the OWAS postures (see Figure 4-11), score the posture adopted in Figure 4-6, C (Physical Agility Tester [PAT], set for low-level task).
   A. 1 (trunk) 3 (upper limbs) 6 (lower limbs)
   B. 2 (trunk) 1 (upper limbs) 3 (lower limbs)
   C. 3 (trunk) 2 (upper limbs) 1 (lower limbs)
   D. 4 (trunk) 1 (upper limbs) 5 (lower limbs)

9. What are the five characteristics of the task that are considered when using ManTRA?
   A. Cycle time, force, speed, awkwardness, and vibration
   B. Trunk posture, upper limb posture, lower limb posture, force, and duration
   C. Intensity of exertion, duration of exertion, exertions per minute, speed of work, and duration of task per day
   D. Head and neck posture, arm and wrist posture, lower limb support, muscle use, and force and load

10. What are the six characteristics of the task that are considered when using the Strain Index?
    A. Cycle time, force, speed, awkwardness, duration per day, and vibration
    B. Head and neck posture, trunk posture, upper limb posture, lower limb posture, force, and duration
    C. Intensity of exertion, duration of exertion, exertions per minute, hand and wrist posture, speed of work, and duration of task per day
    D. Head and neck posture, trunk posture, arm and wrist posture, lower limb support, muscle use, and force and load

REFERENCES

1. Alpert J, Matheson L, Beam W et al: The reliability and validity of two new tests of maximum lifting capacity, *J Occup Rehabil* 1(1):13, 1991.
2. Ang N: Study on the test-retest reliability of the Valpar Component Work Sample 9 (Whole Body Range of Motion), Unpublished Honors thesis, Sydney, New South Wales, 1999, University of Sydney.
3. Barrett T, Browne D, Lamers M et al: Reliability and validity testing of Valpar 19. In Australian Association of Occupational Therapists (AAOT), editor: *Proceedings of the 19th National Conference of the Australian Association of Occupational Therapists*, vol 2, Perth, Western Australia, 1997, AAOT.
4. Beaton DE, Dumont A, Mackay MB et al: Steindler and pectoralis major flexorplasty: a comparative analysis, *J Hand Surg [Am]* 20(5):747, 1995.
5. Beaton DE, O'Driscoll SW, Richards R: Grip strength testing using the BTE work simulator and the Jamar dynamometer: a comparative study. *J Hand Surg [Am]* 20(2):293, 1995.
6. Becht TM, Roberts D: Measured functional trends in military personnel discharged medically due to low back pain. In Worth DR, editor: *Moving in on occupational injury*, Oxford, 2000, Butterworth Heinemann.
7. Bhambhani Y, Esmail S, Britnell S: The Baltimore Therapeutic Equipment work simulator: biomechanical and physiological norms for three attachments in healthy men, *Am J Occup Ther* 48(1):19, 1994.
8. Boadella JM, Sluiter JK, Frings-Dresen MHW: Reliability of upper extremity tests measured by the Ergos Work Simulator: a pilot study, *J Occup Rehabil* 13(4):219, 2003.
9. Brouwer S, Dijkstra PU, Stewart RE et al: Comparing self-report, clinical examination and functional testing in the assessment of work-related limitations in patients with chronic low back pain, *Disabil Rehabil* 27(17):999, 2005.
10. Brouwer S, Reneman MF, Dijkstra PU et al: Test-retest reliability of the Isernhagen Work Systems Functional Capacity Evaluation in patients with chronic low back pain, *J Occup Rehabil* 13(4):207, 2003.
11. Burgess-Limerick R, Dennis G, Straker L et al: Participative ergonomics for manual tasks in coal mining. In *Conference Proceedings of the Queensland Mining Industry Health & Safety Conference 2005*, Townsville, Queensland, 2005, Queensland Mining Industry.
12. Burgess-Limerick R, Joy J, Straker L et al: *Implementation of an ergonomics program intervention to prevent musculoskeletal injuries caused by manual tasks* (Coal Services Health & Safety Trust Research Grant Final Report), Brisbane, Queensland, 2006, University of Queensland.
13. Burgess-Limerick R, Straker L, Pollock C et al: *Manual Tasks Risk Assessment Tool (ManTRA) V 2.0*, 2004. Retrieved August 3, 2006, from http://ergonomics.uq.edu.au/download/mantra2.pdf.
14. Cetinok EM, Renfro RR, Coleman EF: A pilot study of the reliability of the dynamic mode of one BTE work simulator, *J Hand Ther* 8(3):199, 1995.
15. Coleman EF, Renfro RR, Cetinok EM et al: Reliability of the manual dynamic mode of the Baltimore Therapeutic Equipment Work Simulator, *J Hand Ther* 9(3):223, 1996.
16. Cook CJ, Kothiyal K: Influence of mouse position on muscular activity in the neck, shoulder and arm in computer users, *Appl Ergon* 29(6):439-443, 1998.
17. Corlett EN: Assessing the risk of upper limb disorders. In Karwowski W, editor: *International encyclopedia of ergonomics and human factors*, vol 3, London, 2001, Taylor & Francis.
18. Cotton A, Schonstein E, Adams R: Use of functional capacity evaluations by rehabilitation providers in NSW, *Work* 26(3):287, 2006.
19. Coyle A: Comparison of the Rapid Entire Body Assessment and the New Zealand Manual Handling "Hazard Control Record," for assessment of manual handling hazards in the supermarket industry, *Work* 24(2):111, 2005.
20. Curtis L, Mayer TG, Gatchel RJ: Physical progress and residual impairment quantification after functional restoration. Part III: Isokinetic and isoinertial lifting capacity, *Spine* 19(4):401, 1994.

21. de Bruijn I, Engels JA, van der Gulden JWJ: A simple method to evaluate the reliability of OWAS observations, *Appl Ergon* 29(4):281, 1998.
22. Dempsey PG, McGorry RW, Maynard WS: A survey of tools and methods used by certified professional ergonomists, *Appl Ergon* 36:489, 2005.
23. Drinkaus P, Sesek R, Bloswick DS et al: Comparison of ergonomic risk assessment outputs from Rapid Upper Limb Assessment and the Strain Index for tasks in automotive assembly plants, *Work* 21(2):165, 2003.
24. Durand M, Loisel P, Poitras S et al: The interrater reliability of a functional capacity evaluation: the Physical Work Performance Evaluation, *J Occup Rehabil* 14(2):119, 2004.
25. Dusik LA, Menard MR, Cooke C et al: Concurrent validity of the ERGOS work simulator versus conventional functional capacity evaluation techniques in a workers' compensation population, *J Occup Med* 35(8):759, 1993.
26. Eastman Kodak Company: *Kodak's ergonomic design for people at work,* ed 2, Hoboken, NJ, 2004, John Wiley & Sons.
27. Esmail S, Bhambhani Y, Britnell S: Gender differences in work performance on the Baltimore Therapeutic Equipment work simulator, *Am J Occup Ther* 49(5):405, 1995.
28. Fess EE: Correction: instrument reliability of the BTE Work Simulator: a preliminary study, *J Hand Ther* 6(2):82, 1993.
29. Fess EE: Instrument reliability of the BTE work simulator: a preliminary study [abstract], *J Hand Ther* 6(1):59, 1993.
30. Fraulin FO, Louie G, Zorrilla L et al: Functional evaluation of the shoulder following latissimus dorsi muscle transfer, *Ann Plast Surg* 35(4):349, 1995.
31. Gardener L, McKenna K: Reliability of occupational therapists in determining safe, maximal lifting capacity, *Aust Occup Ther J* 46(3):110, 1999.
32. Goldner RD, Howson MP, Nunley JA et al: One hundred eleven thumb amputations: replantation vs revision, *Microsurgery* 11(3):243, 1990.
33. Gouttebarge V, Wind H, Kuijer PP et al: Intra- and interrater reliability of the Ergo-Kit Functional Capacity Evaluation method in adults without musculoskeletal complaints, *Arch Phys Med Rehabil* 86:2354, 2005.
34. Gouttebarge V, Wind H, Kuijer PP et al: Reliability and validity of functional capacity evaluation methods: a systematic review with reference to Blankenship system, Ergos work simulation, Ergo-Kit and Isernhagen work system, *Int Arch Occup Environ Health* 77:527, 2004.
35. Gross DP, Battié MC: Reliability of safe maximum lifting determinations of a functional capacity evaluation, *Phys Ther* 82(4):364, 2002.
36. Gross DP, Battié MC: Construct validity of a kinesiophysical functional capacity evaluation administered within a worker's compensation environment, *J Occup Rehabil* 13(4):287, 2003.
37. Gross DP, Battié MC: The prognostic value of functional capacity evaluation in patients with chronic low back pain: Part 2—Sustained recovery, *Spine* 29(8):920, 2004.
38. Gross DP, Battié MC: Functional capacity evaluation performance does not predict sustained return to work in claimants with chronic back pain, *J Occup Rehabil* 15(3):285, 2005.
39. Gross DP, Battié MC, Cassidy JD: The prognostic value of functional capacity evaluation in patients with chronic low back pain: Part 1—Timely return to work, *Spine* 29(8):914, 2004.
40. Hazard RG, Fenwick JW, Kalisch SM et al: Functional restoration with behavioural support: a one-year prospective study of patients with chronic low-back pain, *Spine* 14(2):157, 1989.
41. Hazard RG, Reeves V, Fenwick JW et al: Test-retest variation in lifting capacity and indices of subject effort, *Clin Biomech* 8:20, 1993.
42. Health & Safety Executive (Health & Safety Laboratory): *Manual handling assessment charts,* 2003. Retrieved August 17, 2006, from http://www.hse.gov.uk/pubns/indg383.pdf.
43. Heinsalmi P: Method to measure working posture loads at working sites (OWAS). In Corlett N, Wilson J, Manenica I, editors: *The ergonomics of working postures,* London, 1986, Taylor & Francis.
44. Hignett S, McAtamney L: Rapid entire body assessment (REBA), *Appl Ergon* 31:201, 2000.
45. Horneij E, Holmström E, Hemborg B et al: Interrater reliability and between-days repeatability of eight physical performance tests, *Adv Physiother* 4(4):146, 2002.
46. Ijmker S, Gerrits EHJ, Reneman MF: Upper lifting performance of healthy young adults in functional capacity evaluations: a comparison of two protocols, *J Occup Rehabil* 13(4):297, 2003.
47. Innes E: *Factors influencing the excellence of work-related assessments in Australia,* Unpublished PhD thesis, Perth, Western Australia, 2001, Curtin University of Technology.

48. Innes E, Straker L: A clinician's guide to work-related assessments: 1—Purposes and problems, *Work* 11(2):183, 1998.
49. Innes E, Straker L: A clinician's guide to work-related assessments: 2—Design problems, *Work* 11(2):191, 1998.
50. Innes E, Straker L: Reliability of work-related assessments, *Work* 13(2):107, 1999.
51. Innes E, Straker L: Validity of work-related assessments, *Work* 13(2):125, 1999.
52. Innes E, Straker L: Workplace assessments and functional capacity evaluations: current practices of therapists in Australia, *Work* 18(1):51, 2002.
53. Isernhagen SJ: Contemporary issues in functional capacity evaluation. In Isernhagen SJ, editor: *the comprehensive guide to work injury management,* Gaithersburg, Md, 1995, Aspen.
54. Isernhagen SJ: Functional capacity evaluation. In Isernhagen SJ, editor: *Work injury: management and prevention,* Gaithersburg, Md, 1988, Aspen.
55. James C, Mackenzie L, Capra M: *Health professionals' attitudes and practices in relation to functional capacity evaluations.* Poster presented at the 14th World Federation of Occupational Therapists' Congress, Sydney, Australia, 2006.
56. Janowitz IL, Gillen M, Ryan G et al: Measuring the physical demands of work in hospital settings: design and implementation of an ergonomics assessment, *Appl Ergon* 37:641, 2006.
57. Kaiser H, Kersting M, Schian HM et al: Value of the Susan Isernhagen Evaluation of Functional Capacity Scale in medical and occupational rehabilitation [Der Stellenwert des EFL-Verfahrens nach Susan Isernhagen in der medizinischen und beruflichen rehabilitation], *Rehabilitation (Stuttg)* 39(5):297, 2000.
58. Karhu O, Harkonen R, Sorvali P et al: Observing working postures in industry: examples of OWAS application, *Appl Ergon* 12(1):13, 1981.
59. Karhu O, Kansi P, Kuorinka I: Correcting working postures in industry: a practical method for analysis, *Appl Ergon* 8(4):199, 1977.
60. Kennedy LE, Bhambhani YN: The Baltimore Therapeutic Equipment work simulator: reliability and validity at three work intensities, *Arch Phys Med Rehabil* 72:511, 1991.
61. Knox K, Moore JS: Predictive validity of the Strain Index in turkey processing, *J Occup Environ Med* 43(5):451, 2001.
62. Kogi K: Basic ergonomics checklists. In Karwowski W, editor: *International encyclopedia of ergonomics and human factors,* vol 3, London, 2001, Taylor & Francis.
63. Kuijer W, Gerrits EHJ, Reneman MF: Measuring physical performance via self-report in healthy young adults, *J Occup Rehabil* 14(1):77, 2004.
64. Lechner DE, Jackson JR, Roth DL, and others: Reliability and validity of a newly developed test of physical work performance, *J Occup Med* 36(9):997, 1994.
65. Lee GKL, Chan CCH, Hui-Chan CWY: Consistency of performance on the functional capacity assessment: static strength and dynamic endurance, *Am J Phys Med Rehabil* 80(3):189, 2001.
66. Lee GKL, Chan CCH, Hui-Chan CWY: Work profile and functional capacity of formwork carpenters at construction sites, *Disabil Rehabil* 23(1):9, 2001.
67. Legge J: Pre-employment functional assessments can be an effective tool for controlling work-related musculoskeletal disorders: a preliminary study. In Burgess-Limerick R, editor: *Back to basics: Proceedings of the 39th annual conference of the Ergonomics Society of Australia,* Canberra, Australian Capital Territory, 2003, ESA Inc.
68. Ljungquist T, Fransson B, Harms-Ringdahl K et al: A physiotherapy test package for assessing back and neck dysfunction—discriminative ability for patients versus healthy control subjects, *Physiother Res Int* 4(2):123, 1999.
69. Ljungquist T, Harms-Ringdahl K, NygrenÅ et al: Intra- and inter-rater reliability of an 11-test package for assessing dysfunction due to back or neck pain, *Physiother Res Int* 4(3):214, 1999.
70. Lo EKS: Demographic study on occupational therapy work rehabilitation programs in Hong Kong Hospital Authority, *Work* 14(3):185, 2000.
71. Lygren H, Dragesund T, Joensen J et al: Test-retest reliability of the Progressive Isoinertial Lifting Evaluation (PILE), *Spine* 30(9):1070, 2005.
72. Lysaght RM: Approaches to worker rehabilitation by occupational and physical therapists in the United States: factors impacting practice, *Work* 23(2):139, 2004.
73. Massaccesi M, Pagnotta A, Soccetti A et al: Investigation of work-related disorders in truck drivers using RULA method, *Appl Ergon* 34:303, 2003.
74. Matheson LN: Evaluation of lifting and lowering capacity, *Vocational Eval Work Adjustment Bull* 19(3):107, 1986.
75. Matheson LN, Danner R, Grant J et al: Effect of computerised instructions on measurement of lift capacity: safety, reliability, and validity, *J Occup Rehabil* 3(2):65, 1993.
76. Matheson LN, Isernhagen SJ, Hart DL: Relationships among lifting ability, grip force, and return to work, *Phys Ther* 82(3):249, 2002.

77. Matheson LN, Mooney V, Grant JE et al: A test to measure lift capacity of physically impaired adults. Part 1—Development and reliability testing, *Spine* 20(19):2119, 1995.

78. Matheson LN, Mooney V, Holmes D et al: A test to measure lift capacity of physically impaired adults. Part 2—Reactivity in a patient sample, *Spine* 20(19):2130, 1995.

79. Matheson LN, Rogers LC, Kaskutas V et al: Reliability and reactivity of three new functional assessment measures, *Work* 18(1):41, 2002.

80. Mattila M, Vilkki M: OWAS methods. In Karwowski W, Marras WS, editors: *Occupational ergonomics handbook*, Boca Raton, Fla, 1999, CRC Press.

81. Mayer TG, Barnes D, Kishino ND et al: Progressive isoinertial lifting evaluation I: a standardised protocol and normative database, *Spine* 13(9):993, 1988.

82. Mayer TG, Barnes D, Nichols G et al: Progressive isoinertial lifting evaluation II: a comparison with isokinetic lifting in a disabled chronic low-back pain industrial population, *Spine* 13(9):998, 1988.

83. Mayer TG, Gatchel R, Barnes D, and others: Progressive isoinertial lifting evaluation: erratum notice, *Spine* 15(1):5, 1990.

84. Mayer TG, Mooney V, Gatchel RJ et al: Quantifying postoperative deficits of physical function following spinal surgery, *Clin Orthop Relat Res* 244:147, 1989.

85. McAtamney L, Corlett EN: RULA: a survey method for the investigation of work-related upper limb disorders, *Appl Ergon* 24(2):91, 1993.

86. McAtamney L, Corlett N: R.U.L.A.—A rapid upper limb assessment tool. In Robertson SA, editor: *Contemporary ergonomics 1994*, London, 1994, Taylor & Francis.

87. McClure PW, Flowers KR: The reliability of BTE work simulator measurements for selected shoulder and wrist tasks, *J Hand Ther* 5(1):25, 1992.

88. Monk V: Postural assessment of building industry tasks using the Ovako Working Posture Analysing System, *J Occup Health Saf Aust NZ* 14(2):149, 1998.

89. Moore JS, Garg A: The Strain Index: a proposed method to analyze jobs for risk of distal upper extremity disorders, *Am Ind Hyg Assoc J* 56:443, 1995.

90. Moore JS, Garg A: The Strain Index. In Karwowski W, editor: *International encyclopedia of ergonomics and human factors*, vol III, London, 2001, Taylor & Francis.

91. Nasl SJ, Hossenini MH, Shahtaheri SJ et al: Evaluation of ergonomic postures of dental professions by Rapid Entire Body Assessment (REBA). In Birjand, Iran [Farsi], *J Dent* 18(1):61, 2005.

92. Ogden-Niemeyer L: *Procedure guidelines for the WEST Standard Evaluation: "Assessment of range of motion under load,"* rev ed, Long Beach, Calif, 1991, Work Evaluations Systems Technology.

93. O'Halloran D, Innes E: Understanding work in society. In Whiteford G, Wright-St Clair V, editors: *Occupation and practice in context,* London, 2005, Churchill Livingstone.

94. Pinder ADJ, Monnington SC: *Benchmarking of the Manual Handing Assessment Charts (MAC),* 2002. Retrieved August 14, 2006, from http://www.hse.gov.uk/research/hsl_pdf/2002/hsl02-31.pdf.

95. Pratt L: *The modification of OWAS and RULA for use in occupational rehabilitation.* Paper presented at the 29th Annual Conference of the Ergonomics Society of Australia, Perth, Western Australia, 1993.

96. Reneman MF, Brouwer S, Meinema A et al: Test-retest reliability of the Isernhagen Work Systems Functional Capacity Evaluation in healthy adults, *J Occup Rehabil* 14(4):295, 2004.

97. Reneman MF, Bults MM, Engbers LH et al: Measuring maximum holding times and perception of static elevated work and forward bending in healthy young adults, *J Occup Rehabil* 11(2):87, 2001.

98. Reneman MF, Dijkstra PU, Westmaas M et al: Test-retest reliability of lifting and carrying in a 2-day functional capacity evaluation, *J Occup Rehabil* 12(4):269, 2002.

99. Reneman MF, Fokkens AS, Dijkstra PU et al: Testing lifting capacity: validity of determining effort level by means of observation, *Spine* 30(2):E40-E46, 2005.

100. Reneman MF, Jaegers SM, Westmaas M et al: The reliability of determining effort level of lifting and carrying in a functional capacity evaluation, *Work* 18(1):23, 2002.

101. Rondinelli RD, Dunn W, Hassanein KM et al: A simulation of hand impairments: effects on upper extremity function and implications toward medical impairment rating and disability determination, *Arch Phys Med Rehabil* 78(12):1358, 1997.

102. Rustenburg G, Kuijer PP, Frings-Dresen MH: The concurrent validity of the ERGOS Work Simulator and the Ergo-Kit with respect to maximum lifting capacity, *J Occup Rehabil* 14(2):107, 2004.

103. Schenk P, Klipstein A, Spillmann S et al: The role of back muscle endurance, maximum force, balance and trunk rotation control regarding lifting capacity, *Eur J Appl Physiol* 96:146, 2006.

104. Schult M, Söderback I, Jacobs K: Swedish use and validation of Valpar work samples for patients with musculoskeletal neck and shoulder pain, *Work* 5(3):223, 1995.

105. Schult M, Söderback I, Jacobs K: Multidimensional aspects of work capability: a comparison between individuals who are working or not working because of chronic pain, *Work* 15(1):41, 2000.

106. Scott GB, Lambe NR: Working practices in a perchery system, using the OVAKO Working posture Analysing System (OWAS), *Appl Ergon* 27(4):281, 1996.

107. Sellars RGM, O'Neill M, Amber-Scott C et al: Assessing pain and disability exaggeration with the functional capacity evaluation process. In Worth DR, editor: *Moving in on occupational injury*, Oxford, 2000, Butterworth Heinemann.

108. Shechtman O, MacKinnon L, Locklear C: Using the BTE Primus to measure grip and wrist flexion strength in physically active wheelchair users: an exploratory study, *Am J Occup Ther* 55(4):393, 2001.

109. Shervington J, Balla J: WorkAbility Mark III: Functional assessment of workplace capabilities, *Work* 7(3):191, 1996.

110. Söderback I, Jacobs K: A study of well-being among a population of Swedish workers using a job-related criterion-referenced multidimensional vocational assessment, *Work* 14(2):83, 2000.

111. Stephens J-P, Vos GA, Stevens EMJ et al: Test-retest repeatability of the Strain Index, *Appl Ergon* 37(3):275, 2006.

112. Stevens EMJ, Vos GA, Stephens J-P et al: Inter-rater reliability of the Strain Index, *J Occup Environ Hyg* 1(11):745, 2004.

113. Straker L, Burgess-Limerick R, Pollock C, Egeskov R: A randomized and controlled trial of a participative ergonomics intervention to reduce injuries associated with manual tasks: physical risk and legislative compliance, *Ergonomics* 47(2):166, 2004.

114. Trevitt N: *A test-retest reliability study on the Valpar Component Work Sample 4.* Unpublished Honours thesis, School of Occupational Therapy, Faculty of Health Sciences, Sydney, New South Wales, 1997, University of Sydney.

115. Trossman PB, Li P-W: The effect of the duration of intertrial rest periods on isometric grip strength performance in young adults, *Occup Ther J Res* 9(6):362, 1989.

116. Trossman PB, Suleski KB, Li P-W: Test-retest reliability and day-to-day variability on an isometric grip strength test using the work simulator, *Occup Ther J Res* 10(5):266, 1990.

117. Tuckwell NL, Straker L, Barrett TE: Test-retest reliability on nine tasks of the Physical Work Performance Evaluation, *Work* 19(3):243, 2002.

118. U.S. Department of Labor Employment & Training: *The revised handbook for analyzing jobs*, Indianapolis, 1991, JIST Works.

119. Valpar International Corp: *Temporal reliability of selected Valpar Component Work Samples: learning curve studies*, 2003. Retrieved September 22, 2003, from http://www.valparint.com/wsstudy.htm.

120. Weigall F, Simpson K: *Manual handling methods in the retail seafood industry: final report, 2002.* Retrieved August 4, 2006, from http://www.workcover.nsw.gov.au/Publications/OHS/ManualHandling/manualhandlingretailseafoodindustry.htm.

121. Wilke NA, Sheldahl LM, Dougherty SM et al: Baltimore Therapeutic Equipment Work Simulator: energy expenditure of work activities in cardiac patients, *Arch Phys Med Rehabil* 74(4):419, 1993.

122. WorkCover Corporation of South Australia: *Occupational therapy fee schedule and guidelines: South Australia workers compensation occupational therapy services*, 2004. Retrieved August 9, 2006, from http://www.workcover.com/NR/rdonlyres/9D90BCDC-EC9E-4CC4-B3C2-6623C186776B/0/proOccTherapyScheduleAmend1104.pdf.

123. Yílmaz F, Yílmaz A, Merdol F et al: Efficacy of dynamic lumbar stabilization exercise in lumbar microdiscectomy, *J Rehabil Med* 35(4):163, 2003.

RESOURCES

Baltimore Therapeutic Equipment Technologies (BTE Work Simulator II, BTE Primus, BTE ER Functional Testing System)
http://www.btetech.com

ERGOS Work Simulator
http://www.simwork.com (North American site)
http://www.wrebv.com (European site)

Ergo-Kit FCE
http://www.fitform.nl/homeec.htm (in Dutch)

Ergoscience Physical Work Performance Evaluation (PWPE)
http://www.ergoscience.com

Isernhagen Work Systems (IWS) FCE (WorkWell FCE v.2)
http://www.workwell.com

EPIC Lift Capacity Test
http://www.epicrehab.com/elc.htm

Valpar Component Work Samples
http://www.valparint.com (North American site)

http://www.valparpacific.com.au (Australian site)

Cornell University Ergonomics Web Workplace Ergonomics Tools—Alan Hedge (many ergonomics tools available via this site, including ManTRA, RULA, REBA and Strain Index)

http://ergo.human.cornell.edu/cutools.html

Analysis Tools for Ergonomists—Thomas E. Bernard (University of South Florida) (many ergonomics tools available at this site, including REBA, RULA, Strain Index)

http://hsc.usf.edu/ ~ tbernard/ergotools

COPE Posture Analysis Tools (free online RULA software)

http://www.cope-ergo.com/assesstools.htm

WinOWAS (free computerized version of OWAS)
http://turva1.me.tut.fi/owas

5

Anthropometry

Nancy A. Baker

Learning Objectives

After reading this chapter and completing the exercises, the reader should be able to do the following:

1. Identify the strengths and weaknesses of the science of anthropometry.
2. Describe factors that influence human size and shape.
3. Use static anthropometric tables to help guide design parameters.
4. Understand the key concepts of reach, clearance, and posture.
5. Identify the effect that the environment plays on the performance components of precision and strength.

Secular trend. General changes in the size and shape of a population from generation to generation.

Sagittal plane. Vertical plane through the longitudinal axis that divides the body into left and right sections.

Coronal (frontal) plane. Vertical plane through the longitudinal axis that divides the body into front and back sections.

Height. Vertical measurement from the floor or seat surface.

Length. Horizontal measurement in the sagittal plane.

Breadth. Horizontal measurement in the coronal plane.

Reach. Imaginary sphere around the worker that can be touched by the worker at all points without shifting the body from the starting point.

Clearance. The space needed to allow free passage of a person or a body segment.

CASE STUDY

A large company is considering redesigning their data-entry department to improve the configuration of each workstation. The company has three shifts of 50 data-entry personnel. All workstations are used by at least three employees during these three shifts, and sometimes floaters (temporary employees) also use the workstations. The therapist hired to consult about the purchase of equipment has ascertained the following information:

- The population of the company is predominantly female (90%).
- The primary ethnicity is white (75%). An equal mix of ethnicities occurs in the remaining 25%.
- The company representatives state that the company is willing to replace the chairs and provide some additional small equipment. No budget is provided for completely redesigning all the capital equipment.
- Each workstation has a standard 30-inch desk and a 4-inch-high central processing unit (CPU) with a 16-inch-tall monitor on top of it. This configuration places the top of the monitor 50 inches from the floor. The keyboard is placed on the 30-inch desk. Each station has a computer wrist rest. The chairs are adjustable up and down from 17.5 to 22.5 inches.
- Most of the data entry is numeric; thus, the employees use the number pad. The mouse and the alphanumeric part of the keyboard are seldom used.

After reading through the chapter, answer the following questions:

1. Describe how the concepts of reach, clearance, and posture influence the therapists' decisions during the design of a computer workstation.
2. How would your recommendations for the computer workstation differ if you designed this setup to accommodate individuals who use wheelchairs for mobility?
3. One of the employees of the company is well below the 5th percentile in height (55 inches). What recommendations could you make to help her customize her workstation to fit her?

Anthropometry, the science of measurement of the human body, provides therapists with building blocks for understanding the complexities of the human form and how it interfaces with its environment. This chapter reviews the principles and methods of static anthropometry. Discussions of reach, clearance, and posture are included, as well as tables of measurements. Methods for the application of these principles to workstation design are also reviewed. Anthropometric concepts will be applied to the case study throughout the chapter.

People have always studied and analyzed the human form. Measurements were often based on human body parts; a foot was the length of the human foot, and a yard was the length from midline to the fingertip. These early methods of evaluating the human form gradually evolved into the modern science of anthropometry. Anthropometry, the measurement of human individuals in order to understand and design for human physical variations, is the cornerstone of the design of all objects and spaces used by humans. Because ergonomics is concerned with shaping the environment to optimize workers' abilities to perform their jobs, an understanding of anthropometry is essential to the application of ergonomics.

When creating a workspace, designers make many complex choices. In addition to the functional use of the space, the parameters of the human form and how it will act within the space must be understood and integrated into the overall design. Designers, therefore, must create a space that is suitable for all potential users, regardless of their size, shape, or capabilities. Often, however, users are envisioned by designers as being the same as they are. Consequently designers design the space to fit their own shape and fail to account for the great variability of the human form.

How can designers understand the population for which they are designing? They could guess as to the general size and shape of the population, but guesses are generally incorrect. They could measure everyone who might use a space or object, but this is often impractical. Alternatively, designers can use the science of anthropometry to develop concrete and scientific information that can be used to design spaces that fit the largest number of people. Anthropometry provides the parameters of human size and shape that allow designers to fulfill the needs of both comfort and function. Anthropometry provides both the understanding of why a workspace fits a worker and the understanding of how a workspace may fail the people who work in it. Anthropometry provides important information on how to shape the environment to fit the greatest number of people.

The term *anthropometry* refers to many types of measurements that are used to completely describe the human form. Along with the dimensions of the human form (stature, breadth, length), anthropometry also describes the mass of the human form (weight, center of gravity), and the parameters of human strength and motion. All of these are important when considering how an individual uses the environment and how to adapt that environment to facilitate each individual's performance. Scientists have developed data that describe many elements of the human form and that are available for estimating the size, shape, and capacities of the population. Anthropometric measurements have been ascertained for children and the elderly, as well as for members of a wide variety of ethnic groups. This chapter reviews static anthropometry as it pertains to workstation design.

STATIC ANTHROPOMETRY

Static anthropometry is the science of measuring length, breadth, and width in the human population. Anthropometrists have reported several universal factors that seem to influence human size and shape: gender, ethnicity, age, and occupation.[11]

Overall the shape of any stable population changes from generation to generation, a phenomenon termed *secular trend*.[11] In general, the overall world population has been becoming larger. Although most researchers are cautious in their explanations as to why the population is getting larger, one theory is that this secular trend of increased size is a result of changes in the environment such as improved diet and the reduction of infectious disease. The recent increase in obesity in the population,[10] in particular, will affect the circumferential and breadth measurements of the population.

Gender Differences

The differences between men and women are more than skin deep. Men generally are larger than women, both overall and in limb length. Less of male body weight is composed of fat tissue, and what fat men have tends to accumulate at the abdomen. A woman's fat tends to accumulate at the hips, thighs, and buttocks. It is interesting to note that obesity in women has not significantly increased since 1999, but obesity has increased in men.[10]

Ethnic Differences

Different ethnic groups have different anthropometric measurements. A general rule of thumb is that ethnic groups that live primarily in tropical climates have a lower body weight than groups that live in colder temperatures.[12] Body proportions vary among ethnic groups; for example, black Africans have proportionally longer lower limbs than Europeans, whereas Asians have proportionally shorter limbs.[11] Differences resulting from ethnicity, however, tend to diminish as populations migrate and commingle.

Aging

It is easy to see the difference age makes in body size and shape when comparing a child with an adult. Anthropometric changes during adulthood, however, are more subtle. As people pass 30, stature decreases and body weight increases. After age 50 for men and 60 for women, body weight again decreases.

Occupational Differences

The tendency for people of different occupations to have different anthropometric proportions is poorly understood. Some occupations, such as soldier or jockey, are self-selective—a specific size or weight is necessary to perform the job. Why other occupations should be stratified by size is a bit of a mystery. Does the job shape the person, or does the correctly sized person select the job?

PERSONS WITH DISABILITIES

The presence of a disability is often an overlooked factor in workstation design. Disability alters not only the size and shape of individuals but also their capacity to perform activities that may be taken for granted by the general population. Consider people who use wheeled mobility devices. Not only do they have to cope with the impairments that placed them in their devices, but the people who use wheeled mobility devices also have the added anthropometric disadvantage of being anywhere from 10 to 18 inches lower than other adults in situations in which standing is needed.[4] In addition, their overall breadth is up to five times that of a person without a device, and thus they are much larger and bulkier. Consider individuals who have an impairment. These individuals may lack full motion or strength because of a mild disability; examples include the frail elderly who cannot rise from a chair because it is too low and individuals with rheumatoid arthritis who cannot open a car door because of weakened hands. In a well-designed environment, these individuals may be able to function fully. However, if placed in a poorly designed environment, these individuals may be totally disabled. Thus, designing an environment that supports the independence of those with disabilities is vital. Using anthropometric measurements to design the optimal environment for people with disabilities often provides an optimal environment for all populations.

When designing for people with disabilities (particularly those with physical challenges such as kyphosis, axial rotation, or limb discrepancies), however, the use of standard anthropometric measurement and techniques is difficult because of the high degree of statistical variability in this population. Type of disability can markedly affect the distributions of body dimensions. A study of the anthropometrics of a population with severe disabilities reported a need for at least four new linear measurements to capture the spatial requirements of those with physical challenges, as well as five angular measurements to account for the inability of many people with disabilities to assume the "standard" seated posture.[7] Therefore individual measurements should always be taken for those with physical challenges.

STATIC ANTHROPOMETRIC MEASUREMENTS

Like most sciences, static anthropometry has conventions. Static anthropometry always looks at human dimensions in either the sagittal plane or the coronal plane. Static anthropometry also uses two standard postures:

Standing posture: The person stands erect and looks straight ahead, with his or her arms in a relaxed posture at the side (Figure 5-1).

Seated posture: The person sits erect and looks straight ahead. The sitting surface is adjusted so that the person's thighs are parallel to the floor and the knees are bent to a 90-degree angle with the feet flat on the floor. The upper arm is relaxed and perpendicular to the horizontal plane, and the forearm is at a right angle to the upper arm and thus also parallel to the floor. Measurements in sitting are made using a horizontal reference point, either the ground or the seat, and a vertical reference point, an imaginary line that touches the back of the uncompressed buttocks and shoulder blades of the subject. Thus, in the standard seated posture, the person is measured with most joints, the ankle, knees, hip, and elbows at 90-degree angles (Figure 5-2).

Table 5-1 describes some common anthropometric dimensions. Use Figures 5-1 through 5-4 to help to clarify each dimension.

These and other dimensions have been measured in thousands of people from different populations. The measurements have been compiled to form tables of anthropometric estimates. These tables can be used to determine the best sizes for aspects of the workspace for different ages, genders, and ethnic populations. These tables can also be used to get a sense of the range and complexity of the human form.

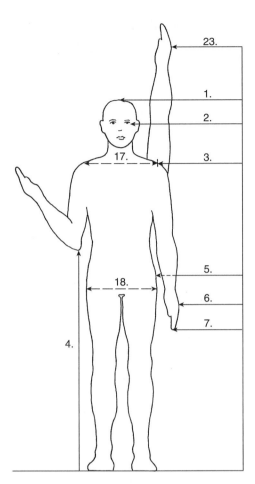

FIGURE **5-1** Static anthropometric dimensions for the standard standing posture. The numbers correspond to data in Table 5-1.

The dimensions in the second and third columns of Table 5-1 refer to the anthropometric estimates for a U.S. population in Table 5-2. The dimensions in the fourth and fifth columns of Table 5-1 refer to the estimates in Tables 5-3 and 5-4 and provide some general estimates for male and female individuals who use wheeled mobility devices. Many of these measurements would be similar in a seated population except that the height and breadth of the wheelchair must be taken into consideration. Table 5-5 provides detailed estimates for the hand and refers to Figure 5-4.

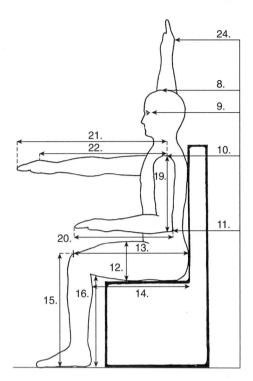

FIGURE **5-2** Static anthropometric dimensions for the standard sitting posture. The numbers correspond to data in Table 5-1.

LIMITATIONS OF THE STATIC ANTHROPOMETRIC ESTIMATES

All the information described is useful for understanding the shape of humans. However, as with any averages, these measurements have some limitations. Remember: anthropometric data offer a guide, not an absolute.

Accuracy

Measuring the human form is a tricky business. Not only is the body composed of round, soft outlines that are prone to compression, but people also tend to slouch. Measurement methods may vary from study to study depending on the researchers. Sometimes, because of the time and expense of anthropometric research, estimates are made using mathematic equations based on stature. Although these provide a very reasonable

Text continued on p. 85.

TABLE 5-1 Anthropometric Dimensions

	Estimates for U.S. Adults (see Figures 5-1 and 5-2, Table 5-2)			Estimates for Wheelchair Users (see Figure 5-3, Tables 5-3 and 5-4)	
	Dimensions	**Descriptions**		**Dimensions**	**Descriptions**
1	Stature	Vertical distance from the floor to the crown of the head	1	Overall height	Vertical distance from the floor to the crown of the head
2	Eye height	Vertical distance from the floor to the inner corner of the eye	2	Eye height	Vertical distance from the floor to the inner corner of the eye
3	Shoulder height	Vertical distance from the floor to the acromion	3	Shoulder height	Vertical distance from the floor to the acromion
4	Elbow height	Vertical distance from the floor to the olecranon process of the elbow	4	Wrist height	Vertical distance from the floor to the wrist crease just below the radial styloid
5	Hip height	Vertical distance from the floor to the greater trochanter	5	Sitting height	Vertical distance from the seat to the crown of the head
6	Wrist height	Vertical distance from the floor to the wrist crease just below the ulnar styloid	6	Knee height	Vertical distance from the floor to the top of the patella
7	Fingertip height	Vertical distance from the floor to the tip of the third digit	7	Overall breadth	Distance between the parallel vertical planes that cross the lateral-most points of the individual or the individual's wheelchair
8	Sitting height	Vertical distance from the seat to the crown of the head	8	Forearm to forearm breadth	Distance between the lateral-most points of the right and left forearms
9	Sitting eye height	Vertical distance from the seat to the inner corner of the eye	9	Hip breadth	Distance between the lateral-most points of the right and left hips
10	Sitting shoulder height	Vertical distance from the sitting surface to the acromion of the shoulder	10	Waist breadth	Distance between the lateral-most points of the right and left sides of the waist
11	Sitting elbow height	Vertical distance from the seat to the olecranon process of the elbow	11	Thigh breadth	Distance between the lateral-most points of the right and left thighs
12	Thigh thickness	Vertical distance from the seat to the top of the thigh at the thickest part	12	Overall depth	Distance between the parallel vertical planes that cross the anterior-most and posterior-most points of the individual or the individual's wheelchair
13	Buttock-knee length	Horizontal distance from the uncompressed buttock to the patella	13	Abdominal extension depth	Shortest perpendicular distance from seat back plane to the most protruding point of the abdominal region

TABLE 5-1 Anthropometric Dimensions—*cont'd*

Estimates for U.S. Adults (see Figures 5-1 and 5-2, Table 5-2)		Estimates for Wheelchair Users (see Figure 5-3, Tables 5-3 and 5-4)	
Dimensions	Descriptions	Dimensions	Descriptions
14 Buttock-popliteal length	Horizontal distance from the uncompressed buttocks to the underside of the knee at the popliteal angle	14 Buttock-knee length	Horizontal distance from the uncompressed buttock to the patella
15 Knee height	Vertical distance from the floor to the top of the patella while in the standard sitting position	15 Buttock-popliteal length	Horizontal distance from the uncompressed buttocks to the underside of the knee at the popliteal angle
16 Popliteal height	Vertical distance from the floor to the underside of the knee at the popliteal angle while in the standard sitting position		
17 Shoulder breadth	Horizontal distance across the shoulder from acromion to acromion		
18 Hip breadth	Horizontal distance at the broadest place on the hips when in the standard sitting position		
19 Shoulder-elbow length	Vertical distance from the acromion to the olecranon process in the standard sitting position		
20 Elbow-fingertip length	Vertical distance from the olecranon process to the tip of the third digit while in the standard sitting position		
21 Upper limb length	Horizontal distance from the acromion to the tip of the third digit with the elbow and wrist extended, and the shoulder flexed to 90°		
22 Shoulder-grip length	Horizontal distance from the acromion to the center of an object gripped in the hand with the elbow and wrist extended and the shoulder flexed to 90°		
23 Standing vertical grip reach	Vertical distance from the ground to the center of an object gripped in the hand with the shoulder flexed to 180° (no stretching)		
24 Sitting vertical grip reach	Vertical distance from the seat to the center of an object gripped in the hand with the shoulder flexed to 180° (no stretching)		

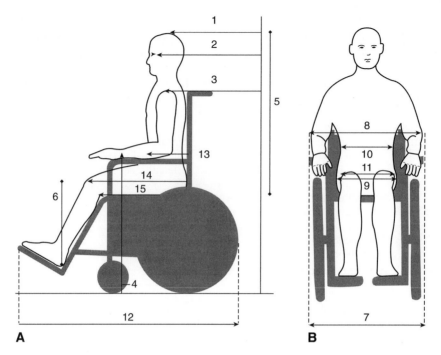

FIGURE **5-3 A,** Static anthropometric dimensions for wheelchair users (side view). The numbers correspond to data in Tables 5-3 and 5-4. **B,** Static anthropometric dimensions for the wheelchair users (front view). The numbers correspond to data in Tables 5-3 and 5-4.

| TABLE 5-2 | **Anthropometric Estimates for U.S. Adults*** |

No. in Figures 5-1 and 5-2	Dimensions	Men Percentile				Women Percentile			
		5th	50th	95th	SD	5th	50th	95th	SD
1	Stature	64.7	69.3	73.9	2.8	59.5	64.0	68.6	2.8
		1644.4	1760.4	1876.3	70.7	1511.6	1626.7	1741.7	70.2
2	Eye height	60.2	64.7	69.2	2.7	55.4	59.7	64.1	2.7
		1528.6	1643.3	1758.0	69.7	1406.1	1517.0	1627.9	67.4
3	Shoulder height	53.3	57.5	61.6	2.5	48.3	52.6	56.9	2.6
		1353.9	1459.7	1565.5	64.3	1226.7	1336.2	1445.6	66.5
4	Elbow height	40.4	43.7	47.0	2.0	37.4	40.5	43.6	1.9
		1025.8	1110.1	1194.5	51.3	949.5	1028.9	1108.4	48.3
5	Hip height	33.5	36.8	40.0	2.0	29.4	32.7	35.9	2.0
		851.3	934.3	1017.2	50.4	747.2	829.9	912.6	50.3
6	Wrist height	30.9	33.8	36.6	1.7	28.6	31.3	34.0	1.6
		785.3	857.5	929.7	43.9	726.6	795.5	864.4	41.9

TABLE 5-2	**Anthropometric Estimates for U.S. Adults*—*cont'd**

No. in Figures 5-1 and 5-2	Dimensions	Men Percentile				Women Percentile			
		5th	50th	95th	SD	5th	50th	95th	S
7	Fingertip height	23.9	26.3	28.7	1.5	22.1	24.4	26.7	1.4
		606.6	*667.4*	*728.1*	*36.9*	*562.3*	*620.3*	*678.4*	*35.3*
8	Sitting height	33.9	36.3	38.7	1.5	31.6	33.9	36.2	1.4
		862.2	*923.0*	*983.7*	*36.9*	*802.0*	*861.1*	*920.2*	*35.9*
9	Sitting eye height	29.3	31.7	34.2	1.5	27.0	29.3	31.7	1.4
		744.2	*805.8*	*867.5*	*37.5*	*685.8*	*745.0*	*804.2*	*36.0*
10	Sitting shoulder height	22.0	24.1	26.1	1.3	20.5	22.6	24.8	1.3
		558.9	*611.3*	*663.7*	*31.8*	*520.9*	*575.1*	*629.2*	*32.9*
11	Sitting elbow height	7.8	9.6	11.4	1.1	7.4	9.2	10.9	1.1
		199.2	*244.5*	*289.8*	*27.6*	*187.8*	*232.7*	*277.5*	*27.3*
12	Thigh thickness	5.2	6.7	8.3	0.9	3.8	6.3	8.8	1.5
		131.7	*171.3*	*211.0*	*24.1*	*95.4*	*159.6*	*223.7*	*39.0*
13	Buttock-knee length	21.7	24.4	27.1	1.6	19.9	23.6	27.2	2.2
		552.0	*620.0*	*688.1*	*41.4*	*506.1*	*598.6*	*691.1*	*56.2*
14	Buttock-popliteal length	18.1	20.6	23.2	1.6	16.6	19.8	23.1	2.0
		458.5	*523.6*	*588.8*	*39.6*	*420.7*	*503.3*	*585.9*	*50.2*
15	Knee height	19.6	21.5	23.4	1.1	17.7	19.5	21.4	1.1
		498.7	*546.1*	*593.5*	*28.8*	*448.4*	*495.9*	*543.4*	*28.9*
16	Popliteal height	15.9	17.7	19.5	1.1	13.9	15.7	17.5	1.1
		404.3	*450.0*	*495.7*	*27.8*	*354.3*	*399.9*	*445.5*	*27.7*
17	Shoulder breadth	14.8	16.3	17.7	0.9	13.2	14.5	15.7	0.7
		376.8	*412.9*	*449.0*	*21.9*	*336.5*	*367.2*	*398.0*	*18.7*
18	Hip breadth	12.3	14.6	17.0	1.4	12.1	15.9	19.7	2.3
		311.8	*371.8*	*431.9*	*36.5*	*307.2*	*403.6*	*500.0*	*58.6*
19	Shoulder-elbow length	13.7	14.9	16.1	0.7	12.3	13.5	14.7	0.8
		347.3	*377.8*	*408.3*	*18.6*	*311.3*	*343.0*	*374.6*	*19.2*
20	Elbow-fingertip length	17.4	18.8	20.2	0.9	15.6	17.0	18.5	0.9
		442.9	*478.5*	*514.1*	*21.7*	*395.0*	*432.9*	*470.8*	*23.0*
21	Upper limb length	29.0	31.4	33.7	1.4	25.6	28.3	31.0	1.7
		736.9	*796.4*	*855.9*	*36.2*	*649.2*	*718.5*	*787.8*	*42.1*
22	Shoulder grip length	23.9	26.2	28.4	1.3	21.8	24.1	26.3	1.4
		608.3	*664.5*	*720.6*	*34.1*	*554.3*	*611.0*	*667.6*	*34.4*
23	Vertical grip reach (standing)	76.6	82.7	88.7	3.7	71.7	76.9	82.0	3.1
		1945.4	*2099.5*	*2253.7*	*93.7*	*1822.1*	*1952.4*	*2082.6*	*79.2*
24	Vertical grip reach (sitting)	48.6	52.0	55.5	2.1	44.6	48.1	51.5	2.1
		1233.3	*1321.5*	*1409.7*	*53.6*	*1133.3*	*1220.5*	*1307.7*	*53.0*

*Data in roman type represent inches; data in italics represent millimeters.
Data are reproduced with permission from PeopleSize anthropometry software, Copyright © Open Ergonomics Ltd., 1999, Melton Road, Hickling Pastures, Melton Mowbray, Leicestershire, LE14 3QG, United Kingdom.

TABLE 5-3 Anthropometric Estimates for Male Wheelchair Users*

No. in Figure 5-3	Dimensions	Overall Sample (n = 75) Percentile					Manual Wheelchair Users (n = 37) Percentile					Power Wheelchair Users (n = 38) Percentile				
		Mean	SD	5th	50th	95th	Mean	SD	5th	50th	95th	Mean	SD	5th	50th	95th
Age (Years)																
1	Overall height	52.0	15.6	23.0	52.0	80.0	57.3	15.6	33.0	57.0	81.0	46.5	13.8	22.0	46.0	70.0
		1309	*60*	*1216*	*1312*	*1394*	*1306*	*47*	*1236*	*1310*	*1379*	*1312*	*71*	*1214*	*1312*	*1494*
2	Eye height	51.1	2.3	47.4	51.2	54.4	50.9	1.8	48.2	51.1	53.8	51.2	2.8	47.3	51.2	58.3
		1312	*60*	*1216*	*1312*	*1271*	*1310*	*47*	*1236*	*1310*	*1379*	*1312*	*71*	*1214*	*1312*	*1373*
3	Shoulder height	46.6	2.2	43.2	46.6	49.6	46.4	1.8	43.7	46.5	49.3	46.8	2.6	43.0	46.8	53.5
		1195	*58*	*1108*	*1194*	*1137*	*1190*	*46*	*1122*	*1193*	*1263*	*1200*	*67*	*1104*	*1200*	*1373*
4	Wrist height	40.7	2.0	36.8	40.8	44.3	40.5	1.6	36.5	40.7	42.8	40.8	2.4	36.7	40.8	46.7
		1043	*52*	*944*	*1046*	*904*	*1038*	*40*	*936*	*1045*	*1098*	*1047*	*61*	*941*	*1046*	*1197*
5	Sitting height	30.3	2.9	25.6	30.2	35.2	29.6	2.5	25.3	29.5	35.4	30.9	3.2	25.9	30.7	35.4
		776	*75*	*658*	*774*	*850*	*760*	*65*	*650*	*756*	*908*	*792*	*81*	*664*	*788*	*909*
6	Knee height	30.1	2.3	26.4	30.7	33.2	31.0	1.8	27.1	31.3	33.8	29.3	2.5	23.4	29.5	33.0
		773	*60*	*678*	*786*	*742*	*796*	*47*	*694*	*803*	*867*	*750*	*63*	*601*	*756*	*845*
7	Overall breadth	24.8	2.5	21.2	24.9	28.9	24.4	2.7	20.2	24.4	30.8	25.2	2.1	21.7	25.1	29.3
		637	*64*	*544*	*639*	*734*	*627*	*70*	*518*	*625*	*791*	*646*	*55*	*557*	*643*	*750*
8	Forearm to forearm breadth	27.8	3.2	23.6	27.7	32.7	27.2	2.7	23.0	26.9	32.7	28.4	3.6	23.7	28.3	34.5
		713	*82*	*604*	*709*	*839*	*698*	*68*	*589*	*690*	*839*	*728*	*92*	*608*	*726*	*885*
9	Hip breadth	23.4	3.2	18.5	23.1	28.7	23.0	2.5	19.2	22.6	27.3	23.9	3.7	15.2	23.7	29.1
		601	*82*	*475*	*593*	*737*	*590*	*65*	*492*	*579*	*701*	*612*	*95*	*391*	*607*	*747*
10	Waist breadth	10.5	1.6	8.1	10.4	13.2	10.3	1.5	8.7	10.9	15.1	10.1	1.6	7.2	9.9	12.8
		270	*41*	*207*	*267*	*339*	*263*	*39*	*224*	*280*	*387*	*258*	*40*	*184*	*255*	*328*
11	Thigh breadth	16.7	2.4	11.9	17.0	20.7	17.3	2.1	12.0	17.4	20.9	16.3	2.6	11.4	16.4	20.7
		429	*61*	*304*	*435*	*530*	*443*	*54*	*308*	*447*	*536*	*417*	*66*	*292*	*420*	*530*
12	Overall depth	47.8	3.9	42.6	48.0	55.3	48.2	4.3	41.8	48.4	57.1	47.4	3.7	42.7	46.4	53.9
		1225	*101*	*1092*	*1230*	*1419*	*1235*	*109*	*1071*	*1240*	*1465*	*1216*	*94*	*1096*	*1189*	*1381*
13	Abdominal extension depth	14.5	2.1	11.0	14.1	18.5	13.9	2.0	10.5	13.8	17.0	15.0	2.2	11.9	14.7	19.0
		371	*55*	*282*	*361*	*474*	*356*	*50*	*270*	*355*	*437*	*385*	*57*	*306*	*376*	*488*
14	Buttock-knee length	24.3	2.8	19.6	24.7	28.6	24.5	2.2	20.6	24.8	27.6	24.2	3.3	17.9	24.6	28.8
		624	*72*	*502*	*633*	*734*	*628*	*56*	*529*	*635*	*709*	*620*	*85*	*460*	*630*	*740*
15	Buttock-popliteal length	20.2	2.8	14.9	20.6	24.5	20.3	2.5	15.5	20.6	23.5	20.2	3.1	13.6	20.5	24.8
		519	*73*	*382*	*527*	*628*	*520*	*63*	*399*	*529*	*604*	*518*	*81*	*349*	*526*	*635*

*Data in roman type represent inches; data in italics represent millimeters.
From Paquet V, Feathers D: An anthropometric study of manual and powered wheelchair users, *Int J Ind Ergon*, 33:198, 2004.

TABLE 5-4   **Anthropometric Estimates for Female Wheelchair Users***

No. in Figure 5-3	Dimensions	Overall Sample (n = 46) Percentile					Manual Wheelchair Users (n = 28) Percentile					Power Wheelchair Users (n = 18) Percentile				
		Mean	SD	5th	50th	95th	Mean	SD	5th	50th	95th	Mean	SD	5th	50th	95th
Age (years)		49.5	15.0	28.0	48.5	74.0	53.1	15.2	33.0	51.0	82.0	44.0	15.0	22.0	41.0	72.0
1	Overall height	48.8 / 1251	2.5 / 63	44.4 / 1139	49.1 / 1258	52.4 / 1343	48.9 / 1254	2.3 / 58	44.4 / 1139	48.9 / 1255	52.4 / 1343	48.6 / 1246	2.7 / 70	44.1 / 1132	49.2 / 1261	52.8 / 1355
2	Eye height	44.5 / 1141	2.5 / 64	40.4 / 1026	44.8 / 1149	48.6 / 1246	44.4 / 1138	2.1 / 55	40.8 / 1047	44.8 / 1148	48.6 / 1246	44.7 / 1145	3.0 / 78	39.3 / 1008	45.1 / 1158	48.7 / 1249
3	Shoulder height	38.9 / 998	2.1 / 53	35.7 / 917	39.0 / 1001	42.2 / 1083	38.8 / 994	2.0 / 50	35.9 / 921	38.7 / 992	42.3 / 1084	39.1 / 1003	2.3 / 58	34.9 / 895	39.3 / 1008	42.8 / 1098
4	Wrist height	30.3 / 777	3.1 / 81	25.0 / 641	30.1 / 772	35.4 / 907	29.4 / 754	2.8 / 73	24.3 / 624	29.7 / 761	34.6 / 887	31.7 / 812	3.1 / 80	26.7 / 684	32.1 / 823	37.5 / 961
5	Sitting height	28.7 / 736	2.5 / 63	24.2 / 621	28.9 / 741	32.5 / 833	29.4 / 753	1.9 / 49	25.9 / 663	29.2 / 749	32.5 / 833	27.7 / 710	2.8 / 73	23.0 / 589	28.5 / 730	33.9 / 868
6	Knee height	62.5 / 276	5.6 / 31	54.3 / 239	61.9 / 269	71.2 / 332	60.8 / 271	5.3 / 30	53.5 / 237	60.2 / 263	70.7 / 329	64.9 / 284	5.2 / 32	56.9 / 240	64.1 / 281	77.6 / 353
7	Overall breadth	70.8 / 234	7.9 / 32	61.3 / 175	68.9 / 233	85.2 / 283	69.6 / 228	7.6 / 30	60.8 / 175	67.5 / 231	84.4 / 283	72.8 / 238	8.2 / 33	61.6 / 165	72.1 / 239	90.6 / 298
8	Forearm to forearm breadth	59.9 / 108	8.1 / 20	44.8 / 84	59.7 / 102	72.6 / 149	58.5 / 109	7.8 / 20	44.9 / 84	59.2 / 105	72.6 / 149	61.0 / 107	8.5 / 21	42.4 / 83	61.2 / 99	76.5 / 163
9	Hip breadth	27.7 / 168	5.2 / 20	21.6 / 143	26.1 / 168	38.3 / 202	27.9 / 168	5.2 / 18	21.6 / 143	26.8 / 167	38.3 / 198	27.4 / 168	5.4 / 23	21.2 / 126	25.3 / 170	41.8 / 210
10	Waist breadth	43.1 / 173	5.1 / 32	36.6 / 132	43.0 / 168	51.9 / 235	43.1 / 170	4.6 / 30	36.6 / 132	42.7 / 167	50.8 / 232	43.2 / 177	6.0 / 35	32.4 / 124	43.7 / 170	53.8 / 255
11	Thigh breadth	44.4 / 464	8.2 / 39	33.8 / 409	43.2 / 464	60.3 / 523	43.6 / 456	7.6 / 36	33.8 / 400	42.8 / 453	59.6 / 518	45.5 / 477	9.1 / 41	31.7 / 417	43.6 / 477	65.5 / 596
12	Overall depth	119.0 / 142	10.0 / 22	104.8 / 111	118.9 / 140	134.0 / 178	116.8 / 141	9.3 / 23	102.5 / 103	116.1 / 136	132.9 / 178	122.4 / 145	10.4 / 21	106.8 / 106	122.2 / 142	152.9 / 181
13	Abdominal extension depth	36.5 / 625	5.6 / 56	28.4 / 543	35.8 / 619	45.7 / 712	36.1 / 608	5.8 / 53	26.4 / 535	34.9 / 602	45.7 / 707	37.2 / 649	5.5 / 52	27.3 / 569	36.5 / 641	46.3 / 776
14	Buttock-knee length	24.4 / 625	2.5 / 65	21.5 / 550	24.5 / 627	29.3 / 752	24.6 / 632	1.7 / 45	21.8 / 559	24.7 / 633	26.6 / 683	23.9 / 614	3.5 / 89	14.3 / 367	23.8 / 612	30.0 / 770
15	Buttock-popliteal length	20.5 / 525	2.4 / 62	16.9 / 433	20.4 / 523	20.5 / 527	20.7 / 532	2.1 / 54	17.6 / 452	20.4 / 524	24.1 / 618	20.0 / 514	2.9 / 74	13.0 / 334	20.4 / 522	25.9 / 663

*Data in roman type represent inches; data in italics represent millimeters.

From Paquet V, Feathers D: An anthropometric study of manual and powered wheelchair users, *Int J Ind Ergon*, 33:197, 2004.

No. in Figure 5-4	Dimensions	Men Percentile				Women Percentile			
		5th	50th	95th	SD	5th	50th	95th	SD
1	Hand length	6.8	7.4	8.1	0.4	6.3	6.9	7.4	0.4
		173	*189*	*205*	*10*	*159*	*174*	*189*	*9*
2	Palm length	3.9	4.2	4.6	0.2	3.5	3.8	4.1	0.2
		98	*107*	*116*	*6*	*89*	*97*	*105*	*5*
3	Thumb length	1.7	2.0	2.3	0.2	1.6	1.9	2.1	0.2
		44	*51*	*58*	*4*	*40*	*47*	*53*	*4*
4	Index finger length	2.5	2.8	3.1	0.2	2.4	2.6	2.9	0.2
		64	*72*	*79*	*5*	*60*	*67*	*74*	*5*
5	Middle finger length	3.0	3.3	3.5	0.2	2.7	3.0	3.3	0.2
		76	*83*	*90*	*5*	*69*	*77*	*84*	*5*
6	Ring finger length	2.6	2.8	3.1	0.2	2.3	2.6	2.9	0.2
		65	*72*	*80*	*4*	*59*	*66*	*73*	*4*
7	Little finger length	1.9	2.2	2.5	0.2	1.7	2.0	2.2	0.2
		48	*55*	*63*	*4*	*43*	*50*	*57*	*4*
8	Thumb breadth (IPJ)	0.8	0.9	1.0	0.1	0.7	0.7	0.8	0.1
		20	*23*	*26*	*2*	*17*	*19*	*21*	*2*
9	Thumb thickness (IPJ)	0.7	0.9	0.9	0.1	0.6	0.7	0.8	0.1
		19	*22*	*24*	*2*	*15*	*18*	*20*	*2*
10	Index finger breadth (PIPJ)	0.7	0.8	0.9	0.0	0.6	0.7	0.8	0.0
		19	*21*	*23*	*1*	*16*	*18*	*20*	*1*
11	Index finger thickness	0.7	0.7	0.8	0.0	0.6	0.6	0.7	0.0
		17	*19*	*21*	*1*	*14*	*16*	*18*	*1*
12	Hand breadth (metacarpal)	3.1	3.4	3.7	0.2	2.7	3.0	3.3	0.2
		78	*87*	*95*	*5*	*69*	*76*	*83*	*4*
13	Hand breadth (across thumb)	3.8	4.1	4.5	0.2	3.3	3.6	3.9	0.2
		97	*105*	*114*	*5*	*84*	*92*	*99*	*5*
14	Hand breadth (minimum)†	2.8	3.2	3.6	0.2	2.5	2.8	3.1	0.2
		71	*81*	*91*	*6*	*63*	*71*	*79*	*5*
15	Hand thickness (metacarpal)	1.1	1.3	1.5	0.1	0.9	1.1	1.3	0.1
		27	*33*	*38*	*3*	*24*	*28*	*33*	*3*
16	Hand thickness (including thumb)	1.7	2.0	2.3	0.2	1.6	1.8	2.0	0.1
		44	*51*	*58*	*4*	*40*	*45*	*50*	*3*
17	Maximum grip diameter‡	1.8	2.0	2.3	0.2	1.7	1.9	2.1	0.1
		45	*52*	*59*	*4*	*43*	*48*	*53*	*3*
18	Maximum spread	7.0	8.1	9.2	0.7	6.5	7.5	8.5	0.6
		178	*206*	*234*	*17*	*165*	*190*	*215*	*15*
19	Maximum functional spread§	4.8	5.6	6.4	0.5	4.3	5.0	5.7	0.4
		122	*142*	*162*	*12*	*109*	*127*	*145*	*11*
20	Minimum square access‖	2.2	2.6	3.0	0.2	2.0	2.3	2.6	0.2
		56	*66*	*76*	*6*	*50*	*58*	*67*	*5*

TABLE 5-5 Anthropometric Estimates for the Hand*

From Pheasant S: *Bodyspace: anthropometry, ergonomics, and design,* ed 2, Philadelphia, 1998, Routledge/Taylor and Francis.

IPJ, Interphalangeal joint (i.e., the articulation between the two segments of the thumb); *PIPJ,* proximal interphalangeal joint (i.e., the finger articulation nearest the hand).

*Data in roman type represent inches; data in italics represent millimeters.

†As for hand breadth (metacarpal), except that the palm is contracted to make it as narrow as possible.

‡Measured by sliding the hand down a graduated cone until the thumb and middle finger just touch.

§Measured by gripping a flat wooden wedge with the tip end segments of the thumb and ring fingers.

‖The side of the smallest equal aperture through which the hand will pass.

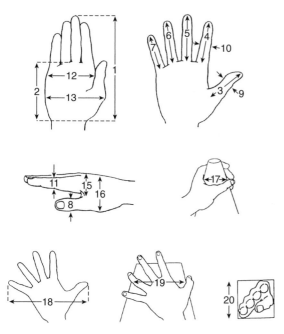

FIGURE **5-4** Static anthropometric dimensions for the hand. The numbers correspond to data in Table 5-5. (From Pheasant S: *Bodyspace: anthropometry, ergonomics, and design*, ed 2, Philadelphia, 1998, Routledge/Taylor and Francis.)

estimate, they may not be totally accurate.[11] Fortunately, unless form-fitting spaces are being designed (such as a space capsule), exact measurements are not always necessary.

Clothing

One of the greatest flaws in anthropometric measurements, at least for workstation design, is that the measurements are often taken of unclothed, unshod persons. Fortunately, most clothing adds only minimal bulk, unless it is protective equipment or bulky outdoors clothing. If workers are likely to be wearing bulky clothing, adjust the measurements accordingly. As a rule of thumb, use the following:

Shoes: Add approximately 1 inch (25 mm) for men and 1 to 2 inches (25 to 45 mm) for women to all measurements involving leg height (these heights do not reflect extremes in fashion).[11]

Heavy clothing can add as little as ½ inch to as much as 2½ inches to measurements.[8]

Population

As mentioned, people in different populations have different sizes. Estimates should correspond with the population type of the people who will use the design. For example, if the population is predominantly Asian, using the information from a western group will result in measurements that are too large. Unfortunately, not all populations have anthropometric estimates that designers can use. In addition, as populations change over time, tables of measurements collected in a population many years previously may not accurately reflect the present-day size of the people in that population.

Averages

All the measurements are averages of a large population. Variations exist for all the measurements when applied to the individual level. Using the average (50th percentile) creates workstations that are too large or too small for most people. Even using the 5th and 95th percentiles, as recommended by ergonomic texts, misses 10% of the population. Data from the 99th and 1st percentiles exclude fewer people but have a greater potential for error. The data may not be reliable because the population used for the measurement is very small.

Although anthropometric data may have flaws, they still provide valuable insights into the overall size and shape of the population. They provide a solid foundation of information that can be used to create a workstation that will fit the largest number of people comfortably. The estimates provided in the tables should be used as a stepping stone to understanding human form when improving or designing the work environment. Use of these estimates should help prevent the mistake of designing for only a few members of a population.

USES OF ANTHROPOMETRIC DATA

The next sections of the chapter build on the static anthropometric estimates and review concepts such as reach and clearance. These concepts are vital to understanding how to construct a workstation. As with all measurements, these are averages. Always consider the overall population and the purpose of the workstation before using any measurement. The numbers included here are for American populations.

Reach

Reach is defined as a sphere around the worker that can be touched by the worker at all points without moving the body from the starting point. The shoulder is the axis or center of the sphere, and the length of the arm is equal to the radius. In some cases, when reach is limited to what is available from elbow to fingertips (as when working on a table), the elbow is the axis and the forearm and hand form the radius. When designing to accommodate reach, consider the smallest user, the 5th percentile woman. If she can reach an object, all larger individuals can reach it, too.

Vertical Reach

Operating buttons on a control panel and getting objects off high shelves are examples of activities that occur during vertical reach.

For a standing reach the 95th percentile man can reach a button that is 94.2 inches (2393 mm) from the ground, whereas the 5th percentile woman would be able to reach a button 75.4 inches (1914 mm) high. To be able to grasp an object, the highest the object can be is 89 inches (2260 mm) for the 95th percentile man and 71.2 inches (1808 mm) for the 5th percentile woman.[9] These reaches assume that the person can stand directly against the control panel.

Figure 5-5 provides the vertical envelope in which a 5th percentile worker can reach an object when sitting. The inner line of the arc represents the 5th percentile female reach, and the outer line represents the 5th percentile man. Individuals can reach further by leaning forward, and the outermost arc represents this occasional extended reach.

For people who use wheeled mobility devices the maximum unobstructed (high) forward reach height is 48 inches (1220 mm) and the minimum unobstructed (low) forward reach is 15 inches

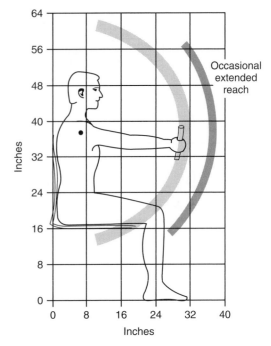

FIGURE 5-5 The vertical envelope in which a 5th percentile worker can reach an object when sitting. The inner line of the arc represents the 5th percentile female reach, and the outer line represents the 5th percentile male. (From Cohen AL, Gjessing CC, Fine LJ et al: *Elements of an ergonomics program*, DHHS [NIOSH] Publication No. 97-117, Washington DC, 1997, U.S. Government Printing Office.)

(360 mm). If access is blocked by a shelf or table that is between 20 and 25 inches (510 to 635 mm) wide, the maximum high forward reach height is 44 inches (1120 mm).[13]

Horizontal Reach

Horizontal height is usually defined by a tabletop or counter; the worker manipulates objects on its surface. Four zones need to be considered (Figure 5-6)[3]:

- Normal work distance is the arc made by the forearm when the body is as close to the table as is comfortable and the elbow is close to the side. This is the area where most precision work is performed. This distance is made up of a radius of approximately 13

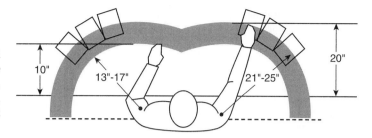

FIGURE 5-6 The four zones of horizontal reach. (From Cohen AL, Gjessing CC, Fine LJ et al: *Elements of an ergonomics program*, DHHS [NIOSH] Publication No. 97-117, Washington DC, 1997, U.S. Government Printing Office.)

inches for the 5th percentile woman and 17 inches for the 5th percentile man (a range of 350 to 450 mm).

- Extended working distance is the area made by the arc of the arm when the elbow is straight. This is best for storing frequently used tools, supplies, and heavy objects. This distance is a radius of approximately 21 inches for the 5th percentile woman to 25 inches for the 5th percentile man (a range of 550 to 650 mm).
- Maximum work distance is established when the body leans forward. This area is best for infrequently used supplies and tools. It is also the area that is considered for the placement of push-buttons and other controls. This distance ranges from 27.6 inches to 31.5 inches (700 to 800 mm).
- Most efficient workspace is defined by a 10-inch (250-mm) square directly in front of the worker and about a hand's span from the edge of the table. This is the area where most people prefer to work, as it places material at the most comfortable distance from the body.

These reaches are optimal when conditions are perfect. Reach distances can be constrained by the following:

- Balance: Greater reach can be achieved by leaning forward and backward. However, this may not be possible if the worker is in a precarious situation or on a slippery surface. It also increases fatigue for repetitive reaching.
- Clothing: Bulky clothing such as coats and other protective suits reduces reach.
- Overall joint mobility: Persons with decreased motion, such as a person with arthritis or in

a wheelchair, may not be able to reach far objects easily.

- Blocking by other surfaces: If a person must reach over or around other objects, reach is decreased.
- Job requirements: Reach can be constrained by needs for precision or strength.

"Visual" Reach (Seeing over Objects)

In the consideration of any workspace, visual contact with important objects is necessary. Workers must be able to see what they are doing, as well as lights, controls, and alarms (Figure 5-7). Some rules for visual reach are as follows[9]:

Objects should not block the normal line of sight.

The most relaxed line of sight when the head is erect is not actually on the horizontal plane; relaxed sight occurs about 10 to 15 degrees below the horizontal. Thus, work that requires continuous visual contact, such as work at a computer, should be placed 10 to 15 degrees below the horizontal eye line.

The eye can comfortably rotate about 15 degrees above and below this imaginary angle. Thus, controls that need to be read frequently should be placed between 30 degrees below the horizontal and 5 degrees above the horizontal. This angle changes if the head flexion angle is increased.

The reading distance of the eye is approximately 15.8 to 27.6 inches (400 to 700 mm) from the eye. The further from the eye the material, the larger and more clearly it must be displayed.

Clearance

Clearance is the space needed to allow free passage of a person or a body segment. Clearance can

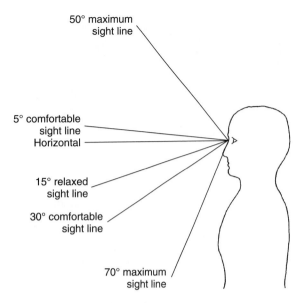

FIGURE **5-7** "Visual" reach.

be as narrow as a hatchway into a submarine or as wide as a doorway in a civic center that allows many people to pass in and out at the same time. Clearance, as with any design, must take into account the uses the area will have, including the traffic patterns and clothing being worn. Historically, clearance has been designed for the biggest user, the 95th percentile man. However, in today's society, clearance must take into account the people who use wheeled devices for mobility, because a wheeled device requires considerably larger spaces in which to maneuver.

The following are some general clearance heights and widths based on a large man or, when appropriate, a user of a wheeled mobility device.

Height

The minimum height of a passageway that will allow a 99th percentile man wearing a helmet and shoes to pass through without ducking is 77 inches (1955 mm).[11]

Width

The minimum width of a passageway depends on potential use.

- The clearance required for one person to walk alone is 25.5 inches (650 mm).[11]
- The clearance required for two persons to walk abreast is 53.1 inches (1350 mm).[11]
- The clearance required for one person in a wheelchair is 36 inches (915 mm).[13]
- The clearance required for a person in a wheelchair to complete a 360-degree turn is a 60-inch (1525-mm) square.[13]

Hand Clearance

Sliding the hand in and out of small spaces can be very important for certain tasks.

The smallest aperture through which a 95th percentile man can slide his hand is a square with each side measuring 5.1 inches (76 mm). If the opening is at least 2.3 inches (38 mm) thick and 4.6 inches (114 mm) wide, the hand can slide in. However, he cannot grasp and remove anything through an opening of this size; he can only press buttons.

If hand access to a place is to be prevented, for example with hand guards, the opening must be less than 2 inches (50 mm) square or no thicker than 1.5 inches (23 mm) and no wider than 3.3 inches (83 mm).[11]

Leg Room

Seated work requires space to stretch and position the legs in a variety of postures. Areas designated for seated work should have enough space for tall people to comfortably place their legs. Generally, workspaces designated for seated work should not have drawers or thick countertops, as this reduces knee space.

The space should be at least 27.2 inches (680 mm) wide and 27.6 inches (690 mm) high.[9]

When they sit, most people like to lean back and stretch their legs under the space; therefore the depth of the space should accommodate this at least at floor level. The space should be 24 inches (600 mm) at knee level and 32 inches (800 mm) at floor level.[9]

Posture

Essentially the orientation of body parts in space, posture is believed to have a profound effect on the health and well-being of the worker. Working in one unchanging position, or static posture, has been associated with the development of musculoskeletal disorders. Postures that position the body or body parts so that muscles must work strongly against gravity, such as holding the arms out at shoulder height or working with the torso bent, often cause discomfort in the worker.[1]

Anthropometric data are commonly used to place the body in the best posture for the job. But what is the best posture? In general, maintaining the limbs and torso as close to the neutral posture as possible is considered to place the least strain on the body. When a person is standing, the neutral posture can be achieved by having the head upright over the torso, the torso upright with the center of gravity over the hips, the knees slightly bent, and the arms in a relaxed position at the sides. Working positions that allow the worker to maintain or return to this posture frequently are considered to put the least amount of stress on the body. For sitting, the posture is similar, except it is shaped by the chair on which the worker is sitting.

The position in which an individual sits can place a great deal of stress on the lower back. The so-called "correct" sitting posture in which the individual is positioned at 90-degree hip flexion, 90-degree knee flexion, and 90-degree elbow flexion, with ramrod-straight back and erect head, is a myth that may have caused some harm. Research on discal pressure during sitting suggests that this position places greater pressure on the lower back than sitting in a relaxed posture in the chair.[2] Observations of workers suggest the posture most often selected is one that allows them to lean back in the chair at about an angle of 105 degrees.[6] This position allows the back to be supported by the chair, taking some of the weight off the spinal disks and musculature. The best chair allows the worker to recline slightly.

One often asked question: Is it better to sit or stand on the job? Both have good points. Whether a person should sit or stand on the job depends on the requirements of the task. The advantages of standing to work are that it increases mobility, allows the worker to cover a larger work area, makes large control motions possible, allows the

worker to exert body weight as force, and saves space. The advantages of sitting to work are that it minimizes operator fatigue, increases operator stability, provides support to exert force, permits the use of pedals, and accommodates a wide range of operator sizes.[5]

Several rules should be kept in mind to help decrease the effects posture may have on the body:

- Position should be changed frequently. Prolonged static postures place a great deal of stress on the worker.
- Positions that cause forward inclination of the head should be avoided. The torque caused by the weight of the head (approximately 8 pounds) increases dramatically the further from midline the head is placed. Make sure visual work is high enough to keep the head balanced over the spine.
- Upper arms should be kept next to the body, and raising arms overhead should be avoided. As with the neck, the torque on the shoulders increases as the arms move toward 90-degree angles.
- Body parts should be kept aligned; twisting and asymmetry should be avoided. Asymmetry tends to place muscles in positions of weakness.
- Neutral postures should be maintained and extremes of range avoided. This is especially true for the wrist and hands, which can be in some very awkward postures.
- A back support should always be provided, preferably one that can be inclined to greater than 90 degrees.
- Body parts should be placed in the positions of greatest strength.

Precision and Strength

Anthropometrics directly affect a worker's ability to do work that requires precision or strength. As with posture, an understanding of anthropometrics can help correctly position workers to perform such tasks.

Precision

Precision is strongly influenced by the need to see work; the smaller the work, the closer it must be held to the eyes. Precision is enhanced by the worker's ability to hold the work close to the body and to support his or her arms or hands while working. In general, precise work should be positioned about 2 to 4 inches (50 to 100 mm) above elbow height.[9] This does not necessarily refer to work-surface height. The actual surface may be lower or higher than this, as tools and job demands may require the worker to position the job above or below the work surface. For example, when considering how to position the work for a welder, the therapist must take into account the height of the welding wand and position the work low enough that the hand holding the wand is 2 to 4 inches (50 to 100 mm) above elbow height. Figure 5-8 demonstrates the approximate work heights for differing precision requirements.

Strength

Strength is directly influenced by posture and therefore anthropometrics. All muscles have an optimal muscle-tension length at which they are strongest.[2] When the body part is positioned at this optimal length, greater strength is achieved. Strength alone, however, is not all that is necessary for a job. Some tasks are more dependent on leverage, body equilibrium, and friction. Pulling often requires the use of body weight to counter-

balance the task. In general, however, jobs that require strength should be performed with the object 6 to 16 inches (150-400 mm) lower than the elbow.[9]

After the basics of anthropometry are understood, the therapist will have to integrate the information into actual workstation design. Let's go back to our case study to apply what we have just learned. The therapist realizes she is unable to design each workstation to fit individuals. Instead, she concentrates on making the workstation fit the greatest variety of workers by using the static anthropometric tables to determine the optimal sizes for the greatest number of people. She decides to use the static measurements for U.S. adults (see Table 5-2) to help determine equipment for a group of office workers. The therapist creates a table to help estimate the variety of sizes likely to occur within this population (Table 5-6). She makes the following recommendations based on the table:

1. Purchase adjustable chairs. A review of available models suggests that most chairs adjust between 16 and 21 inches. These meet the height requirements of taller men and women; however, footrests for shorter men and women will need to be available. The chairs should have adjustable armrest

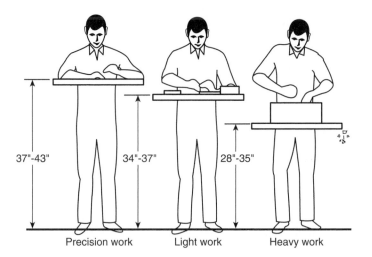

Standing work:
Workbench heights should be
—above elbow height for *precision work,*
—just below elbow height for *light work,* and
—4-6 in. below elbow height for *heavy work.*

37"-43"   34"-37"   28"-35"

Precision work   Light work   Heavy work

FIGURE **5-8** Approximate work heights for differing precision requirements. (From Cohen AL, Gjessing CC, Fine LJ et al: *Elements of an ergonomics program,* DHHS [NIOSH] Publication No. 97-117, Washington DC, 1997, U.S. Government Printing Office.)

TABLE 5-6	**Case Study Using Static Anthropometric Estimates to Help Determine Equipment Requirements for Office Workers**		
Anthropometric Segment	**Smallest Estimate (inches)**	**Largest Estimate (inches)**	**Corresponding Workstation Measurement**
Popliteal height	13.9 (5th percentile woman)	19.5 (95th percentile man)	Chair seat height
Elbow height from chair	7.4 (5th percentile woman)	11.4 (95th percentile man)	Armrest height
Hip breadth	12.3 (5th percentile man)	19.7 (95th percentile woman)	Seat pan width
Buttock popliteal length	16.6 (5th percentile woman)	23.2 (95th percentile man)	Seat pan depth (subtract 2 inches for actual seat pan depth)
Sitting elbow height (popliteal height + elbow height from chair)	13.9 + 7.4 = 21.3	19.5 + 11.4 = 30.9	Keyboard height
Eye height (popliteal height + sitting eye height)	13.9 + 27.0 = 40.9 (5th percentile woman)	19.5 + 34.2 = 53.7 (95th percentile man)	Top of monitor

heights from 7 to 9.5 inches. The armrests should also be adjustable in and out to allow for hip breadth. The seat pan should be no more than 18 inches deep, and the back of the chair should adjust forward so that the seat pan depth can be reduced by 4 inches.

2. Provide all desks with adjustable keyboard holders. The holders should be adjustable from between 2 and 7 inches below the desk height (because no chair is going lower than 16 inches, the measurement of the elbow height from the ground is adjusted to a 16-inches height for 5th percentile women). A keyboard holder with space for a mouse is recommended.

3. The CPU should be placed to one side on the desk, or on the floor. The monitor should be removed from the computer and placed on an adjustable monitor holder that rises from desk level to 9 inches above the desk.

These three recommendations provide enough versatility to meet the needs of 95% of the workers. The therapist also provides educa-

tion on how to adjust the workstation to meet individual needs.

CONCLUSION

This chapter has reviewed the uses of static anthropometric tables for designing workstations for large populations. Static anthropometry provides the essentials for understanding the variability of the human form. It can greatly reduce time and effort while greatly increasing the accuracy of design by providing the designer with information concerning the broadest ranges of measurements in a population, including individuals with disabilities. These estimates can provide the designer with information about clearance, reach, and posture that is essential to good design. Although these methods do have limitations, such as high variability, lack of measurements with clothes, and a missing percentage of the population, they do provide the best estimates of human size now available. Taken as a whole, static anthropometric measurements are invaluable tools for the ergonomist and therapist.

Learning Exercise
Applied Anthropometry—Designing for One

Overview

Apply the principles of ergonomics in your work environment.

Purpose

The purpose of this exercise is to evaluate your own work environment. You will determine if there are factors in your environment that may be enhancements to your work. You will also try to determine any characteristics of your work that could be altered using ergonomic principles.

Exercise

Collect anthropometric measurements of yourself. Measure the parameters of your workstation. Identify potential risk factors (hazards). Prioritize controls. (Resource: Spaulding S: *Meaningful motion: biomechanics for occupational therapists,* London, 2005, Churchill Livingston).

Learning Exercise
Applied Anthropometry–Designing for a Group

Overview

Apply the principles of ergonomics to a population of people.

Purpose

The purposes of this exercise are to practice techniques of measuring a population and to apply those measurements to workstation design.

Exercise

Measure all the students in the class. Identify the average, 5th, and 95th percentile measurements for the classroom population. Using these measurements, identify how to design chairs, desks, and the general layout of the classroom to facilitate learning for the population as a whole.

ACKNOWLEDGMENT

The author would like to thank Somaya Malkawi for her help with the drawings and the tables.

Multiple Choice Review Questions

1. Which factor does not influence the size and shape of the human form?
   A. Gender
   B. Occupation
   C. Education
   D. Clothing

2. The horizontal distance from the acromion to the tip of the third digit, with the elbow and wrist extended and the shoulder flexed to 90 degrees, is the:
   A. shoulder grip length.
   B. fingertip height.
   C. popliteal height.
   D. upper limb length.

3. You are designing a utensil with a built-up handle that you plan to adapt for many different clients. You know that you can make it larger by adding padding. What should the starting circumference of this handle be?
   A. 1.69 inches
   B. 1.77 inches
   C. 2.32 inches
   D. 3.25 inches

4. Through the use of anthropometric estimates, an accurate prediction of the exact size and shape of any individual is possible.
   A. True
   B. False

5. Which of the following are anthropometric measures?
   A. Height
   B. Weight
   C. ROM
   D. All of the above

6. With regard to workspace design, the material currently being manipulated by the worker should be no more than how many inches from the edge of the work table?

A. 3 inches
B. 10 inches
C. 17 inches
D. 27 inches

7. When considering the overall height of a person who uses a wheelchair for mobility, the height of the wheelchair is not included in the measurement.
A. True
B. False

8. The hip angle that puts the least pressure on the discs while a person is seated is:
A. 90 degrees.
B. 95 degrees.
C. 100 degrees.
D. 105 degrees.

9. Which of the following percentiles is best for determining reach requirements?
A. 5th percentile men
B. 5th percentile women
C. 50th percentile women
D. 95th percentile women

10. If a push button is placed at 56 inches above the ground, what is the furthest horizontal distance it can be (measured in the same plane as the backrest of the chair) and still be accessible to 95% of the population?
A. 12 inches
B. 16 inches
C. 20 inches
D. 24 inches

REFERENCES

1. Bernard BP, editor: *Musculoskeletal disorders and workplace factors,* DHHS (NIOSH) Publication No. 97-141, Washington DC, 1997, U.S. Department of Health and Human Services.
2. Chaffin DB, Andersson GBJ: *Occupational biomechanics,* ed 2, New York, 1991, Wiley.
3. Cohen AL, Gjessing CC, Fine LJ et al: *Elements of an ergonomics program,* DHHS (NIOSH) Publication No. 97-117, Washington DC, 1997, U.S. Government Printing Office.
4. Das B, Kozey JW: Structural anthropometric measurements for wheelchair mobile adults, *Appl Ergon* 30:385, 1999.
5. Diffrient N, Tilley AR, Harman D: *Humanscale 7/8/9,* Cambridge, Mass, 1981, MIT Press.
6. Grandjean E, Hunting W, Pidermann M: VDT workstation design: preferred settings and their effects, *Hum Factors* 25:161, 1983.
7. Hobson DA, Molenbroek JFM: Anthropometry and design for the disabled: experiences with seating design for the cerebral palsy population, *Appl Ergon* 21:43, 1990.
8. Human Factors Engineering Technical Advisory Group: *Human engineering design data digest,* MIL-STD-1472, Washington DC, 2000, Department of Defense.
9. Kroemer KHE, Grandjean E: *Fitting the task to the human,* Philadelphia, 1997, Taylor and Francis.
10. Ogden CL, Carroll MD, Curting LR et al: Prevalence of overweight and obesity in the United States, 1999-2004, *JAMA* 295:1549-1555, 2006.
11. Pheasant S: *Bodyspace: anthropometry, ergonomics, and design,* ed 2, Philadelphia, 1998, Taylor and Francis.
12. Roberts DF: *Climate and human variability. An Addison-Wesley module in anthropology,* No. 34, Reading, Mass, 1973, Addison-Wesley.
13. United States Access Board: *Revised ADA-ABA Guidelines,* 2004. Retrieved June 12, 2006, from www.access-board.gov/ada-aba/index.htm.

SUGGESTED READING

Diffrient N, Tilley AR, Bardagly JC: *Humanscale 1/2/3,* Cambridge, Mass, 1974, MIT Press.
Food and Nutrition Technical Assistance (FANTA): *Anthropometric Indicators Measurement Guide,* 2003 Edition. Available online at www.fantaproject.org/publications/anthropom.shtml.
Peebles L, Norris B: *Adultdata: the handbook of adult anthropometric and strength measurements—data for design safety,* Nottingham, United Kingdom, 1998, University of Nottingham. Available free at www.dti.gov.uk/publications.
Smith S, Norris B, Peebles L: *Older adultdata: the handbook of measurements and capabilities of the older adult,* Nottingham, United Kingdom, 2000, University of Nottingham. Available free at www.dti.gov.uk/publications.

Web Sites
Ergoweb: www.ergoweb.com
Strength data for design safety: www.dti.gov.uk/files/file21827.pdf

6

Basic Biomechanics

Sandi J. Spaulding

Learning Objectives

After reading this chapter and completing the exercises, the reader should be able to do the following:

1. Understand biomechanical principles that are vital to practice in ergonomics, with emphasis on the principles implicit in assessments such as the NIOSH manual lifting equation.
2. Use biomechanical principles when working in the area of ergonomics.
3. Apply biomechanics principles in ergonomic practice.

Force. Force is defined as mass (m) times acceleration (a) ($F = ma$, with the units in Newtons). For example, a person may try to pound a nail into a piece of wood and increase the force used, relative to an earlier attempt. The person can either use a heavier hammer with the same acceleration or can use the same hammer but with an increase in the speed (with respect to time) with which he or she hits the wood.

Torque. Torque is force (F) times distance (d) ($T = Fd$, with the units in Newton-meters). To increase the torque, for example, when trying to loosen a lug nut, a person can either increase the force he or she is using or place his or her hand farther away from the point of application. To increase this distance a person can either move the hand farther down the wrench or use a longer wrench.

Friction. Friction is the product of the characteristics of two surfaces relative to one another (coefficient of friction) and the normal force exerted on the upper surface (a normal force is one that is exerted straight downward). The greater the roughness of one or both of the two surfaces, the greater the coefficient of friction. The greater the normal force, the greater will be the friction ($F = \mu F_N$, where F is the force of friction, μ is the coefficient of friction, and F_N is the normal force).

CASE STUDY

Ms. Marion Stonehouse is the owner and sole proprietor of a small pet food store, which is one of a chain in the country in which she lives. She is in her 40s, is about 5 feet 6 inches tall, and is quite fit.

Her work appears, from the customer's perspective, to be sedentary because someone buying something in her store will find her behind the cash register. However, when the store is closed, she does a great deal of heavy lifting. She lifts 40-pound bags of pet food and birdseed, as well as all the other merchandise that she sells in the store. Stacking shelves and maintaining extra inventory in the back of the store involves not only lifting but also carrying large objects to heights above her shoulders, as well as climbing ladders to stock merchandise for storage above the shelves from which the customers take their purchases.

One aspect of the job for Ms. Stonehouse and her worker is unloading the products once a week from a large truck that comes from a central warehouse. The worker on the truck and Ms. Stonehouse have many good techniques to ensure that they undergo the least amount of stress possible. Lifting techniques that demonstrate good practices include using a mechanically driven lift to move pallets of supplies, using a wide base of support when reaching for objects, using a portable cart with wheels to increase ease of moving products, and having two people move the cart when it is fully loaded.

Ms. Stonehouse has no physical difficulties at present because she is using good equipment for moving heavy loads, but given the extensive lifting and shifting of product that she does, she is concerned that she might have problems in the future. Ms. Stonehouse and the ergonomist she is consulting are evaluating her work and making suggestions for change so that she can avoid work-related injuries.

This chapter will explain the units of measure for biomechanical principles and discuss important biomechanical principles that are used in the study of ergonomics. The material about biomechanics will be incorporated into considerations of the work Ms. Stonehouse is doing.

SYSTEMS OF MEASUREMENT

There are two systems of units for mechanical terms: the international system of units (SI) and the British system of measurement (BTU). The international system is most commonly used, but both are currently in practice in different places in the world. See Table 6-1 for some of the biomechanical terms, their definitions, and units in the SI system.

BIOMECHANICS

Biomechanics, or the study of human movement using mechanical principles, consists of two main categories: kinematics and kinetics. Kinematics is the study of movement without the involvement of the forces used in the movement. Kinetics is the discipline of including the forces acting to create motion. Biomechanics can also be considered to be divided between statics and dynamics. The study of statics includes the forces on an object or person without the occurrence of movement. Dynamics includes the forces as well as movement. This chapter will begin with a discussion of kinematics and kinetics and then will cover some other mechanical principles that are required by ergonomists.

Kinematics

Kinematics includes movement without considering the source of the movement. There are different aspects of kinematics: displacement, velocity, and acceleration. Displacement is distance with a direction (meters [m]). Velocity is a change in displacement or speed with direction (meters per second [m/s]). Acceleration is an increase in velocity (meters per second squared [m/s²]) and deceleration is a decrease in velocity (also m/s²). Kinematics can occur in a straight line (linear kinematics), in curves, or in a combination of both linear movement and curves, which is called *curvilinear kinematics.*

Kinetics

Kinetics is the discipline of engineering and biomechanics that considers the effects of forces acting on a person, object, or system.

Force

Force is a term that is used in everyday life. For example, someone may talk about a jar taking a

TABLE 6-1   Definition of Some Mechanical Terms and Their Units of Measurement

Mechanical Concept	Definition of Concept	Units of Measure (SI Units)
Displacement	Displacement is distance with a direction.	m
Velocity	Velocity is displacement divided by time or the distance an object moves in a certain amount of time.	m/s
Acceleration	Acceleration is velocity divided by time or is how quickly or slowly an object can increase in speed.	m/s^2
Force	Force is the mass of an object times acceleration.	kgm/sec^2 or newtons (N)
Mass	Mass is the physical property of matter that gives it weight and inertia.	kg
Moment of force	A moment of force is the distance times time.	kgm^2/s^2
Weight	Weight is mass times the force of gravity (9.8 m/s²).	kgm/s^2
Momentum	Momentum is mass times velocity.	kgm/s

lot of force to open or having to force open a door in winter because of frost. However, force also has a mechanical definition. By understanding the concept of force we can understand one of the basic issues of ergonomics, because force can aid or be a problem for a worker. Force is equal to mass times acceleration:

Force = mass times acceleration
Where mass is expressed in kg and acceleration in m/sec² (SI)
or mass is expressed in slugs and acceleration in ft/sec² (BTU)

Now, what does that mean? It implies that if there is a greater mass, then the force will be greater. For example, if Marion Stonehouse were to spend much of her time lifting 40-kilogram (kg) bags of food, rather than 20-kg bags, she might have less difficulty. It also suggests that the faster she tries to lift and move the wares, the greater the force that will be required by her. Therefore, when evaluating a worker, the therapist should be aware of the weight lifted and whether or not this can be altered to make the task easier.

Another issue concerning force is important for Marion. The reason she is able to lift objects at all is because her muscles produce force within her body. That muscle force produces movement. She

has strong enough muscles to do her work. Sometimes the force of the muscles is not great enough, or the number of repetitions a person does is too many, so the muscles become fatigued or injured. Ms. Stonehouse must be concerned about keeping her lifting within her strength range; otherwise she could be subjecting herself to injury if she either has to use too much force to lift or has to create a force too frequently. Those two factors, the mass of the object and the acceleration inherent in the movement, can be manipulated so that less force is required. These factors are taken into account in the National Institute of Occupational Safety and Health (NIOSH) Manual Lifting equation, which is discussed in Chapter 11, Lifting Analysis.

Lever Systems

Forces often do not work in isolation; there is often resistance to force. A lever system exists when there are one or more active forces and one or more resistive forces working against the action. Levers involve an active and a resistive force, as well as an axis of rotation. There are three categories of levers. Where the forces and axis are placed and the magnitude or size of the forces will affect how a lever operates. Levers can often be used to make work easier.

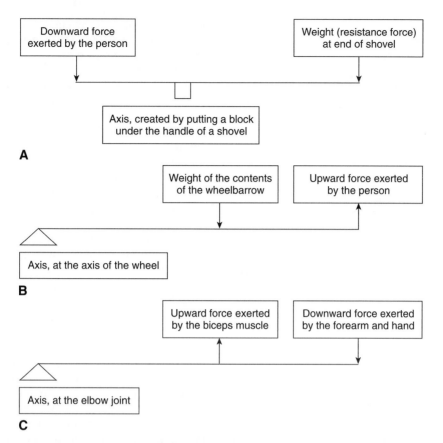

FIGURE 6-1 **A,** First-class lever. If the downward force exerted by the person is greater than the resistive force of the weight, then the weight will move upward. **B,** Second-class lever. The resistance is between the axis of rotation and the effort force, for example, a wheelbarrow. The axis is at the center of the wheel; the weight, or resistance, is in the wheelbarrow; and the effort is in the hands of the person. **C,** Third-class lever. The effort is between the resistance and the axis.

First-Class Lever

A first-class lever is one in which the active or motive force is at one end and the resistive force is at the other end, with the axis in the middle (Figure 6-1, *A*). A first-class lever example would be lifting a load of concrete by hand. If a person uses a shovel as a lever, rather than trying to lift it by hand, the shovel can be put under the object, an axis could be created by putting a block under the handle of the shovel, and the person could push down on the shovel and rotate the load to where it is needed. If the lever arm between the axis and the hand is greater than the lever arm between the axis and the weight, then the person has a mechanical advantage. The mechanical advantage is the length of the effort arm divided by the length of the weight or resistance arm. If that number is greater than one, there is a mechanical advantage for the person doing the lifting. If Ms. Stonehouse has to move an object off the floor onto a pallet, she can put a shovel or other implement under the object, create an axis with another object such as a block of wood, then push down at the other end of the lever and rotate the object. The longer her distance from the axis relative to the distance from the object to be lifted, the easier it will be for her to lift.

Second-Class Lever

In a second-class lever, the weight is between the axis and the effort (Figure 6-1, *B*) Always, in a second-class lever, the mechanical advantage is greater than one, but again it can be increased by increasing the distance from the effort to the axis or decreasing the distance from the weight to the axis.

Third-Class Lever

A third-class lever has the effort between the axis and the resistance (Figure 6-1, *C*). Most muscles in our bodies are third-class levers. Think of the insertion of the biceps tendon. It attaches on the forearm, near the elbow, but is one of the movers of the forearm and the hand. Third-class levers are useful in that the effort can have a short lever arm, but they always have a mechanical advantage less than one.

Torque

Torque is force created through a distance:

$$Torque = force \times distance$$
Where force is expressed in kgm/s^2
and distance in m
Therefore torque is expressed in kgm^2/s^2

Torque is also called a *moment of force,* which usually is a term related to rotation. If one wants to increase torque, consider the equation: one can either increase the force of an object or increase the distance from the object. An increased torque can be useful. Moments of force are often evaluated in research for people performing tasks with equipment and affect the ability to perform activities.[6] If Marion wants to rotate a display cabinet using a metal bar to help her, she can increase the amount of torque she can produce on the cabinet without increasing the amount of force that she has to produce, just by increasing the length of the bar.

You can think about the torques produced when lifting. Some work has been done to determine the effects of actually moving objects farther from a person in the attempt to force him or her to move closer. However, this research suggests that people do not take a step under such circumstances.[7] For example, if Marion is holding a box of canned goods out 30 cm in front of her, her muscles must work harder than if the box were only 10 cm in front of her.

Within the body, the muscles contract to produce force. Those muscles are attached at specific places on bones, so there is also a torque component because there is always a distance between the point of attachment and the joint or axis about which the body part moves. The biceps muscle is attached very close to the elbow joint. Because it is so close, most of the torque will come from the muscle strength rather than the distance from the rotation point.

A number of other biomechanical principles become important when considering the interaction between a person and his or her environment.

Friction

If you have ever stepped out onto a wet ceramic step while wearing shoes without tread, you are very aware of the effects of having a very low level of friction between two surfaces. Research suggests that friction needs to be taken into account in many work environments, including the hospital environment in which lifting patients must occur.[13] The force of friction (F_f) is equal to the characteristics of two surfaces in relation to one another (the coefficient of friction, or μ) times the downward, or normal, force (F_N) that is exerted on the surfaces. The formula for friction is as follows:

$$F_f = \mu \times F_N$$

The coefficient of friction does not have any units because it involves one surface relative to another. The friction force has the same units as any other force: kgm/s^2. Shoe sole properties and ground surfaces can be analyzed to determine how much slip may occur with them.[9-12] Marion can be helped by an increase in friction if she begins to wear shoes that have rough soles and keeps the floor dry or chooses floor material that is rougher than the one she has. Then the coefficient of friction will be increased, so she is less likely to slip. She may decide that rather than carrying or dragging large bags of food from one area to another, she will put them on a wheeled cart. Then she will reduce both the amount of effort she expends and also the effect of friction on her. Antislip devices should be considered for individuals.[4,5] However, it has been found by some researchers that for loads to be pushed on the floor, a high enough coefficient of friction may be needed.[4] Often, floor slipperiness is considered in a laboratory environment, but research suggests that analyses should be conducted in the workplace.[3]

Dynamic friction is the friction that exists when one object is moving on another one. Dynamic friction is always less than static friction if all other aspects of the situation are constant. Therefore, if Ms. Stonehouse starts sliding one product on another she will find it easier to keep moving the product once it has started to move.

Rolling friction, or the friction generated within wheel configurations, may also need to be taken into account when evaluating ergonomics.[1]

Slip potential is always increased when friction is reduced. For example, applying the base of a ladder to dry surfaces has been shown to increase friction, but when the ladder is used on an oily surface, friction is reduced and slip potential is increased.[2]

Stress and Strain

Two mechanical principles, stress and strain, play an integral part in how the body responds to forces. Stress is the internal deformation in response to an externally applied load. For example, a person who has a spastic upper extremity that moves toward flexion can be using a splint to reduce potential flexion contractures. The person's muscle strength can push against the splint but not bend it. The splint may experience stress, or internal deformation, without any outward sign of change. The unit of measure for stress is N/m^2.

Strain is the change in dimension that occurs because of an external load. For example, if a person is using a mechanical lift, such as a forklift, on a worksite to carry a large load on a pallet, there may be no problem for the forklift. However, if the weight to be lifted exceeds the strength of the material in the lift component of the equipment, the metal material of the fork may bend under the load. This is extremely unlikely, because equipment is designed to withstand appropriate loads, but is an example of what might occur if the equipment were not designed in a manner that can withstand loading. Stress and strain as well as other mechanical phenomena can occur within the human body. See Chapter 11 for examples of mechanical principles related to the spine and lifting.

Elasticity

Elasticity is related to the length an object is stretched relative to its resting length. If a person stretches an elastic band, the longer it is stretched, the more force is present when it is released. It has stored elastic energy. If the material is stretched and then released, it returns to its original length. If two elastics are put side by side, their strength is added together; to increase strength of elastics, this configuration would be useful. If elastics with the same properties in terms of strength and material are combined, one to the end of the other, then the force they exert together is half the force that would be exerted if one were working alone.

Materials can be brought to a state of failure by either too much or too frequent stretching. Carpal tunnel syndrome (CTS), a problem in the area of the wrist, might occur if someone stretches or holds the wrist and hand in awkward positions for too long over a period of time. Extensive research has been conducted into repetitive strain injuries (RSIs). An article by Keller, Corbett, and Nichols provides insight into the pathogenesis and problems related to repetitive strain injuries. The authors determined that a large number of computer users experience high rates of repetitive strain injury related to work and discussed the assessment and treatment of RSI.[8]

Many other biomechanical principles can be and are applied to ergonomics. Some of these principles are discussed in Chapter 9, Physical Environment. Other principles can be found in the resource materials noted at the end of this chapter. It is important for the therapist working in ergonomics to be very familiar with these principles because they are the underpinning of the physical aspects of the worker and his or her environment.

Learning Exercise

Overview

The learning exercises provided are designed to increase your practical understanding of some basic biomechanics concepts.

Purpose

The purpose of these learning exercises is to consider the case of Ms. Stonehouse and how biomechanical principles would be coming into effect in her work in more ways than have been alluded to in this chapter. You will try to determine how she could change aspects of her work, based on the knowledge of basic biomechanics you have learned in this chapter.

Exercise

Create a list of 10 discrete tasks you think someone in a job such as the one held by Ms. Stonehouse could be asked to do. Once you have created the list, write down any biomechanical principles that would be applicable to the task. For example, if one of the tasks you have imagined is that she is using a ladder to lift dog beds up to a storage area, consider the biomechanical aspects of this—for example, she would have to be on a ladder. When you have created the 10 tasks, determine the biomechanical principles, then determine how you might make each task easier based on biomechanical principles. Perhaps the ladder used could be a stepladder, rather than a straight ladder, which could slip because of the ladder-floor characteristics.

Multiple Choice Review Questions

1. If a person is trying to push an object along the floor and it suddenly gives way and moves along, the following principle of mechanics has come into play:
   A. Dynamic friction
   B. Static friction
   C. A first-class lever
   D. Stress tension

2. Ms. Stonehouse is trying to carry a large bag of food and do it with as little force on her arms as possible. To keep the effect of the weight low, she might try to:
   A. keep her feet as close together as possible.
   B. move quickly.
   C. keep the food as close to her body as she can.
   D. be sure that the ground friction force is high.

3. Ms. Stonehouse has found that if she stretches the stretchable ropes holding the food on the shelves, when she releases the ropes the food is held tightly on the shelves. She is using the property of:
   A. strain, in which the force is proportional to the relaxed state.
   B. viscosity, in which the force is related to the thickness of the material.
   C. stress, in which the force is increased with the distance from the origin.
   D. elasticity, in which the force is proportional to length relative to the resting state.

4. Lifting an object that is in a crate by using a lever will be harder if:
   A. the axis is closer to the hands than to the object in the crate.
   B. the handles are increased in length to increase the lifting force.
   C. the object in the crate is increased in weight.
   D. the person doing the lifting bends to increase the lever arm.

5. An individual who is trying to increase the torque applied to an object is attempting to:
   A. make the task more difficult.
   B. work around a corner that protrudes into the work space.
   C. increase the efficiency with which he or she is working.
   D. decrease the difficulty of the task.

6. Ms. Stonehouse is attempting to increase the force she is exerting on a carton of cleaning products. To increase this force she can:
   A. increase the acceleration of her movement.
   B. decrease the velocity of her pushing.
   C. increase the displacement of the object.
   D. increase the static friction between herself and the object.

7. Velocity:
   A. is the speed of a movement in a direction.
   B. is measured in kgm/s^2.
   C. is noted by whether or not there is displacement occurring.
   D. cannot be measured by an ergonomist.

8. Momentum is measured in:
   A. feet per second.
   B. kilograms times meters per second.
   C. kilograms times meters per second squared.
   D. force times distance.

9. In a second-class lever:
   A. the force is between the axis and the working force.
   B. the effort force is farther from the axis than the resistance.
   C. the axis is between the effort and the resistance.
   D. the forces are equal and opposite.

10. Ms. Stonehouse has noted that she has slipped a couple of times in her storeroom. Although she has not hurt herself, she is afraid that she might in the future. She has asked you to help her avoid further slips, if possible. One of the first things you might consider examining is:
    A. the height to which she is lifting boxes.
    B. the width of the shelving units.
    C. the lighting conditions in the room.
    D. the material that has been used for the floor surface.

REFERENCES

1. Al-Eisawi KW, Kerk CJ, Congleton JJ et al: Factors affecting minimum push and pull forces of manual carts, *Appl Ergon* 30:235, 1999.
2. Chang WR, Chang CC, Matz S: Available friction of ladder shoes and slip potential for climbing on a straight ladder, *Ergonomics* 48:1169, 2005.
3. Chang WR, Li KW, Huang YH et al: Assessing floor slipperiness in fast-food restaurants in Taiwan using objective and subjective measures, *Appl Ergon* 35:401, 2004.
4. Ciriello VM: Psychophysically determined horizontal and vertical forces of dynamic pushing on high and low coefficient of friction floors for female industrial workers, *J Occup Environ Hyg* 2:136, 2005.
5. Gard G, Berggard G: Assessment of anti-slip devices from health individuals in different ages walking on slippery surfaces, *Appl Ergon* 37:177, 2006.
6. Greig M, Wells R: Measurement of prehensile grasp capabilities by a force and moment wrench: methodological development and assessment of manual workers, *Ergonomics* 47:41, 2004.
7. Jorgensen MJ, Handa A, Veluswamy P et al: The effect of pallet distance on torso kinematics and low back disorder risk, *Ergonomics* 48:949, 2005.
8. Keller K, Corbett K, Nichols D: Repetitive strain injury in computer keyboard users: pathomechanics and treatment principles in individual and group intervention, *J Hand Ther* 11:9, 1998.
9. Kim IJ, Smith R, Nagata H: Microscopic observations of the progressive wear on shoe surfaces that affect the slip resistance characteristics, *Int J Ind Ergon* 28:17, 2001.
10. Koningsveld E, van der Grinten M, van der Molen H et al: A system to test the ground surface conditions of construction sites—for safe and efficient work without physical strain, *Appl Ergon* 36:441, 2005.
11. Li KW, Chen CJ: The effect of shoe soling tread groove width on the coefficient of friction with different sole materials, floors, and contaminants, *Appl Ergon* 35:499, 2004.
12. Lipscomb HJ, Glazner JE, Bondy J et al: Injuries from slips and trips in construction, *Appl Ergon* 37:267, 2006.
13. McGill SM, Kavicic NS: Transfer of the horizontal patient: the effect of a friction-reducing assistive device on low back mechanics, *Ergonomics* 48:915, 2005.

SUGGESTED READING

Brand PW, Hollister A: *Clinical mechanics of the hand,* ed 3, St Louis, 1999, Mosby.

Chaffin DB, Andersson GBJ, Martin BJ: *Occupational biomechanics,* ed 4, Hoboken, NJ, 2006, John Wiley & Sons.

Dvir Z: *Clinical biomechanics,* London, 2000, Churchill Livingstone.

Hall S: *Basic biomechanics,* ed 4, Boston, 2002, McGraw-Hill Higher Education.

Hall S: *Basic biomechanics with dynamic human CD and PowerWeb/OLC bind-in passcard,* Boston, 2002, McGraw-Hill Humanities/Social Sciences/Languages.

Kreighbaum E, Barthels K: *Biomechanics: a qualitative approach for studying human movement,* ed 4, 1995, Benjamin Cummings.

Kumar S, editor: *Biomechanics in ergonomics,* Philadelphia, 1999, Taylor & Francis.

Nordin M, Frankel VH: *Basic biomechanics of the musculoskeletal system,* ed 3, Philadelphia, 2001, Lippincott Williams & Wilkins.

Robertson GE: *Introduction to biomechanics for human motion analysis,* Canada, 2004, Waterloo Biomechanics.

Spaulding SJ: *Meaningful motion: biomechanics for occupational therapists,* London, 2005, Churchill Livingstone.

Winter DA: *Biomechanics and motor control of human movement,* ed 3, 2004, John Wiley & Sons Canada, Ltd.

7

Cognitive and Behavioral Demands of Work

Lynn Shaw, Rosemary Lysaght

Learning Objectives

After reading this chapter and completing the exercises, the reader should be able to do the following:

1. Discuss the cognitive and behavioral demands of work occupations.
2. Describe how cognitive and behavioral risks are measured.
3. Discuss external factors that influence optimal cognitive and behavioral performance in the workplace.
4. Evaluate the cognitive requirements and behavioral demands of work needed to inform return-to-work strategies.

Cognitive demands. Demands associated with work tasks that require thinking, information processing, learning, imagining, and anticipating.

Behavioral demands. The actions, efforts, and interactions required to conduct work tasks.

Workplace contextual factors. Aspects of the workplace environment that affect the way work may be performed, when it is performed, and under what conditions it is performed.

Work occupations. Productive occupations, career, profession, or jobs that workers perform for monetary reimbursement.

CASE STUDY

Kara has worked as a laboratory technician and area supervisor for 10 years. She is a petite, soft-spoken woman in her late 50s and has been off work for 12 months. Currently she is on long-term disability leave for depression. Three months before she left work, her performance started to decline. Her co-workers noticed that she was not completing her work, and they frequently had to perform some of her duties before the end of her shifts. Her co-workers liked Kara. To them, Kara was a mother figure who had trained them in some of the essential tasks needed to be a successful laboratory technician in the hospital. Her pace at work was less than moderate, yet the work demanded a consistently high pace in order to keep up with the testing required in the laboratory.

When she was no longer able to function at work, she went on short-term disability leave and then advanced to long-term disability. For 4 months she was suicidal and unable to manage self-care. With medication and treatment, she was able to regain a sense of functional competency in daily self-care activities.

As an occupational therapist, you received a referral from the insurance company to assist Kara in determining her capacity for returning to work and to set up an RTW plan. After meeting with Kara and reading her file, you begin to get a sense that Kara has low self-esteem, lacks confidence in her ability to return to the workplace for fear of poor performance, and is somewhat anxious about her relationship with co-workers. Kara reported that she feels she has lost her sense of identity because she has been out of the workplace for so long. She also lacks a sense of power to make changes that could improve things for her in the workplace. She is afraid that the employer will not let her come back to work.

As the occupational therapist, you contact the staff ergonomist, who agrees to meet with you to conduct an evaluation of the work demands. Although the workplace has provided you with a physical demands analysis of a laboratory worker job, you note that most of the information about the job relevant to Kara's return to work is not evident on the form.

You require the following information before developing an RTW plan:

- What are the cognitive and behavioral demands of the job that Kara will need to resume on her return to work?
- How can these job demands be measured? What tools and processes exist? Are they valid and reliable?
- What job specific information does the employer have—for example, job descriptions or procedure manuals?
- What job demands are cognitively or behaviorally complex?
- How do situations or factors in the workplace influence the temporality or frequency of these demands?
- How do I match Kara's functional capacities with work demands and requirements?
- How can Kara be included in this evaluation process?

Understanding and differentiating cognitive and behavioral demands of work is a complex endeavor. It is often difficult to separate the cognitive and behavioral demands required of work occupations from the human capacity to execute those demands. Some of the confusion is caused by the inconsistent use of terms such as *skills*, *tasks*, *demands*, *workload*, *capacities*, and *potential*, as well as the overlap of factors described within the psychosocial, cognitive, and behavioral domains of work. The aim of this chapter is to provide therapists with information and a process for evaluating cognitive and behavioral demands of work that can, in turn, be used to develop disability prevention programs and inform return-to-work (RTW) programs for workers with injuries or disabilities. Information in this chapter may also assist therapists in working with employers, workers, worker representatives, and engineers to develop strategies for managing or adjusting work demands when cognitive and behavioral demands of work are high relative to worker capacity.

BACKGROUND

A number of disciplines and fields of knowledge are contributing to the emergence of classifications, taxonomies, and tools for evaluating cognitive components of work. Researchers in psychology have examined cognitive workload from a human information processing perspective,[1] and organizational psychologists have recently begun to focus on positive psychology, studying "human strengths and optimal functioning" and their impact on the health and productivity of workers.[5] Occupational health researchers have also advanced knowledge about the behavioral and cognitive demands that influence mental health and functioning of workers. For example, both the Job Demands and Control model[2,3] and the Effort-Reward Imbalance model[7] provide measures used to examine the impact of work demands and work capacities on health. These tools are designed to study the relationship of workplace strain to outcomes such as back pain and cardiovascular disease, and human resource issues such as worker motivation and job satisfaction. Cognitive science, a field within human factors, has contributed to the development of a cognitive taxonomy that elaborates on cognitive attributes and actions required to process, synthesize, and use information in performing jobs.[10] A process for consistently evaluating cognitive demands was proposed by Wei and Salvendy to assist in job evaluation, job design, and job rotation, as well as in personnel selection and training.[10]

Clinical occupational health providers such as ergonomists, occupational health nurses, occupational therapists, physicians, and social workers have used evidence-based tools in the evaluation of cognitive and behavioral work demands to assist in the matching of workers with mental or behavioral health problems to appropriate job tasks during the RTW process. The clinical community has also contributed to assessments of cognitive function and neurologic trauma or impairments. These developments across disciplines have contributed to the depth and breadth of information available to therapists to address a multitude of issues central to cognitive and behavioral job demands and worker functioning.

In clinical practice there is growing acceptance for the use of a holistic approach to understanding factors that influence worker health and performance, including workplace factors (e.g., psychosocial and physical work environments), individual factors (e.g., engagement and support), and aging factors (e.g., cognitive and physical effects of aging). As a result, therapists are required to provide advice and expertise to enable optimal worker performance through strategies that might prevent injury or support successful transitions back to work for persons with cognitive or behavioral impairments. To generate solutions, the therapist must know what information is relevant to the case, situation, or problem, how to measure the demands of work, and how to anticipate potential risks and challenges in the workplace. The case study about Kara will be used throughout this chapter to demonstrate the information and process needed to provide recommendations for RTW programs.

UNDERSTANDING COGNITIVE AND BEHAVIORAL WORK DEMANDS

In conducting job demands analyses, it is important to distinguish between the requirements for competent job performance and work capacity. *Job demands* and *requirements* refer to the tasks and components of work, or the specific requirements of a work occupation. *Worker skills* and *abilities* refer to the capacities and expertise of the person that are used in performing or executing job demands. Although these elements are related, especially if the worker's skills are a good match for the job demands, each must be evaluated separately using appropriate tools and measures. In the same way that we would evaluate the physical demands of a job (e.g., a worker is required to lift 50-pound boxes to a surface at shoulder height up to 10 times a day) separately from a worker's physical capacity (e.g., maximum lifting capacity and tolerances), we must consider cognitive and behavioral demands as separate from the incumbent worker's abilities. This chapter will address how to rate and measure cognitive and behavioral job demands. For information on assessment of human cognitive performance and behavioral skills, abilities, and expertise, therapists should consult appropriate texts and literature. Further information about these sources is located in the reference list at the end of this chapter.

Cognitive Demands

Typically, therapists view cognitive skills at the level of the person. The domain of human cognitive abilities is often understood and expressed through terms such as *short-term* or *long-term memory, problem solving, attention span, communication skills,* and *computational ability.* Cognitive functioning is essential to occupational competence at a personal level but is also important in the workplace, as it enables workers to be productive and fulfill the demands of work. For instance, cognitive functioning is a multilevel process that enables a person to perceive, imagine, organize, assimilate, analyze, communicate, sense problems, and manipulate information and knowledge[9] in order to understand, reason, make decisions, create ideas, problem solve, and take actions in the context of doing a work activity. The execution of job tasks that require cognitive functions also requires human cognitive resources such as memory, vision, hearing, attention, concentration, literacy skills, communication, and an increasing reliance on electronic and technologic skills. Wei and Salvendy suggest that cognitive work tasks or job elements can be classified into the *cognitive skills* required to carry out work tasks and the *cognitive resources* needed to execute those cognitively based performance skills.[10] We drew on the work of Wei and Salvendy[10] and others[2,3,9] to compile a list of cognitive (skill) requirements and a list of cognitive resources needed to perform cognitive work tasks (Box 7-1).

Each job can be thought of as having a particular physical or cognitive load, and often one of these elements is in higher demand than the other. All work requires cognitive skills, but the cognitive load may be high or low, and the profile of cognitive skills required is unique for each job. The role of the therapist is to identify and describe the work demands or tasks that require specific application of cognitive functioning and to identify the nature and level of the cognitive demands. In this process, therapists must be careful to evaluate and define the nature of the cognitive work task requirements, not the worker. To do this, therapists can draw on their knowledge of human cognition, their awareness of the complexities of occupation-environment interactions, and their

skills in task analysis to identify and analyze cognitively based work demands. Box 7-1 can assist the therapist in framing the cognitive demands of work. Cognitive requirements of work must be fully understood in terms of their complexity, then translated into terms to which the end-user, such as the worker, the employer, the supervisor, or the insurer, can relate.

Once the cognitive work requirements are understood, the therapist may then take steps

---

Box 7-1	*Cognitive Demands of Work*

Cognitive Requirements of Job Tasks

Critical thinking (judgment, analysis, reasoning, calculation, manipulation, generation of knowledge and ideas)

Creative thinking using imagination and generating creative ideas

Information acquisition, searching, and retrieval

Information processing: assimilate, organize

Mental planning and scheduling

Learning

Communicating

Comprehending

Translating knowledge

Perceiving and interpreting interpersonal information

Using intuition—sensing or anticipating problems

Cognitive Resources

Memory (short-term, long-term)

Attention, visual and auditory concentration

Imagination

Communication skills (verbal, nonverbal), interpersonal skills, graphic expression, written skills

Vision

Visual processing

Visual perception

Auditory processing

Hearing and listening skills

Literacy and reading, writing, and documentation skills

Computer and technologic skills

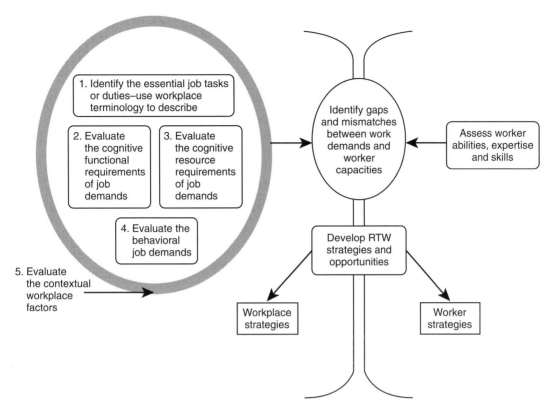

FIGURE 7-1 Process for evaluating cognitive and behavioral demands and the workplace context in developing an RTW plan.

to identify cognitive performance strengths and weaknesses of the worker, acknowledge gaps or mismatches between the worker and the work requirements, and develop a comprehensive RTW intervention that matches a worker's abilities to suitable job demands. Therapists need to adopt a consistent approach to defining and describing cognitive demands through translating information about cognition into understandable language when requesting procedural changes or accommodations to a worker's cognitive workload. The range of cognitive work demands and the workplace dynamics must also be determined to assist the therapist in identifying contextual factors that might hinder performance, as well as opportunities for creating a successful transition and resumption of duties as a person recovers from an illness

or injury. This process of evaluating the cognitive requirements of a job and the cognitive resources required to execute job demands in consideration of workplace influences is shown in Figure 7-1.

For Kara's job as a supervisor, the first step is to identify the job demands or tasks that are required. In this case example, scheduling staff is one of Kara's responsibilities. Step two is to identify and evaluate the cognitive demand. The job demand of scheduling staff in the laboratory requires the mental functions of planning and scheduling. Step three is considering the cognitive resource requirements. This cognitive demand is enacted using cognitive resources such as short- and long-term memory, concentration, prior knowledge and experience, reading literacy, writing, and technologic skills because scheduling is done on the computer.

Many tools or lists of cognitive skills may serve as resources when evaluating these demands of work occupations. Existing tools commonly used to measure cognitive components of work, discussed later in this chapter, do not capture or measure all cognitive demands. Thus, the therapist must use judgment in attempting to comprehensively appraise the diversity of and interrelationship between the cognitive skills and resources required to execute job demands. Specific tools for evaluating and rating these demands are provided later in this chapter.

Behavioral Demands

Behavioral demands of work occupations refer to the actions and interactions a worker may encounter that require a specific response or subsequent set of actions to manage or perform duties and tasks in the workplace. These include the enactment of social processes and relationships with others, performance of management responsibilities, enactment of worker responsibilities, general competencies, and accountabilities, and enactment of specific competencies. An overview of the specific behavioral demands that may be associated with work is provided in Table 7-1. These demands require a person to be able to demonstrate specific social and interpersonal skills or competencies that often combine or draw on prior experience, specific training, cognition, and affective skills in order to successfully exercise these behaviors. For the most part, these demands are defined as actions and are thus conceptualized using a gerund, or "-ing" word. The role of the therapist is to identify which demands are required and to determine the nature of these demands and how they unfold when work occupations are executed. Again, this list of behaviors is not complete; however, it is meant to organize an array of behavioral demands that therapists can draw on when considering the types of behaviors and demands required in the workplace.

Step 4 of the process illustrated in Figure 7-1 indicates that the therapist identifies the behavioral demands and appraises the salient interactions required to perform work.

In order to begin development of a plan to return Kara to the workplace, use the behavioral demands from Table 7-1 and identify the demands that Kara can be expected to perform in her role as a laboratory supervisor. Based on the information from the case, prioritize the demands that may be challenging for Kara and require consideration in developing a modified RTW strategy. What demands would you consider modifications for, or address in a progressive work conditioning process?

Develop a set of questions for Kara and for Kara's manager to assist you in obtaining information you will need to implement an RTW plan that offers a gradual resumption of full duties. Next, consider what each stakeholder will need to do in order for a feasible and client-centered plan to be developed. Consider Kara's role (worker strategies), as well as what the manager needs to do (workplace strategies). What is your role as a therapist in creating the return-to-work plan?

CONTEXTUAL INFLUENCES ON COGNITIVE AND BEHAVIORAL WORK DEMANDS AND WORKER PERFORMANCE

Workplace factors include the governance structures in a workplace, workplace culture, exposure to change, and risk concerns such as physical security and safety. All of these factors can affect the nature of cognitive and behavioral demands and influence the success of the worker-job match. Box 7-2 includes some of the workplace factors that need to be considered in evaluating the impact of contextual factors on worker productivity and performance. Governance and position status factors can affect the degree of power or responsibility a worker can exercise at work. Workplace culture can influence the acceptance and belonging needs of a worker.[8] In addition, productivity dynamics such as the urgency, speed, degree of interruptions, and unplanned or unexpected tasks can, in turn, influence the cognitive and behavioral requirements and demand an adaptive response from the worker. For therapists, the consideration of the environment and how it shapes the way work unfolds in a given environment is essential for designing a successful

TABLE 7-1 **Behavioral Components of Work**

Component	Examples

Enactment of social processes, interactions, and relationships with others	Interacting with supervisor
	Interacting with others
	Providing supervision
	Managing conflict
	Working cooperatively with other employees or customers
	Working in isolation from others
	Interpreting and responding to nonverbal cues and gestures
	Providing social support to co-workers
	Implementing a social interaction approach when working with others:
	    Using a friendly, congenial customer-oriented approach
	    Using a caring approach
	    Using a professional, expert-oriented approach
	    Using a collaborative-partnership, team-oriented approach
	    Using a business-oriented, networking approach

Enactment of worker responsibilities and requirements	Exercising supervision Receiving supervision Exercising self-supervision Training self and others Taking initiative Working safely Socializing with others Networking with others Working independently Working interdependently Working cooperatively with others; using team work Exercising independent control and autonomy over decisions and problem solving Exercising control over work pace Self-directing schedule and prioritizing work tasks Solving problems Making decisions
Executing emotional job demands	Exercising self-awareness; demonstrating a high self-regard and self-confidence Exercising autonomy through reflection and action in midst of practice or performing duties Exercising self-regulation of emotions (e.g., be calm in emotionally charged situations) Exercising sensitivity toward others Exercising or conveying compassion, empathy, sympathy Executing a positive attitude Conveying hopefulness Acting in a courteous manner Acting in a kind and thoughtful manner Exercising emotional intelligence Motivating self Managing emotions of others

Continued

TABLE 7-1	Behavioral Components of Work—*cont'd*

Component	Examples
Enactment of management responsibilities and requirements	Managing material, financial, human resources, quality, and production of work Managing negative attitudes of others Managing and resolving conflict Managing cultural sensitivities Managing through training, instructing, negotiating, or persuading, giving feedback, coaching, mentoring Managing social and emotional needs Engaging a directive, supportive, participative, or achievement-oriented supervisory or leadership approach Solving problems Making decisions
Enactment of general competencies and accountabilities	Paying attention to detail Performing multiple tasks
Enactment of specific competencies	Operating lift truck Using statistical software Dispensing pharmaceuticals

Box 7-2	*Emotional, Cognitive, Security-Related, and Environmental Tasks*

Time pressures
Deadline pressures
Safety pressures
Security pressures
Life and death pressures
Exposure to emotional situations
Exposure to confrontational situations
Exposure to high risk with regard to safety and physical well-being
Exposure to environmental stimuli (noise, people, machines, distractions)
Position status
Union status
Type of governance (style):
    Authoritative
    Directive
    Supportive
    Participative
    Achievement-oriented

RTW program. The workplace environment can have a significant impact on a person in terms of feedback regarding performance when returning to work, but returning to work also requires a person to be ready to accept changes and adapt activities and actions based on the pressures exerted by the workplace environment. Other environmental considerations such as noise, heat, cold, physical space, location, tools and equipment, and resources and supports may also influence a worker's capacity to fulfill cognitive and behavioral demands.

Step 5 in the process outlined in Figure 7-1 requires that the contextual factors that influence the performance of work in this workplace be considered. In this case, for example, the schedules are done biweekly to make adjustments for changes in shift resulting from employees who are ill or absent, holidays, and vacation planning.

Based on our case, create a description that captures the essence of the workplace. What are the challenges and facilitators that might inform the implementation of the RTW plan? How might contextual factors affect Kara's ability to adapt to modified work and accept and respond to changes and pressures in the workplace? How can this information be used to support the RTW process? Consider how the worker or others involved in the workplace might be included to support a transitional RTW process for Kara.

What contextual information do you need that cannot be assumed from the case information provided? Develop a list of additional information you need, and develop a set of strategies for obtaining this information. Then follow through with the process to identify the areas requiring consideration and create a plan to address these issues.

MEASURING THE COGNITIVE AND BEHAVIORAL DEMANDS OF WORK

Numerous challenges are involved in assessing workload, because many cognitive and behavioral demands are less observable than physical demands. By focusing on the behavioral aspects of cognitive skills, however, it is possible to identify and rate demand levels. For example, recording the degree to which one is exposed to emotional situations on a job is arguably more objectively determined than is measuring the level of sensitivity required. Another challenge lies in the fact that cognitive and behavioral ratings are often done by or with workers themselves so that a broad and inclusive spectrum of the job demands is considered. Individual worker perceptions of the inherent cognitive demand of a job may vary greatly, however, based on their personal qualities, such as the worker's ability to function in the presence of multiple stimuli or with high or low supervision.

Document Review

Job descriptions provided by a company or work unit can provide useful background information on the position in question, including responsibilities, physical risks, hours of work, and specific knowledge or preparation required. The latter can provide insight into the nature of the work. For example, if a worker is required to have many years of experience in the use of technical equip-

ment, one may anticipate that a high level of attention to detail and accountability are required. A worker who is required to pass numerous police screenings will likely have some level of self-supervision, as well as personal accountability. Other sources outside of the workplace, such as government job descriptions and ratings, like the National O*Net Consortium: Occupational Information Network (O*Net) (http://online.onetcenter.org), also provide good background information, but it may not be directly relevant to the demands of work in a particular workplace. For example, the cognitive and behavioral demands of a cleaning job may be quite different for a worker who works on a crew with other workers than for one who is independently responsible for an entire building, although the physical demands may be quite similar.

Observation

An impartial rater, such as a therapist or occupational health nurse, may observe job performance and note the variety of demands required in the cognitive and behavioral spectrum. Use of a structured format or checklist helps observers attend to key factors and to consistently record demand levels. In order for analyses to be complete, it may be necessary to observe for extended time periods or to sample time segments from different times of the day or week. Observational analysis is generally done in conjunction with other information sources (e.g., review of job descriptions, interviews) in order to guide time sampling to ensure that the review is comprehensive.

Worker Interviews

Job incumbents possess the most in-depth knowledge of a job and are an invaluable source of information concerning job demands. Although some workers will lack the experience to critically evaluate the level of job demand, many contemporary workers have been employed in a number of different positions over the course of their working life and will have keen insight into the key risks or demands associated with the current job. Use of behaviorally based scales and examples is helpful in identifying the level of demand.

Supervisor Interviews

Supervisor input is useful for understanding job duties and how they fit with the overall flow of the workplace. Expectations of worker performance in such functions as customer service, emergency preparedness, and cooperation with other workers may be best identified by a person with a broad, supervisory perspective. Supervisor interviews alone typically provide insufficient information on which to base job demands analysis (JDA), however, as often the supervisor is removed from a job and its detailed requirements.

As with any measurement system, cognitive and behavioral job rating tools must satisfy basic standards for reliability and validity. Validity issues in rating forms are typically addressed in the developmental stages by including vocational and occupational health experts in the creation and refinement of tools such that the items included are meaningful, relevant, and comprehensive. The reliability of a measure, which is the reproducibility of the score over time or across raters, is enhanced by the following:

- Clear definitions: The levels of an item and their meaning must be clearly stated and defined for the rater. Ambiguous definitions lead to wide variance in scoring, based on differences in interpretation from one job setting to another and from one rater to another.
- Training: Job raters require both thorough orientation to rating tools and experience in using the tool under supervision in order to eliminate misconceptions. This is particularly important in the case of tools measuring the cognitive and behavioral aspects of work, because of the less observable nature of many of the items. Training is generally enhanced by providing detailed documentation as to how to use the tool, along with sample cases.
- Experience: As in other areas of JDA, familiarity with a measurement tool and exposure to a wide variety of job types help to situate observations in a broader context. Observers are more able over time to differentiate among levels of cognitive and behavioral

demand than when few reference points are available.

Rating Systems

A number of approaches to identifying the cognitive and behavioral demands of work are available in the literature and from corporate and government sources. Functional demands are examined in different ways depending on the group conducting the analysis and the group's purpose. Government agencies (such as the U.S. Department of Labor, Employment and Training Administration [DLET] and Statistics Canada) maintain databases of jobs and their corresponding training and skill requirements. These systems include ratings related to the knowledge level required and other cognitive components of work. For example, O*Net, the job database maintained by DLET, includes ratings on more than 40 cognitive and behavioral skills for each job (Table 7-2). These skills range from the basic skills required to perform a job to required aptitudes in areas such as complex problem solving, resource management, and social, technical, and systems skills. Skill ratings are done by incumbent workers who are assumed to have in-depth knowledge of jobs, and the resulting scales are used primarily for vocational guidance and planning and for public policy development.

Unions typically perform job demands analyses for the purpose of delineating the responsibility level of work in order to determine the relative value of the job, with the goal of creating fair and equitable compensation scales. The Uniform Classification Standard developed by the Treasury Board of Canada for classification of public sector jobs has been used or adapted by major unions in that country. It rates four key elements of jobs: Responsibility, Effort, Skills, and Working Conditions. Table 7-3 demonstrates how the Universal Classification has been modified for use by one major union, the Canadian Union of Public Employees (CUPE). Many of these demands address the cognitive and behavioral aspects of performing work. A sample rating scale is shown in Figure 7-2. In order to allocate point values to jobs using the various scales, determinations are typically done by job evaluation committees that

| TABLE 7-2 | O*NET Skill Requirements Categories |

Skills	Developed Capacities
Basic Skills	**Capacities That Facilitate Learning or the More Rapid Acquisition of Knowledge**
Active learning	Understanding the implications of new information for both current and future problem solving and decision making
Active listening	Giving full attention to what other people are saying, taking time to understand the points being made, asking questions as appropriate, and not interrupting at inappropriate times
Critical thinking	Using logic and reasoning to identify the strengths and weaknesses of alternative solutions, conclusions, or approaches to problems
Learning strategies	Selecting and using training or instructional methods and procedures appropriate for the situation when learning or teaching new things
Mathematics	Using mathematics to solve problems
Monitoring	Monitoring and assessing performance of one's self, other individuals, or organizations to make improvements or take corrective action
Reading comprehension	Understanding written sentences and paragraphs in work-related documents
Science	Using scientific rules and methods to solve problems
Speaking	Talking to others to convey information effectively
Writing	Communicating effectively in writing as appropriate for the needs of the audience
Complex Problem-Solving Skills	**Capacities Used to Solve Novel, Ill-Defined Problems in Complex, Real-World Settings**
Complex problem solving	Identifying complex problems and reviewing related information to develop and evaluate options and implement solutions
Resource Management Skills	**Capacities Used to Allocate Resources Efficiently**
Management of financial resources	Determining how money will be spent to get the work done and accounting for these expenditures
Management of material resources	Obtaining and seeing to the appropriate use of equipment, facilities, and materials needed to do certain work
Management of personnel resources	Motivating, developing, and directing people as they work, identifying the best people for the job
Time management	Managing one's own time and the time of others
Social Skills	**Capacities Used to Work with People to Achieve Goals**
Coordination	Adjusting actions in relation to others' actions
Instructing	Teaching others how to do something
Negotiation	Bringing others together and trying to reconcile differences

Continued

TABLE 7-2 O*NET Skill Requirements Categories—*cont'd*

Skills	Developed Capacities
Persuasion	Persuading others to change their minds or behavior
Service orientation	Actively looking for ways to help people
Social perceptiveness	Being aware of others' reactions and understanding why they react as they do
Systems Skills	**Capacities Used to Understand, Monitor, and Improve Sociotechnical Systems**
Judgment and decision making	Considering the relative costs and benefits of potential actions to choose the most appropriate one
Systems analysis	Determining how a system should work and how changes in conditions, operations, and the environment will affect outcomes
Systems evaluation	Identifying measures or indicators of system performance and the actions needed to improve or correct performance, relative to the goals of the system
Technical Skills	**Capacities Used to Design, Set up, Operate, and Correct Malfunctions Involving Application of Machines or Technologic Systems**
Equipment maintenance	Performing routine maintenance on equipment and determining when and what kind of maintenance is needed
Equipment selection	Determining the kind of tools and equipment needed to do a job
Installation	Installing equipment, machines, wiring, or programs to meet specifications
Operation and control	Controlling operations of equipment or systems
Operation monitoring	Watching gauges, dials, or other indicators to make sure a machine is working properly
Operations analysis	Analyzing needs and product requirements to create a design
Programming	Writing computer programs for various purposes
Quality control analysis	Conducting tests and inspections of products, services, or processes to evaluate quality or performance
Repairing	Repairing machines or systems using the needed tools
Technology design	Generating or adapting equipment and technology to serve user needs
Troubleshooting	Determining causes of operating errors and deciding what to do about them

TABLE 7-3 Work Characteristics Included in the Canadian Union of Public Employees Gender-Neutral Job Evaluation Plan

Characteristic	Examples	Characteristic	Examples
Responsibility	Accountability Safety of others Supervision of others Contacts with others	Skill Working conditions	Knowledge Experience Judgment Disagreeable working conditions
Effort	Concentration Physical effort Dexterity		

Subfactor 4 - Concentration

DEFINITION:	This subfactor measures the period of time wherein mental, visual, and/or aural concentration is required on the job. Both the frequency and duration of the effort are to be considered.

DEGREES:

1. Occasional periods of short duration.

2. Frequent periods of short duration; OR
   Occasional periods of intermediate duration.

3. Almost continuous periods of short duration; OR
   Frequent periods of intermediate duration; OR
   Occasional periods of long duration.

4. Almost continuous periods of intermediate duration; OR
   Frequent periods of long duration.

5. Almost continuous periods of long duration.

NOTES TO RATERS:

1. Attentiveness is required for all jobs; rate tasks requiring concentration.

2. Concentration includes activities such as listening, interpreting, reading, watching, driving, inputting data, or when a combination of the five senses, sight, taste, smell, touch, and hearing, is required in the course of doing the job that result in mental/sensory fatigue.

3. Consider components such as interruptions and the requirements for simultaneous processing of information (i.e., maintaining concentration despite frequent interruptions or changes in work priorities).

4. **Duration** of uninterrupted time is measured as follows:
   Short — Up to and including 1 hour.
   Intermediate — Over 1 hour, and up to and including 2 hours.
   Long — In excess of 2 hours.
   Frequency relates to work carried out on a regular basis throughout the year.
   Occasional — Once in a while, most days.
   Frequent — Several times a day or at least 4 days per week.
   Almost Continuous — Most working hours for at least an average of 4 days per week.

5. Subfactor Chart

FREQUENCY	DURATION		
	Short	**Intermediate**	**Long**
Occasional	1	2	3
Frequent	2	3	4
Almost Continuous	3	4	5

FIGURE **7-2** Sample rating format from the Universal Classification Standard.

base job ratings on job questionnaires completed by workers and supervisors.

Measures emerging from psychology, as previously mentioned, are used primarily in research in order to measure the relationship between job demands and various outcomes of interest. An example of a scale used for this purpose is the Job Content Questionnaire,[3] a standardized, self-administered tool that measures a number of cognitive, behavioral, and contextual job factors including decision authority, choice and variety in work, psychologic demands and mental workload (including general psychologic demands, role ambiguity, concentration, and mental work disruption), job security, and supports available. The subject is asked to indicate on a scale ranging from "Never" to "Extremely Often" the extent to which the job requires him or her to work fast, how often the worker must expend excessive effort, whether the job is hectic, and other similar factors. This tool has well-established predictive validity and reliability but is available only from the authors for use in research.

From a rehabilitation perspective, the cognitive and behavioral demands of jobs are of increasing interest to therapists and occupational health personnel, given their relevance to successful job performance. The goal of JDA in rehabilitation is to understand and objectify the requirements of the work for use in work conditioning and modified return-to-work programs. Many JDA tools in use provide only global ratings of cognitive and behavioral demands and lack sufficient detail to match jobs to the functional capacities of the worker. In addition, only a few JDA tools identify the demands of work versus the capabilities of the worker.

USING JOB DEMANDS ANALYSIS TOOLS: CITY OF TORONTO JOB DEMANDS ANALYSIS INSTRUMENT

One example of a JDA tool that addresses physical, cognitive, and behavioral aspects of work is the City of Toronto Job Demands Analysis Tool (CoT).[6] This instrument was developed by therapists, ergonomists, occupational health personnel, and a consulting psychiatrist based on their experiences with a broad spectrum of jobs and workers

over several years. A four-point rating scale is provided for each item, with "4" representing the highest level of demand, and unique descriptions are provided for each rating level within each item. Figure 7-3 shows the section of this tool that is used for evaluating the responsibility and accountability demands of work. The full list of cognitive and behavioral demands addressed in this tool is shown in Figure 7-4 as it would be completed for Kara's job. It includes factors ranging from relationships with others (e.g., supervision, cooperation with other workers, communication) to independent cognitive demands (e.g., memory, literacy, attention to detail, exposure to distracting stimuli) and emotional control (e.g., working with deadline pressures, exposure to emotional and confrontational situations).

The CoT established content validity of this tool[6] and more recently inter-rater reliability was established through a study using student and expert raters.[4] The second part of the CoT tool provides therapists with a means to record the worker's functional capacity, based on separate clinical assessments. A parallel process of rating of the worker's capacity to perform these job demands is completed to identify areas of potential mismatch. These mismatches are then used as a basis for developing an RTW plan.

CONCLUSION

This chapter draws attention to the need for a broader evaluation of the demands and requirements of work occupations. Measuring the cognitive and behavioral demands of work in addition to the physical elements of the job will lead to a more complete and comprehensive JDA. Efforts of therapists to rate these demands and identify inherent challenges will assist them in the development of RTW plans for clients. In addition, through the JDA process therapists may identify potentially highly complex or behavioral work requirements that may lead to risks such as stress and anxiety. Thus, therapists may use this information to make recommendations for changes in work processes, procedures, or the workplace context to help workers and employers reduce the onset of problems and improve workplace health.

Responsibility and accountability required "Responsibility and accountability required" refers to the extent of liability or safety risk that could result if the employee does not exercise appropriate judgment or attention during the performance of job tasks. A high rating indicates that the job is a safety-sensitive position with the potential for grave consequences if errors or inattention occur.		**Responsibility and accountability** The ability to exercise appropriate judgment and behave in a responsive manner during the performance of work. A low rating indicates a potential error or inattention that could have grave consequences if the worker is required to perform safety-sensitive work.
Job Demands Analysis Definitions	**Rating**	**Functional Abilities Definitions**
Error in judgement or attention would have insignificant consequences	1	May be prone to errors in judgment and/or lapses of attention and therefore should only perform work in which such errors or lapses would have insignificant consequences
Error in judgment or attention would create inconvenience	2	Able to exercise some judgment and responsibility, but occasional lapses may occur; the worker should be assigned to work in which such lapses would not create serious difficulties
Error in judgement or attention could create serious difficulty or significant expense	3	Able to exercise a moderate degree of judgment and responsibility, but not to a sufficient extent to assume responsibility for safety of others
Error in judgment or attention could have grave or life-threatening consequences	4	Able to exercise sufficient judgment and responsibility to perform well in safety-sensitive positions in which the worker is responsible for the safety of others

FIGURE **7-3** City of Toronto JDA sample of behavioral demand.

Job Demands Analysis Definitions	Ratings		Functional Abilities Definitions
Degree of Self-Supervision Required			**The Ability to Self-Supervise**
Predominantly self-supervised through-out the shift (may contact supervisor to obtain work direction as needed)	4	3	Can tolerate infrequent supervision
Degree of Supervision Exercised			**The Ability to Supervise Others**
Has full supervisory responsibility for other employees	4	3	Able to provide work direction and some elements of managing work performance with the exclusion of disciplinary action
Deadline Pressures (time pressure)			**The Ability to Tolerate Deadline Pressures (time pressure)**
Time pressure is high: the majority of work is performed under rigid time constraints and the volume of work is high (assumes that the work pace is high OR the worker must extend the workday to manage the volume of work)	4	2	Capable of moderate work pace and can occasionally work under time constraints
Attention to Detail			**The Ability to Attend to Detail**
Significant attention to detail or concentration required for many tasks or intense attention to detail or concentration required for some tasks	3	2	Able to concentrate on or attend to details for some tasks, although not at an intense level
Performance of Multiple Tasks			**The Ability to Perform Multiple Tasks**
Responsible for multiple tasks, with some time-management skill and judgment required to determine priorities	3	2	Can handle more than one task, but requires clear cues to indicate when each task should be performed
Exposure to Distracting Stimuli			**Tolerance to Distracting Stimuli**
Moderate degree of distracting stimuli during some tasks or portions of the shift	3	3	Able to work effectively with a moderate degree of distracting stimuli
Need to Work Cooperatively with Others			**The Ability to Work Cooperatively with Others**
The majority of work requires close cooperation with others	4	3	Can work cooperatively with others on some tasks
Exposure to Emotional Situations			**Ability to Tolerate Emotional Situations**
Occasional exposure (approx. weekly) to emotionally stressful circumstances or emotionally distressed individuals with whom the worker must interact in order to complete job requirements	3	2	Able to tolerate infrequent exposure (e.g., monthly) to emotionally stressful circum-stances or emotionally distressed individuals

FIGURE 7-4 Sample behavioral and cognitive job rating using the CoT JDA tool applied to Kara's job demands.

Exposure to Confrontational Situations			Ability to Tolerate Confrontation
Occasional exposure (up to weekly) to confrontational situations in which assistance is immediately available	2	2	Able to tolerate occasional exposure (up to weekly) to confrontational situations in which assistance is immediately available
Responsibility and Accountability Required			**Responsibility and Accountability**
Errors in judgment or attention could have grave or life-threatening consequences	4	3	Able to exercise a moderate degree of judgment and responsibility, but not to a sufficient extent to assume responsibility for safety of others
Reading Literacy			**Ability to Read**
A high degree of reading literacy is required to read reports, manuals, or other documents with a high degree of comprehension	4	4	Able to read at an advanced level without difficulty
Written Literacy			**Ability to Write**
Required to create reports, complex documents, or any communications that require a high degree of grammatical form and/or careful wording	4	3	Able to compose memos or letters with accurate spelling, grammatical construction, and clarity.
Numerical Skills			**Ability to Perform Numerical Skills**
Required to use more complex arithmetical operations such as division, multiplication, percentages, or ratios	3	3	Able to use more complex arithmetical operations such as division, multiplication, percentages, or ratios
Verbal Communication			**Ability to Communicate**
Moderate communication skills are required to comprehend and communicate information fluently (e.g., to work crews)	3	3	Has sufficient communication skills to comprehend and communicate information fluently
Memory			**Memory**
Moderate memory ability is required to recall information that is harder to remember because it is recalled infrequently, or because there are time constraints within which to recall the	3	3	Has moderate memory ability; can recall information that is harder to remember because it is infrequently used or because of time pressures
Computer Literacy			**Ability to Use Computers**
Required to use one or more computer programs at a competent level (e.g., most office workers using word processing and e-mail applications)	3	3	Able to use one or more computer programs at a competent level expected for most office workers

FIGURE **7-4** cont'd.

Learning Exercise

Overview

This learning exercise is designed to make the student aware of various aspects of the cognitive and behavioral demands of work.

Purpose

The purpose of this exercise is to encourage the student to use a critical and thorough approach in evaluating the cognitive and behavioral demands of work.

Exercise

To apply the information from this chapter and enhance practical skills in identifying cognitive and behavioral demands, choose a commonly understood job such as a resource or reference librarian in the local university or college library. This exercise may be approached as a casual observation or as a formal worksite visit.

1. Using a casual observation only: Visit the library and observe the librarian performing his or her job. Use Boxes 7-1 and 7-2, Table 7-1, and/or the CoT JDA form to observe, identify, and record the cognitive and behavioral requirements of a resource librarian. Choose a rating scale, then try to rate the demands you observe as well as categorizing them into simple complex requirements. Identify demands that you cannot observe and about which you require further information. What questions might you pose to the librarian to get the information you need and to justify your rating of these demands?
   - Hold a small group discussion about the experience of conducting the observation. Identify what was easy and what was difficult to observe, and create a list of strategies you would use to evaluate the cognitive and behavioral components that you remain unsure about.
   - As a group, describe the contextual factors you observed in the workplace. Identify the factors in the workplace context that are constant and those that are variable. Create a list of questions you would ask the librarian to enhance your understanding of the nature of the contextual factors.
   - Identify potential people you would involve if you were developing an RTW plan for an employee.
2. Alternative exercise for the same job: Conduct a formal worksite visit (one in which you ask the employer's permission to perform an evaluation as part of a learning exercise) with opportunity for interviews and use of other collateral information. First, review a job description and conduct an Internet search to identify some key behavioral or cognitive demands of the position. Next, conduct an observation and identify demands as above. From your observations, try to rate the behavioral and cognitive demands. Work in a small group and identify a list of questions you want to ask to further your understanding of these tasks. Ask to meet with the librarian to interview him or her for more detailed information, or invite the librarian to a class. In class, conduct a group interview to further refine your understanding of these demands. Write up a description of the cognitive and behavioral demands. Identify and record the simple and highly complex demands of this workplace.

Multiple Choice Review Questions

1. Measuring cognitive and behavioral demands of work requires a therapist to:
   A. interview the supervisor.
   B. discuss job demands with the insurer.
   C. collect information from a variety of sources.
   D. use a form that the union endorses.

2. Cognitive and behavioral job demands are:
   A. the skills and abilities of workers.
   B. requirements of the work itself.
   C. easily understood by supervisors.
   D. outcome measures of human performance.

3. In order to create an effective RTW plan for clients who have experienced injury or disability, the therapist should:
   A. measure or evaluate the physical demands of work.
   B. measure or evaluate the behavioral and cognitive demands of work.
   C. identify client characteristics.
   D. conduct a job demands analysis and evaluate worker capacity.

4. Managing and resolving conflict is an example of a:
   A. cognitively based job requirement.
   B. behavioral job requirement.
   C. physical job requirement.
   D. cognitive skill.
   E. contextual influence on performance.

5. After worker characteristics and limitations are assessed, an initial step in planning a return-to-work intervention is to:
   A. identify gaps and mismatches between the work demands and the worker's capabilities.
   B. evaluate the cognitive functional requirements of the job.
   C. evaluate the behavioral job demands.
   D. determine what contextual factors are involved.

6. Evaluating cognitive and behavioral demands of work is conducted for:
   A. planning return to work.
   B. evaluating risks in the workplace.
   C. rating jobs for compensation.
   D. All of the above

7. Making numeric calculations at work is an example of a:
   A. highly complex behavioral demand.
   B. highly complex cognitive demand.
   C. cognitive demand.
   D. behavioral demand.

8. Interviewing the supervisor as part of the JDA process is:
   A. the easiest way to gather information about cognitive demands.
   B. the best way to gather information about cognitive demands.
   C. necessary for assuring the insurer that the information collected is accurate.
   D. one way to gather information.

9. The goal of job demands analysis in rehabilitation is:
   A. to involve the worker in evaluating his or her work modification process.
   B. to satisfy the employer that all areas of work are considered in RTW planning.
   C. to provide an objective evaluation of work demands for RTW planning.
   D. to provide a health and safety risk assessment for all work tasks.

10. Consideration of factors in the workplace context is important in the JDA process because:
    A. these factors affect the way work is conducted.
    B. these factors are very similar in every worksite.
    C. these factors always positively support the return-to-work process.
    D. these factors include the essential duties of work occupations.

REFERENCES

1. Giannini AJ, Giannini JN, Melemis SM: Visual symbolization as a learning tool, *J Clin Pharmacol* 37:559, 1997.
2. Karasek R: Job decision latitude, job demands and mental strain: implications for job redesign, *Adm Sci Q* 24:285, 1979.
3. Karasek R, Brisson C, Kawakami N et al: The job content questionnaire (JCQ): an instrument for internationally comparative assessments of psychosocial job characteristics, *J Occup Health Psychol* 3:322, 1998.
4. Kirley W, Shaw L, Jogia A: Evaluating inter-rater accuracy and consistency in conducting job demands analysis, *Proceedings of the University of Western Ontario Occupational Therapy Conference on Evidence Based Practice,* 5:33, 2005.
5. Maslach C, Schaufeli W, Leiter M: Job burnout, *Annu Rev Psychol* 52:397, 2001.
6. Raybould K, McIwain L, Hardy C, Byers J: *Improving the effectiveness of the job demands analysis tools,* Unpublished article publicly available from the author.
7. Siegrist J: Effort-reward imbalance at work and health. In Perrewe PL, Ganster DC, editors: *Historical and current perspectives on stress and health,* Amsterdam, 2002, JAI Elsevier.
8. Strong S, Rebeiro K: Creating a supportive work environment for people with mental illness. In Letts L, Rigby P, Stewart D, editors: *Using environment to enable occupational performance,* Thorofare, NJ, 2003, Slack.
9. Venesy BA: A clinician's guide to decision making capacity and ethically sound medical decisions, *Am J Phys Med Rehabil* 73:219, 1994.
10. Wei J, Salvendy G: The utilization of the Purdue Cognitive Job Analysis methodology, *Hum Factor Ergon Man* 13:59, 2003.

SUGGESTED READING

Raskin SS, Mateer CA: Neuropsychological management of mild traumatic brain injury, New York, 2000, Oxford Press.

Sohlberg MM, Mateer CA: Introduction to cognitive rehabilitation: theory and practice, New York, 1989, Guilford Press.

Zoltan B: Vision, perception, and cognition: a manual for the evaluation and treatment of the neurologically impaired adult, ed 3, Thorofare, NJ, 1996, Slack.

Web Sites

Human Resources and Skills Development Canada—National Occupational Classification Career Handbook:
www23.hrdc-drhc.gc.ca/ch/e/docs/ch_welcome.asp

Job Stress Network: www.workhealth.org

National O*Net Consortium: Occupational Information Network (O*Net) Online: http://online.onetcenter.org

8

Psychosocial Factors in Work-Related Musculoskeletal Disorders*

Asnat Bar-Haim Erez

Learning Objectives

After reading this chapter and completing the exercises, the reader should be able to do the following:

1. Increase awareness of the need to assess psychosocial risk factors in ergonomic intervention.
2. Increase understanding of which factors are the most relevant for evaluation and intervention.
3. Have basic ergonomics tools for analysis of psychosocial risk factors.

Psychosocial factors. Ergonomic risk factors that describe how the work organization is perceived by workers and managers[10] and that can be roughly divided into three categories: factors associated with the work environment, factors associated with the extra-work environment, and individual characteristics of the worker.[36] The assumption is that conflicts in one of these categories precipitate a process of mental stress that affects the worker's physical health.

Demand-control-support model. A theoretic model for identifying the relationship between psychosocial

factors and work-related musculoskeletal disorders.[24] According to this model, psychologic demands have adverse effects on a worker if they occur jointly with low decision latitude (i.e., the opportunity to use and develop skills at work). The social support component in this model is the support available in the workplace that is thought to mediate between the demands and the appearance symptoms.

Cognitive-behavioral strategies. Strategies based on the cognitive-behavioral psychotherapy frame of reference. Such strategies include focusing on the

*Portions of this chapter are retained from the previous edition chapter written by Karen Lindgren.

source of the stress and paying close attention to its interpretation, examining the attribution style after symptoms and stress occur, and adopting alternative methods for addressing problems. The techniques used include relaxation (including use of biofeedback), activity pacing, cognitive restructuring, and mental imagery.[25]

CASE STUDY

"I gave my employees the best chairs and they are still unhappy."

Sara has been an operator in the obituary department of a large national newspaper for the last 3 years. Her job is to take telephone calls from people who are interested in placing an obituary in the newspaper. She came to therapy with complaints of headaches and pain in her upper extremities and wrist and was diagnosed with de Quervain's tendonitis in the hand. She has been in therapy for 4 weeks and has made good physical progress, but efforts to place her back at work failed even though light duty status was offered. Sara is single (with no children) but has a friend who accompanies her to therapy and appears to be a good support for her. She has a college education (a bachelor's degree in general world history) but has never really used it for higher-levels jobs.

Sara was reluctant to complete formal questionnaires, so an informal interview was conducted to get to the bottom of her feelings toward going back to work. It became clear that several issues bother her at work. Apparently she does not have control over how many calls she gets per shift, and she cannot stop for a break between calls (she is permitted only a formal break for lunch and two more short breaks). On the lower side of the screen, a message telling her how many calls are waiting for her is constantly running. She has hardly made any friends at work because she and her co-workers are constantly working, each person in his or her own cubicle. She feels she is considered a troublemaker because she tried to change some of the conditions and her superiors did not back her up. She feels that the job itself is stressful enough, because it involves talking with bereaved people all day with lack of time to relate to them.

Sara does have biomechanical risk factors (sitting in front of the computers all day); however, the psychosocial risk factors appear to be the significant ones with regard to helping her return to work. As you read the chapter, try to identify the psychosocial stressors that might be relevant for Sara and how did they affect both her symptoms and her return to work.

Psychosocial issues in the workplace are one of the areas included in risk factors analysis during an ergonomic assessment. This chapter defines psychosocial risk factors, including those proposed by the National Institute of Occupational Safety and Health (NIOSH) and the International Labor Office (ILO), and reviews research regarding the relationship of specific risk factors and work-related musculoskeletal disorders (WRMSDs), along with methodologic problems. The chapter also discusses four pathways that explain this relationship, interventions for clinicians, and future directions for intervention.

Understanding the role of psychosocial risk factors is important in the intervention and prevention of disability. NIOSH called for researchers to address the variety of risk factors thought to contribute to job stress and work-related disability in the work environment.[35] Consequently, researchers began to study the relationship between psychosocial factors and disability. Evidence has verified the importance of the relationships between psychosocial stressors and psychologic dysfunction and between psychosocial and musculoskeletal problems.

Although the occurrence of WRMSDs is generally considered multifactorial, past research has focused mainly on physical load. More recent research, however, has included an examination of the relationship between psychosocial factors and WRMSDs. For example, in the Netherlands these health problems (i.e., psychologic dysfunction and musculoskeletal problems) are the main causes of disability in two thirds of occupation-related disability cases.[15] Despite this research, no consensus has been reached regarding the definition of psychosocial factors and how such factors relate to WRMSDs.[36,39]

PSYCHOSOCIAL RISK FACTORS

Several definitions of psychosocial factors have been proposed. Most definitions suggest that psychosocial factors depend on workers' perceptions, a point emphasized by Hagberg and colleagues: "Psychosocial factors at work describe how the work organization is perceived by workers and managers; work organization is the objective nature of the work process and it deals with the way in which work is structured and processed" (p. 11).[10]

NIOSH defines *psychosocial factors* as a general term that identifies many variables that can be roughly divided into three categories: factors associated with the work environment, factors associated with the extra-work environment, and individual characteristics of the worker.[36] The assumption is that conflicts in one of these areas precipitate a process of mental stress that affects the worker's physical health. The psychosocial risk factors in each category are detailed in the following sections.

Work Environment

Psychosocial work environment (or work organization) risk factors include the following: (1) characteristics of the job (e.g., workload, job control, repetition and monotonous tasks, mental and cognitive demands, clear job definitions), (2) organizational structure (e.g., communication issues), (3) interpersonal relationships at work (e.g., relationships with employer, supervisor, co-workers), (4) temporal aspects of work (e.g., shift work, cycle time of tasks), (5) financial and economic aspects (e.g., salary, benefits), and (6) community aspects of occupation (e.g., prestige, status).

Extra-Work Environment

Extra-work environment includes factors that come from outside the work. These include psychosocial factors that relate to the worker's other life-roles, such as responsibilities and function with the family.

Individual Worker Characteristics

Individual worker characteristics include the genetic factors (e.g., anthropometric characteristics, gender, intelligence), acquired aspects (e.g., social class, culture, educational factors), and disposition (e.g., personality, characteristic traits, attitudes toward life and work). Disposition often

affects the way workers perceive or react to the same work situation.[17]

In contrast to NIOSH, the World Health Organization and ILO[35], in a joint report, organized work-related psychosocial factors into five categories: the physical environment; factors intrinsic to the job (e.g., workload, work design); arrangement of work time (e.g., hours of work, shifts); management or operating practices (e.g., roles of the worker, relationships at work); and technologic changes. This definition is similar to the NIOSH description but does not identify individual worker differences or extra-work environments.

PSYCHOSOCIAL FACTORS AND WORK-RELATED MUSCULOSKELETAL DISORDERS

NIOSH examined the research and literature related to all aspects of psychosocial risk factors and reported that there is evidence for five psychosocial factors potentially related to WRMSDs (mainly in areas of the back and upper extremity disorders).[36] These variables are job satisfaction, intensified workload, monotonous work, job control, and social support. NIOSH reports stronger support for the relationship between these psychosocial factors and WRMSDs in the back, neck, and shoulder area than in the hand and wrist area.[36] This may be because a larger number of studies concentrated on the back, neck, and shoulder area rather than on the hand and wrist area or because most studies done on the hand and wrist area did not consider psychosocial variables. Studies examining these relationships are reviewed in Table 8-1.

Job Satisfaction

Low levels of job satisfaction may be associated with high levels of upper extremity musculoskeletal symptoms.[14,47] Several researchers have reported that low levels of job satisfaction correspond to the development and duration of musculoskeletal symptoms, although these results did not hold true in a longitudinal study with Finnish workers in which job satisfaction did not predict neck and shoulder symptoms in a follow-up 1 year later.[7,13,49] Hughes and colleagues[16] reported low job satisfaction (and decision latitude) to be important

TABLE 8-1   Psychosocial Factors Associated with Upper Extremity and Back Musculoskeletal Disabilities

Study (Year)	Occupational Population	Control Used	Body Area Studied	Job Satisfaction	Workload	Monotonous Work	Job Control	Social Support
Ahlberg-Hulten (1995)	Health care workers (female)	Longitudinal (study of same group)	Back				+ (with high demands)	+
Bernard et al (1992, 1994)	Newspaper workers	None	Upper extremity		+		+ (for data-entry workers)	+
Bigos et al (1991)	Aircraft plant workers	History of back injury	Back	+			+	+
Bongers et al (1994)		Longitudinal	Back	+	+			
Hales et al (1994)	Telecommunications workers	Extra-job factors	Upper extremity		+		+	+
Head et al (2006)	Civil service employees	Longitudinal (study of same group)	Sickness absence		+		+	+
Himmelstein et al (1995)	General population		Upper extremity	+			+	+
Hopkins (1990)	Keyboard clerks		Upper extremity	+		+	+	+
Houtman et al (1994)	General population	Physical stressors	Back, upper extremity		+*	+*†	+*†	
Hughes et al (1997)	Aluminum smelter workers		Back	+				
Jensen et al (2002)	Computer workers	Repetitive movements and time of work at the computers	Neck, hand, and wrist MSD symptoms		+			
Johansson (1995)	Home care workers		Upper extremity				+ (with physical load)	

Study	Population/occupation	Study design/exposure	Outcome						
Kaila-Kangas et al (2004)	Cohort of metal industry	Longitudinal data	Back				+	+	
Karasek et al (1987)	White collar workers		Upper extremity		+		+	+	
Leino and Hanninen (1995)	Factory workers (blue and white collar)	Physical load			+			+	
Linton (1990)	General population								
Nielson et al (2004)	Pharmaceutical, municipality, services	Two-year longitudinal study (of same group), physical load	Sickness absence			+	+	+	
Ostergren et al (2005)	General population	Cohort study with 1-year follow up	Shoulder and neck		+ (in women)		+ (in women)		
Svensson and Anderson (1983)	Health care workers	Physical load, life and job satisfaction	Back		+				
Thorell et al (1991)	Six different occupational groups	Physical load	Upper extremity		+		+		
Tola et al (1988)	Mechanics, carpenters, office workers	Upper extremity		+					
Toomingas et al (1997)	Furniture movers, general workers		Upper extremity		+ (with mental load)			+	
Viikari-Juntura et al (1991)	General population	Longitudinal	Upper extremity		+				+ (women)

MSD, Musculoskeletal disorder.
*Upper extremity.
†Back.

predictors of increased back pain in heavy-industry workers. The variation in results may be a result of population differences. Going back to our case study, Sara is an educated woman who found herself in a job that appears to be not up to her cognitive skills; does this factor play a role in her symptoms?

Intensified Workload

Intensified workload is most consistently associated with WRMSDs and is usually measured by perceived time pressure, workload (and workload variability), and work pressure.[2,7,11,46] Houtman and colleagues[15] reported that a fast pace of work had a significant relationship to WRMSDs and primarily caused back symptoms, even when data were adjusted for the degree of physical load. A study that controlled for physical load found an association between workload and upper back and limb symptoms.[29] Others have found that increased workload (time pressure and greater time at a computer) was related to symptoms in the neck, shoulder, hand, and wrist.[3,4,19,38]

To help distinguish among various elements of workload, Lindstrom[30] identified two types: *quantitative workload* (large amount of work, long hours, or haste at work) and *qualitative workload* (tasks too simple or too difficult). Both types affect workers' health negatively but through different mechanisms. Quantitative workload affects biomechanical factors and stress, whereas qualitative workload affects mental overload and thus overall physical well-being. Similarly, Toomingas and colleagues[48] differentiated physical workload from mental workload. They discovered that high mental demand was related to general musculoskeletal sensitivity, especially in the neck and low back.

Think about Sara's work. It is basically defined as quantitative: "Take as many ads as you can." However, as Sara commented, she mostly deals with bereaved individuals and has to be strict with them. This approach appears to go against her personality; she takes her customers' situations to heart. This means her therapist and employer need to take into account the qualitative elements that affect Sara.

Monotonous Work

Monotonous work is associated with neck symptoms and low back pain.[14,15,31,44] Some theorize that the rate of detection of symptoms is higher in "less-interesting" jobs because boring work fails to distract attention from symptoms.[39]

Job Control

Job control, one of the most consistently researched psychosocial factors, is frequently linked to musculoskeletal symptoms.[11,44,46] Bernard and colleagues[4] speculated that the introduction of computers caused a lack of control over specific aspects of work, reduction of task diversity, and increased isolation. These psychosocial factors were more important predictors of hand and wrist symptoms in newspaper departments with a high concentration of data-entry workers (thought to have low-control jobs) compared with editorial workers (thought to have jobs involving more decision making and varied tasks). Ahlberg-Hulten and colleagues[1] reported that lower back symptoms are associated with lack of job control and the presence of extremely demanding work, whereas upper back symptoms appear to be associated with emotional and interpersonal factors. A longitudinal study of the role of psychosocial factors on neck and shoulder and low back pain among Finnish men and women reported that a poor sense of job control was associated with neck and shoulder pain and that fewer years of education corresponded with low back pain.[49] In an investigation of home care workers, decreased job control combined with high physical workload increased the prevalence of musculoskeletal symptoms in the neck and shoulders.[20] A more recent study also found low job control to be one of the main factors to be associated with hospitalization resulting from back disorders other than intervertebral disk disorders.[21]

Another way of examining the effect of job control on workers is to look at the time they are absent from work. One of the more recent studies investigated the impact of job control on absence from work and reported that high levels of decision authority predicted low absence rates.[34] In reference to our case study of Sara, this risk factor is obviously the greatest.

As can be seen from the review, job control has been linked to musculoskeletal symptoms, but the locations of injuries have varied from study to study. In addition, major methodologic differences exist among studies (e.g., differences in the populations studied and definitions of job control). Individual factors, such as gender or education, may affect psychosocial factors and physical symptoms, making definitive conclusions difficult.

Social Support

Social support from co-workers or supervisors has been studied in a variety of populations with fairly consistent results. Perception of poor social support is associated with increased reports of symptoms, although the direction of this relationship is unclear. Himmelstein and colleagues[13] differentiated individuals who worked with WRMSDs from those who did not by noting that the individuals who did not work because of WRMSDs expressed more anger toward their employers (although both groups had a similar perception of the work environment). In a rare longitudinal study, Bongers and colleagues reported that high physical demands combined with poor social support increased symptoms.[7] Feuerstein reported that decreases in co-worker cohesion correlated with higher pain ratings (but not with distress).[9] Other research supports the theory that decreased social support from co-workers and supervisors correlates with increased musculoskeletal symptoms in the upper extremities (neck and shoulder area, wrist and hand area) in a variety of occupations (e.g., furniture movers, secretaries)[3,4,11,14,48] and is a cause for sickness absence from work.[12,32]

Despite these fairly consistent results, several studies have not found an association between social support and symptoms such as the neck and shoulder pain or general musculoskeletal aches.[23,46] In addition, the relationship between social support and symptoms is unclear; perhaps symptoms lead to decreased social support. Bigos and colleagues[5] and Leino and Hanninen[29] have attempted to clarify this relationship. Both groups reported that dissatisfaction with social relationships at work predicted the report of musculoskeletal symptoms.

THEORIES EXPLAINING THE RELATIONSHIP BETWEEN PSYCHOSOCIAL FACTORS AND WORK-RELATED MUSCULOSKELETAL DISORDERS

Several theories attempt to explain the influence of psychosocial factors on the development of musculoskeletal symptoms. Most of these theories assume that psychosocial factors help cause symptoms, although some suggest other relationships. Four main theories are reviewed in this section.

One of the most popular explanations suggests that psychosocial factors increase muscle tension and exacerbate existing biomechanical strain on the musculoskeletal system through increased mental stress.[4,36,50] In one study, increased electromyographic activity was recorded from the muscles of the neck (trapezius) and the erector spine muscles during mentally stressful activities.[48] Electromyographic activity increased with ergonomic loads and increased further when psychologic loads were added, which supports the theory of increased muscular tension resulting from mental stress. Absence of relaxation mediates the effects of poor psychosocial work conditions.[33] Bongers and colleagues[7] suggest that psychosocial factors directly influence mechanical loads through changes in posture caused by stress. For example, people tend to change posture when pressured by deadlines (e.g., hunched trunk, elevated shoulders). In addition, stress originating from the combination of few variables, such as poor job control or poor social support joined with a poor capacity to cope, may increase muscle tone and, in the long run, lead to musculoskeletal disorders. Theorell and colleagues demonstrated that increased mental demands are associated with increased worry, fatigue, and difficulty sleeping.[45] These symptoms correspond with behavior that increases muscle tension, which is associated with back, shoulder, and neck discomfort.

Sauter and Swanson[39] suggest an ecologic model describing a pathway leading from work organization to musculoskeletal outcome in office workers. The pathways included in this model are based on research with a specific population (computer workers). The model identifies a direct path between work technology (tools and work system) and both physical demands (including ergonomics) and work organization. A direct path also exists between physical demands and work organization, suggesting that physical demands are exacerbated by organizational demands (i.e., increased job specification increases repetition). Another path identified in the model exists between work organization and psychosocial strain (i.e., stress). This path is suggested to affect musculoskeletal outcomes in two ways. First, stress increases muscle tension and autonomic processes and adds to the biomechanical strain that already exists. Second, cognitive processes mediate the relationship between biomechanical strain and musculoskeletal symptoms (i.e., the process of detecting and interpreting symptoms can further influence stress at work). Stress-related arousal may increase sensitivity to normal musculoskeletal sensation; the worker becomes aware of any small sensation that in other situations would be suppressed. Workers involved in stressful work conditions may also attribute normal musculoskeletal sensation to work conditions and believe such sensations to be a sign of injury and illness. Musculoskeletal disorder is influenced by environmental forces that include medical, societal, and cultural factors; legal and compensation systems; and workplace relationships. The cognitive-perceptual process may lead to interpretation of discomfort as an underlying injury and may develop into sickness and lead to disability.

The demand-control-support model[22,24] provides another view for identifying the relationship between psychosocial factors and WRMSDs and is a widely accepted model for work-related stress. According to this model, psychologic demands have adverse affects on a worker if they occur jointly with low decision latitude. Low decision latitude is identified by the absence of authority to decide what to do and how to do it and by the lack of intellectual discretion (i.e., the opportunity to use and develop skills at work). The social support component in this model is the support available in the workplace that is thought to mediate between the demands and the appearance of symptoms. Research on this model supports the assumption that these components are relevant to the development of musculoskeletal disorders.[46]

Research examining this model showed that these factors are significant at work, but their association with specific physical complaints is mixed. Kopek and Sayre[26] used longitudinal data from a national survey in Canada and found that high psychologic demands and low skill discretion were independently associated with pain and discomfort but not in diagnosed back pain. They concluded that work-related stress is a significant risk factor for nonspecific complaints of pain or discomfort among workers. Ostergren and colleagues[38] assessed the impact of mechanical exposure and the work related psychosocial factors on specific pain, in the neck and shoulder. They found that high psychologic demands and low job decision latitude correlated with increased risk for developing neck and shoulder pain, although it was true for women and not for men even after controlling for high mechanical exposure and sociodemographic factors.

Another model on which more recent research is based is Siegrist's Effort-Reward Imbalance model.[40,41] This model rests on the hypothesis that a combination of high level of effort expended and little reward received (money and career opportunities) have pathologic effects on health.

METHODOLOGIC PROBLEMS

Interpretation of the research is complicated by the different designs used, populations studied, and type of psychosocial factors and WRMSDs examined. Several methodologic problems are included here to clarify research techniques. Most of the research examining the relationships between psychosocial risk factors and WRMSDs use cross-sectional designs, making causality impossible to determine.[7,13] Few studies have considered the confounding effect of physical stressors (static load and repetitive work) when assessing the relationships between psychosocial risk factors and WRMSDs.[7,15,39] An exception is the study by Theorell and colleagues,[46] who did control for physical stressors when assessing factors such as social support. NIOSH notes that changes in physical and biomechanical demands frequently occur simultaneously with changes in psychosocial demands, making it difficult to delineate the causal relationships between them.[36]

Another problem arises from the tools used to measure psychosocial factors. Psychosocial factors are difficult to measure with objective measurements and are usually subjective, assessed through surveys or self-report techniques. Cognitive theorists suggest that the individual is a filter through which the environment is observed; for instance, Lazarus[28] emphasizes the cognitive and affective functions of the individual identifying work demands. Thus determining whether risk factors are colored by one's perception or are reflective of the "true" situation is difficult.

Although many studies found the relationships to be significant, the strength of these relationships is modest.[36,39] This prevents definitive conclusions or solutions when creating and using programs for workers suffering from WRMSDs. Sauter and Swanson[39] suggested ways to improve research by (1) developing longitudinal studies, (2) improving the tools used to assess health and psychosocial factors, (3) improving analytic methods to separate the effects of the psychosocial factors, and (4) examining the suggested pathways and explaining the relationships. Siegrist suggests analyzing combined models of stress and its effect on work and moving beyond a single assessment of occupational exposure to study its dynamics over time.[42]

ASSESSMENT: THE OCCUPATIONAL STRESS INVENTORY

The occupational stress inventory (OSI) was designed to measure occupational stressors and to provide measures for the theoretical model linking work-related stress with the psychological strains experienced by the worker.[37] It also aims at identifying coping resources available to the worker to deal with the stressors and the psychologic strain. The OSI measures three dimensions in occupational adjustment: occupational stress, psychologic strain, and coping resources.

Occupational Stress

Occupational stress is measured with six scales of the occupational roles questionnaire that include

role overload (how much job demands exceed resources and whether the worker can accomplish the expected workloads); *role insufficiency* (appropriateness of the worker's training, education, skills, and experience to job requirements); *role ambiguity* (the level of the worker's understanding of the expectations and evaluation criteria); *role boundary* (the extent to which the worker experiences conflicts in role demands or loyalties); *responsibility* (the amount of responsibility perceived by or given to the worker to ensure the performance and welfare of others on the job); and *physical environment* (the frequency with which the worker is exposed to extreme conditions [e.g., high levels of environmental toxins]).

Psychologic Strain

Psychologic strain is measured with four scales of the personal strain questionnaire that include *vocational strain* (the amount of difficulty the worker is having in work quality or output); *psychologic strain* (the effect of any emotional problems); *interpersonal strain* (the amount of disruption in interpersonal relationships); and *physical strain* (physical illness or poor self-care habits).

Coping Resources

Coping resources are measured with four scales of the personal resources questionnaire that include *recreation* (pleasure and relaxation derived from regular recreational activities); *self-care* (the frequency with which the worker engages in personal activities that reduce or alleviate chronic stress); *social support* (the extent to which the individual feels support and help from those around him or her); and *rational and cognitive coping* (how frequently the individual uses cognitive skills to deal with work-related stress).

These three categories indicate the dynamics among work-related stressors, strain experiences, and coping resources.

INTERVENTIONS

Psychosocial factors alone cannot account for disability. Excluding them in the evaluation and prevention processes, however, may inhibit successful intervention. The nature of the psychosocial risk factors and their distribution among workers may suggest the direction and level of intervention (i.e., individual or organizational). Three levels of intervention are used to improve the work environment: prevention that aims at reduction in work constraints; prevention that aims to increase individuals' ability to cope with stress and change; and individual rehabilitation of employees who have already shown consequences of occupational stress.[27] It has been suggested that intervening at the first level of prevention is the most efficient.[6]

Himmelstein and colleagues suggested that early intervention to prevent work disability might benefit from focusing on reducing employer-employee conflicts, improving medical management of pain, and enhancing the ability to cope with residual pain and distress and avoiding unnecessary surgery.[13] Lindstrom describes a research-based model for creating a good work organization based on psychosocial intervention.[30] The need to optimize quantitative workload and qualitative workload is emphasized, and the level of autonomy and freedom at work is maximized because they are thought to decrease stress and hence musculoskeletal symptoms. Improving interpersonal relationships among workers and improving communication between employees and supervisors is encouraged. Coping skills are improved either through mental exercises or increased mastery of work. The organization of the entire workplace is evaluated and altered by occupational health professionals. Workers at risk are provided with support and skills to deal with the work demands through group workshops, new skills-development workshops, and individual support from occupational psychologists.

Other intervention programs use cognitive-behavioral methods, such as relaxation and cognitive restructuring, to provide the worker with coping skills.[8,43] Cognitive strategies include focusing on the source of the stress and paying close attention to its interpretation, examining the attribution style after symptoms and stress occur, and adopting alternative methods for addressing problems. Cognitive-behavioral strategies also help improve pain management by altering cognitive,

behavioral, and affective responses. The techniques used include relaxation (including using biofeedback), activity pacing, cognitive restructuring, and imagery and distraction to deal with pain.[25] These techniques require a clinical psychologist who is able to assess and treat within the framework of cognitive-behavioral therapy.

Lavoie-Tremblay and colleagues[27] implemented a different concept of intervention to improve the psychosocial work environment of health care workers. Based on combined models of Karasek and Siegrist (mentioned previously), they used a five-step program in which the organization and employees were active participants. The first step was getting the organization to commit. The second step was identifying job constraints by using evaluation forms used in the two models and grouping them into known psychosocial factors (the most frequent identified factors were workload and social support). Step 3 involved developing action plans to improve work environment in the areas that were identified as stressful. Step 4 involved implementation of the action plans. Step 5 involved evaluation of the action plans' success and follow-up. The process was not an easy one, and the readers are referred to this paper for more elaboration.[27] However, the importance of this study lies first in its theoretic framework (basing the assessment and implementation on known models) and second in the process itself—mainly the involvement of the employees and management in the program and including a follow-up to assess long-term effect.

Changing the psychosocial environment in the workplace is essential but may be difficult.[27] Think about the newspaper Sara is working for; the company would like both to serve the people who want to place obituaries and to make a profit. How do we create an environment that fits both the employer and the employee? How would you approach the psychosocial factors presented by Sara to help her return to work?

CONCLUSION

The role of psychosocial factors in WRMSDs has received increased attention from researchers and clinicians. However, the field needs standardized instruments to measure psychosocial factors to further cross-study comparisons. In addition, clinical tools should be developed to assess work-related psychosocial factors and treatment outcomes.

Learning Exercise

Overview

This exercise is designed to help you learn to incorporate psychosocial factors into routine ergonomic evaluation and intervention.

Purpose

The purposes of this exercise are to identify risk factors that might affect workers in your workplace and to suggest ways to reduce factors you find to be harmful to various employees.

Exercise

Choose various departments to which you have access. Interview employers and employees from various departments in order to assess the existence of psychosocial risk factors that they view as significant to them. Prioritize which risk factors might be the most influential on the workers' health. Think about possible solutions that may be applicable (and acceptable) in this place. Do a follow-up visit to reassess both the risk factors and how the employees view the risk factors and solutions.

Multiple Choice Review Questions

1. The difference between the NIOSH and the ILO definitions of work-related factors is that:
   A. ILO includes the physical and ergonomics environment.
   B. NIOSH includes extra-work factors and ILO does not.
   C. NIOSH includes organizational factors and ILO does not.
   D. Both A and B

2. The psychosocial factor most consistent with WRMSD is:
   A. social support.
   B. job satisfaction and job control.
   C. social support, workload, and job control.
   D. monotony at work.

3. What is the most common explanation for the relationship between psychosocial factors and WRMSDs?
   A. Physical demands increase the biomechanical stress on muscles, leading to WRMSDs.
   B. Cognitive processes cause musculoskeletal symptoms to be magnified.
   C. Psychosocial factors increase mental stress, which in turn increases muscle tension that exacerbates existing biomechanical strain on the musculoskeletal system.
   D. Work organization affects social support.

4. Why is it difficult to find a causal relationship between psychosocial factors and WRMSDs?
   A. Most studies use a cross-sectional design, making it difficult to determine causality.
   B. Changes in physical and biomechanical demands frequently occur together with changes in psychosocial demands, making it difficult to determine causality.
   C. Both A and B
   D. Not enough research exists to determine causality.

For questions 5 to 10, look at the case study. Would the following approaches help Sara get back to work?

5. To get Sara back to work, her employer should provide her with incentives such as bonuses, etc.
   A. True
   B. False

6. Her employer should assess with Sara the areas that she feels hinder her productive work and set priorities and an action plan.
A. True
B. False

7. Her employer should advise Sara to take a relaxation technique course so she can practice during and after work.
A. True
B. False

8. Her employer should provide the employees in Sara's department opportunities to socialize, such as special days out, lunchtime, etc.
A. True
B. False

9. Her employer should provide the employees with seminars aimed at stress management.
A. True
B. False

10. Sara's condition stems from work overload only.
A. True
B. False

REFERENCES

1. Ahlberg-Hulten GK, Theorell T, Sigala F: Social support, job strain and musculoskeletal pain among female health care personnel, *Scand J Work Environ Health* 21:435, 1995.
2. Bernard B, Sauter S, Fine L: *Hazard evaluation and technical assistance report.* NIOSH Report No. HHE 90-013-2277, Cincinnati, 1993, U.S. Department of Health and Human Services, Public Health Service, Centers for Disease Control and Prevention, National Institute for Occupational Safety and Health.
3. Bernard B, Sauter S, Fine L et al: Job task and psychosocial risk factors for work-related musculoskeletal disorders among newspaper employees, *Scand J Work Environ Health* 18(suppl 2):119-120, 1992.
4. Bernard B, Sauter S, Fine L et al: Job task and psychosocial risk factors for work-related musculoskeletal disorders among newspaper employees, *Scand J Work Environ Health* 20:417, 1994.
5. Bigos SJ, Battie MC, Spengler DM et al: A prospective study of work perceptions and psychosocial factors affecting the report of back injury, *Spine* 16:1, 1991.
6. Bond F, Bunce D: Job control mediates change in a work reorganization intervention for stress reduction, *J Occup Health Psychol* 6:290, 2001.
7. Bongers PM, Winter CR, Kompier MA et al: Psychosocial factors at work and musculoskeletal disease, *Scand J Work Environ Health* 19:297, 1993.
8. Feuerstein M: Workstyle: definition, empirical support, and implications for prevention, evaluation, and rehabilitation of occupational upper-extremity disorders. In SD Moon, SL Sauter, editors: *Beyond biomechanics: psychosocial aspects of musculoskeletal disorders in office work,* Bristol, Penn, 1996, Taylor & Francis.
9. Feuerstein M, Sult SC, Houle M: Environmental stressors and low back pain: life events, family, and work environment, *Pain* 22:295, 1985.
10. Hagberg M, Silverstein B, Wells R et al, editors: *Work related musculoskeletal disorders (WMSDs): a reference book for prevention,* London, 1995, Taylor & Francis.
11. Hales TR, Sauter SL, Peterson MR et al: Musculoskeletal disorders among video display terminal users in a telecommunications company, *Ergonomics* 37:1603, 1994.
12. Head J, Kivimaki M, Martikainen P et al: Influence of change in psychosocial work characteristics on sickness absence: the Whitehall II study, *J Epidemiol Community Health* 60:55, 2006.
13. Himmelstein JS, Feurstein M, Stanek EJ et al: Work-related upper-extremity disorders and work disability: clinical and psychosocial presentation, *J Occup Environ Med* 37:1278, 1995.
14. Hopkins A: Stress, the quality of work, and repetitive strain injury in Australia, *Work Stress* 4:129, 1990.
15. Houtman IL, Bongers PM, Smulders PG et al: Psychosocial stressors at work and musculoskeletal problems, *Scand J Work Environ Health* 20:139, 1994.
16. Hughes RE, Silverstein BA, Evanoff BA: Risk factors for work-related musculoskeletal disorders in an aluminum smelter, *Am J Ind Med* 32:66, 1997.
17. Hurrell JJ, Murphy LR: Psychological job stress. In Rom WN, editor: *Environmental and occupational medicine,* ed 2, New York, 1992, Little, Brown.
18. International Labor Office (ILO): *Psychosocial factors at work: recognition and control,* Geneva, 1986 ILO.
19. Jensen C, Ryholt CY, Burr H et al: Work-related psychosocial, physical and individual factors associ-

ated with musculoskeletal symptoms in computer users, *Work Stress* 16:107, 2002.

20. Johansson JA: Psychosocial work factors, physical workload and associated musculoskeletal symptoms among home care workers, *Scand J Psychol* 36:113, 1995.

21. Kaila-Kangas L, Kivimaki M, Riihimaki H et al: Psychosocial factors at work as predictors of hospitalization for back disorders, *Spine* 29:1823, 2004.

22. Karasek RA: Job demands, job decision latitude, and mental strain: implications for job redesign, *Adm Sci Q* 24:285, 1979.

23. Karasek RA, Gardell B, Lindell J: Work and non-work correlates of illness and behavior in male and female Swedish white collar workers, *J Occup Behav* 8:187, 1987.

24. Karasek RA, Theorell T: *Healthy work,* New York, 1990, Basic Books.

25. Keefe FJ, Egert JR: A cognitive-behavioral perspective on pain in cumulative trauma disorders. In SD Moon, SL Sauter, editors: *Beyond biomechanics: psychosocial aspects of musculoskeletal disorders in office work,* Bristol, Penn, 1996, Taylor & Francis.

26. Kopek JA, Sayre EC: Work-related psychosocial factors and chronic pain: a prospective cohort study in Canadian workers, *J Occup Environ Med* 46:1263, 2004.

27. Lavoie-Tremblay M, Bourbonnais R, Viens C et al: Improving the psychosocial work environment, *J Adv Nurs* 49:655, 2005.

28. Lazarus RS: Psychological stress and adaptation and illness, *Int J Psychol Med* 8:225, 1974.

29. Leino PI, Hanninen V: Psychosocial factors at work in relation to back and limb disorder, *Scand J Work Environ Health* 21:134, 1995.

30. Lindstrom K: Psychosocial criteria for good work organization, *Scand J Work Environ Health* 20:123, 1994.

31. Linton SJ: Risk factors for neck and back pain in a working population in Sweden, *Work Stress* 4:41, 1990.

32. Lund T, Labriola M, Christensen KB et al: Psychosocial work environment exposures as risk factors for long-term sickness absence among Danish employees: results from DWECS/DREAM, *J Occup Environmental Med* 47:1141, 2005.

33. Lundberg U, Kadefors R, Melin B et al: Stress, muscular tension and musculoskeletal disorders, *Int J Behav Med* 1:354, 1994.

34. Nielsen ML, Rugulies R, Christensen KB et al: Impact of the psychosocial work environment on registered absence from work: a two-year longitudinal study using the IPAW cohort, *Work Stress* 18:323, 2004.

35. NIOSH: *Proposed national strategy for the prevention of musculoskeletal injuries,* Washington, DC, 1986, U.S. Department of Health and Human Services.

36. National Institute for Occupational Safety and Health (NIOSH): *Musculoskeletal disorders and workplace factors,* Washington, DC, 1997, U.S. Department of Health and Human Services, Public Health Service, Centers for Disease Control and Prevention, NIOSH.

37. Osipow SH, Spokane AR: *Manual for the occupational stress inventory,* Odessa, Fla, 1987, Psychological Assessment Resources.

38. Ostergren P-O, Hanson BS, Balogh I et al: Incidence of shoulder and neck pain in a working population: effect modification between mechanical and psychosocial exposures at work? Results from a one year follow up of the Malemo shoulder and neck study cohort, *J Epidemiol Community Health* 59:721, 2005.

39. Sauter SL, Swanson NG: An ecological model of musculoskeletal disorders in office work. In SD Moon, SL Sauter, editors: *Beyond biomechanics: psychosocial aspects of musculoskeletal disorders in office work,* Bristol, Penn, 1996, Taylor & Francis.

40. Siegrist J: Adverse health effects of high-effort/low-reward conditions, *J Occup Psychol* 1:27, 1996.

41. Siegrist J: Reducing social inequalities in health: work-related strategies, *Scand J Public Health* 30:49, 2002.

42. Siegrist J: Psychosocial work environment and health: new evidence, *J Epidemiol Community Health* 59:888, 2004.

43. Spence SH: Cognitive behavior therapy in the treatment of chronic, occupational pain of the upper limbs: a two-year follow-up, *Behav Res Ther* 29:503, 1991.

44. Svensson H, Anderson GBJ: Low-back pain in 40- to 47-year-old men: work history and work environment factors, *Spine* 8:272, 1983.

45. Theorell T: Possible mechanisms behind the relationship between the demand-control-support model and disorders of the locomotor system. In SD Moon, SL Sauter, editors: *Beyond biomechanics: psychosocial aspects of musculoskeletal disorders in office work,* Bristol, Penn, 1996, Taylor & Francis.

46. Theorell T, Harms-Ringdahl K, Ahlberg-Hulten G et al: Psychosocial job factors and symptoms from the locomotor system: a multicausal analysis, *Scand J Rehabil Med* 23:165, 1991.

47. Tola S, Riihimaki H, Videman T et al: Neck and shoulder symptoms among men in machine operating, dynamic physical work and sedentary work, *Scand J Work Environ Health* 14:299, 1988.

48. Toomingas A, Theorell T, Michelsen H et al: Association between self-rated psychosocial work conditions and musculoskeletal symptoms and signs, *Scand J Work Environ Health* 23:130, 1997.

49. Viikari-Juntura E, Vuori J, Silverstein BA et al: Lifelong prospective study on the role of psychosocial factors in neck-shoulder and low-back pain, *Spine* 16:1056, 1991.

50. Waersted M, Bjorklund RA, Westgaard RH: Shoulder muscle tension induced by two VDU-based tasks of different complexity, *Ergonomics* 34:137, 1991.

9

Physical Environment

Sandi J. Spaulding

Learning Objectives

After reading this chapter and completing the exercises, the reader should be able to do the following:

1. Discuss issues in the physical environment that can have an impact on work performance.
2. Understand the components of the physical environment that are inherent in workplaces.
3. List methods to ameliorate problems in the physical environment.

Lighting. "Light is a wave, similar to a wave on the surface of the ocean. The quantity that characterizes the color is the wavelength, or the distance between adjacent crests of the wave. For red light this distance is about twice as great as for violet light . . . a light wave can travel through empty space, as it does between the sun and the earth."[1] Light seems to have a wave structure, and it appears to have discrete components because of the manner in which it stimulates visual receptors.[3]

Sound. Sound consists of waveforms, either simple or complex, that are heard by a person or are recorded with a microphone that picks the sound waves out of the air.

Vibration. Vibration is a motion that repeats over and over. Vibration can vary both in size (amplitude) and in how often it repeats (frequency). A hand tremor in a person who has Parkinson's disease occurs at a low frequency of about 8 cycles per second, and the individual cycles can usually be seen by someone watching. A vibration from equipment can occur at a much higher frequency and, although the overall movement can sometimes be seen, it is often occurring so quickly that is impossible to see individual movements up and down.

CASE STUDY

Mark du Toit owns a large landscaping business. He works outside using equipment such as forklifts (Figure 9-1, *A*), jackhammers, bulldozers, excavators (Figure 9-1, *B*) and large trucks. His work consists of removing concrete; digging foundations for large landscaping projects; delivering large loads of gravel, plants, and trees; and doing other types of outdoor work that is contracted to him by homeowners and businesses. To do this work he must use all the equipment he has, as well as employing people in the summer to help him. He works outside approximately 8 to 10 hours a day during the spring, summer, and fall. He lives in a climate in which outside work is not possible during the winter months, so that is usually when he takes his vacation and repairs his equipment.

He has other people working with him and will hire occasional workers if he finds that his work is more than he and his assistants can handle. However, both he and his assistants work very long hours when there is work, which is for about 10 months of the year. Additional help does not preclude him or his permanent employees from using the equipment all day; it simply permits him to meet his deadlines by having more of his equipment in use at one time.

Mr. du Toit has two physical environments. The first environment is the outside environment. In this environment, he is coping with high light conditions and high heat, in the 30° C (86° F) range on sunny days, or he could be working in relatively cool conditions, such as between 5° and 10° C (41° to 50° F) with rain or frost in the early spring and late fall. So the outside physical environment varies greatly for him and depends on the season of the year. The inside of the larger pieces of equipment that he drives is the second environment. Most of his equipment, other than the jackhammer, is equipment in which he sits and operates controls to move and work with heavy materials. The inside of such equipment often can be noisy, can vibrate, and can move around erratically while a person is working. Mr. du Toit is very aware of safety considerations, incorporates many safety features into his equipment, and provides protection against noise by ensuring that there is ear protection equipment in each piece of machinery (Figure 9-2).

Presently, Mr. du Toit does not have any health concerns, but many aspects of his physical environment might lend themselves to someone in his position having difficulties in the future. Some solutions, such as buying appropriate equipment, can make the job less physically demanding for the workers. This chapter addresses some of the components of the physical environment that can present long-term difficulties for workers and that can be controlled through the use of ergonomics.

The physical environment is the context in which an individual works. The person may work outside, as is the case for Mr. du Toit, where natural environmental characteristics affect performance. A worker might be in an indoor environment, in which other issues come into play. For example, equipment that is used or how much and what type of artificial lighting is used to

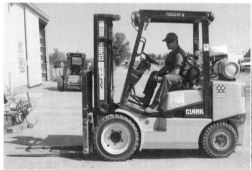
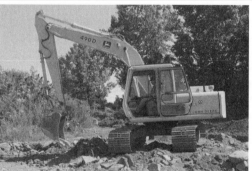

A   **B**

FIGURE **9-1 A,** A front-end loader forklift. **B,** An excavator.

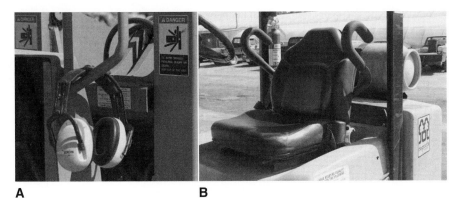

A   **B**

FIGURE 9-2 **A,** Ear protection equipment and danger notices. **B,** Forklift with cushioned seat and fire extinguisher.

replace ambient lighting may be problematic. A third environment in which some workers find themselves is an enclosed machine, such as a front-end loader, a truck, or a backhoe, each of which has its own environmental issues.

Some environmental issues can be the same regardless of whether the worker is outside, inside, or operating machinery. This chapter, rather than being divided into where work occurs, focuses on environmental components including vibration, lighting, sound, and physical characteristics of work and the environment such as friction and load-carriage. Attributes of each environmental feature are discussed, with the differences among environments noted.

VIBRATION

Vibration can be present in an environment either because of equipment that a person is handling, such as a chainsaw, or because it is translated to the person in a "whole body" sense (i.e., vibration that affects the whole body). Whole-body vibration (WBV) occurs often in enclosed-machine environments, such as in the type of equipment that Mr. du Toit uses, unless vibration-reducing design features, such as keeping the seat as separate from the cab as possible, are incorporated.

Concepts of wave patterns are used to describe vibrations. Wave characteristics are used to de-

scribe many environmental characteristics, including both light and sound. To understand any of these environmental features, it is helpful to understand some of the concepts of waveforms. The therapist should refer to a book on signal processing, advanced mathematics, or engineering aspects of waves to gain a more extensive understanding of waves.

A motion that repeats itself is called a *vibration.*[25] Three waveforms are shown in Figure 9-3. The waveforms in Figure 9-3, *A* and *B,* are periodic waveforms that will continue oscillating, with the waveform looking the same. These figures were created from mathematic formulas. The waveform in Figure 9-3, *C,* is a random waveform created with a random number–generation program. Its behavior cannot be determined.

Several definitions are used in the understanding of waves and vibrations:

- *Cycle:* The movement of a body from an undisturbed position, to a maximum position in one direction, through equilibrium, and to the other extreme or minimum position. A pendulum demonstrates a cycle. If a ball on a string is hanging straight down then is pulled to one side and let go, it will go from that position, down through the resting position and up to a maximum level on the other side. It will continue to do this until it is slowed by the pull of gravity and possible

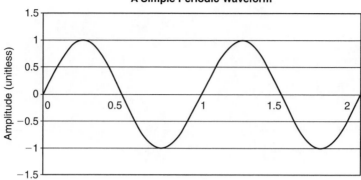

A Simple Periodic Waveform

A

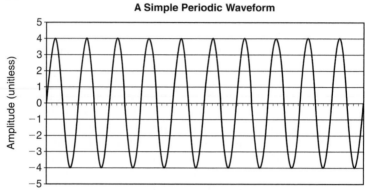

A Simple Periodic Waveform

B

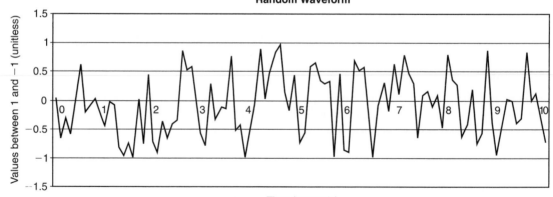

Random Waveform

C

wind resistance. Figure 9-3, *A*, shows two complete cycles of a waveform.

- *Amplitude:* The maximum displacement of the object (in Figure 9-3, *A*, this amplitude is 1, whereas in Figure 9-3, *B*, it is 4).
- *Frequency:* The number of times that an object completes one cycle in a given amount of time. The frequency of the wave in Figure 9-3, *A*, would be 1 cycle per second if the *x* or horizontal axis were in seconds, with one second occurring when the wave crosses zero the second time (or 1 Hertz [Hz]). The frequency of the wave in Figure 9-3, *B* would be 10 cycles per second, or 10 Hz. The frequency of sound vibrations that a healthy, young adult can hear can range up to approximately 20,000 Hz.
- *Resonant frequency:* If the frequency of an object, including tissues in a person, has a natural frequency, and this frequency is the same as an external excitation, then the object or tissues in a person are said to *resonate,* which means that there will be excessive amplitudes present in the object. Harm can occur in a person who is constantly subjected to external physical vibrations in a work environment.
- *Random vibrations:* The value of a signal at any time cannot be predicted (see Figure 9-3, *C*).[25] It is more difficult for people to prepare for a random event than it is for them to stabilize themselves for a predictable, periodic vibration. For example, Mr. du Toit can anticipate the vibration of a machine, despite the fact the vibration can be detrimental to him. Contrarily, it is difficult for him to anticipate random situations, such as driving into a pothole in the road in the spring in a cold climate, especially if that pothole is not easily visible to the driver of the machine.

Vibrations are often present in machines, usually as cyclic physical phenomena. Workers such as Mr. du Toit who come in contact with these vibrating machines will also vibrate. These externally induced vibrations can cause negative repercussions for the worker.[21]

Measurement of Vibrations

Vibration can be measured using biomechanical equipment. For example, an accelerometer (a piece of equipment that measures acceleration), when used with data collection and analysis hardware and software, can determine the amplitude and frequency of vibrations (Figure 9-4). Sources for more information about measuring vibration and obtaining equipment to measure vibration are listed in Box 9-1.

It is not always easy to reduce vibration. Engineers often try to understand the causes of vibration, then design equipment with reduced vibratory amplitude. Solutions for the worker may be difficult to manage; however, it is important, when possible, to have the individual exposed to as few vibratory incidents as possible. Vibrating environments such as a moving vehicle, and particularly, heavy machinery, can cause degenerative changes

---

FIGURE **9-3 A,** A simple periodic waveform that repeats over and over. This type of waveform can represent the vibration of a piece of equipment, such as a jackhammer. **B,** A simple periodic waveform that has a higher frequency because it goes up and down more often in the same length of time as the wave shown in *A*. It also has a larger amplitude, so if it were being used to describe a similar piece of equipment as that shown in *A*, the equipment would be moving up and down more and would be moving more quickly. Mr. du Toit will experience vibration during his work, through his body when he is in the machines and up through his arms when he is using handheld equipment. The amplitude of the vibration will be manifested in how much the equipment moves up and down. The frequency will be shown by how often the equipment moves through the cycle. **C,** With a random waveform the characteristics of the wave are not simple and cannot be described. If a person were driving a car on a dirt road and hit holes in the road randomly, a random waveform could describe the movement of the car and the people bouncing around in it. For Mr. du Toit, this type of vibration may affect him when he is going from job to job or when he is collecting gravel from a site in which the roads are not well maintained.

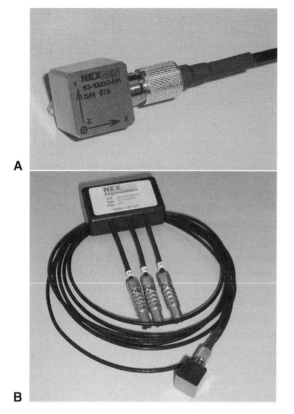

Box 9-1 *Sources for Purchasing Vibration Monitoring Equipment*

Canadian Centre for Occupational Health and Safety—
www.ccohs.ca/oshanswers/phys_agents/vibration/vibration_measure.html
National Instruments—
http://sine.ni.com/nips/cds/view/p/lang/en/nid/12049
NexGen Ergonomics—
http://nexgenergo.com/ergonomics/vats.html
Response Dynamics—
www.responsedynamics.com
Reliability Direct—
www.reliabilitydirect.com/vibrationmeterproducts/vibrationmeterindex.htm

FIGURE 9-4 An accelerometer can determine the amplitude and frequency of vibrations. **A** and **B,** Series 3 accelerometers. (Courtesy NexGen Ergonomics, Inc., Pointe Claire, Quebec.)

to the body.[7] Exposure to WBV may cause a variety of health difficulties.[24,26] WBV exposure varies with type of terrain and with type of load in a vehicle, with the highest magnitudes demonstrated during traveling, suggesting that exposure assessments should include several measurements, taking into consideration the terrain type and adjusting the method of driving a vehicle when it is loaded.[26] Biomechanical models used to simulate the responses of the body[12,13] help in simulating and designing vibration isolators, which can separate the driver from the effect of vibrations. Vibrations measured at levels of the vertebrae in heavy haul truck operators[15] and framesaw operators[9] can exceed International Standard Organization (ISO) standards during operation. However, researchers are beginning to understand the anthropometric characteristics that affect WBV[30] and design seating to reduce WBV,[19] and it is hoped that this knowledge, as it is acquired, will decrease the vibration to which individuals are exposed.

SOUND

Sound is also a combination of either simple or complex waveforms. Sounds are all around us, but when sound is interfering, either because it is unwanted and disrupts concentration or because it is too loud (which would be considered *noise*), it can interfere with a worker's functioning. Factors that affect noise risk include noise level, duration of exposure, frequency of the sound, individual susceptibility, vulnerability resulting from environmental factors, and vulnerability resulting from biologic factors.[20]

Sound is the result of wave activity in the air that reaches a person's ear. Figure 9-3 not only applies to vibration but can be used to describe sound as well. Noise, which could be considered to be a random waveform (Figure 9-3, *C*) is a subset of sound that is either annoying to the

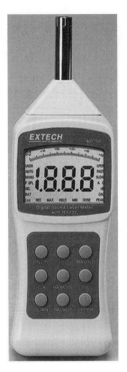

FIGURE **9-5** A sound level meter, used by ergonomists to measure noise. (Courtesy Extech Instruments, Waltham, Mass.)

person and may interfere with performance of tasks or is so loud that it is injurious to a person's hearing.

A person can be negatively influenced by sound in a variety of ways. Sound then can be considered noise. For example, researchers have found that reaction time on a visual display terminal task can be prolonged. The authors suggested that even low-intensity background noise can be associated with impaired performance in spatial attention and can cause an increase in energy consumption.[29] Workers report that concentration was impaired by office noise.[2] Box 9-2 lists some sources for purchasing sound meters (Figure 9-5).

LIGHTING

Lighting can facilitate a worker's sight if it is at the right level but can impede function if it is

either too high or too low.[4] Not only can it impede performance, it can also eventually damage the worker's vision.

Illumination

Lighting in an indoor environment includes both ambient light from the outside (usually visible through windows) and artificial light. The quality and quantity of light can vary in work environments, and it can vary over time of day or time of year.

Measurement

Light can be measured by examining the light reflected off a surface. This type of measurement is used by photographers who use light meters that are within a camera. The second method of measuring light is to examine the light hitting an object, rather than reflecting off it. Measuring the light directed toward a person or an object gives a better estimate of the light source; however, in work situations reflected light can be a major issue. For example, if the worker is working in an indoor environment on an assembly line that conveys shiny metal objects, the worker is affected by the ambient light (light in the environment) as well as the light reflecting off the equipment, thus increasing the amount of light reaching the eyes of the worker. Some of that light might be detrimental, in that it can cause glare. Conversely a person can be working in an environment in which the walls are painted a dark color, which absorbs light rather than reflects it, creating a light environment very different from one that includes

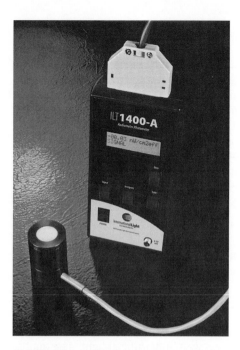

FIGURE 9-6: A light measurement device. (Courtesy International Light Technologies, Peabody, Mass.)

Box 9-3	*Sources for Purchasing Light Meters*
D.A.S. Distribution— www.dasdistribution.com/products/ lm-economical_models.htm International Light Technologies— www.intl-light.com/product/meter Sekonic— www.sekonic.com/main	

reflected light (Figure 9-6). Sources for measurement devices are included in Box 9-3.

Visual difficulties have been reported not only by individuals with poor vision but also by older individuals without visual impairment, suggesting that environments might be designed to take changes in vision throughout the life cycle into account.[23]

Luminance

Researchers suggest that low luminance levels around a computer display should be avoided but that individuals are more comfortable with levels at or a little below that of the central task.[27]

Contrast Sensitivity

Contrast sensitivity is the ability to see differences between different tonalities of surfaces. Contrast sensitivity can be measured using a Pelli-Robson chart, in which letters show increasing similarity to the background and a person will be able to distinguish the letters only to a certain level of sensitivity. There can be very high contrast in the environment. For example, many workshop floors or stairs have stripes on the edges to either denote the boundaries within which the worker can work or to denote a change in surface characteristics. These stripes are usually a very different color from the background. If one were to look at them in terms of contrast only, there would be high contrast so that most people should be able to see them whether or not they have normal color vision.

Studies have been conducted to explore the effect of lighting and medium on a person's function.[28] The results of these authors' work suggests that using either the display medium of a screen or paper does not change memory performance or electroencephalographic response; however, the individuals preferred paper to screen. Individuals also demonstrated better performance under lower contrast ratios. This work suggests that luminance contrast can affect performance. New lighting in a workplace may influence the workers' performance, from visual performance to problem solving. To estimate the influence of lighting change, it may be appropriate to separate the mechanisms affected by the changes.[11]

Mr. du Toit must contend with many different lighting situations. If it is bright outside and he is manipulating levers within one of his pieces of equipment, he may have difficulty distinguishing the levers because of glare. He might be wise to use protective eyewear and give consideration to how much ultraviolet light is entering his equipment through the windows.

STRUCTURAL FEATURES

Structural features of the environment are extremely important and can be designed to lighten the workload and improve performance. If the structure of the environment is not considered, the opposite may occur—the worker may have difficulty, and performance may be degraded.

Ground Characteristics

Ground characteristics such as soil or ground conditions and other working surfaces may influence the safety of a worker.[14,18] The interrelationship between a worker's footwear and the ground is dependent on friction. Friction, both static and dynamic, was discussed in Chapter 6. The reader is referred to that chapter for details about the concepts. Friction could be an issue for Mr. du Toit in terms of the footwear he uses when handling equipment outside. He might also consider whether gloves would be appropriate to use when holding equipment, using levers in the larger pieces of equipment, or turning the steering wheel of his truck.

The issue for the worker is that the friction between the ground and the foot be adequate so that slipping is improbable. However, antislip devices on the bottoms of shoes[8] and tread grooves on shoes[17] may provide a good foothold, safety, and improved balance when a worker walks on slippery surfaces. It has been suggested that focusing on work surfaces may reduce the trips and slips on the worksite.[18]

Equipment Related to Posture (Sitting or Standing)

Workstation height and orientation, when adjusted optimally for the worker, can help both wrist and upper extremity posture.[22] Workplace layout, specifically the path of moving objects to be lifted[6] and the distances they should be lifted,[10] affect kinematics and loads of workers' spines.

Temperature

Temperature surrounds the worker. If the temperature of the environment is out of the safe range for the person and the task that he or she is performing, the body will be under stress. Mr. du Toit must be cognizant of the environment in which he is working, to be sure that it is comfortable for him. Temperatures can be too high or too low. Controlling temperature can be difficult if a person is changing his or her activity level and thus changing how much internal heat is produced. It can also be influenced by movement of machinery that in itself can generate heat.

CHEMICALS AND TOXINS

Some workers may be in situations in which they have to handle chemicals or come into contact with them in their work. Workers may need specialized knowledge to handle chemicals in small quantities. If a person is in physical contact with small doses of acetylsalicylic acid (the active ingredient in aspirin), there may be no specialized knowledge for handling the chemical. However, chemicals can be extremely toxic and capable of causing injury.[16] Toxic chemicals can enter the environment in many ways, including the air, water, soil, or food, and may enter the body by inhalation, ingestion, or skin absorption, be absorbed into the bloodstream, and undergo metabolism or be delivered to organs.[16] Chemicals, depending on their composition, can cause injury because they are toxic when inhaled, cause burns if the person comes in contact with them, can be highly flammable (burn easily), or have a flash point such that they can burn spontaneously under certain conditions. The effects on an individual after toxic chemical exposure can be progressive, permanent, or reversible.[16] The reader is referred to Levy and colleagues[16] for a detailed analysis of chemical toxins, their effects, and methods of dealing with them.

There are specific requirements for handling chemicals safely. The worker must be trained in reading and understanding warning labels on containers or in rooms that hold chemicals. People must be protected from toxic chemicals. This protection can range from simple precautions, such as wearing protective gloves, to handling chemicals only when totally isolated from them, either through use of protective clothing including a breathing apparatus that brings air from outside a potentially toxic air situation or through working in a highly controlled environment. See the resources listed in Box 9-4 for further understanding of toxic chemical issues.

ALLERGIES

Some workers have allergies to aspects of their working environment. Glove use has increased in the health care professions to protect the professionals from diseases such as acquired immunodeficiency syndrome (AIDS). One of the allergies that has become a problem for many individuals, often related to glove use, is an allergy to latex.[5] Latex-related symptoms include a localized contact urticaria (a localized flare reaction after contact between a substance and the skin or mucous membranes) to asthma and anaphylaxis.[5] Individuals can be advised to avoid natural rubber latex and to recognize and manage allergic reaction. Local symptoms can be dealt with using anitihistamines, but systemic symptoms require major intervention, including rescue medication for anaphylaxis.[5] Obviously, the potential for latex allergies should not be considered lightly. Further reading in the comprehensive text edited by Chowdhury and Maibach[5] would be appropriate for employers and employees who may be consid-

ering the presence and potential impact of latex materials within a worker's environment.

AIR QUALITY

Air quality is a global environmental concern. Air quality can be more specifically an issue for workers in particular environments. For example, individuals who were active in coal mining before there was an understanding of the effect of coal dust inhaled into a worker's lungs could have developed a lung disease that may have been fatal. A less devastating example of the effects of poor air quality is exemplified in a poorly ventilated university classroom in which students may feel drowsy but recover quickly after leaving the room.

Air pollution can be present either in the ambient environment or in an indoor environment. Ambient air pollutants are thought to be derived mainly from fuel combustion and include many different pollutants. Progress to control air pollution must be made at a societal level. For example, the United States' Clean Air Act of 1970 mandated that the government develop air-quality standards.[16] Adverse health effects of exposure to such pollutants can include excess cardiorespiratory mortality, asthma, increased respiratory difficulties, decreased lung function, and reduced immune function.[16] It appears, then, that it would be appropriate to keep workers away from ambient air pollution wherever possible.

It is possible that indoor air quality can be better controlled by the employer and/or building designer. Many people work indoors and may be engaged in many types of jobs, from highly physically active work on a shop floor to sedentary work, such as a job performed while sitting at a desk.

WATER QUALITY

Water quality, like air quality, is a global environmental issue. Very little of the world's water is usable, but it must be available to people for their survival. The quality and availability of water can both be issues that must be specifically addressed for some workers.

Learning Exercises

Overview

The learning exercise is designed to make the student aware of various aspects of a work environment that may affect the worker.

Purpose

The purpose of these exercises is to encourage the student to become a good observer of various environments. Once the student is able to observe the environment, when called on to evaluate an environment he or she will be able to focus on aspects of the environment that are important to the worker.

Exercises

1. Consider your own work environment. Think about each of the concepts discussed in this chapter and see if any of them affect the tasks you do. For example, if you use a computer, what is the ambient light level around you relative to the light emitted by the computer screen? If you are sitting at a desk, are the heights of the chair and the table correct? What sort of ground characteristics do you encounter as you are going to classes? Do you ever find yourself in situations in which friction is less than desirable?

2. Consider Mr. du Toit and his occupations. What aspects of his work environment might you want to consider evaluating?

3. Consider watching someone at a construction site. While you are watching, think about the various environmental characteristics that affect the worker. Consider how, if you were asked to evaluate the environment, you might go about doing so. Can you see anything at the worksite that could be a potential hazard for the worker, either in a brief period of time, or over a long work time? Remember to think about the physical environment, lighting, vibration, and all the other concepts considered here. Are there other aspects of the environment that you notice that have not been discussed in this chapter but that may have an impact on the worker? Compare your observations with those of other people who are doing the same observations in a different setting. Are there differences in the environments that will affect the worker? Compare protective equipment that you saw in use, and also surmise from your observations other types of protection, such as vibration-damping techniques that may be being used but that would be difficult for you to see.

Multiple Choice Review Questions

1. The following issue will probably be a problem for someone trying to concentrate in a crowded room full of computer users:
   A. Vibration
   B. Noise
   C. Friction
   D. Lighting

2. If Mr. du Toit reports that he is experiencing difficulty feeling objects with his index fingertip and has a feeling of tingling, you might suspect that the following is the most likely environmental cause of his problem:
   A. The truck he drives does not have enough heat during the colder days.
   B. The equipment he is using is going over rough roads.
   C. The jackhammer he is using is causing a sinusoidal vibration.
   D. The weight of the levers in his front-end loader is excessive.

3. If a student is setting up a workstation for his or her computer and asks you to help make the environment as comfortable as possible, you will focus much of your attention on:
   A. the noise level that is created by the student listening to music while working.
   B. the vibration that is being caused by the constant motion of the internal hard drive of the computer.
   C. the lighting of the room in relation to the ambient outdoor lighting.
   D. the height of the chair and desk, relative to the student.

4. Mr. du Toit wants to upgrade his heavy machinery, specifically his front-end loader, which is used to dig and move dirt. He asks you for some of the specific features that might be ergonomically appropriate to improve his working environment. The one issue you might focus most highly on could be:
   A. the damping of vibration from the machine to the seat.
   B. the noise in the cab of the machine.
   C. the position of the handles in the equipment.
   D. the temperature control of the cab.

5. Mr. du Toit finds that his eyes are becoming fatigued on the job. You will need to evaluate the lighting situation. Your first approach might be to:
   A. test Mr. du Toit's eyes using a contrast sensitivity chart.
   B. evaluate the glare coming from the ground surrounding his worksite.
   C. consider the time of year he is working.
   D. determine whether the lighting conditions in his equipment are adequate.

6. The floors of the pieces of machinery that Mr. du Toit is using are made of a type of sheet metal that is easy to clean. The issue that could arise because of the floor type is:
   A. contrast sensitivity issues with his vision.
   B. low static friction between the floor and his shoes.
   C. increased lighting in the cab of the equipment.
   D. vibration increase caused by the flexibility of the floor.

7. Light can be measured:
   A. at the source of the light, especially out of doors.
   B. at the object absorbing the light because of black surfaces.
   C. at the object reflecting the light.
   D. at the source with a meter to determine contrast sensitivity.

8. The peak amplitude of a wave is:
   A. the distance between the peaks of the waveform.
   B. the frequency of the waveform.
   C. the distance between the top and the bottom of the waveform.
   D. the highest point on the waveform.

9. The physical environment that is most likely to have a physical impact on Mr. du Toit's health over time is:
   A. the outside environment, because of the temperature fluctuations.
   B. the inside of his equipment, because of the potential for vibration.
   C. the indoor environment, because of the desk work he has to do.
   D. the environment related to the equipment that he has to use with his hands.

10. One of the factors of noise risk is:
    A. duration of noise.
    B. repeated sinusoidal properties of noise.
    C. vulnerability resulting from size of machinery.
    D. random access to the noise.

REFERENCES

1. Atkins KR: *Physics,* ed 2, New York, 1970, John Wiley & Sons.
2. Banbury SP, Berry DC: Office noise and employee concentration: identifying causes of disruption and potential improvements, *Ergonomics* 48(1):25, 2005.
3. Bennett AG, Rabbetts RB: *Clinical visual optics,* ed 2, Boston, 1989, Butterworths.
4. Boyce PR: *Human factors in lighting,* New York, 2003, Taylor & Francis.
5. Chowdhury MMU, Maibach HI: *Latex intolerance: basic science, epidemiology, clinical management,* Boca Raton, 2006, CRC Press.
6. Davis K, Marras W: Load spatial pathway and spine loading: how does lift origin and destination influence low back response? *Ergonomics* 48(8):1031, 2005.
7. Fritz M, Fischer S, Brode P: Vibration induced low back disorders—comparison of the vibration evaluation according to ISO 2631 with a force-related evaluation, *Appl Ergon* 36(4):481, 2005.
8. Gard G, Berggard G: Assessment of anti-slip devices from healthy individuals in different ages walking on slippery surfaces, *Appl Ergon* 37:177, 2006.
9. Goglia V, Grbac I: Whole-body vibration transmitted to the framesaw operator, *Appl Ergon* 36(1):43-48, 2005.
10. Jorgensen MJ, Handa A, Veluswamy P, Bhatt M: The effect of pallet distance on torso kinematics and low back disorder risk, *Ergonomics* 48(8):949, 2005.
11. Juslen H, Tenner A: Mechanisms involved in enhancing human performance by changing the lighting in the industrial workplace, *Int J Ind Ergon* 35(9):843, 2005.
12. Kim IJ, Smith R, Nagata H: Microscopic observations of the progressive wear on shoe surfaces that affect the slip resistance characteristics, *Int J Ind Ergon* 28(1):17, 2001.
13. Kim TH, Kim YT, Yoon YS: Development of a biomechanical model of the human body in a sitting posture with vibration transmissibility in the vertical direction, *Int J Ind Ergon* 35(9):817, 2005.
14. Koningsveld E, van der Grinten M, van der Molen H et al: A system to test the ground surface conditions of construction sites for safe and efficient work without physical strain, *Appl Ergon* 36:441, 2005.
15. Kumar S: Vibration in operating heavy haul trucks in overburden mining, *Appl Ergon* 35(6):509, 2004.
16. Levy BS, Wegman DH, Baron SL et al, editors: *Occupational and environmental health: recognizing and preventing disease and injury,* ed 5, Philadelphia, 2006, Lippincott Williams & Wilkins.
17. Li KW, Chen CJ: The effect of shoe soling tread groove width on the coefficient of friction with different sole materials, floors, and contaminants, *Appl Ergon* 35:499, 2004.
18. Lipscomb HJ, Glazner JE, Bondy J et al: Injuries from slips and trips in construction, *Appl Ergon* 37:267, 2006.
19. Makhsous M, Hendrix R, Crowther Z et al: Reducing whole-body vibration and musculoskeletal injury with a new car seat design, *Ergon* 48(9):1183, 2005.
20. Maltby M: Occupational audiometry: monitoring and protecting hearing at work, London, 2005, Butterworth-Heinemann.
21. Mansfield NJ: *Human response to vibration,* Washington DC, 2005, CRC Press.
22. McGorry RW, Dempsey PG, O'Brien NV: The effect of workstation and task variables on forces applied during simulated meat cutting, *Ergonomics* 47:1640, 2004.
23. McGregor LN, Chaparro A: Visual difficulties reported by low-vision and nonimpaired older adult drivers, *Hum Factors* 47:469, 2005.
24. McPhee B: Ergonomics in mining, *Occup Med (Lond)* 54(5):297, 2004.
25. Rao SS: *Mechanical vibrations,* Upper Saddle River, NJ, 2004, Pearson/Prentice Hall.
26. Rehn B, Lundstrom R, Nilsson L et al: Variation in exposure to whole-body vibration for operators of forwarder vehicles—aspects on measurement strategies and prevention, *Int J Ind Ergon* 35(9):831, 2005.
27. Sheedy JE, Smith R, Hayes J: Visual effects of the luminance surrounding a computer display, *Ergonomics* 48:1114, 2005.
28. Shieh KK, Chen MH, Wang YW: Effects of display medium and luminance contrast on memory performance and EEG response, *Int J Ind Ergon* 35(9):797, 2005.
29. Trimmel M, Poelzl G: Impact of background noise on reaction time and brain DC potential changes of VDT-based spatial attention, *Ergonomics* 49(2):202, 2006.

30. Wang W, Rakheja S, Boileau PE: The role of seat geometry and posture on the mechanical energy absorption characteristics of seated occupants under vertical vibration, *Int J Ind Ergon* 36(2):171, 2006.

SUGGESTED READING

Kroemer K, Kroemer H, Kroemer E: *Ergonomics—how to design for ease and efficiency,* Englewood Cliffs, NJ, 1984, Prentice-Hall.

Putz-Anderson V, editor: *Cumulative trauma disorders—a manual for musculoskeletal diseases of the upper limb,* Bristol, Penn, 1988, Taylor & Francis.

Stanton NA, Salmon P, Walker G et al: *Human factors methods: a practical guide for engineering and design,* Hampshire, England, 2005, Ashgate.

Tochihara Y, Ohnaka T: *The ergonomics of human comfort: health and performance in the thermal environment,* London, 2005, Churchill Livingstone.

10

Human Factors in Medical Rehabilitation Equipment: Product Development and Usability Testing

Valerie J. Berg Rice

Learning Objectives

After reading this chapter and completing the exercises, the reader should be able to do the following:

1. Understand the definition, principles, and use of usability testing for rehabilitation product design.
2. Describe the role of therapists in assisting in usability testing of rehabilitation equipment and products.
3. List basic principles of usability testing and how they contribute to product design.
4. Understand each of the three phases and each of the nine steps suggested for conducting usability evaluations of products.

User-centered design. The process by which a product is designed so that the user is given the most important influence.

Prototype testing. The evaluation of a newly developed trial product by the end-users who represent the target market.

Efficacy testing. A more formal process of performance testing in a controlled setting to determine the effectiveness of the product.

Magnitude estimation. An experimental technique used in psychophysical experiments that involves having a subject compare his or her current sensation with a reference sensation.

CASE STUDY

The New Equipment Company calls you and asks you to help them as they develop a new walker. They have other walkers in their line of products, but they think they can create a new series of walkers specifically designed for various populations. Although they understand many of the basic components of walkers and know about the extra accoutrements that can be attached, they are less certain about how to design walkers that might benefit specific populations, such as those who have experienced a stroke versus those who have cerebral palsy or are elderly (Figure 10-1). They know the basic principle of ergonomics—that is, that products should be designed to fit the individuals who use them—but they don't work with those who might benefit from using a walker on a daily basis. You do, as you work with clients with varying degrees of physical disabilities. What will you, as a consultant, do for this company? Where does your expertise fit in with that of a usability expert (an ergonomist or human factors engineer)? Can you consult with them and do all the testing on your own, or do you need to form a team? Do they have the necessary team members already on their staff? Would they even know who would be needed, or are they looking to you to supply that information? You've received the call. They need help. Where and how do you begin . . . or do you get involved at all?

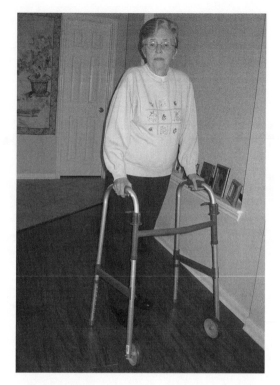

FIGURE **10-1** Different designs of walkers may benefit one population more than another.

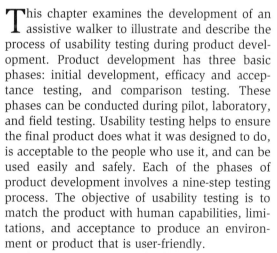

This chapter examines the development of an assistive walker to illustrate and describe the process of usability testing during product development. Product development has three basic phases: initial development, efficacy and acceptance testing, and comparison testing. These phases can be conducted during pilot, laboratory, and field testing. Usability testing helps to ensure the final product does what it was designed to do, is acceptable to the people who use it, and can be used easily and safely. Each of the phases of product development involves a nine-step testing process. The objective of usability testing is to match the product with human capabilities, limitations, and acceptance to produce an environment or product that is user-friendly.

Three groups use medical and rehabilitation equipment: health care personnel, clients, and caregivers. Equipment should be evaluated for effectiveness, ease-of-use, comfort, and acceptability for all three user groups. This process is called *usability testing* (also known as *evaluative testing, development research,* or *operational testing*) (Box 10-1). Introducing changes to a product line is easier during the initial development of the product, with small changes made throughout the development process as required. If necessary, however, usability testing can be implemented during any of the stages of product development, and products can even be retrofitted.[22] Usability testing provides valuable information for equipment design, and knowledge of usability testing can help therapists make recommendations for equipment purchase by their patients. Usability testing that helps provide an appropriate equipment design or work process can help prevent injuries, reduce human error during product use, and increase product sales.

Box 10-1 | *What Is Usability Testing?*

Usability measures the quality of a user's experience when interacting with a product or system—whether a website, a software application, mobile technology, or any user-operated device.

In general, usability refers to how well users can learn and use a product to achieve their goals and how satisfied they are with that process. Usability may also consider such factors as cost-effectiveness and usefulness.

Two international standards further define usability and human-centered design:

- [Usability refers to] the extent to which a product can be used by specified users to achieve specified goals with effectiveness, efficiency and satisfaction in a specified context of user (ISO 9241-11).
- Human-centered design is characterized by the active involvement of users and a clear understanding of user and task requirements; an appropriate allocation of function between users and technology; the iteration of design solutions; multi-disciplinary design (ISO 13407).

From the U.S. Department of Health and Human Services, www.usability.gov.

Box 10-2 | *What Is User-Centered Design?*

User-centered design (UCD) is the structured process for product development that includes users throughout each phase of the design process. In addition, a macroergonomic approach is often used that includes the overall business mission, goals, and culture, as well as the target audiences' preferences, abilities, and requirements.

OVERVIEW

Usability testing is the systematic evaluation of the "interaction between people and the products, equipment, environments, and services they use" and "is the fundamental principle that underpins all ergonomics."[20] Usability testing also has been called *user-acceptance testing, user trials,* and *usability engineering* and is usually conducted by human factors engineers or ergonomists.

Some products are developed by designers or engineers who assume their products are functional, easy to use, and acceptable. This assumption is often based on the designer's own knowledge or on the fact that the designer (and his or her colleagues) can easily use the product. Usability testing makes no such assumptions; it makes the user (within the target audience) the most

important influence on product design. This is referred to as *user-centered design* (Box 10-2).

Usability testing is most well known when used to evaluate the interface between the user and a machine or technology, such as in the computer industry. Examples include evaluating controls and displays on automobile consoles or in aircraft cockpits, designing user-friendly software, and designing human-computer interfaces and websites. However, usability testing also applies to products that are not considered machines, such as workstations.[14] Both complex equipment (e.g., anesthesia monitors and mammography machines) and simple equipment (e.g., walkers and dynamic splints) can benefit from experimental evaluation that concentrates on users.

User testing may or may not be conducted by the equipment manufacturer. However, in an effort to reduce user errors and improve safety, the U.S. Food and Drug Administration (FDA) initiated requirements in 1997 that manufacturers of Class II and III medical devices (and certain Class I devices) adhere to design practices that include addressing the needs of the users. This includes all users—practitioners, clients, clients' caregivers, and even corporate users—if the device might be used by workers in a work setting. Some of the concerns include human-machine interface design, understandability of labeling and instructions, effective operation of the device, and proper storage, maintenance, and calibration. Obviously, this can be accomplished only through human factors evaluations and targeted user testing. The Association of Medical Instrumentation (AAMI)

Human Factors Engineering Guidelines and Preferred Practices for the Design of Medical Devices addresses human factors evaluations, including appropriate steps to user-friendly, error-resistant design and scaling of human factors efforts to the match the device.* The FDA monitors manufacturers though field inspections, product reviews, and postmarket surveillance.[30] In fact, the distinction has been made between clinical trials and targeted usability testing when demonstrating user-effectiveness. During clinical trials, users follow strict protocols. However, during targeted usability testing, all target user groups are included and testing includes understanding of instructions, product use, the potential for product misuse, and use under less-than-optimal conditions.[27] Although human factors engineers or ergonomists may be the lead in such evaluations, health care professionals can contribute substantially as team members during evaluation of medical or rehabilitation equipment.

CONSIDERATIONS

Users of health care equipment have different skills, abilities, knowledge, and requirements[4-6]; they range from physicians, technicians, and rehabilitation specialists to clients and nonprofessional providers, such as friends and family members. Caregivers caring for an older individual (such as spouses) may have impairments themselves. The physical and cognitive characteristics of each user group, along with any symptoms of disease processes, must be considered in the design of the equipment they will use. For example, diabetic retinopathy may impair the ability of a person with diabetes to read the small pen and credit card design displays on blood glucose meters.[5] If the product is to be used internationally, usability evaluations must be conducted in a variety of settings or conditions. In many cases, adequate information about the target population is not available,

especially for special populations such as those with lifelong disabilities.[17] Usability evaluations involving the intended users are crucial in the design of medical and rehabilitation equipment to ensure safety and efficacy.

Usability testing applies equally to the design of procedures, processes, and systems. A macroergonomic systems perspective addresses the entire problem, rather than a small part (see Chapter 3). Standard operating procedures (SOPs) for client treatment written for worst-case scenarios must address issues of comprehension, linear versus multitrack processes, availability of personnel and equipment, levels of employee training, levels of client education, and sometimes even clients' cultural background. For example, if a U.S. rehabilitation facility is located in a region with a significant Hispanic population, emergency SOPs should be printed in both Spanish and English and employees should be able to communicate and understand emergency messages in Spanish. Procedures guiding medical decision making can do much to prevent human error. Considering errors as evidence of the failure of a system rather than the failure of an individual is a more effective alternative in reducing human error,[12] including medically related human errors.[6,19,25]

The context of device use is important,[23] and ecologic validity (how closely the testing environment resembles the actual environment) is a significant consideration during usability testing. For example, if users are expected to operate equipment in adverse conditions, such as providing emergency medical care while on board an aircraft, the design should take into account factors such as lighting, font size and shape on any instructions, and equipment layout. Precision guides might even be considered, in case of turbulence. Inadequate staffing, shift work, double shifts, or using contractors who are unfamiliar with particular devices or SOPs are relatively common and can result in failure to follow proper instructions, inadvertent operation of controls, failure to recognize critical circumstances, poor decision making, or lack of attention.[16] Failsafe designs may have multiple safety features to help avoid improper use of equipment, such as preventing the improper attachment of two pieces of equipment, which

---

*The AAMI guidance document entitled Human Factors Engineering Guidelines and Preferred Practices for the Design of Medical Devices (HE48-1993) as well as Human Factors Design Process for Medical Devices (ANSI/AMI HE74-2001) are available from AAMI at www.aami.org or within the U.S. at 1-800-332-2264, ext. 217.

could occur in emergency (i.e., hurried) situations. Human factors or ergonomic considerations in the design of equipment and processes should be preventive. Demands of equipment setup and adjustment, durability, maintainability, and interaction with other devices should be considered.

Iatrogenic injuries or illnesses are adverse effects resulting from medical procedures or medications that are not a direct or indirect complication of a client's injury or illness.[24] Sometimes, iatrogenic injuries are the result of errors facilitated by inadequate labeling of a device or medication, inherent defects in the design of the device, or improper use of the equipment. Medical equipment associated with user problems and errors ranges from the relatively simple (syringes) to the complex (computer-controlled diagnostic equipment).[13] Well-designed usability testing is important, as the design of the equipment and the instructions for using the equipment may influence the occurrence of errors. Appropriate design may assist in preventing human error. Design interventions can assist with relatively simple "devices" such as home pill dispensers just as well as with complex devices such as anesthesia machines or diagnostic equipment. The proper design of rehabilitation equipment can encourage independence, boost self-esteem, and broaden abilities in activities of daily living.[3] Basic principles of usability testing are shown in Box 10-3.

PROCESS

If therapists decide to take on the task of consulting regarding the development of a new walker (as in the case study mentioned at the beginning of the chapter), they must first become familiar with the equipment. This includes the current design and any prior difficulties with this or similar products. Some of this information can be obtained through the FDA, as the team can request copies of any negative reports regarding the equipment. This requires sufficient lead time to order and read through the reports before beginning testing. Once familiar with the equipment, the purpose of the equipment, the situations and environments in which the equipment would be used, and the target populations, the team can move on to usability testing.

The first step in the usability testing process is to identify subject matter experts (SMEs) and the user population (Figure 10-2, step 1, p. 159). An SME is any person who can be a valid judge of a design by virtue of his or her experience, education, or research of system operations, job performance, or task dimensions. SMEs and representatives from the user group meet to define the project and ask questions about the product (see Figure 10-2, step 2). During this meeting the groundwork is laid for development of design objectives and task and function analysis (steps 3 and 4). Therapists might serve in this capacity rather than being part of the overall (ongoing) usability testing team. Certainly, therapists' expertise on life skills and expectations throughout the life span, human development milestones, disease, and future expectations of the disease process will assist with developing the test objectives and tasks. Techniques used during meetings with user groups can include focus groups and user workshops, informal discussions, interviews (structured or open-ended), questionnaires, brainstorming, checklists, and observations.[18,28]

The next two steps, which can occur simultaneously, are to identify design objectives more explicitly and to conduct a task and function analysis (see Figure 10-2, steps 3 and 4). Design objectives focus on product features that affect performance, safety, expense, acceptance, comfort, ease of use, and aesthetics. Inclusion of these objectives in initial product development helps confirm that the product is effective, safe, and accepted by user groups before expensive investments are made in product creation and large-scale production. Changes are not as easy to implement and are more expensive when attempted after final creation, production, and dissemination. Design should be closely related to task and function analysis provided by investigators, users, and SMEs as a team. These are the critical success factors. Establishing critical success factors for the users and the producers of the equipment identifies usability as essential to ensuring a successful product. This lets the user and producer know that their problems and concerns are the focus of the design. During a task and function analysis, the task and subtasks to be performed are selected in terms of those that are most

Text continued on p. 160

Box 10-3 *A Few Basic Principles*

1. Testing should resemble the actual situation in which the item will be used, as closely as possible.
   A. That is, participants should complete a task simulation that closely resembles their normal activity or activities. It is important to know whether the item being tested is easy and helpful to use during the tasks for which it was designed. After this is known, adding additional tasks can be useful, such as more complicated tasks or alternate scenarios. Some researchers will test using a more difficult task or scenario, with the idea that if the worker can do the more difficult task, then surely they can accomplish the easier tasks. Although this may be true, if the target audience participants cannot do the additional task, the essential question will remain: Can this person use this device or process in the way it was intended to be used, with the intended consequences, easily?
   B. Care should be taken when adding additional tasks, as this could prolong a test session beyond the length of time the target population would normally engage in an activity. This is especially true in situations in which the individual is able to work at his or her own pace. This is another area in which therapists can provide valuable information. For example, certain diseases and disabling conditions are especially likely to cause fatigue, such as multiple sclerosis, amyotrophic lateral sclerosis, and even recent stroke. Therapists can help researchers design tasks and scenarios that are realistic and will not unduly challenge the participants. This will reduce frustration for participants and should result in more accurate test feedback in terms of the number and pattern of errors, as well as subjective responses.

2. Worst case scenario testing reveals worst case information.
   A. As mentioned in the preceding section, at times it is beneficial to use additional tasks during usability testing, sometimes even using a "worst case scenario." There are good reasons for doing this. First, with the introduction of difficult tasks the maximum capabilities of the participants can be defined. This type of testing is often done when it is imperative to design a task within a person's capabilities in order to reduce human error. An example would be testing airplane pilots on dual task performance; as their primary task becomes more difficult, they spend less time on secondary tasks. By carefully annotating where and when this happens, designers gain knowledge about designing the equipment and tasks in a cockpit so the pilot is not overtaxed.
   B. A second reason for this type of testing is to identify the maximum number and diversity of problems associated with a product or procedure. This is important so designers can use the information to redesign the product or procedure to address the identified problems. The difficulty can be in the interpretation of this information. Although a carefully designed study that slowly introduces more and more difficulty can tell you about a participant's basic capabilities, a study that simply has a participant do very difficult tasks does not answer the same question. For example, if a person can lift and carry 50 pounds (i.e., accomplish the most difficult task scenario), he or she can probably lift and carry 30 pounds (i.e., accomplish the less difficult "basic" task). However, if testing shows the participant cannot lift and carry 50 pounds (i.e., accomplish the most difficult task scenario), the tester has no idea if the participant can lift and carry

Box 10-3 *A Few Basic Principles—cont'd*

30, 25, or even 20 pounds (i.e., accomplish the less difficult "basic" task). In other words, using a worst case scenario does not answer the question of whether the participant can do a particular job or task other than the one tested.

3. Usability testing should be unobtrusive.

   A. Although participants will be aware they are taking part in a study and will typically sign a consent form to participate, it helps if task accomplishment is paramount during testing and the test process is invisible to the user. For example, camera setup should be done before arrival and tested, so that participants can perform the task as normally as possible during testing. Minimal adjustments should be made after the participant arrives, such as raising or lowering the camera to capture the full individual or pertinent actions on camera.

   B. During data collection, extraneous variables that could influence the outcome need to be controlled as much as possible. This means that the individuals conducting testing should offer no coaching, no additional instructions during the task (unless those instructions are part of the normal process), and no feedback to the participant. In addition, no additional distractions should be present, other than those that are normally part of the task or situation.

4. During testing, all instructions need to be precise and exactly the same for each participant.

   A. This is a basic tenet of all research and data collection, as to do otherwise can bias the results (as mentioned in 3B, above). "Instructions" include all information (verbal or written) on how to use a product or do a procedure. It also includes any verbal feedback to participants. Positive feedback, negative

feedback, and coaching during testing have been shown to influence the test results. This means that all feedback to participants should be exactly the same.

   B. Potential methods to control the influence of the individual testers include following a specific protocol, including all verbalizations and/or having each tester brief and evaluate an equal number of participants from each disability group. That is, if a tester gives instructions to and evaluates an equal number of persons in each testing situation, then this potential influence on outcome can be controlled.

5. Usability testing should be free of bias.

   A. All instructions and comments by reviewers must be free of bias. This can be more difficult than it seems, and it is always beneficial to have individuals experienced in writing surveys and questionnaires to help in their design. Even the wording of a survey question, if different from wording typically used by the target group, could bias the results.

   B. All recording of data must be precise and free from bias. That is, when recording subjective data from participants, the individuals conducting the evaluation should not record the information in their own words. Instead, participants can select their responses from a given list or a Likert Scale or their comments should be recorded verbatim. If data collection is done in a focus group, having one or two recorders, as well as a tape recorder, can help.

6. Measures must reflect the target audience, the product, and the actual situation in which the person would act.

   A. Usability testing should simulate the actual situation in which the item will be used (as mentioned in 1), use the appropriate target audience(s), and demonstrate product use in the way the product is intended to be used.

Continued

| Box 10-3 | *A Few Basic Principles—cont'd* |

B. When conducting usability testing with health care products, the target audience can include the client, client's family members or caregivers, and health care professionals. If the client is elderly, the caregiver may be a spouse who is also elderly and could have associated difficulties, such as reading small print (presbyopia) or having difficulty with precision tasks. All of these considerations must be taken into account.

C. If the product is likely to be used in numerous situations and environments, some of those may need to be added to the testing schedule. For example, people with diabetes do not test their blood sugar only at home and under excellent lighting conditions. They may also test their blood sugar just before eating at a restaurant or while on a picnic at the beach with their family. Therefore, the ability to read the digital signal must be evaluated in differing lighting and environmental conditions.

7. Ease-of-use is partially determined by user feedback.

A. Acceptance testing must be accomplished, in part, by having participants report on how easy a product was to use and what problems they had. However, if they have no reference point of comparison, their feedback cannot be taken in context. This means that a member of a target audience who has never previously used the product or attempted to do the task in question may have difficulty providing useful feedback. In these situations, participants may be asked to accomplish a task with and without a particular device, thus providing contextual information.

B. If participants have performed the task previously, it is helpful to understand the conditions in which they completed the task, whether assistance was provided, or whether an additional, but somewhat different, tool was used to assist with task completion. This information is essential to determine whether the present product or procedure offers advantages or disadvantages.

8. Concomitant verbalization is a good technique during usability testing but must be accomplished with care.

A. Concomitant verbalization means that the participant verbalizes aloud what he or she is doing, and why, while taking action. The purpose of this technique is to have the participant "think out loud," so the tester can understand why a process or device is a problem or one is better than another. Without this information, an evaluation may discover that a mistake has been made (an error), but not why—that is, the evaluators may not understand whether the product design or an errant thought process might have contributed to the error.

B. There are difficulties with this process, however. Verbalizing what you are doing, while you are doing it, requires additional cognitive effort. Therefore the participant must be permitted to do the task and verbalize what he or she is doing and why, without interruptions. Additional instructions, coaching, or feedback will disrupt the process. If the participants have to listen to and process additional feedback while verbalizing what they are doing, they are likely to lose track of what they are doing as they seek to listen to, remember, and act on the new instructions. Therefore, as previously stated, this technique requires the monitor to quietly observe (or film) without disrupting the process or distracting the participant. In addition, this technique introduces additional time, as the respondent will take longer to verbalize what he or she is doing than if he or she were to simply perform the actions.

9. Each process should clearly be evaluated with regard to the impact on the system.

<table>
<tr><td colspan="2">Box 10-3   A Few Basic Principles—cont'd</td></tr>
</table>

A. If the process or product being tested includes reading, understanding, and following instructions, these portions may need to be evaluated separately from the task itself. The participant's ability to remember the instructions and the need for repeated exposure such as looking back or asking questions are also important.

B. In the same way, if a task has several subtasks, they may also need to be incorporated into testing.

10. The target audience needs to be well-defined and appropriately represented.

A. This is necessary for accuracy of representation and generalizability of results. As mentioned previously, the target audience for health care and rehabilitation equipment may include the client, family member caregivers, or medical professionals. Members of each group may have a very different experience with the equipment based on their own abilities and needs, and each experience is equally valid.

B. Without sufficient representation, the end users may be misrepresented. For example, having five members of a target group may not provide sufficient information to generalize the results: statistical assessments cannot reach an appropriate level of significance, and designers may be left to draw conclusions from insufficient descriptive data. Although it is possible to conduct assessments with a low number of participants, and indeed, the target audience may be so small that finding a large enough representation is difficult, care should be taken to ensure a well-defined target audience and sufficient representation. Regardless, the population should be thoroughly described in any consequent reports.

This information was compiled, in part, during consultation with Vote-PAD, Inc., www.vote-pad.us.

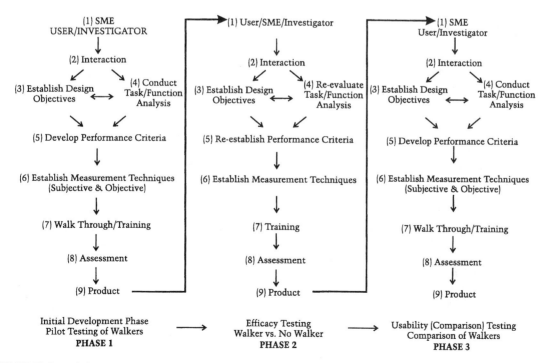

FIGURE **10-2** Usability test procedures. *SME,* Subject matter expert.

demanding, frequent, and essential for the user population. These need to be balanced in accordance with the normal activities of the user group. The analysis also identifies the pattern and sequence of tasks and subtasks.

The design objectives and the information from the task and function analysis are used for the fifth step, the development of performance criteria. Performance criteria should closely resemble the requirements of the task and should be performance oriented (action oriented). For example, a task analysis of an assembly job might indicate that fine-motor coordination is important for performance.

Measurement techniques to quantify performance are chosen (see Figure 10-2, step 6). These techniques include both objective and subjective measurements. Typical objective measurements include reaction time, number of errors, and type of error. Subjective measurements include user ratings of comfort, convenience, ease of use, and aesthetics.

Once the measurement techniques are chosen, subjects are recruited and trained (see Figure 10-2, step 7). Completing steps 1 to 6 before recruiting subjects is important to guarantee full disclosure of the evaluation process. A walk-through or trial of the evaluation process should be conducted at this time.

Finally, the evaluation process is conducted as either a formal or an informal research project (see Figure 10-2, step 8). The results are used to critique or redesign the product (see Figure 10-2, step 9).

The process is repeated as new information becomes available or the design is changed. A design is proposed, tested, rejected (or accepted), and revised repeatedly.[21] During the initial design and development a number of prototypes may be developed and tested. Designs can be assessed using product description, mock-ups, prototypes (partial or full), or complete functional products. One or two design options are then chosen for rigorous evaluation. The evaluations can be categorized as experimental or nonexperimental, formal or informal, two-dimensional or three-dimensional, and nonperformance or performance oriented.[21]

An experimental evaluation requires measurement of subject performance under contrasting conditions in a controlled environment and use of experimental and statistical controls. A nonexperimental evaluation does not require contrasting conditions or strict controls. For example, evaluating a subject's reaction time and subjective reaction to several versions of a product in a laboratory is experimental. Having subjects complete a subjective rating scale while using a single product on the job is nonexperimental. Formal assessments have definite procedures and are well defined; informal assessments have less well-defined objectives and procedures. For example, a questionnaire is formal, but an open-ended group discussion is informal. Two-dimensional evaluations examine a product's attributes through checklists, whereas three-dimensional evaluations may use mock-ups or prototypes and can incorporate either nonperformance or performance measurements.[21]

An experimental evaluation of two or more prototypes determines which design is better or best according to user performance and preference. If only one product is evaluated, the assessment addresses the same design questions of effectiveness, ease of use, accomplishment of the mission, and deficits or areas that need improvement, but only for that one product.

As mentioned, an important aspect of usability testing is that it is performed during each stage of development. Even after the product is on the market, usability assessment can be conducted to ensure the product remains useful and effective. If product development occurred without usability testing, evaluation may be the first step in determining whether change is needed. The user population, especially clients, may not voice their concerns about the effectiveness of a product. This leaves the responsibility with the developers and SMEs. The information gained from a usability evaluation after the product is on the market can determine the need for product redesign and assist medical personnel in making recommendations. Information regarding the effectiveness, efficiency, and ease-of-use of a product is important in the recommendation of a product for purchase by a client, a client's family, or a medical facility.

PRODUCT DEVELOPMENT, EFFICACY TESTING, AND COMPARISON TESTING OF AN ASSISTIVE WALKER

Given that therapists have accepted the job as consultants and members of the ergonomic evaluation team, they first review the literature and construction of walkers and refamiliarize themselves with the types of clients who use them. They review the accoutrements that users may want, such as baskets, pouches for carrying small items, and drink holders. They examine the balance characteristics of walkers. Some are balanced at the center handle; these walkers are designed for clients with hemiplegia and thus with limited use of one hand. Wheeled walkers may be especially beneficial during the early rehabilitation process, but it is difficult to know whether one with front wheels only or one with three wheels will best serve a client. Other important features are the weight, portability, and stability of the walker and the height, shape, and size of the grip handles. Some clients may want a walker with an attached seat.

Given that the New Equipment Company has an idea for a new walker design, the team decides to start there. They plan for three iterations of the usability process. During the first iteration (product development), several variations of the new walker design will be constructed and evaluated. This is *prototype* or *pilot testing,* which involves the evaluation of a newly developed trial product by the end-users who represent the target market. Both the walker design and the testing process are evaluated. The information gained from the pilot test is used in the second iteration of the usability process, in which the best walker design (as determined during the pilot test) is evaluated (efficacy testing). This phase involves a more formal process of performance testing in a controlled setting to determine the effectiveness of the new walker. The final phase (comparison or field testing) involves a field study to determine user acceptance and performance. This testing is conducted in a setting similar to the environment in which the walker will be used (see Figure 10-2, phase 3).

Each phase is considered part of the usability testing. *Usability testing* means that the product

is evaluated by obtaining information from representative users, often while they use the product. To reiterate, the goals of usability testing are to develop a product that accomplishes the purpose for which it was designed, is easy and safe to use, and will be used.

Creating a product that will be utilized involves other factors, such as aesthetics, that influence whether a person chooses to use the product. In addition, the best design is one that does not require the user to study an instruction manual; instead, the design should guide the user's actions so that use of the product is intuitive.

First Iteration: Product Development

The goal of product development is to produce several design alternatives and to select one for additional evaluation. The first step is to identify the SMEs, users, and investigators (see Figure 10-2). This group could include product developers, medical personnel who have prescribed walkers for clients, therapists and nurses who work closely with clients who use walkers, family members of clients who use walkers, and the clients themselves. A target group of clients should be identified, because the needs of various groups, such as those with hemiplegia and those with cerebral palsy, differ. For example, a client who has problems with balance and coordination may not want wheels on his or her walker, and a client who quickly becomes fatigued may need an attachable seat that folds while he or she is walking. Identification of a target group should be based on demographics; knowledge, skills, and experience; attitude; lifestyle; cognitive and physical abilities; and cultural background. In the case study, New Equipment Company wants to create several walkers for different populations; therefore more than one target group would be identified and involved in testing. It may be that New Equipment Company has already had their marketing department identify the groups that will have the largest population that could benefit from, and would be likely to purchase, their walkers over the next 25 years.

The second step is the interactive process between the investigators and the SMEs and users (see Figure 10-2). During this interaction, defi-

Box 10-4	*Design Objectives for Product Development*

Primary

Walker

Lightweight
Adjustable height
Adjustable width
Stability

User

Appropriate weight distribution
Ability to maintain erect posture during use

Secondary

Comfort
Ease of use
Ease of adjustment
Ease of storage
Portability
Optimum grip height
Shape
Size

Tertiary

Attractiveness
Convenience

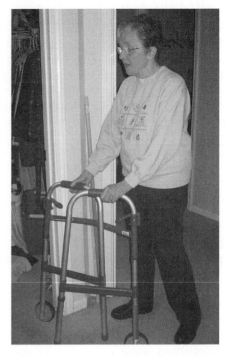

FIGURE **10-3** Being able to fold a walker for storage may be important to a person who does not need to use it to walk for short distances or on a daily basis.

ciencies in existing walker designs are identified and consequent research questions are developed. Positive aspects of existing walker designs may also be identified and incorporated into the design objectives (see Figure 10-2, step 3). If the producers of the equipment have different aims, these also need to be identified. Such aims could include high sales, marketability, production location or costs, and user education or manual development.

Design objectives are developed as a result of the observations, replies to questionnaires, and discussions among SMEs, users, and investigators (Box 10-4). Design objectives should include any items considered important to enable full, practical use of the walker. The development of design objectives should answer the question, "What design features are important for a walker to be used by this target population?" The purpose of a walker is to assist people in walking by allowing them to stabilize themselves by putting some of their weight on the walker handles. Thus, the first objective should be stability. Secondary characteristics of the design are those that are important to a user but that may not influence the primary purpose of the product. An example is making the walker easily collapsible for placing into a car or storage area (Figure 10-3). Tertiary items include attractiveness and convenience. Convenience characteristics of a walker might include baskets or pouches for personal items and attachable trays to hold food or drinks.

Labeling design objectives as primary, secondary, and tertiary does not mean one level is more important than another. Secondary and tertiary items are important because they influence whether the product will be accepted and used. A product may help clients accomplish a task but be so difficult, inconvenient, or unattractive to use that people choose to do without it. The importance of individual design objectives should be determined by the combined interaction of the SMEs, users, and investigators.

While design objectives are being defined, a task and function analysis should be accomplished (see Figure 10-2, step 4). Information gained from establishing the design objectives should be used in conducting the task and function analysis and vice versa. The task and function analysis is based on input from users and SMEs. The investigator who conducts the assessment should observe the user performing a typical task and break the task into its component parts. These components should be described using action phrases. The design objectives and the information gained from the task and function analysis are used to develop performance criteria (see Figure 10-2, step 5).

Representative tasks are identified on the basis of criticality, frequency, and difficulty. The selected tasks can be used as independent variables (the different walkers are also independent variables). For this situation, the tasks chosen could include walking and maneuvering around items that block the user's path; entering, using, and exiting a restroom; and using a small set of stairs. The first task is used to test the walker prototypes. Performance criteria are developed from the selected task or tasks.

The sixth step is to establish subjective and objective measurements. Because the first iteration is the development phase, the investigator may decide to use only one task to select the new design for the walker. Similarly, the investigating team may choose to use only the design objectives deemed most important. The breadth and depth of the evaluation during the product-development stage are determined by the investigator or investigating team. Consideration of costs and benefits assist the investigator in making the determination. For example, if construction of the walkers for additional testing is expected to be expensive, the testing should be thorough. If construction and possible alterations are relatively inexpensive, the prototype study may be smaller in terms of breadth and depth (or complexity).

Box 10-5	*Dependent Measurements for Product Development*

Objective

Walker weight
Height adjustment
Percentage of the target population that can use the walker
Distance between walker legs
Biomechanical analysis of weight distribution
Material strength

Subjective

Perceived stability
Perceived comfort
Perceived pain or strain
Perceived exertion
Perceived ease of use
Perceived ease of adjustment
Perceived portability
Forced-choice rankings

Design objectives (dependent measurements) require both objective and subjective measurements. Dependent measurements for the sample situation are listed in Box 10-5. In addition to the measurements listed, the base and depth of the walker should be measured to determine walker stability. Many manufacturers list the weight capacity of walkers. If more information is required, however, material strength can be determined through consultation with an engineer familiar with the materials and construction of walkers. Subjective measurement techniques may include interviews, questionnaires, rankings, Likert scale ratings, or ratings by means of techniques such as magnitude estimation (Box 10-6).[1,11] Group interviews, rather than open-ended individual interviews, are often used to promote discussion.[20] Forced-choice rankings, especially useful in the comparison of several designs, require the user to rank the designs in order of preference. Observations and ratings by the investigator can be helpful, but the investigator must take care not to bias the results.

Box 10-6	*What Is Magnitude Estimation?*

Magnitude estimation is an experimental technique used in psychophysical experiments. Magnitude estimations involve having a subject compare a current sensation with a reference sensation. For example, a subject might be asked to handle a box of a particular weight and then be asked to judge other weights as weighing more or less than the reference weight. Another example would be the comparison of tactile pressures administered by a monofilament as being of greater or lesser sensation.

Subject training and a walk-through of the testing process constitute the seventh step (see Figure 10-2, step 7). Enough training should be done to eliminate a learning (or practice) effect. Subjects should not continue to improve with time, regardless of experimental condition.

The eighth step is the actual assessment; in this case it involves a comparison study of several prototype walkers. Subjects perform one or more of the reference tasks, and the investigator collects and analyzes objective and subjective information. On the basis of the analysis, one design is usually selected for the next phase, efficacy testing. In the example, the walking task is evaluated in a nonexperimental, formal-informal, three-dimensional, and performance-oriented context. *Nonexperimental* means no statistical controls, even though contrasting conditions are used (one walker design compared with another). The comparison study contains both *formal* and *informal* elements: A formal procedure and questionnaire are used in addition to an informal interview session. The process is *three-dimensional* because prototypes of the walkers are used in a realistic task or series of tasks.

The goal of the evaluation (to identify one walker for additional testing) can be met with a relatively small number of participants. Subjects receive a detailed briefing, undergo a medical screening, and sign an informed-consent form.

Each hospital or nursing facility usually has a human-use committee that determines the requirements for briefing, screening, and the format and contents of the consent form.

The experimental design is a repeated-measurements design, counterbalanced for order. The term *repeated-measurements design* means that each subject serves as his or her own control and completes the task under each of the experimental conditions (various walker designs). Counterbalancing for the order in which each walker is used can be accomplished by using a balanced Latin-square design. This means each treatment condition (each walker design) is immediately preceded and followed once by each of the other conditions.[31] (This is often the preferred method to counterbalance a design without having to conduct tests of all possible ordering combinations.) Another method of controlling for order effects is to randomize the order of administration.

Analysis of the subjective data can be accomplished by the use of nonparametric statistical analysis.[26,31] Nonparametric statistical analysis is a useful tool for usability studies that collect subjective data and use small sample sizes. Parametric statistical analysis can be used for objective data when proper experimental design and sufficient population sampling are used. Considerable debate exists about using parametric statistics with subjective data.[2,15,29]

The results should clearly indicate the preferred design on the basis of user preference and performance data. The investigator may give a weighting factor to items considered to be of primary importance. For example, object load, adjustability, use by the greatest percentage of the target population, and biomechanical advantage may be weighted more than convenience and aesthetics.

As a result of the first iteration, design 1 is selected for additional testing. As seen in Table 10-1, the design is selected because it has the largest height range and is considered the most stable, adjustable, and portable. Its use caused the least pain and strain, and it was ranked the preferred walker. Note that design 1 was selected despite being the most difficult to use.

TABLE 10-1	Hypothetical Results from Product Development		
	Design 1	**Design 2**	**Design 3**
Load	6 lb	7 lb	16 lb
Height	17-37 in	32-37 in	30-38 in
Weight distribution	Good	Good	Good
Material construction	350-lb capacity	375-lb capacity	500-lb capacity
Posture	Good	Good	Good
Stability	17.5*	12.2	14
Comfort	14.5	15.8	16
Pain or strain	12.1*	14.2	14.6
Ease of use	10.3	12.2	16.8*
Ease of adjustment	18.7*	16	14.8
Portability	16.5*	13.9	9.8
Ranking	1.25*	2.25	2.5

*Significantly different from other two walkers ($P < .05$).
Note: All ratings (except ranking) used a Borg-type scale with anchored subjective ratings of 0 to 20.[8] The lower number indicates less and the higher number indicates more of the given quality. Rankings were 1 to 3.

Second Iteration: Efficacy Testing (Controlled Setting)

The goal of efficacy testing is to determine whether the walker improves the user's ability to walk and maneuver through the activities of daily living—that is, it answers the question of whether the walker is effective for completing the tasks the user needs to complete. Therefore, testing consists of having subjects use the walker, as opposed to not using a walker, while performing several representative tasks. If the investigator believes that walkers have been shown to be effective ambulation tools and that such an evaluation would be superfluous, this phase can be eliminated. If this phase is eliminated, usability testing begins with a comparison between the new design and existing designs (usability [comparison] testing; see Figure 10-2, phase 3).

Identification of the SMEs and users was accomplished in the beginning of phase 1 (pilot testing); the experimental subjects now are added to the group as SMEs (see Figure 10-2, phase 2, step 1). The interaction among SMEs, users, and

the investigator should focus on the results of the pilot test accomplished during phase 1.

The design objectives for the walker most likely will remain the same as those identified in the development phase (see Figure 10-2, phase 2, step 3; Box 10-4). However, additional objectives can be identified in the pilot testing and in the interactions among the subjects, SMEs, and users.

The task and function analysis should be re-evaluated (see Figure 10-2, phase 2, step 4). The representative tasks can be altered on the basis of information gained during the development phase. For the second iteration of the process (efficacy testing), all three representative tasks are used to ascertain whether the new walker meets the functional goals. The tasks identified during the task or functional analysis are walking and maneuvering around items that block the user's path; entering, using, and exiting a restroom; and using a small set of stairs. Each task is completed in a controlled laboratory setting. In each task, performance criteria should provide information essential to successful performance and include

TABLE 10-2	Hypothetical Results from Efficacy Testing: Walking and Maneuvering Task	
	Walker	No walker
Total time	9.2 min	15.6 min
Get up	1 min	2 min
Turn right	0.45 min	1.2 min
Walk 5 ft	1.5 min	2.6 min
Walk around chair	0.6 min	1.5 min
Walk 4 ft	1.3 min	2 min
Avoid toy	1 min	1.9 min
Walk 5 ft	1.77 min	2.9 min
Sit in chair	1.4 min	1.5 min
Heart rate	145 beats/min	155 beats/min
Perceived exertion	15.8*	18.3
Stability	19.7*	5.1
Comfort	18.5*	6.7
Pain or strain	5.5*	14.2

*Significantly different from no walker ($P < .05$).
Note: All ratings (except ranking) used a Borg-type scale with anchored subjective ratings of 0 to 20.[8] The lower number indicates less and the higher number indicates more of the given quality.

objective and subjective data (see Figure 10-2, phase 2, step 5). When the same criteria are used for product development, efficacy testing, and comparison testing, performance standards can be developed and product improvement can be monitored. Additional dependent measurements in the example include time to complete each element of the task, time to complete the entire procedure, heart rate, and perceived exertion (Table 10-2).[7-9]

In the example, the same objective and subjective measurement techniques used during the development phase are used during efficacy testing (see Figure 10-2, phase 2, step 6; Box 10-5). The first task is walking and maneuvering around items that block the user's path and involves the following procedures: rising from

an easy chair, turning right, walking 5 feet and maneuvering to the left of a chair that blocks the path, walking 4 feet and maneuvering right to avoid a child's toy, walking another 5 feet, and sitting in a kitchen chair.

In addition to the primary task of walking, important secondary tasks should be included in the testing procedure. For example, if the walker is used to enable someone to move between a desk and a filing cabinet, such a task pattern should be incorporated into the testing procedure.

Again, subjects should be trained in each task used in the test procedure (see Figure 10-2, phase 2, step 7). Because more than one task is being studied (walking, maneuvering in a restroom, and using stairs), the order of the tasks should be balanced to control for order effects, such as transfer of learning or a conditioning effect. Training of test subjects in testing procedures also decreases the likelihood that learning effects will influence the study results.

After training, the actual assessment (experimental evaluation) takes place. Task performance should be evaluated by timing and accuracy data. In the example, efficacy testing is experimental, formal, three-dimensional performance testing. As with any research method, consistency in experimental testing must be ensured in subject training, measurement techniques, and data compilation. Two excellent resources on these topics are Winer and colleagues[31] for laboratory studies and Cook and Campbell[10] for field studies.

During efficacy testing, the number of subjects will probably be greater than the number who participated in the pilot test. Adequate results can be obtained with a relatively small number of subjects, especially because this is a repeated-measurements study. Statistical analysis can include a repeated-measurements analysis of variance and post hoc testing.

The results should give the investigator clear information about the efficacy of use of the walker (as opposed to no walker) in terms of both the subjects' performances and their preferences. Efficacy testing provides information on the benefits and limitations of using the walker in three different situations for men and women. Initial results suggest that the walker is beneficial (see Table 10-2). The subjects performed the task more quickly, experienced less subjective exertion, less pain and strain, more stability, and more comfort, and had a lower heart rate when they used the walker than when they did not use the walker. The final output is the product (see Figure 10-2, phase 2, step 9), which is reevaluated by the research team.

Third Iteration: Comparison Field Testing

The second iteration of the usability cycle (efficacy testing) revealed that the walker was helpful in improving ambulation and maneuvering in using a restroom. However, the following concerns were identified during testing:

- The gripping edge of the walker was uncomfortable and caused pain on the thenar eminence during ambulation.
- Subjects requested a handle material that does not feel cold to the touch and comes in different colors.
- Subjects requested detachable accessories, such as a tray for holding objects, a recessed cup holder, and a basket with adjustable sections.
- The fold-up seat was weak and unstable and did not have appropriate contour or padding.

The concerns must be discussed by SMEs, subjects, users, and investigators (see Figure 10-2, phase 3, steps 1 and 2). The cost of product development and the purchase price must be considered, along with the preferences expressed. The changes that can be made are incorporated, and a new walker is constructed (see Figure 10-2, phase 3, step 3). The new design must then be reevaluated in the type of environment in which it is to be used. In addition, the investigator should compare this design with that of other walkers available on the commercial market (usability [comparison] testing; see Figure 10-2, phase 3).

A review of the task and function analysis reveals that the assistance provided by the walker is most pronounced during the walking task. Because both the old and the new design objectives can be tested by walking, this task is chosen as representative (see Figure 10-2, phase 3, step 4). The purpose of the comparison field testing is to compare one or more designs with one another in a realistic environment. The investigator can compare the findings obtained when a subject uses the new walker design with the findings obtained when no walker is used to verify the results of the efficacy test in a realistic environment.

The task in comparison testing should be similar to the task used during efficacy testing in the laboratory. The tests can be conducted in nursing homes, rehabilitation centers, or even in a home environment in which throw rugs, narrow halls, and wheelchairs are obstructions. It can also be conducted in a work setting in which storage cabinets are located in the halls, ramps are located between split-level floors, and low-level ambient light is used. The most appropriate setting for the target group is determined by the users, SMEs, and the investigator. If users are required to perform additional tasks or carry objects, these tasks are included in the evaluation (see Figure 10-2, phase 3, step 5). The objective and subjective measurement techniques are the same as those used during efficacy testing to verify results (see Figure 10-2, phase 3, step 6). In this case, the investigating team might decide to have individuals who use walkers to use each of the candidate walkers in their own home environments and observe them performing each of the identified tasks (maneuvering around objects, going to the restroom, and going up and down a small stair [Figure 10-4, A-D]). Because each subject is using each of the candidate walkers, the subjects serve as their own comparison, and the task does not have to be identical for each subject.

Training and walk-through of the test situation are conducted because the conditions have changed from a laboratory-based evaluation to a field test. Training helps prevent mistakes during testing and eliminates a learning effect (see Figure 10-2, phase 3, step 7). The assessment is the eighth step, and applying the data obtained to the product design is the ninth step.

The results of the comparison test in the example were as follows: The new design was ranked as the preferred walker compared with the other two walkers. The subjects' heart rates were

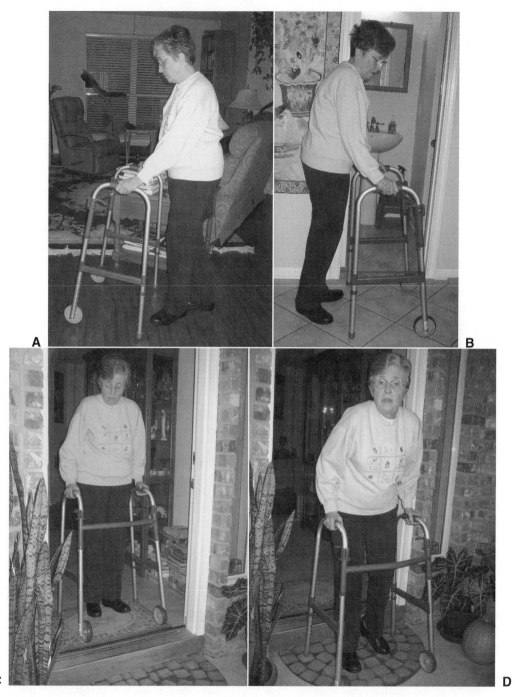

FIGURE 10-4 Evaluating the use of each walker in several tasks within the users' home environment allows the investigators to get accurate measures of ease-of-use, effectiveness, and efficiency. **A,** In this case, Mary Jo maneuvers around furniture and into her living room, where there is a large rug. **B,** She goes to the bathroom, but the walker does not fit through the doorway, so she must approach sideways and then hold onto the doorway itself. **C** and **D,** She exits her home down a single small step, which calls for balancing herself, lifting the walker, and placing it down the step—not an easy process!

TABLE 10-3 Hypothetical Results of Walker Subjective Ratings		
	New design	Walker A	Walker B
Stability	18.8	17.7	19
Comfort	15.3*	12.3	14
Pain or strain	8.9*	17.3	16.2
Ease of use	15	15.9	16.5
Perceived exertion	16.4	15	15.2
Ranking	1.25*	2.5	2.25

*Significantly different from other two walkers ($P < .05$).
Note: All ratings (except ranking) used a Borg-type scale with anchored subjective ratings of 0 to 20.[8]
A lower number indicates less and a higher number indicates more of the indicated quality. Rankings are 1 to 3.

lower with the new design. Subjects completed the task faster when they used the new design; however, time to stand and sit was slower. Subjects found the new design easier to use. Use of the new design increased comfort and decreased pain and strain. No differences were found for ratings of stability, perceived exertion, or performance of ancillary tasks. These results showed the new design to be superior for ambulatory assistance as measured by user preference and performance (Table 10-3).

CONCLUSION

Usability testing of medical or rehabilitation equipment is an essential component of product development but is often neglected. This neglect becomes obvious when practitioners or clients attempt to use the product. Without user testing, products are often difficult to use, cannot be used intuitively, and are not comfortable. Unfortunately, it becomes obvious they are not made for all categories of users, such as technicians, medical practitioners, and clients. The importance of usability testing of medical equipment has become widely recognized, as evidenced by its consideration as one criterion for approving products and

Learning Exercises

The best way to understand usability testing is to conduct a user-centered evaluation of a product. Imagine you are a consultant and you have been asked to evaluate a product. This can be a rehabilitation device, a toy, a consumer product, or even a "health aid" such as a therapeutic back scratcher. Once you have selected a product, conduct the following exercises.

1. Develop a "panel of experts" to include members from a user group or groups, a researcher/ergonomist, and a therapist. Each person should agree to speak (and think) from their perspective.
2. Have the panel discuss the product, past concerns with the product, what they would like to see in a "perfect" product, and the environments in which they might use it.
3. Write down some objectives relating to what the product should do, what design features should be included, and what types of task(s) would be most common for its use.
4. Decide which scenario(s) you will use for testing the product; include the environment, the tasks, and the target population(s).
5. Decide what performance you want to measure. Remember that you may want to include the user's ability to read and follow the instructions for product use, if there are any.
6. Decide how you will measure the performance in number 5. Will you count errors, time completion of a task, or merely observe the product use and ask questions? Remember, children may not be able to easily verbalize their likes and dislikes.
7. If the evaluation process requires it, conduct a walk-through of the evaluation process. Sometimes this is not desirable as you want to see how the individual uses the product for the first time. Have a colleague assume the role as a member of the target population and use the product as you have designed the evaluation. If there is more than one target population, have colleagues assume those roles.
8. Evaluate the product, obtain feedback from the target population, and then meet as a group to evaluate and interpret the results.
9. Write a synopsis of your findings and recommendations for product design changes.

setting international and national standards. Fortunately, testing and designing evaluative and treatment equipment, devices for special populations, and technology for groups that consider themselves technically challenged have gained the attention of a number of human factors or ergonomics practitioners.

Medical professionals often design equipment based on their experience with clients or according to individual client needs but fail to complete the design sequence by conducting systematic user tests. Rather than have complete knowledge of the success of the product, they have two sets of opinions: their own and those of the clients with whom they work. Little attempt is made to make the product effective for a broad client population.

Usability testing provides a mechanism to evaluate a product from a user's perspective. The procedure should be used to assess all rehabilitation and medical equipment. Usability testing should include factors such as ease of operational learning, effectiveness, efficiency, flexibility, maintainability, durability, safety, and task matching with user characteristics. Manufacturers, practitioners, and instructors in professional programs should begin introducing the concepts and procedures of usability testing to improve client care.

Multiple Choice Review Questions

1. Select the true statements among the following:
   A. Usability testing is the systematic evaluation of the "interaction between people and the products, equipment, environments, and services they use."
   B. Usability testing "is the fundamental principle that underpins all ergonomics."
   C. Usability testing has been called *user-acceptance testing, user trials,* and *usability engineering.*
   D. Choices A and C are true.
   E. Choices A and B are true.
   F. Choices A, B, and C are true.

2. In usability testing of medical and rehabilitation equipment, what user groups should be considered? (Select the single best answer.)
   A. All health care professionals and health care technicians who use the equipment
   B. All health care professionals, health care technicians, and family members of clients who might benefit from the equipment, as well as the clients themselves
   C. Anyone who is around the client on a regular basis
   D. Any person who is expected to use the equipment
   E. All family members of and health care providers for clients who might benefit from the equipment

3. Which of the following statements are true with regard to user-centered design (UCD)? (More than one may be selected.)
   A. User-centered design is synonymous with usability testing.
   B. User-centered design is a structured process for product development and includes users throughout each phase of the design process.
   C. User-centered design often involves a macroergonomic approach that includes the mission, goals, and culture of the business, as well as the likes, abilities, and requirements of the target audience.
   D. User-centered design is design that benefits not only persons with disabilities, but those who are able-bodied.

4. The U.S. Food and Drug Administration has standards that address the need for user-testing of medical devices and products.
   A. True
   B. False

5. Which of the following are true with regard to ecologic validity? (More than one may be selected.)
   A. Ecologic validity is important because a person's environment can influence his or her performance.
   B. Ecologic validity refers to how closely the testing environment resembles the actual environment.
   C. Ecologic validity refers to making the person's environment "user-friendly."
   D. An experiment has ecologic validity if investigators are actually evaluating what they think they are evaluating.

6. Which of the following are true with regard to this basic principle of usability testing: Testing should resemble as closely as possible the actual situation in which the item will be used"?
   A. This means that those members of the target audience who are participating should complete a task simulation that closely resembles their normal activity or activities.
   B. The investigator decides on his or her own which tasks are important to include.
   C. The best idea is to use the most difficult task the target audience has to do, because if they can do that task, they can do all of the other tasks.
   D. All pertinent tasks the users have to do should be included in usability testing, regardless of how long the testing takes.

7. Usability testing is considered an "iterative" process.
   A. True
   B. False

8. The phases of usability testing occur in the following order:
   A. Efficacy testing, comparison testing, acceptance testing, and initial development

   B. Initial development, comparison testing, efficacy, and acceptance testing
   C. Initial development, efficacy testing, comparison testing, and acceptance testing
   D. Initial development, efficacy and acceptance testing, and comparison testing
   E. Any of the phases can occur in any order; it depends on the product and the process desired by the manufacturer.

9. Select the statements below that are not true with regard to concomitant verbalization. (More than one answer may be selected.)
   A. Concomitant verbalization is a good technique during usability testing but must be accomplished with care.
   B. Concomitant verbalization means that the participant verbalizes aloud what he or she is doing, and why, while performing actions.
   C. Concomitant verbalization requires no additional cognitive effort.
   D. Concomitant verbalization helps the investigator understand why a user does what he or she does. It helps the investigator understand whether the product design or an errant thought process might have contributed to the error.
   E. Providing feedback or asking questions during user testing and concomitant verbalization is acceptable, as long as the investigator gets the additional information necessary to ascertain the usability of the product.

10. Prototype testing involves the evaluation of a newly developed, trial product, most often involving end-users of the product as participants in the evaluation of the product.
   A. True
   B. False

REFERENCES

1. Allard F: Information processing in human percentual motor performance, Kin 356 course notes, Waterloo, Ontario, 2001, Department of Kinesiology, University of Waterloo.
2. Anderson NH: Scales and statistics: parametric and nonparametric, *Psychol Bull* 58:305, 1961.
3. Bamforth S, Brooks N: Effective design methodologies for rehabilitation equipment: the cactus project. Design applications for industry and education. In *Proceedings of the 13th Annual Conference on Engineering Design,* London, 2001, Professional Engineering Publishing.
4. Bogner MS: An introduction to design, evaluation, and usability testing. In VJB Rice, editor: *Ergonomics in health care and rehabilitation,* Boston, 1998, Butterworth-Heinemann.
5. Bogner MS: *Human error in medicine,* Mahwah, NJ, 1994, Lawrence Erlbaum Associates.
6. Bogner MS: *Misadventures in health care: inside stories (Human error and safety series),* Mahwah, NJ, 2003, Lawrence Erlbaum Associates.
7. Borg GA: *Physical performance and perceived exertion,* Lund, Sweden, 1962, Gleerup.
8. Borg GA: Perceived exertion as an indicator of somatic stress, *Scand J Rehabil Med* 2:92, 1970.
9. Borg GA: Subjective aspects of physical and mental load, *Ergonomics* 21:215, 1978.
10. Cook TT, Campbell DT: *Quasi-experimentation: design and analysis issues for field settings,* Boston, 1979, Houghton Mifflin.
11. Cordes RE: Use of magnitude estimation for evaluating product. In Grandjean E, editor: *Ergonomics and health in modern offices,* New York, 1984, Taylor & Francis.
12. Dekker S: *The field guide to human error investigations,* Burlington, Vt, 2002, Ashgate Publishing.
13. Dhillon D: *Medical device reliability and associated areas,* NY, 2000, CRC Press.
14. Erickson BJ, Kossack MF, Blaine JG et al: Application of usability testing for improving PACS workstation design. *Proceedings of the International Society for Optimal Engineering,* San Diego, Calif, 2000. Available from the Society of Photo-Optical Instrumentation Engineers, Bellingham, Wash.
15. Gaito J: Measurement scales and statistics: resurgence of an old misconception, *Psychol Bull* 101:159, 1987.
16. Hyman WA: Errors in the use of medical equipment. In Bogner MS, editor: *Human error in medicine,* Hillsdale, NJ, 1994, Erlbaum.
17. Kumar S, Rice VJB: Ergonomics for special populations: an introduction. In VJB Rice, editor: *Ergonomics in health care and rehabilitation,* Boston, 1998, Butterworth-Heinemann.
18. Kuniavsky M: *Observing the user experience: a practitioner's guide to user research,* San Francisco, 2003, Morgan Kaufmann Publishers.
19. Leape LL: The preventability of medical injury. In Bogner MS, editor: *Human error in medicine,* Hillsdale, NJ, 1994, Erlbaum.
20. McClelland I: Product assessment and user trials. In Wilson JR, Corlett EN, editors: *Evaluation of human work: a practical ergonomics methodology,* Boca Raton, Fla, 2005, CRC Press.
21. Meister D: *Behavioral analysis and measurement methods,* New York, 1985, Wiley.
22. Meister D: *Conceptual aspects of human factors,* Baltimore, 1989, Johns Hopkins University Press.
23. Moray N: Error reduction as a systems problem. In Bogner MS, editor: *Human error in medicine,* Hillsdale, NJ, 1994, Erlbaum.
24. Perper JA: Life-threatening and fatal therapeutic misadventures. In Bogner MS, editor: *Human error in medicine,* Hillsdale, NJ, 1994 Erlbaum.
25. Rice VJ, Gable C: A combined macroergonomic and public health approach to injury prevention: two years later. In *Proceedings of the Human Factors and Ergonomics Society Annual Conference,* New Orleans, 2004.
26. Siegel S, Castellan NJ: *Nonparametric statistics for the behavioral sciences,* New York, 1988, McGraw-Hill.
27. Swain E: FDA to emphasize human factors, *Med Device Diagn Ind Mag* September:20, 2005.
28. Vink P: *Comfort and design,* Florida, 2005, CRC Press.
29. Westermann R: Interval-scale measurement of attitudes: some theoretical conditions and empirical testing methods, *Br J Math Statistic Psychol* 36:228, 1983.
30. Wiklund ME: Is your human factors program ready for FDA scrutiny? *Med Device Diagn Ind Mag* January:100, 2003.
31. Winer BJ, Brown DR, Michels KM: *Statistical principles in experimental design,* New York, 1991, McGraw-Hill.

SUGGESTED READING

Crocker P: *Focus group research for marketers,* 2001, Xlibris.
Krueger RA, Casey MA: *Focus groups: a practical guide for applied research,* Belmont, Calif, 2000, Sage Publishing.
Rice VJB: *Ergonomics in health care and rehabilitation,* Boston, 1998, Butterworth-Heinemann.
Wilson JR, Corlett N: *Evaluation of human work,* Boca Raton, FL, 2005, CRC Press.

11

Lifting Analysis*

Daniel Focht

Learning Objectives

After reading this chapter and completing the exercises, the reader should be able to do the following:
1. Use biomechanical principles when analyzing a lift.
2. Critically analyze three lifting techniques.
3. Develop an abatement protocol to prevent commonly encountered lift-related injuries.

Low back. The lumbar spine and its anterior/posterior components. Iliosacral area may also be included.
Pain. Subjective, often nocuous response to stressors that overwhelm the tissues being exposed.

Prevention. The use of accepted scientific principles in the obviation of risk factors that may predispose an individual to injury.

---

*Portions of this chapter are retained from the previous edition chapter written by Diane Aja and Krystal Laflin.

CASE STUDY

You have received notification that one of the employers you work with, Boston Packaging, Inc., is experiencing an inordinate amount of new injuries, primarily low back. Apparently the employer, which specializes in the binding, packaging, and distribution of reference textbooks, has installed a new line. The area in which the majority of the injuries are occurring is in the packaging department. You have been asked to assess the area and recommend controls.

The essential functions of an employee working in the packaging department are that he or she packages the books in boxes ranging in size from $50 \times 50 \times 30$ cm ($20 \times 20 \times 11$ in). The textbooks vary in size and weight, which results in boxes ranging in mass from 20 to 30 pounds. The books are packaged and sealed on a roller line that stands approximately 75 cm (30 inches) from the floor. Once packaged the boxes are placed on pallets directly behind the employee. Each pallet raises the palletized material approximately 9 cm ($3^1/_2$ inches) from the floor. Boxes are stacked three deep and four high. When full the pallet is transported via fork truck to shipping, and a new pallet replaces the old.

This chapter covers the present evidence on lifting and discusses the various lifting techniques that are used in the study of ergonomics. Because the lower lumbar region has been the joint complex that has received the most scrutiny, it will be the focus of the chapter. Our case study at Boston Packaging, Inc. will be incorporated into the chapter contents.

Lifting is an activity that is an essential part of everyday life. Unfortunately, it has been implicated as a contributing factor in the development of a variety of musculoskeletal injuries, particularly those that involve the lumbar spine.[1,8] To illustrate the gravity of this pervasive problem, a review of contemporary data shows that of the 1.4 million occupational injuries reported to the Bureau of Labor Statistics in 2002, 11.7% involved injury to the lower back. Of these, 38.8% correlated positively with a mechanism of injury related to lifting.[3] This results in a staggering financial cost that has been estimated in terms of work days lost per year, and the combined direct and indirect

medical costs have led to an aggressive movement by industry as a whole, medical professionals, and ergonomists to focus on prevention via workplace education and design.[51] This combined effort has resulted in some exciting and novel approaches to counter these work-related injuries, as you will see in the following review.

THE BIOMECHANICS OF LIFTING

Since Nachemson's landmark 1964 study,[37] myriad studies have been conducted to accurately assess the internal and external stressors that influence spinal function and contribute to injury. Chapter 6 on Basic Biomechanics provides an excellent overview of biomechanics, and the reader is asked to review this information before reading this chapter. Please pay particular attention to the terms *compression*, *shear*, and *torsion*.

LIFTING TECHNIQUES

Traditionally, one of the first and most easily applied administrative controls to prevent the high incidence of low back injuries at the work site is training the workers to lift in a biomechanically safe manner. There has been, however, considerable controversy as to which of the most commonly used lifts (stoop, squat, or semi-squat) is most effective in protecting the worker.[45] For this reason a critical analysis of each lift is warranted.

Stoop Lift

The stoop lift (Figure 11-1) is a maneuver that typically requires maximal flexion of the trunk and as near to terminal extension of the knees (without locking) as possible.

Squat Lift

The squat lift (Figure 11-2) requires knee flexion >90 degrees and trunk flexion <30 degrees.

Semi-Squat Lift

The semi-squat lift shares characteristics of the stoop and squat. As can be seen in Figure 11-3, the semi-squat uses a posture calling for knee flexion >45 degrees and trunk flexion at approxi-

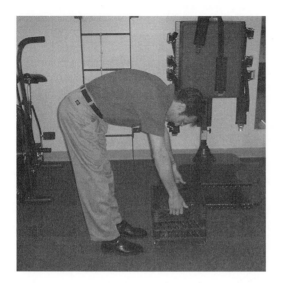

FIGURE **11-1** A stoop lift.

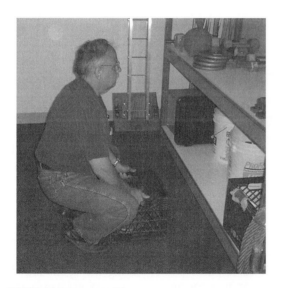

FIGURE **11-2** A squat lift.

mately the same angulation. Note the greater anterior tilt of the pelvis with this approach in comparison with the other lifts, promoting a lumbar lordosis.

Research studies suggest that hand placement should avoid the more precarious floor or near-

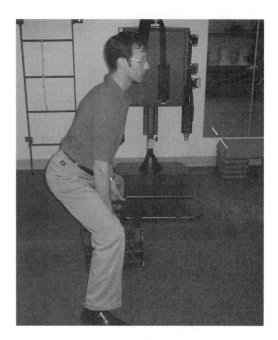

FIGURE **11-3** A semi-squat lift.

floor grasp.[14] If the near-floor hand couple is adopted in an attempt to maintain the integrity of the lift, the squat lift soon becomes a semi-squat when the subject attempts to negotiate the lower lift-surface.[45]

Freestyle Lift

Additional lifting styles deserve attention, as they have been reported in the literature. These include the freestyle lift. This lift resembles in most respects the semi-squat but can differ from person to person. It is this variability that makes it difficult to examine during controlled studies.[51]

Trunk Kinetic Lift

The trunk kinetic lift is characterized by a sudden extensor moment of the knees before the lift.[48]

Load Kinetic Lift

The load kinetic lift requires a closer approximation of the load to the body just before the initial acceleration moment. This lift, too, is seen as a variation of the three more standard lifts.[48]

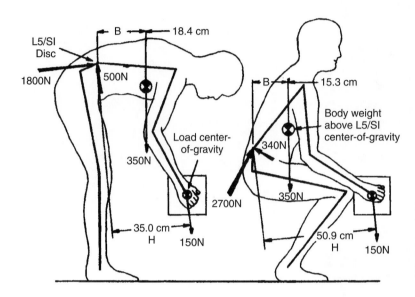

(Dead load) 130N — .07g Horizontal acceleration

3.3° Acceleration vector angle

Vertical acceleration 1.15g   150N (Live load)

FIGURE **11-4** An approximate 50% variance in lumbar moments at the L5/S1 segment when comparing squat and stoop lift. (From Chaffin DB, Andersson GB: *Occupational biomechanics*, ed 2, New York, 1991, John Wiley & Sons.)

CRITIQUE OF LIFTING TECHNIQUES

Biomechanical Analysis

Toussaint and colleagues[47] determined that the lumbar moment at L5/S1 and compressive forces were equal for the stoop and squat lifts when testing young and middle-aged male subjects lifting barbells weighing 8 kg and 15 kg. Van Dieen demonstrated a slight difference, with the stoop lumbar moments being 2% to 8% less than for the squat lift.[49]

Kumar reported that lumbar moments were similar in nine male subjects who performed maximum isometric and isokinetic exertions when using the squat and stoop lift.[27] When analyzing all three lifts, Mittal and Malik[36] and de Looze and co-workers[10] found that the semi-squat demonstrated higher lumbar moments, but that the difference among all three lifts was only 5%.

It is generally accepted that the closer the load is placed to the body, the more significantly di-minished the resultant compressive forces to the lumbar spine (Figure 11-4).[2] This is a strategy that is employed more effectively in the semi-squat lift (load between the feet and knees) than with the stoop or squat lift.

When assessing the relative effects of both compression and shear forces, the data remain contentious. Although increased compression appears to be present with the stoop versus the squat lift, the shear forces are significantly higher (in some cases 180%) during the squat lift.[16,40] This finding was further supported by Kingma and co-workers,[23] who reported that low back loading was significantly higher during squat lifting than with the stoop lift when lifting from the floor (0.05 m). It is speculated that this is a result of the longer moment arm created by the more posterior fulcrum of L5/S1 in relation to the load being lifted during the squat lift. These stressors can be ameliorated, however, by decreasing the moment arm with placement of the load between the feet, as noted during the modified or semi-squat lift,[12] rather than behind, as noted during the pure squat or stoop lifts.

Foot placement, however, is contingent on the size of the load. If the container is too wide (large) to allow for proper foot placement (greater than shoulder width—approximately 30 cm [12 in]), then the ideal lift would be the stoop, since it would result in less compressive forces.

Soft tissue compliance, another consideration (e.g., lumbothoracic paraspinals and spinal ligaments), follows standard length-tension relationships during the various lifts. It was reported that the supraspinous and interspinous ligaments more effectively countered the lumbar moment (be it as a result of shear or compressive forces) during the stoop rather that the squat and semi-squat lifts.[34] This phenomenon is extremely important to keep in mind because it can modify the shear force at the lumbar disc by up to 700 N purely by supporting the activation of the erector spinae.[35]

Physiologic Response

Oxygen uptake/consumption, %VO$_2$ max, the gold standard of energy expenditure, was found to be greater with the squat lift than with the stoop.[22] This was a result of the increased effort requirements of the quadriceps and hip extensors and the resultant increased blood perfusion noted during the squat and semi-squat lifts versus the lesser demands of the erector spinae and trunk musculature during the stoop lift.[17] In a study measuring overall lifting endurance, 12 subjects were tested while lifting a 10-kg load at a rate of six times per minute using both the squat and stoop lift. There was a 38% disparity in oxygen consumption, with the stoop requiring less effort.[27]

Lifting capacities did show slight but contradictory differences when the various lifts were compared. Granata and colleagues reported that the squat, semi-squat, and stoop lifting potentials were similar.[21] Conversely, Magnusson and co-workers reported squat capacities to be on average 10% greater than those of the stoop lift.[30] This propensity, however, was neutralized as repetition, exposure rate, and time increased, with the stoop lift winning out.[30] In fact, it has been found that with repetition and increased exposure, sub-

jects tend to switch from the squat and semi-squat to the stoop lift because of the increased energy demands of the squat lifts.[49]

Perceived Exertion

Rating of perceived exertion (RPE), a subjective measure, rates the individual's own awareness of the effort required to perform a particular activity. Straker and Duncan reported that subjects rated the squat lift at a higher RPE than both the semi-squat and the stoop lifts.[46] In a separate study 90% of the subjects rated the squat lift as more fatiguing than the stoop lift.[41] Another more subjective measure of individual lifting tolerances uses maximum allowable weight (MAW) as a determining factor. In these cases a psychophysical factor is used, characterized by the subject's holistic perceptions as to his or her maximal effort.[42] With this in mind, researchers reported that 17 females selected a MAW 20.5% greater for the stoop than for the squat lift.[46] When comparing the squat and semi-squat exclusively, subjects chose a greater 25.4% MAW, preferring the semi-squat over the squat.[17]

Finally, and most compelling, is the response of an individual experiencing low back pain and what adjustments are made to negotiate a lift from floor to waist. A survey of asymptomatic individuals and individuals with low back pain promulgated by Damkot and colleagues revealed that the asymptomatic group showed no preference between the squat or stoop lift but that more than two thirds of those with back pain (symptomatic group) had adopted the squat or semi-squat as their preferred lift.[9]

Table 11-1 shows that none of the lifts demonstrate a clear advantage over the others. In fact, all lifts, to some extent, have the potential to create stressors not only to the spine but to a number of other structures (e.g., knees, hips, shoulders). It is important for therapists to critically appraise lifting techniques and recommend those that match the client's capacities to the task that is to be performed.

Knowing that increased angulation of the lumbar spine—through flexion—causes both increased compression and shear forces to the intervertebral disc, it would make intuitive sense

TABLE 11-1   Comparison of Lifts

Criteria	Squat	Semi-squat	Stoop
Maximum allowable weight (MAW)	*	***	**
Oxygen consumption	*	**	***
Heart rate	*	**	***
Ventilation	*	**	***
Relative load	**	**	**
Lumbar movement	**	**	**
Lumbar compression	**	**	**
Lumbar shear	***	**	*
Fatigue kinematics	*	**	***
Strength capacity	**	**	**
Effect of pain	***	**	*

The number of stars denotes the preferred lift:
3 = best, 1 = worst.
Data from Straker LM: A review of research on techniques for lifting low-lying objects: 2. Evidence for a correct technique, *Work* 20(2):83, 2003.

to prescribe the semi-squat or squat technique when an individual is required to lift heavy objects on an occasional basis.[38] The semi-squat lift allows for closer placement of the load to the body, thus creating a smaller moment arm and less compressive force.[2] The preferred lift between the semi-squat lift and the pure squat would be the semi-squat. In addition, the squat requires more energy expenditure, thus making the semi-squat the preferred lift for occasional heavy effort (four work cycles per minute). Van Dieen and colleagues suggest that the physical plant may not allow for such a lift (because of cramped spaces and so on).[49] For this reason a variation can be prescribed, with all practical considerations kept in mind. If lighter loads are to be handled but at a higher frequency than four per minute, the stoop lift would be a viable option. The caveat here would be whether or not the stoop requires a multiplanar effort, which would then put the lower lumbar segments at increased risk.

Marras and colleagues demonstrated that there are additional risk factors to be considered when assessing the injury potential of various lifting and high exertion efforts above and beyond what we have already discussed.[32] This section identifies a number of these factors and provides recommendations that the therapist can use.

The rate at which any lift is performed is extremely important. It has been well documented that lumbar compressive forces increase by 15% when lifting is performed quickly, as compared with using a steady, smooth approach when lifting identical loads.[4] The frequently seen phenomena of the "jerk lift" generally results from lifting a load in which the mass of the object to be lifted is unknown. Butler and colleagues compared the lifting strategies of subjects exposed to unmarked loads weighing 0, 150, 250, and 300 N.[5] They found that the majority of subjects were more prone to overestimate the mass of the unmarked load and braced for a heavy lift. This resulted in a rapid ascent and acceleration when lifting the lighter 0 and 150-N loads, which caused an unbalanced effort, hyperextension of the lumbar spine, and subsequent higher compressive lumbosacral moments. These findings imply that appropriate marking or "weight coding" may be an inexpensive and effective control to obviate this tendency.

The National Institute for Occupational Safety and Health (NIOSH) revised lifting formula of 1991 identified the important role of an effective hand grip and couple in the practice of safe lifting.[39] An additional consideration is the benefit of a secure grasp when handling an unstable load. Instability resulting from the lack of an effective grasp can adversely affect stability (of the load), which can and frequently does result in the involuntary increased recruitment of the core-trunk muscle groups (rectus and external and internal obliques). This greater coactivation of antagonistic muscles during the lift generally leads to increased lumbar compressive forces.[31]

The accepted design, although not always used in practice, is to have hand holes and handles on the object to reduce the incidence of unstable and "jerky, uncontrolled" efforts when lifting from a variety of work surface heights and when negotiating loads of differing mass. It was reported that acceleration times, vertical ground reaction forces, and L5/S1 compression were higher for boxes with handles than without in Freivalds' study of 1984.[14] These findings, albeit noteworthy, expressed only a small variance of 5 N (329 versus 324) and most probably were a result of the subjects being aware of the obvious hazard when lifting an object without handles and taking the necessary precautions.

OTHER CONSIDERATIONS

In the past numerous intangibles were not considered when researching the risk factors associated with lifting. Marras and Sommerich[33] and Granata and Marras[19] reported the benefit of using three-dimensional dynamic models when assessing the biomechanics of the lumbar spine during multiplanar movements outside of the sagittal plane. They postulated that the two-dimensional dynamic and static models grossly underestimated the true stress to the lower lumbar segments that typically occurred during a "real world effort."

Granata and Marras reported that compression at the L5/S1 joint was a poor indicator of the potential for injury.[20] Their findings concluded that accurate predictions, correlating effort and the potential for injury, would also have to take into consideration a number of other factors including the following:

- Load rate
- Lateral shear and torsion (side bending and twisting in coupled and uncoupled movements)
- Velocity
- Acceleration
- Worker experience and attitudes toward the job

Table 11-2 depicts the correlation coefficients r^2 between maximum spinal compressive-shear forces and the probability of a high-risk classification.

Other situations common to some occupations, but rarely seen in others, may have considerable

TABLE 11-2 **Correlation Coefficients r^2 between Maximum Spinal Compressive-Shear Forces and the Probability of a High-Risk Classification**

	Lateral Shear	AP Shear	Compression
Static load	—	—	0.135
Dynamic load	0.191	0.195	0.441
Load rate	0.343	0.345	0.428

AP, Anterioposterior.

impact on the potential for injury. Poor footing and ground slope were investigated to assess the potential for risk and resulted in the following conclusions. Kollmitzer et al reported that there was a definite advantage in a parallel vs. step-forward (staggered) stance when attempting to minimize the involuntary, often hazardous, postural adjustments that typically occur during a front load knee-to-chest lift.[24] The center of mass (COM) was maintained more efficiently, and compressive forces and lateral and anteroposterior shear involving the L5/S1 joint were significantly less.

Incline

Shin and Mirka suggested that lumbosacral moments were considerably larger when lifting from an inclined slope compared with a declined surface.[44] The explanation was that as the slope increased from −20 degrees to 0 degrees to +20 degrees, so did the flexion angle of the lumbar segments. This subsequent increase in angulation resulted in an increased moment arm of the trunk, hydrostatic pressure of the disc, and torque at the L5/S1 segment. This finding was consistent with all lift variations (stoop, squat, and semi-squat). It is interesting to note, however, that although there was a discernible difference in moment at the low back with varying slope surfaces, there was no appreciable difference in lifting capacities.[50] When assessing equal numbers of male and female subjects, there was less than a 2% variance between 40 degrees of slope angle (25.1 to

25.5 kg [55.3 to 56.2 lb] in male subjects and 19.9 to 20.3 kg [43.9 to 44.8 lb] in female subjects).

Stability of the Load

Stability of the load to be lifted will be our final analysis of extraneous physical factors influencing a subject's lifting capacity. The untoward results of negotiating a lift during which the subject's perception of effort is blinded have been discussed, but Lee and Lee took it one step further in their 2002 endeavor.[28] When comparing their subjects' response to lifting a stable load with one that has been manipulated to shift both anterior to posterior and vice versa, they found that the unstable loads carried significantly higher risks for poor mechanics and low back injury.

Postural data demonstrated that the lumbar spine flexes more during the unstable situation than when one is maneuvering a load that does not shift.[28] The tendency was to preserve a stable center of gravity (COG) by flexing the trunk and lowering the load and body as a unit. This resulted in a more kyphotic lumbar spine and exposed the intervertebral disc to even greater hydrostatic pressure. The lesson to be learned by these findings, and the application to the work site, would include the implementation of appropriate packaging processes and further education of those employees handling the material in a more biomechanically efficient manner.

A major goal for the therapist is to reduce the risk of lift-related injuries at both the work site and at home. The primary concern is to recognize the presence of risk factors and understand how each factor influences the pathologic process. Many risk factors that can predispose an individual to a lift-related injury have been identified in this chapter. A number of others have been researched, including the correlation between injury and anthropometrics, age, gender, smoking, obesity, and even parity.[29] These are factors, however, that either are inherited or reflect a personal choice and are not easily influenced by our interventions.

Factors that can be manipulated are the physical plant and worker attitude, if managed properly. The biomechanical analyses that have been enumerated provide us with very basic but proven standards that can be used to implement such an effort. These standards include the following:

- *Keep the load close.* Evidence overwhelmingly identifies the benefit of maintaining the load close to the body while lifting from a variety of work surface heights. The reduction in lumbar stress has been documented, and the behavior can be easily addressed in injury-prevention protocols.

- *Ensure the placement of a secure hand couple.* The presence of an effective grasp assist (handle or hand hole) minimizes trunk instability during a lift involving asymmetric handling and load shift. Studies have shown that handling an unstable load results in extrasagittal moments (lateral bending and torsion), causing increased compression, shear, and torque on the intervertebral disc. The uncontrolled and "jerky" movements that typically ensue also result in the recruitment of antagonist muscle groups, which adds to the co-activation factor and can further stress the lower lumbar components.

- *Maintain a degree of lumbar lordosis at the initiation and during the lift.* Granata and Bennett[18] and many other researchers have proven that the curvature (flexion beyond neutral) of the lumbar spine can exponentially increase the compressive and shear forces to the disc, particularly during lifting of loads in excess of 50 pounds. What is to be considered heavy is of course relative and should take a number of factors into account. However, the premise is sound; maintain as much lordosis as the situation will allow.

- *Use the lifting technique that is most applicable to the situation.* Although controversy exists as to which lifting technique is the most beneficial, there does appear to be some agreement as to which of the three most accepted lifts is more appropriate under what circumstances.

  Semi-squat. Frequently seen as the safest lift in terms of resultant forces to the intervertebral disc, but it does carry a high energy cost, which will limit applicability during highly repetitive efforts. Convention would dictate that this would be the ideal lift for heavy loads performed on an occasional basis (10% to 33% of the work day).

    Squat lift. To be used as an alternative to the semi-squat when space is limited and load size does not allow for foot placement to the side of the object to be lifted. This also is the lift preferred by individuals experiencing acute and chronic low back pain.

    Stoop lift. Although this lift is the antithesis of what is usually professed by the therapist as being the ideal lift, it apparently has an application. Lifting scenarios requiring light loads (20 pounds and below) on a frequent basis (defined as 33% to 66% of the workday by the Department of Labor's Dictionary of Occupational Titles) are more efficiently managed using this technique.

- *When lifting on an uneven-sloped surface, face down the slope to negotiate the lift.* Although the ideal would be to seek a level surface, when these circumstances do arise this approach has been proven to be the less hazardous.
- *When lifting, do so as much as is possible in the sagittal plane.* Although we live in a three-dimensional world, we need to be cognizant of the degree of deviation into multiplanar fields while lifting.

Pushing and Pulling

This chapter would be remiss if pushing and pulling activities were not discussed in the examination of material handling and injury potential. With the increasing evidence correlating lifting and carrying with low back and other musculoskeletal disorders, engineering controls have focused on converting these processes to ones that are seemingly less menacing and more biomechanically efficient, namely pushing and pulling.[42,43] What was found, however, was that the magnitude and type of forces acting on the spine, and the resultant vectors changed from the vertical to the horizontal axis, added the component of frictional resistance to the equation when pushing or pulling.[42]

De Looze and co-workers examined subjects who performed pushing and pulling tasks while walking on a treadmill.[11] One stage of the assessment monitored their performance when pushing or pulling against a stationary bar, and the other involved pushing and pulling a four-wheeled cart on the same treadmill. Both experiments were conducted at the same rate of speed.

Both the low back and shoulder complexes were examined. Results demonstrated that the net joint torques at the shoulder were minimal during pushing maneuvers but greatly increased during pulling efforts. Horizontal force, as opposed to torque, at the shoulder was significant during both activities. The mediating factor was that of handle height and hand placement, with the correlation being positive as the height increased from 50% to 80% of shoulder height. Vertical forces were most prominent with the handle and hand placement at the lowest positions, whereas horizontal forces remained constant or slightly increased as the handle placement became higher.

Compressive forces to the shoulder while pushing changed as the approach became more vertical, implying that handle heights at or below 50% of shoulder height may predispose the shoulder to impingement.[11] No inferences were made relative to the potential for injury while pulling, but it would make intuitive sense that with increased loads, torque at the shoulder, particularly through internal rotation, would increase, subjecting the soft tissue of the subacromial region to insult. However, more research in this area is warranted.

Optimal pushing height for the best performance appeared to be at or about waist level. The greatest potential to overcome inertial forces and sustain the effort occurred at handle heights between 100 and 109 cm, approximately 70% of shoulder height.[18] Chaffin and colleagues have determined this optimal zone to be quite similar, between 91 and 114 cm.[7]

Although there is an optimal zone to generate maximal pushing efforts, the effect such efforts may have on the lower lumbar region reveals that different vectors of force result as the lumbar moments change. Using the more horizontal approach was found to increase lumbar moments substantially as compared with a more vertically oriented effort.[18] The tendency of those subjects participating in this study was to change from a more forward, flexed-at-the-waist, extended-elbow position to a more extended trunk and flexed-elbow strategy as the load increased. This appeared to be an automatic strategy to protect lower lumbar structures from increased stress.

Comparing pulling with pushing, the vector of force is substantially higher at the L5/S1 joint when pulling as compared with pushing. This comes as a direct result of the increased moment and flexed posture (at the waist) inherent with pulling as opposed to pushing.[18] De Looze and co-workers also found that torque at the L5/S1 was significantly higher with pulling as opposed to pushing, further illustrating that, if possible, pushing should be the preferred method of material transport over pulling.[11]

The final consideration when evaluating pushing and pulling tasks is foot placement and the avoidance of slippage resulting from a poor coefficient of friction (COF). Injuries secondary to these conditions can be serious and usually result from the loss of balance and uncontrolled acceleration of the whole body.

The optimal COF while pushing appears to be 0.6. In their landmark study of 1971, Kroemer and Robinson reported that pushing force potential decreased significantly when the COF fell below this mark.[26] Gao and Abeysekera reported that walking on a dry, level surface results in an acceptable COF of 0.5.[15] Adding water, oil, or other contaminants to the surface, however, greatly decreased the COF and resulted in decreased balance and sway patterns. The need, then, for careful analysis of the flooring type and tripping and slipping hazards cannot be overstated.

COF considerations are also a factor when considering potential force production. It was found that subjects were capable of efforts in excess of 66% higher when pushing objects on surfaces carrying a COF greater than 0.5.[6] This agreed with previous studies affirming the need for a level, dry surface when any pushing or pulling activity is being evaluated.[13,25]

Once the risk factors have been identified, it is the therapist's mission to control the frequency, severity, and, if possible, the very presence of the risk. For this reason standardized material handling guidelines have been developed by a number of authors and agencies. The gold standard, to date, is that which has been developed by NIOSH. A review and critique follow.

MANUAL LIFTING ANALYSIS

NIOSH developed the *Work Practices Guide for Manual Lifting* as the first comprehensive tool to assist in the process of risk factor identification and subsequent ergonomic abatement to correct those factors identified as being potential problems. Terms such as *action limit* (AL) and *maximum permissible limit* (MPL) became synonymous with this first true work practices guide.[38]

The requirements for the analysis were that the lift to be analyzed be two-handed, be smooth, provide unrestricted posturing, and involve the handling of a container whose width did not exceed 76.2 cm—basically, an ideal lift. The goal was to establish the AL, which was defined as the calculated-average load for a lift that could be managed safely by 99% of the working male population and 75% of the working female population. The MPL then would be the product of three times the AL.

The equation that was developed looked like this:

$$AL = 90 \times (6/H) \times (1 - [0.01|V - 30|]) \times (0.7 + [3/D]) \times (1 - [F/F_{max}])$$

Where:

H = The horizontal distance of the load from the worker

V = The vertical distance of the load from the floor or work surface to the hand couple before the lift

D = The vertical displacement of the lift from start to finish

F = The frequency of the lift

F_{max} = The frequency coefficient based on the length of the work day (1 to 8 hours)

The calculation then resulted in determining the AL. If the actual weight of the object being lifted in the analysis exceeded the MPL ($3 \times$ AL), then the lift was deemed hazardous.

The ergonomic community initially applauded the guideline as precedent setting and a welcomed standard from which to conduct accurate measures of potential risk. It wasn't long, however, before the instrument came under fire for being impractical and not applicable to endeavors that required asymmetric lifting efforts. This resulted in the revision of the guideline in 1991.

The revised guideline took into consideration two new, but very important, real-world variables that occurred during most lifting activities, those being an angle of asymmetry and the quality of hand couple.[39] As the original guideline assessed the lift only in the sagittal plane, the new guideline made provisions for the angle of displacement from the line of load center to the center of the ankle from beginning to end point. This was measured relative to the midsagittal plane.

The other added feature was efficacy of hand couple. This was classified using the following three criteria: (1) good—fingers wrapped completely around the object or handle; (2) fair—not all but a few of the fingers could grasp the object or handle; and (3) poor—partial or fingertip grasp of the object or handle.

The revised equation would now result in the determination of a recommended weight of lift (RWL). This value would represent the MAW recommended to pose a minimal amount of risk to 90% of the working population as a whole.

CASE STUDY

Job Description

Harold works as a cook and order-taker at a fast-food restaurant. He is 6 feet 4 inches (193 cm) tall, of slender build, and the primary provider for his family. After suffering sporadic lower back pain for several years, Harold received the diagnosis of acquired spinal stenosis with shooting pain in the right leg. Harold experiences the most pain when he repetitively hands trays of food to customers during a busy lunch hour. The counter is 36 inches (91 cm) wide, 48 inches (122 cm) high at the customer service end, and 36 inches (91 cm) high where the worker fills the trays with food. The filled trays of food weigh as much as 5 pounds (2.3 kg), and the worker is not allowed to slide the tray of food across the counter.

Job Analysis

The calculations using the 1981 formula are as follows:

$$AL = 90 \times (6/H) \times (1 - [0.01 \, |V - 30|]) \times (0.7 + [3/D]) \times [1 - (F/F_{max})]$$

H origin = 18 inches (46 cm); V origin = 42 inches (107 cm)

H destination = 30 inches (76 cm); V destination = 50 inches (127 cm)

D = 8 inches (20 cm); F = four lifts per minute

$F_{max} = 18$ (from F_{max} table, NIOSH 1981)

$$AL \text{ (destination)} = 90 \times (6/30) \times (1 - [0.01 \, |50 - 30|]) \times (0.7 + [3/8]) \times (1 - [4/18])$$
$$= 90 \times 0.2 \times 0.8 \times 1.075 \times 0.78$$
$$= 12 \text{ pounds (5.4 kg)}$$

The calculations using the 1991 lifting formula are as follows:

$$RWL \text{ (destination)} = 51 \times (10/H) \times (1 - [0.0075 \, |V - 30|]) \times (0.82 + [1.8/D]) \times (1 - 0.0032 \, A) \times FM \times CM$$

H origin = 18 inches (46 cm); V origin = 30 inches (76 cm)

H destination = 30 inches (76 cm); V destination = 50 inches (127 cm)

D = 8 inches (20 cm); A = 0

FM = 0.84 (from table; using the criteria of four lifts per minute, duration of ≤1 hour, V ≥ 30 in. [76 cm])

CM = 1 (from table; using the criteria of good coupling and V ≥ 30 inches [76 cm])

$$RWL = 51 \times (10/30) \times ([1 - (0.0075 \, |50 - 30|]) \times (0.82 + [1.8/8]) \times 1 \times 0.84 \times 1$$
$$= 51 \times 0.33 \times 0.85 \times 1.045 \times 0.84$$
$$= 12.56 \text{ pounds (5.7 kg)}$$

Discussion

The actual weight of the object being lifted is 2.3 kg (5 pounds), well below the 5.4-kg (12-pound) AL calculated using the 1981 formula and the 5.7-kg (12.56-pound) RWL calculated using the 1991 formula. Clearly, more risk factors are present for Harold than just lifting food trays. For someone with Harold's diagnosis, activities that involve repetitive forward flexion should be avoided. This example demonstrates an important concept for evaluators of work sites. The NIOSH formula was designed to be used as a guideline only and is not the only factor to be considered in the evaluation of a workstation. The lifting formula does, however, provide a way to break the lifting task into components. Analysis of the task variables of both calculations shows that the horizontal multiplier causes the greatest reduction in each LC (0.2 in the 1981 formula and 0.33 in the 1991 formula). Figure 11-5 shows that the horizontal reach of the job is of primary importance.

This lifting task can be analyzed with the 1981 formula because no asymmetric twisting is involved in the lift. When the 1991 formula is used, the asymmetric and coupling multipliers are not a factor ($A = 0$; $CM = 1$). For this job, the difference between the 1981 AL (12 pounds [5.4 kg]) and the 1991 RWL (12.56 pounds [5.7 kg]) is negligible.

Harold never successfully returned to work as a fast-food employee. He did benefit from education in proper body mechanics and learned how to stabilize his back when performing the tray-lifting job. However, Harold could not tolerate the constant standing and repetitive movements involved in all aspects of fast-food work. He moved from a cold to a warm climate and assumed a job as a bookstore manager. He reported that he finds the warm climate better for his back.

Although the revised version of the NIOSH lifting formula was more flexible in its scope, it still lacked the pragmatic application that most clinical staff would require in their everyday practice.

NIOSH has made a number of additional attempts to upgrade the model, but to date, their application far exceeds what most therapists would consider practical in the quick but discerning evaluation of workplace risk factors. To this end the search for an expeditious but effective screening tool that could identify a potentially hazardous work practice led to my endorsement of the Utah Assessment of Back Compressive Forces.

UTAH ASSESSMENT OF BACK COMPRESSIVE FORCES (BLOSWICK ESTIMATION OF BACK COMPRESSIVE FORCE)

The Utah Assessment of Back Compressive Forces is a relatively simple and concise tool to evaluate the compressive forces encountered by the lower lumbar spine during various lifting efforts. As can be seen by reviewing Figure 11-6,

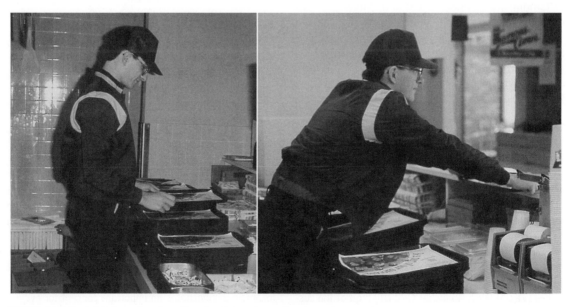

FIGURE 11-5 Fast-food worker handing food tray to customer.

Estimation of Back Compressive Force
A representation of the model by Donald S. Bloswick at the University of Utah.

Job		Analyst	
Task		Date	

Measure			Symbol	Value
Body weight [lb]			BW	[lb]
Load [lb]			L	[lb]
Horizontal distance [in] (Hands to lower back {L5-S1 joint})			HB	[in]
Back posture (angle from vertical)	Θ [°]	sin Θ	Θ	[°]
Vertical	0	0.0		
Bent 1/4 of the way	23	0.4	sin Θ	[–]
Bent 1/2 of the way	45	0.7		
Bent 3/4 of the way	67	0.9		
Horizontal	90	1.0		

Contributor	Computation	Value
Back posture $A = 3(BW) \sin\Theta$	3 * ( ) * ( )	
Load moment $B = 0.5(L * HB)$	0.5 * ( ) * ( )	
Direct compression $C = 0.8[(BW)/2 + L]$	0.8 * {( ) / 2 + ( )}	
Estimated compressive force $F_c = A + B + C$	Sum computed values in last column. Comparison value: 700 lb	

If the estimated compressive forces exceeds 700 lb, consider a more detailed analysis or make changes. Note: This is just an estimate and its accuracy varies with posture, especially as the hands move forward of the shoulders.

FIGURE 11-6 Bloswick's revised estimation of back compressive force. (From Bloswick DS: Ergonomics. In Harris RL, editor: *Patty's industrial hygiene and toxicology*, ed 5, vol 4, New York, 2000, John Wiley & Sons.)

the examiner determines the values listed on the worksheet and addresses the variables of body weight, load, horizontal distance, and back posture. These then become the components of an equation that can predict the potential or actual existence of excessive lower lumbar compressive forces. At this juncture the therapist can manipulate any of the variables to provide the necessary ergonomic abatement. This can be done on site and in many cases affect the situation immediately.

Although the issue of asymmetry is not addressed in this quick screen, all of the most frequently encountered risk factors are identified and measured. If, again, the activity is deemed poten-tially hazardous by this preliminary assessment tool, then a more elaborate biomechanical analysis taking into account multiplanar movement patterns can be applied.

Let's review our case study of Boston Packaging, Inc. The first step for the therapist was to assess, via a quick screen, the risk potential of the job. At the time of the ergonomic assessment, two employees were working the line, one male and one female. The man weighed 210 pounds, and the woman weighed 130 pounds.

The Bloswick Estimation of Back Compressive Force was chosen as the quick reference guide. To illustrate the differences between potential and actual compressive forces, both individuals were assessed. Figure 11-6 has the following computations:

	Male Employee	Female Employee
Body weight	210 lb	130 lb
Load	20 lb	20 lb
Horizontal distance (hands to lower back)	50 inches	24 inches
Trunk angle	0.9 (¾ bend)	0.4 (¼ bend)

The reason for the considerable differences between the male and female employees' horizontal and trunk angle distances was the male's tendency to stack the pallets back row first with a front-oriented approach. This resulted in his adoption of a stooped posture while lowering the load to the pallet, thus increasing the lever and moment arm and angle of trunk flexion (Figure 11-7, *A*).

Conversely the female employee chose a different approach. She preferred to walk behind the pallet to load the back row. This allowed for the box to be maintained closer to the body and for her to employ the squat lift, one more appropriate for heavier loads (Figure 11-7, *B*). This in turn reduced the lever and moment arm and decreased the angle of trunk flexion. The comparative analysis of the two approaches, using the equation in Figure 11-6, demonstrated the following.

	Male Employee	Female Employee
Back posture	567	156
Load moment	500	240
Direct compression	100	68
Sum	1167 lb (5134 N)	464 lb (2042 N)

It is quite clear that the male employee's extremely forward bent posture, in addition to the excessive moment arm created by reaching over the length of the pallet, created forces to the lower lumbar structure far in excess than has been deemed safe by NIOSH's lifting guidelines. In contrast, the female employee handled the same object in a much more efficient manner, exposing her to significantly less compressive force.

The therapist's first recommendation would be to train all employees assigned to this packaging line in the proper loading of the pallet, in addition to demonstrating the proper lifting technique.

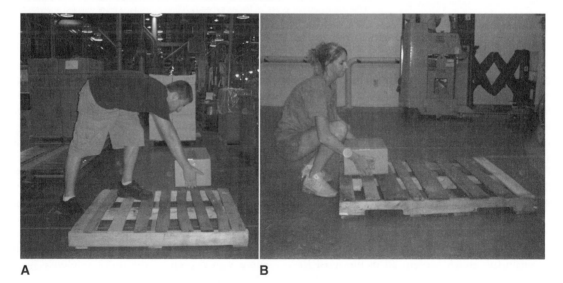

A   **B**

FIGURE **11-7 A,** Male worker—stoop lift. **B,** Female worker—squat lift.

Further considerations would include recommendations regarding pallet height assistive devices such as scissor or other hydraulic lifts that would limit the horizontal distance that would have to be negotiated. These, again, are examples of knowing what variables contribute to the risks and how the variables can be manipulated to mitigate the risks.

After reflecting on the case study, answer the following questions:

1. Identify the most critical aspects of the subject's work characteristics as outlined in this case study that predispose him or her to injury.
2. Which risk factors can be addressed immediately, and which can be minimized through work site design modification?
3. How are you, as the consulting therapist, going to justify to the company's administrators the expenditure of nonbudgeted monies to rectify the potential risks?

CONCLUSION

The analysis of lifting, and the inherent risk factors associated with it, is an ongoing process. The review of evidence literature reveals that there is no particular lifting technique that is superior to another, but there are a number of principles that need to be observed when an individual is exposed to a potentially difficult and injury-producing endeavor. To reiterate, these include the following:

- Maintain the load as close to the body as possible
- Ensure adequate hand couple
- Maintain the lumbar spine in as much of a lordotic curve as possible
- Lift in the sagittal plane, and avoid extraneous multiplanar movement patterns
- Ensure proper footing
- Lift slowly
- Use the lifting technique (stoop, squat, semi-squat) best suited for the situation

These principles can easily be applied to any number of occupational scenarios that require moderate or heavy lifting. From the shipping and receiving dock floor to the nursing unit, common everyday stressors can be mitigated if these criteria are followed.

Occupational and physical therapists possess a breadth of knowledge relative to the factors that influence human performance. It is our responsibility as therapists to incorporate this knowledge into common processes to prevent the maladies associated with aberrant lifting practices through education, early intervention once an injury has

---

Learning Exercise

Overview

Can the biomechanical analysis of a potentially injurious lift be captured by observation alone?

Purpose

The purpose of this exercise is to determine, through observation, what happens at various joint structures (particularly the low back, hips, knees, neck) at and approaching an individual's stated or perceived maximum lifting effort. If your observations are reliable and can be replicated, they can serve as means by which a work situation can be identified as potentially hazardous. From that point a more empirically based analysis can be performed.

Exercise

Observe classmates during a floor-to-waist lift using a standard milk crate as the container. Increase the load to be lifted by regular increments (5 to 10 pounds) until the individual reaches his or her safe lifting maximum. Observe for the following:

1. At what point does the subject's lifting style change?
2. What lifting style (squat, stoop, semi-squat) does the subject adopt at the outset, and what style is employed at the maximal effort?
3. What changes in joint angulation (estimate only) occur at the hip versus the low back, knees, and head and neck as the subject advances from an easily managed load to one that is subjectively perceived as difficult?

occurred, and postinjury maintenance programming.

A critical component of our involvement is to become familiar with the nuances of our patients' lifestyles, be it at work or at home, and what practices may put them at risk for lift-related low back injury or the aggravation of an ongoing condition. This requires observation not only in the clinic but also at the work site and at times at home. We must become mobile therapists, because practice demands may require that we treat offsite, at the work place, or in the clinic and that we follow the patient once he or she has returned to full duty. As a result I have been able to devote this comprehensive care model for the worker with an injury. It is through this ongoing involvement with our clients and the commitment to further research that we can make a positive impact on the occurrence and prevalence of lift-related injuries.

Multiple Choice Review Questions

1. The spinal motion segment consists of:
   A. the apophyseal joint and lumbar paraspinals.
   B. adjacent vertebral bodies and the intervertebral disc.
   C. the junction of the sacrum and the ilium.
   D. interspinous ligaments and vertebral endplates.

2. The motion segment is exposed to which force vectors(s)?
   A. Compression, torsion, shear
   B. Flexion, extension, sidebending
   C. Sagittal, transverse, frontal
   D. Ascending, descending, lateral

3. The three most researched lifting techniques include:
   A. squat, semi-squat, and stoop.
   B. stoop, kinetic, and crouch.
   C. squat, quad, and astride.
   D. golfer's, lateral, and semi-squat.

4. The lifting technique that requires greatest aerobic cost is:
   A. the stoop.
   B. the squat.
   C. the semi-squat.
   D. the kinetic lift.

5. Per the NIOSH lifting guide, the maximum allowable force that the L5/S1 segment can withstand is:
   A. 2000 N.
   B. 3400 N.
   C. 5000 N.
   D. 1000 N.

6. Which of the following lifting techniques would be ideal for a task that requires lifting frequent, light loads from the floor?
   A. Stoop
   B. Squat
   C. Semi-squat
   D. Kinetic

7. Which is the preferred lift of those who are experiencing chronic or acute low back pain?
   A. Stoop
   B. Squat
   C. Semi-squat
   D. Kinetic

8. The optimal height range from which to overcome inertial forces while pushing is:
   A. 90 to 115 cm.
   B. 50 to 65 cm.
   C. 100 to 125 cm.
   D. 70 to 90 cm.

9. The variable that was used in the 1991 NIOSH lifting guide that set it apart from its predecessor (i.e., the 1981 lifting guide) was:
   A. vertical displacement.
   B. horizontal distance from the load.
   C. type of hand couple.
   D. frequency of the lift.

10. The Bloswick Evaluation of Low Back Compressive Forces uses what benchmark as its maximum allowable aggregate?
   A. 500 pounds
   B. 800 pounds
   C. 1000 pounds
   D. 700 pounds

REFERENCES

1. Andersson GBJ: Epidemiologic aspects on low back pain in industry, *Spine* 6(1):53, 1981.
2. Bendix T, Eid SE: The distance between the load and the body with bi-manual lifting techniques, *Appl Ergon* 14(3):185, 1983.
3. Bureau of Labor Statistics: *Lost-work time injuries and illness: characteristics and resulting time away from work, USDL 04-460*, Washington, DC, 2002, U.S. Department of Labor.
4. Bush-Joseph C, Schipplein O, Andersson GB et al: Influence of the dynamic factors on the lumbar spine moment in lifting, *Ergonomics* 31(2):211, 1988.
5. Butler D, Andersson GB, Trafimow J et al: The influence of load knowledge on lifting technique, *Ergonomics* 36(12):1489, 1993.
6. Chaffin DB: A biomedical model for use in industry, *Am Ind Hyg Assoc J* 3(3):79, 1988.
7. Chaffin DB, Andersson GB, Bernard MJ: *Occupational biomechanics*, ed 4, New York, 2006, John Wiley & Sons.
8. Chen Y-L: Optimal lifting techniques adopted by Chinese men when determining their maximum acceptable weight of lift, *Am Ind Hyg Assoc J* 61(8):642, 2000.
9. Damkot DK, Pope MH, Lord J et al: The relationship between work history, work environment and low back pain in men, *Spine* 9(4):395, 1984.
10. de Looze MP, Kingma I, Thunnissen V et al: The evaluation of practical biomechanical model estimating lumbar moments in occupational activities, *Ergonomics* 37(9):1495, 1994.
11. de Looze MP, van Greuningen K, Rebel J et al: Force direction and physical load dynamic pushing and pulling, *Ergonomics* 43(3):377, 2000.
12. Dolan P, Earley M, Adams MA: Bending and compressive stresses acting on the lumbar spine during lifting activities, *J Biomech* 27(10):1237, 1994.
13. Fox WF: Body weight and coefficient of friction determinants of pushing capability. In *Human Engineering Special Studies Series*, No 17, Marietta, Ga, 1967, Lockheed.
14. Freivalds A, Chaffin DB, Garg A et al: A dynamic biomechanical evaluation of lifting maximum acceptable loads, *J Biomech* 17(4):251, 1984.
15. Gao G, Abeysekera J: A systems perspective of slip and fall accidents on icy and snowy surfaces, *Ergonomics* 47(5):573, 2004.
16. Garg A: What basis exists for training workers in correct lifting technique? In Marras WS, Karwowski W, Smith JL et al, editors: *The ergonomics of manual work,* London, 1993, Taylor & Francis.
17. Garg A, Saxena U: Physiological stresses in warehouse operations with special reference to lifting technique and gender: a case study, *Am Ind Hyg Assoc J* 46(2):53, 1985.
18. Granata KP, Bennett BC: Low-back biomechanics and static stability during isometric pushing, *Hum Factors* 47(3):536, 2005.
19. Granata KP, Marras WS: An EMG-assisted model of loads on the lumbar spine during asymmetric trunk extensions, *J Biomech* 26(12):1429, 1993.
20. Granata KP, Marras WS: Relation between spinal load factors and the high-risk probability of occupational low-back disorder, *Ergonomics* 42(9):1187, 1999.
21. Granata KP, Marras WS, Davis KG: Variation in spinal load and trunk dynamics during repeated lifting exertions, *Clin Biomech* 14(6):367, 1999.
22. Hagen KB, Harms-Ringdahl K, Hallen J: Influence of lifting technique on perceptual and cardiovascular responses to submaximal repetitive lifting, *Eur J Appl Physiol Occup Physiol* 68(6):477, 1994.
23. Kingma I, Bosch T, Bruin L et al: Foot positioning instruction, initial vertical load position and lifting technique: effects on low back loading, *Ergonomics* 47(13):1365, 2004.
24. Kollmitzer J, Oddsson L, Ebenbichler GR et al: Postural control during lifting, *J Biomech* 35(5):585, 2002.
25. Kroemer KHE: *Push forces exerted in 65 common work positions, AMRTL-68-143,* Wright-Patterson Air Force Base, Ohio, 1969, Aerospace Medical Research Laboratory.
26. Kroemer KHE, Robinson DE: *Horizontal static forces exerted by men standing in common working postures on surfaces of various tractions, AMARL-TR-70-114,* Wright-Patterson Air Force Base, Ohio, 1971, Aerospace Medical Research Laboratory.
27. Kumar S: Lumbosacral compression in maximal lifting efforts in sagittal plane with varying mechanical disadvantage in isometric and isokinetic modes, *Ergonomics* 37(12):1975, 1994.
28. Lee YH, Lee TH: Human muscular and postural responses in unstable load lifting, *Spine* 27(17):1881, 2002.

29. Levangie PK: Association of low back pain with self-reported risk factors among patients seeking physical therapy services, *Phys Ther* 79(8):757, 1999.

30. Magnusson M, Granqvist M, Jonson R et al: The loads on the lumbar spine during work at an assembly line. The risks for fatigue injuries of vertebral bodies, *Spine* 15(8):774, 1990.

31. Marras WS, Davis KG, Kirking BC et al: A comprehensive analysis of low-back disorder risk and spinal loading during the transferring and repositioning of patients using different techniques, *Ergonomics* 42(7):904, 1999.

32. Marras WS, Lavender SA, Leurgans SE et al: The role of dynamic three-dimensional trunk motion in occupationally-related low back disorders. The effects of workplace factors, trunk position, and trunk motion characteristics on risk of injury, *Spine* 18(5):617, 1993.

33. Marras WS, Sommerich CM: A three-dimensional motion model of loads on the lumbar spine: I. model structure, *Hum Factors* 33(2):123, 1991.

34. McGill S: *Low back disorders: evidence-based prevention and rehabilitation,* Champaign, Ill, 2002, Human Kinetics.

35. McGill SM, Norman RW: Effects of an anatomically detailed erector spinae model on L4/L5 disc compression and shear, *J Biomech* 20(6):591, 1987.

36. Mittal M, Malik SL: Biomechanical evaluation of lift postures in adult Koli female labourers, *Ergonomics* 34(1):103, 1991.

37. Nachemson A: In vivo measurements of intradiscal pressure, *J Bone Joint Surg Am* 46:1077, 1964.

38. NIOSH: *Work practices guide for manual lifting,* U.S. Department of Health and Human Services, NIOSH Technical Report No. 81122, Cincinnati, 1981, NIOSH.

39. NIOSH: *Scientific support documentation for the revised 1991 NIOSH lifting equation: technical contract reports,* Springfield, Va, 1991, U.S. Department of Commerce, Technical Information Service.

40. Potvin JR, McGill SM, Norman RW: Trunk, muscle and lumbar ligament contributions to dynamic lifts with varying degrees of trunk flexion, *Spine* 16(9):1099, 1991.

41. Rabinowitz D, Bridger RS, Lambert MI: Lifting techniques and abnormal belt usage: a biomechanical, physiological and subjective investigation, *Safety Sci* 28:155, 1998.

42. Resnick ML, Chaffin DB: Kinematics, kinetics, and psychophysical perceptions in symmetric and twisting pushing and pulling tasks, *Hum Factors* 38(1):114, 1996.

43. Schibye B, Skogaard K, Laursen B et al: Mechanical load of the spine during pushing and pulling. In Seppalla P, Luopajarvi T, Nygard CH et al, editors: *Proceedings of the 13th Triennial Congress of the IEA,* vol 4, 1997.

44. Shin G, Mirka G: The effects of a sloped ground surface on trunk kinematics and L5/S1 moment during lifting, *Ergonomics* 47(6):646, 2004.

45. Straker LM: A review of research on techniques for lifting low-lying objects: 2. Evidence for a correct technique, *Work* 20(2):83, 2003.

46. Straker L, Duncan P: Psychophysical and psychological comparison of squat and stoop lifting by young females, *Austr J Physiother* 46(1):27, 2000.

47. Toussaint HM, van Baar CE, van Langen PP et al: Coordination of leg muscles in backlift and leglift, *J Biomech* 25(11):1279, 1992.

48. Troup JD, Leskinen TP, Stalhammar HR et al: A comparison of intraabdominal pressure increases, hip torque, and lumbar vertebral compression in different lifting techniques, *Hum Factors* 25(5):517, 1983.

49. van Dieen JH, Hoozemans MJ, Toussaint HM: Stoop or squat: a review of biomechanical studies on lifting technique, *Clin Biomech* 14(10):685, 1999.

50. Wickel E, Reiser RF: *Effect of floor slope on submaximal lifting capacity,* Presented at the Rocky Mountain Bioengineering Symposium & International ISA Biomechanical Sciences Instrumentation Symposium, Ft. Collins, Colo, 2004.

51. Wrigley AT, Albert WJ, Deluzio KJ et al: Differentiating lifting technique between those who develop low back pain and those who do not, *Clin Biomech* 20(3):254, 2005.

SUGGESTED READING

The resources below may be obtained through the following website: www.hsc.usf.edu/~tbernard/ergotools:

- Liberty Mutual Manual Materials Handling Tables (1991)
- Utah Back Compressive Force by Donald S. Bloswick
- NIOSH Work Practices Guide for Lifting (www.cdc.gov/niosh/94-110.html)
- Static Work Analysis, based on Rohmert methods.
- Estimation of Metabolic Rate

12

Seating

Ellen Rader Smith

Learning Objectives

After reading this chapter and completing the exercises, the reader should be able to do the following:

1. Appreciate the importance of the seated worker's need for good chair support.
2. Appreciate the natural conflicts between the body's need for dynamic movement and the need for support while seated.
3. Apply basic ergonomic and biomechanical principles and job or task analysis to make appropriate chair recommendations.

Adjustability. The ability to change; with reference to chairs, features should allow, rather than inhibit, postural changes.

ANSI/HFES. The American National Standards Institute/Human Factors and Ergonomics Society, the organizations that are jointly developing new ergonomic guidelines for computer workstations.

Static muscle loading. A continuous state of muscle contraction without active movement; as related to maintaining one fixed work posture; associated with depleting muscles of oxygen and fresh blood supply and the accumulation of waste products.

*Portions of this chapter are retained from the previous edition chapter written by Diane C. Hermenau.

CASE STUDY

Jim is a dental technician and the owner of a full-service dental laboratory. He sustained injuries to the cervical spine in a motor vehicle accident. Following C4-5 surgical fusion, Jim was initially unable to resume work duties because of his inability to maintain the required work posture or sustain his upper body in a position to allow the performance of fine precision required to finish dental crowns, paint and glaze teeth, or sit at a computer and perform the administrative aspects of his business. Occupational therapy and ergonomic intervention were initiated to facilitate Jim's return to work. This involved a review of his specific work duties at two dental benches and at his desk so that the appropriate chairs could be selected in conjunction with other ergonomic interventions.

Concomitant with the growth of computers throughout industrial and traditional offices and the changed nature of workplace from multidimensional to unidimensional is the importance of supportive chairs for workers who are required to sit the majority of the day. The workday no longer has many of the natural breaks that used to be related to the diverse job tasks that allowed workers greater opportunities to get up and move around. For this reason, chair design and selection are at the core of ergonomic workstation design and are critical to the comfort, well-being, and productivity of all seated persons, whether they be office workers, assembly line workers, production workers, students, administrative assistants, or office executives, because poorly designed workstations put users at risk for musculoskeletal injuries.

Increasingly, therapists with expertise in seating and ergonomic workplace design are working as industrial consultants for seating issues. This chapter discusses the biomechanics of sitting, the risks related to prolonged sitting and poor posture, the features of ergonomic chair design, and the importance of a proper worker-workstation fit as part of an ergonomically correct work environment.

CONSIDERATIONS OF SITTING

It has long been known that movement is essential to health, well-being, and levels of alertness. People are designed for activity and not sitting. The body's need for movement is common knowledge even to laypersons, who, for example, begin seeking more comfortable positions and making postural adjustments during extended car rides, after initially being able to sit comfortably. While true for both passengers and drivers, this is particularly true for the driver who is "glued" to the steering wheel and needs to remain focused on the road. Changing the seat inclination and stopping the car to take a stretch break are other comfort-driven actions with which lay persons are familiar. Take this real-life situation a step further and consider the effects of prolonged sitting on a long-distance truck driver, who is also exposed to jarring shocks and vibration and who is limited in his freedom to stop because of his need to reach his destination in a timely manner. Similarly, employees at light assembly, inspection, and conveyor workstations are captives in their chairs and work areas and lack the free-dom to get up[45] or move around because they are performing one step in a work process that depends on each worker in the production process. Office workers in nonelectronic offices used to have many built-in breaks, such as retrieving files or reference information, faxing, copying, and face-to-face communication with co-workers. In today's electronic office workers are no longer afforded many of the traditional breaks from prolonged sitting, because these tasks can now be routinely performed at self-contained workstations, minimizing workers' need to get up.[13]

Researchers began studying the effects of sitting on the body in the 1940s. *Sitting* has been defined as a position in which the weight of the body is transferred to a supporting area, mainly by the ischial tuberosities of the pelvis and their surrounding soft tissues.[49] In sitting, most of the body weight is on the buttocks, back, and feet. Biomechanical and ergonomic research has flourished since the 1970s when back pain and other musculoskeletal issues related to sitting and static muscle loading were identified as a larger part of health and wellness issues, particularly as work in many sectors, such as textiles and laboratories, has become more sedentary. Jobs that once involved a variety of tasks that allowed workers the opportunity to freely move around their work areas now require sitting for prolonged periods in fixed postures at computer terminals.

Occupational and physical therapists who address well populations, young and old, working and nonworking, realize that the issues related to sitting comfortably are not restricted to the workplace. Consider students from preschool through college who are using computers more and more. What type of chairs do they have? On what type of work surfaces are the computers placed? Are changes made to one or the other or both as a child grows? Have the schools recognized the role of ergonomic furnishings for computers that are now used throughout the system, and in particular placed side by side in limited areas at tables that are not always intended for computers? Consider students who sit in the classroom all day and who then sit at their home computers to do homework or in front of electronic game systems. Whether doing research at home or in the library, students, professionals, and nonprofessionals alike can do more from one sedentary posture by clicking on the Internet than by actively exploring bookshelves or files. It is clear that healthy sitting habits need to be instilled in students from a young age and that they need to integrate movement into their regular lifestyle and way of life, to reduce the risk for any of the conditions that are well known to a generation of "couch potatoes" (see Chapter 14).

THE BODY'S NEED FOR MOVEMENT

We often sit because of the fatigue that results from standing, as sitting requires about 20% less energy in comparison with standing.[25] Sitting is also a more efficient way to perform many occupational and nonoccupational tasks, as the chair offers the necessary support and stability that is a prerequisite to performing purposeful coordinated movement or work tasks. Sitting in many jobs makes good sense, as it relieves the body's supporting muscles (e.g., those of the trunk and legs), offers them a chance to rest, and is less demanding on the blood circulation to the legs. Sitting

allows the chair, along with the floor or a footrest, to support the seated person's body mass. With all this said, it must be realized that the body was designed not to sit, but rather to move. This presents a dichotomy: Should we sit or stand, as neither is entirely restful for our bodies, or should we find some balance between the two?

Most sitting or sedentary work tasks require the use of the hands and arms to accomplish meaningful tasks or work. However, with little active or dynamic movement of larger muscle groups, these muscles are in a prolonged state of contraction and a state of heightened tension.[23] Because the muscles are not afforded the benefits of active pumping of blood that transports sugar and oxygen to dynamically contracting muscles, they must depend on their own reservoirs. This results in the buildup of waste products such as CO_2 and lactic acid, which then causes muscle spasms and fatigue.

Movement helps increase blood flow throughout the body to the muscles and relieves pressure on the discs. A lack of active movement while sitting and working in relatively flexed postures also results in static muscle loading, which can lead to venous pooling, causing the legs to swell. Another consideration in assessing the effect on seated posture is how the maximal voluntary contraction (MVC) relates to the onset of muscle fatigue and the recovery time from static work loads.[12] Cortlett compares the limits of static work to the experience of muscle pain, similar to how elevated heart rates or shortness of breath are indicators of the limits of physical activity. Grandjean notes that MVCs of <20% of the maximal muscle contraction, and in particular those not greater than 8% of the maximum, can be held for longer periods without fatigue, in contrast to shorter tolerances to sustain static work when a high percent of a person's maximum force is required.[23] Rodgers has done extensive research on the interrelationships of static work loads, required rest periods, job design, and job enlargement to minimize the effects of these issues for seated workers.[44]

At the computer, keyboarding involves both static and dynamic work, as does light assembly work when the work object is near the operator.

Static muscle work is required by the shoulders and arms to hold the hands at the required work position, and dynamic finger and hand motions are required to key or manipulate objects. Use of a mouse is often associated with higher static loading factors, as the mouse is not always adjacent to the keyboard, resulting in arm postures associated with extended forward or lateral arm reaches. It will become more evident throughout this chapter that the chair must provide users with optimal support, enabling them to best interface with their work tools. At the same time, workers need regular dynamic movement interspersed throughout the day to relieve the cumulative musculoskeletal strain that results from sustained, static body postures. We may even know this subconsciously when we squirm in our seats or get up to take breaks. In a sense, we are listening to the body's cues that it is time to relieve the static posture and change positions. The tenet of movement must be included as a regular part of all ergonomics training, including that for new chairs, because workers may inadvertently think that they can sit without breaks in their new chairs.

ANATOMIC AND BIOMECHANICAL CONSIDERATIONS

A review of anatomy is helpful to fully appreciate the biomechanics of sitting. Thirty-three vertebrae comprise the spine, including the cervical, thoracic, and lumbar vertebrae; the sacrum; and the coccyx. In standing the spine forms three natural curves: the cervical and lumbar curves are inward (lordosis), and the middle or thoracic curve is outward (kyphosis). The cervical and lumbar portions of the spine are mobile in relation to the thoracic spine. The intervertebral discs are located among the vertebrae, act as shock absorbers, and provide flexibility to the spine. Ligaments provide stability to the vertebrae and are located on the anterior and posterior walls of the spine. Muscles along the spine maintain posture and provide stability to the trunk. The nerves that comprise the spinal cord are protected by the vertebrae and pass to the extremities, allowing motor and sensory information to pass to and from the brain.

Although blood flows along the spine, there is a limited blood supply to the discs.

Lower Body

When sitting, the pressure falls onto the two small "sit bones" or the ischial tuberosities. Compressive stresses exerted on areas of the buttocks beneath the tuberosities are high and have been estimated as 85 to 100 psi, with the forces almost doubled when sitting cross-legged.[51] Studies of persons sitting upright on flat seating, such as bleachers, have found significant buildups of pressure that can exceed those that have been determined to cause blood circulation problems in users of wheelchairs.[11] This can easily explain why this type of sitting posture cannot be sustained more than briefly and why most of the chairs we sit in offer more padding and support. When one sits upright, approximately two thirds of the body's weight is distributed to the chair seat, with the backrest, armrest, and floor supporting the remainder.[11] Research suggests that maintaining one third or less of the body weight on the feet is necessary to minimize leg discomfort.[12]

The sacrum is essentially fixed and moves in relation to the pelvis. A forward or anterior rotation of the pelvis causes the lumbar spine to move toward increased lordosis to maintain an upright trunk. When the pelvis tilts backward, the lumbar spine tends to flatten, causing kyphosis. Radiographic studies have verified that the pelvis rotates backward and the lumbar spine flattens during sitting.* Disc pressures also change dramatically when a person moves among standing, upright, and slouched seated postures (Figure 12-1). Nachemson and Elfström[36] and Andersson and Ortengren[5] found that disc pressure is greater during sitting than during standing and that disc pressures drop with an inclination of the chair backrest (the angle formed between the seat and the backrest), especially when it is tilted from vertical to 110 degrees. Nachemson and Morris published data on in vivo disc pressure measurements in people who stood and sat without support. They reported that the pressures mea-

---

*References 1, 4, 7, 8, 29, 48, 49, 52.

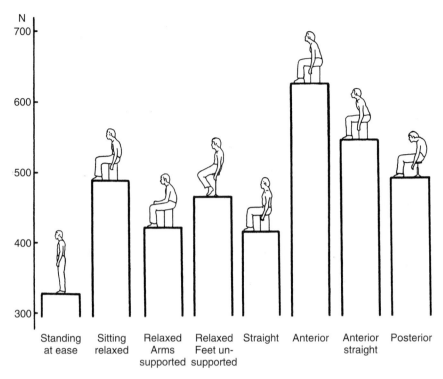

FIGURE 12-1 Variations in disc pressure among various unsupported seated postures, in comparison with a person standing at ease. (From Chaffin D, Andersson G: *Occupational biomechanics*, New York, 1984, Wiley & Sons.)

sured in standing subjects were approximately 35% lower than those measured in seated subjects.[37] Research also demonstrates that increased disc pressure means that the discs are being overloaded and will wear out more quickly.[24]

There are several reason why preserving the lumbar lordosis is critical to healthy sitting. With a change to kyphosis, the body's center of gravity shifts from over the lumbar spine to in front of it. With the shift of upper body weight, the space between lumbar discs is compromised, causing low back muscle fatigue and pressure on the lumbar discs, disrupting the normal equilibrium.[13] Various sitting positions also reflect changes in the seated person's center of gravity (Figure 12-2). In *reclined postures,* the seat and backrest are tilted backward and the center of body mass is behind the ischial tuberosities. Although this posture reduces the pressure on the discs, it is not necessarily functional for working because it also increases the viewing distance and arm reach to the work area. It can also increase strain on the neck if the user flexes his or her head forward for viewing, without the benefits of a high backrest or even a headrest. *Upright postures* involve the trunk being upright and straight, with the seat and backrest at an approximate 90-degree angle and the center of body mass over the ischial tuberosities. In *forward postures,* the seat and backrest are tilted forward, placing the center of mass in front of the ischial tuberosities. These postures are usually assumed in relation to the task, for example, fine detail work often involves leaning forward, telephone conversations can be conducted while reclined, and work at a keyboard is usually performed in an upright posture (or the so-called "traditional series" of 90-degree body links).

Muscle activity has been extensively researched through electromyography (EMG) of the back mus-

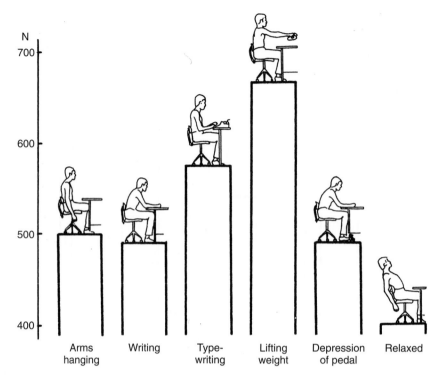

FIGURE 12-2 Disc pressure has been compared in various seated postures while the person with low back support performs usual desk activities. (From Chaffin D, Andersson G: *Occupational biomechanics*, New York, 1984, Wiley & Sons.)

cles during standing and sitting. Studies by Lundervold[31-33] and Floyd and Roberts[22] reported that myoelectric activity decreases when the back support is located in the lumbar region rather than in the thoracic region. This confirmed a finding by Åkerblom,[1] who performed the first comprehensive study of the biomechanics of sitting, that a support in the lumbar region is as effective as a full back support. Fifty years later, however, the needs of many seated workers and, in particular, computer operators also require upper body support to address the static muscle demands posed by the nature of work today.

Zacharkow's research supports the theory that supporting the sacrum and lower thoracic spine is necessary to achieve proper sitting posture.[56] The rationale behind sacral–lower thoracic support when sitting is that the proper axial relation between the thorax and the pelvis must be restored by bringing the upper trunk over the hips. Zacharkow points out that because sitting is a dynamic activity, people sit on their ischial tuberosities, causing the pelvis to rock. Without sacral support to produce an anterior pelvic tilt, the sacrum rotates posteriorly, bringing the lumbar spine into a flattened or kyphotic position. A forward seat-pan tilt, advocated by Mandal,[34] can also reduce pressure on the discs and increase the lordosis. An issue for many workers in this posture is a feeling that they are sliding from the seat. This issue can, however, be adjusted for by proper seat height adjustments, which usually require increasing the overall seat height and providing the proper support beneath the feet.

EMG supports the finding that sitting in a slouched or reclined position relaxes the trunk muscles and requires minimal muscle activity to hold the body weight in balance. However, disc pressures are greatest when a person sits with a slouched posture. This represents another dichotomy between postures that are best for minimizing disc pressures and those that involve less muscle exertion. Similarly, although the reclined sitting posture is associated with lesser amounts of disc pressure, this cannot be a functional work position, and the associated extended reaches to the work area will again throw off the body's equilibrium.

When someone is seated, the legs need to be supported so that they do not dangle, allowing the muscles to pull on the hip and in turn the low back. Prolonged sitting can also cause compression of the sciatic nerve, resulting in paresthesias. Proper positioning and support are also important when sitting because of circulatory issues related to the lower extremities being in a dependent position and vulnerability of the popliteal area behind the knee. This can result in restricted blood circulation if the two major veins in this area are compressed by the weight of the body or from a seat pan that is too deep and does not provide 1 to 2 inches of clearance between the seat edge and back of the knees. Winkel notes that increases in lower extremity volume of 4% occur over a workday, that supporting the legs with either the floor itself or a footrest can help minimize this effect, and that movement every 15 minutes can reduce swelling up to 2.3%.[54,55]

Upper Body

When one is sitting, the lower spine provides basic support and the upper or cervical spine supports the head for viewing, whether looking forward to a computer screen or down to written text or the work item. Neutral postures of the head (e.g., without extreme flexion, rotation, or side bending) and maintaining the arms near the torso are associated with less musculoskeletal stress.

The movement of flexing and extending the head can be considered an anatomic first-class lever, where the approximate position of the axis (the second cervical vertebra) acts as the fulcrum, the effort is supplied by the extensors of the head, and the resistance is the weight of the head.[53] Further biomechanical analysis related to changes in head position, reflected by changes in the movement distance between the axis of motion and the head's center of gravity, can show a five-fold increase acting on the erector spinae muscle and an almost two-and-one-half–fold increase in the reaction force on the C5 disc when comparing erect postures with 45-degree flexed postures for screen viewing.[43] In addition, when the head is held forward for extended periods of time, increased posterior cervical muscle activity is required to support the weight of the head, resulting in increased muscle fatigue.

The line of vision dictates head and neck posture. If the work surface is too low or the computer screen is too far away from the user, neck and trunk flexion result. If work items are located to the sides, there is increased strain on the lateral support muscles, as the head rotates to allow viewing of the work item (e.g., a monitor that is not positioned in-line relative to the keyboard). Studies of computer operators reveal that while the small muscles of the forearms and hands are undergoing near constant dynamic contractions, the proximal muscles of the shoulders and neck statically contract to provide postural support. Onishi and co-workers reported that EMG activity of the trapezius muscle reached 20% to 30% of its maximal level of contraction during keyboard operations.[40] Having the arms supported has been found to decrease activity levels of the trapezius muscle, but this is not always a feasible work posture. Improper visual correction is another factor that can result in compensatory cervical spine and upper back postures contributing to neck and shoulder pain, as does improper screen positioning for persons who wear bifocals or trifocals.

COMMON CHAIR ISSUES

Workers often complain of discomfort while seated. Does this relate to the chair itself, the appropriateness of the chair for that person or task, incorrect chair adjustments, poor worker posture or work habits, or any combination of the above? It is easy to look at the once-traditional metal industrial chair that has a hard seat, hard and small backrest, and no adjustability. It is no wonder that employees have been noted to become creative in the ways they tape their chairs; they are responding to their bodies' messages that the chair is uncomfortable and needs to be padded to allow enhanced comfort that can help workers' well-being and ability to be productive.

Chairs in office settings appear to better address seated workers' needs when compared with those in industrial settings. The sitting and support needs of sedentary industrial workers has not been given the same attention as those of their office counterparts. Many chairs found on production floors are associated with not only ergonomic but also safety issues. For example, chairs with four legs rather than a five-legged base of support pose inherent safety concerns that place users at risk for falling, because these chairs can easily tip as a result of decreased stability. Many shop chairs are actually old office chairs that have been replaced with newer chairs and have similar stability issues. Typically, these chairs have a continuous seat pan and backrest, have minimal to no lumbar support, and often have broken parts, including their one adjustable feature—the pneumatic seat height. Of course the need for ergonomic chairs varies with the work area. Old chairs placed in areas where sitting is required only occasionally is acceptable. It is, however, inappropriate to use a recycled chair where sitting is the preferred posture for the majority of the work shift. Box 12-1 provides a list of the many problems associated with office and industrial chairs.

Equally important to the design aspects of the chair is the lack of worker training in how to properly adjust the chair. Often when a company does invest in a good chair, they do not provide the necessary education to users on how to use the chair's features and/or explain the rationale for why the various adjustments are important to the seated worker's comfort. It is not uncommon to see even the most basic chair adjustment feature of pneumatic height not being properly used. For example, a chair height that is too low causes the hips and knees to flex beyond 90 degrees, resulting in the knees being higher than the hips, a posterior pelvic tilt, lumbar flattening, and a decrease in diaphragmatic breathing. A chair that is too high causes the worker to lean forward to obtain support from the floor, preventing use of

> **Box 12-1** **_Typical Problems Associated with Many Office and Industrial Chairs_**
>
> - The backrest is not easily adjustable and offers limited range of adjustment to provide adequate low back support.
> - Older industrial chairs lack padding, have sharp edges that may pose pinch points, and have a four-legged base of support.
> - The seat height adjustment on manually adjusted (rather than pneumatic) chairs is controlled by spinning the seat clockwise to raise and counterclockwise to lower the seat. This adjustment cannot be made by the seated worker, and this mechanism tends to break over time.
> - The tension control knob is often difficult to reach because it is under or behind the seat. Furthermore, most workers are unfamiliar with the purpose of this knob and rarely use it.
> - The seat may be too deep for shorter people, causing their feet to dangle and their legs to swell. To avoid pressure behind the legs, these users lean forward to access the work area and do not receive the benefits of back support.
> - Chair armrests are often too wide, too low, or too high to be used at a given work surface. Armrests that are too high can interfere with the user's ability to pull the chair under the work surface, forcing the worker to sit forward on the seat, foregoing the benefit of the backrest.
> - Some of the newer ergonomic chairs have more features than are necessary, and the use of their controls (and/or interrelationships among them) becomes confusing, resulting in little use of the adjustment features that added to the chair's cost.

the chair backrest for support. The importance of chair height adjustments takes on increased significance if workers work at more than one location and need to move their chair between locations (e.g., between a dedicated computer area and writing area or multiple work benches).

ERGONOMIC CHAIR DESIGN AND SELECTION

Good ergonomic chair design provides easily adjustable and accessible features for seat height, backrest and level of lumbar support, and seat inclination. High backrests, armrests, and footrests are optional features; the need for these must be determined after tasks are analyzed to ensure compatibility between the chair selected and the tasks performed and individual user needs. Ergonomic chairs need to confer stability by providing good support to the buttocks via the seat pan and to the back via the backrest. Concurrently the chair must also allow the seated person the opportunity to freely move within the seated position.

Dainoff refers to three basic chair designs.[13] *Fixed posture chairs* tend to lock the person into the one so-called "ideal" or "preferred" posture by means of static posture settings. *Dynamic chair designs* move with the person, are free-flowing or move continuously with the user, and have easily adjusted changes in backrest inclination. *Combination chairs* allow the user to both lock the chair into select positions of support and keep it "free-floating for others." As an example, users in combination chairs can keep the backrest essentially locked in an upright posture (offering back support) when typing and keep it free-floating or allow for freedom of back movement while on a conference call that does not involve simultaneous viewing of the screen, data input, or retrieval. Several combination features are afforded by various ergonomic chairs; these include dynamic forward seat-pan tilt and backrest inclination acting as a unit, an adjustable backrest inclination with seat tilt, or independent adjustments of the backrest and seat. There is no one chair that is appropriate for all applications or users.

In today's competitive marketplace, nearly all office chairs are touted as being ergonomically designed, often just because they have pneumatic seat-height adjustments. This labeling can be deceptive and does not assure buyers that the selected chair is ergonomically correct for intended users or a specific job application. Taking this a step further, although a chair may meet ergonomic design criteria as set forth by the American National Standards Institute/Human Factors and Ergonomics Society (ANSI/HFES) or the Business and Institutional Furniture Manufacturer's Association (BIFMA), a trade association of furniture manufacturers and suppliers, the chair may still not be comfortable or appropriate for all users.

The chair is only one element of a system or workstation setup. Chairs cannot be viewed in isolation from the person and task; they must be viewed in the broader context for which they are intended and be integrated into the total task, equipment, and workstation design, while the organizational elements are also addressed.[10] Consideration must also be given to the personal habits and preferences of diverse users. As people sit in different postures to perform various work tasks (e.g., to perform dentistry, laboratory work, accounting, or secretarial work or to operate a sewing machine), the ergonomic chair selected for each job should allow the worker to comfortably perform his or her specific occupational activities. When seated, workers improve their posture via good chair support; they also minimize the cumulative stresses to the musculoskeletal system that can result from an 8-hour workday or roughly one third of each day. This can have a significant impact on one's overall well-being.

When designing equipment and chairs, industrial designers and furniture manufacturers must account for the combined variations in size and posture of users, so that the human-machine match can be optimized to the extent possible. This helps avoid mismatches between users and equipment, which can lead to musculoskeletal discomfort, inefficiencies in the work process, and reduced worker productivity.[14,39] A number of recommendations have been published with regard to anthropometric (body size) data related to seating design (e.g., seat-pan and backrest dimensions, backrest and seat-height adjustability).[2,9,16,17,46] Traditionally, anthropometric design accommodates people as small as the 5th-percentile woman to as large as the 95th-percentile man. There is a wide variation in the

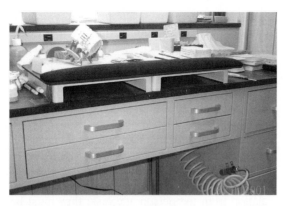

FIGURE **12-3** Ergonomic interventions need not be costly. Therapists can often find nontraditional applications for many items used on a daily basis and/or work aides. In this case, two monitor risers were placed side by side to provide 2 inches of height, atop which an old keyboard tray with a wrist rest was placed.

physical size of the working population, such as the 34-cm (almost $13^1/_2$-inch) difference between the tall man and small woman in the anthropometric database used in the ANSI standard (see Chapter 5).[27]

Jim's work at his lab bench requires controlled hand, arm, and head postures and eye-hand coordination. Given his 6-foot, 1-inch height, height modifications to his traditional 29-inch-tall bench are needed to provide him with the necessary forearm support (Figure 12-3).

Anthropometric data also differ from country to country, within populations and/or subpopulations. These variations in physical dimensions of individuals need to be accommodated when furniture is being purchased for particular users. For example, if a company employs mainly women who are of short stature, it does not make sense to purchase chairs designed to accommodate up to the 95th-percentile man, but rather those with overall smaller dimensions. If larger chairs were purchased, the buyer or manager might be very upset to see these women sitting without the benefit of the back support because they need to sit forward to access their work areas. In contrast, in a diverse workforce, having one chair that can accommodate both smaller and larger employees is appropriate. Another alternative is having several sizes of the same chair to help accommodate variations in worker size. Seat depths that adjust in the anterior-posterior plane can make a huge difference in helping support the legs and buttocks of small and tall persons alike, increasing the percentage of workers who can comfortably sit in chairs with this feature. Big and tall model chairs are indicated for men who exceed the 95th percentile. To make seating issues more complex, variations in size related to overall stature, limb lengths, breast size, and overall strength and fitness are further qualifiers in applying anthropometric data to proper chair selection. From an aesthetic point of view, manufacturers make different styles of chairs that complement one another so that a diversity of styles and sizes can be visually pleasing.

The basic features of a well-designed ergonomic chair include the following:

- A seat height that is easily adjustable and has a pneumatic pedestal base
- Ability of the user to easily make all adjustments while seated
- Good lumbar support
- A backrest that adjusts vertically to support the lumbar spine as well as in an anterior-posterior direction and that is narrow enough to allow freedom of arm movement without chair interference
- Dynamic movement options of the backrest and seat pan, preferably with independent movement of the two
- A seat pan with a curved front or waterfall edge to reduce pressure behind the knees
- A tension adjustment that affects the ease of forward and backward inclination of the backrest
- A five-prong base of support to prevent the chair from tipping
- Casters that are sturdy and allow for both mobility and stability
- Seat padding that is soft but not too soft, to allow even distribution of pressure; the upholstery should reduce heat transfer in warm climates and static electricity in cold weather and should be easy to clean

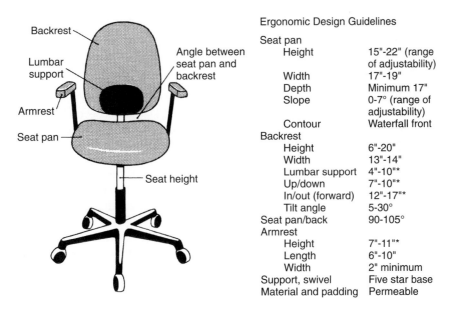

Ergonomic Design Guidelines

Seat pan	
Height	15"-22" (range of adjustability)
Width	17"-19"
Depth	Minimum 17"
Slope	0-7° (range of adjustability)
Contour	Waterfall front
Backrest	
Height	6"-20"
Width	13"-14"
Lumbar support	4"-10"*
Up/down	7"-10"*
In/out (forward)	12"-17"*
Tilt angle	5-30°
Seat pan/back	90-105°
Armrest	
Height	7"-11"*
Length	6"-10"
Width	2" minimum
Support, swivel	Five star base
Material and padding	Permeable

FIGURE **12-4** Ergonomic design guidelines for a chair. (*Measured relative to chair seat.)

Guidelines for an ergonomically well-designed chair are specified in Figure 12-4, with additional information provided in the selection of seating standards.

Armrests and Footrests

Armrests and footrests are optional features that can facilitate comfort. Armrests, if present, should be adjustable, should be small and low enough to fit under the work surface, should not interfere with the task, and should be able to offer body support when the worker is close to the work area. Armrests come in different lengths relative to the seat pan (e.g., half, full, or two thirds) and should be cushioned to eliminate sharp edges or pressure on the ulnar nerve at the elbow level. Nonadjustable armrests are often too wide for the average person and too high for a person with long arms, causing increased shoulder elevation. In tight workspaces, armrests can interfere with chair rotation and may be contraindicated. Some chairs allow for the removal of only one armrest and this can be helpful in tight work areas. Some armrests can move in the horizontal planes (e.g., closer or further from the worker's sides) and be angled inward or outward. When the armrest on the side of the mouse-using arm is angled to support the forearm, this adjustment can be associated with comfort benefits as related to reduced static muscle loading. It is important to realize, however, that armrests are not intended for use while typing, as the resultant posture to access the keyboard then involves shoulder abduction and wrist ulnar deviation. Armrests are appropriate for assembly tasks in which the arm has to be held away from the body and is not moved extensively during the work cycle.[16] EMG studies substantiate lowered trapezius muscle activity when armrest support is used; research has also shown reductions in disc pressure when armrests are used.[5] Overall, it is safe to say that armrests can be useful in some jobs and a detriment in others.

Footrests are often indicated to foster the positioning of shorter workers. The use of footrests prevents the user's feet from dangling or being without support, thereby helping to maintain lower body circulation and keeping the knees at about the same level or slightly lower than the hips. Without support, the weight of dangling legs can contribute to low back strain. Footrests can also add another level of adjustability to the work area, particularly if the work surface height cannot be adjusted and the employee needs to raise his or her seat height to meet this level.

Footrests come in a variety of styles: fixed or portable, horizontal or tilted. Portable footrests must be large enough to support the soles of both feet. The recommended size of a footrest is 30 cm × 41 cm (12 inches × 16 inches) with angles of 25 to 30 degrees and a nonskid surface.[47] Most users tend to prefer footrests that allow movement; a dynamic ergonomic design is preferable, although not required. Telephone books or other makeshift footrests can also provide the necessary support and can be readily implemented as an interim solution. Integrating a footrest, particularly one that adjusts in small vertical increments, into the design of an industrial workstation can also be helpful; this also helps maintain a neat under-desk area and avoids the possibility of trip hazards that can result from misplaced footrests. Footrails that run along the length of one or several adjacent workstations are another option that offers similar support.

Some industrial chairs and stools have foot rings. The foot ring can either be adjustable and move independently of the seat height or be fixed and move in conjunction with the seat height as it adjusts. Nonadjustable foot rings can present an issue for shorter workers whose feet cannot reach the ring, particularly when they need to raise the chair to access the work area. Workers who rotate to different stations must be trained to take the time to adjust the footrest, the foot ring, or overall chair height to support their individual needs. Taking these few seconds is paramount to the comfort and musculoskeletal health of workers who rotate for 2- to 3-hour periods or a full 8-hour shift rotation. Some workers say that the tactile reminder of a footrest serves as a postural reminder to help them sit up straighter, regardless of the chair.

Lumbar Supports and Wedges

A wide variety of lumbar supports is available to supplement the back support offered by existing chairs. These range from half or full rolls, to rounded or oblong pillows, to full-length molded plastic frames that feature lower back and lateral support (e.g., Obus Forme Lowback or Highback Backrest support). In many workers' attempts to enhance their seating comfort, they often add a lumbar support that is inappropriate for their needs (e.g., it may be too deep, resulting in increased leg depth beyond the seat pan, which can also contribute to back pain). Often, users simply do not know how to increase or decrease the lumbar support on chairs that have moveable supports (e.g., Herman Miller Aeron and Steelcase Leap chairs). Training seated workers in the proper uses of and indications for lumbar or even upper back supports is necessary to avoid additional seating issues. Towel or pillow rolls from home can also be used in an evaluative capacity before purchasing any support.

Another chair enhancement that can be used in select chairs, particularly those with a hard, flat seat such as a classroom chair or a simple task chair that does not have a lot of seat padding, is a seat wedge. Wedges offer ischial support and tip the pelvis anteriorly, encouraging upward postures with good spinal alignment. Seat wedges can also be useful in chairs that lack forward tilting features and offer the seated person the opportunity to get closer to his or her work by use of this cushion. Therapists can assess if this seating modification is appropriate for their clients in promoting an anterior pelvic tilt by placing a small towel roll under a person's ischial tuberosities. Rubber wedges and discs have been used for children with nonseating issues. The school-based therapist may want to address ergonomics in the classroom; this issue is the focus of the International Ergonomics Association's (IEA) Ergonomics for Children and Educational Environments Technical Committee. Proper seating and developing good habits in children at a young age is important so that a generation of slouchers is not created.[35]

Special Situations and Nonconventional Chairs

Some jobs are performed more easily while standing. These jobs are generally associated with the need for repeated forward arm reaches of >41 cm (16 inches) or vertical reaches of >15 cm (6 inches).[16] Because standing requires 20% more energy than sitting,[25] this can be fatiguing to workers who need to assume this posture throughout the work day. Sit-and-stand stools or prop seats offer standing workers an in-between option: they are afforded buttock support by a stool that is higher than a conventional chair and that has a forward-sloping seat that allows the user to achieve a semi-sitting posture. When sitting or standing with this support, the lumbar lordosis can be maintained, most of the user's weight is on the buttocks, leg fatigue is reduced, and users can freely move their upper extremities. These chairs can be beneficial to workers in the food industry, at manufacturing workbenches, and in the laboratory where adequate foot cut-out space is lacking, preventing the use of traditional chairs. Many of these chairs are light enough that they can be easily moved among workstations.

A chair design that has become commercialized in the past decade is the Balans chair. This chair features a half-sitting, half-kneeling posture, with a forward-tilted seat and knee support. This design results in a wider hip angle and maintains the three natural curves of the spine, preserving lumbar lordosis. Studies by Krueger reported that the load on the knees and lower legs is too great in this seated posture and becomes painful.[30] Use of this design is also contraindicated when users need to get up and down frequently to perform diverse work tasks. This design can be helpful when sitting at a dedicated workstation (or even at the television) that does not require frequent upper body movement and in persons without knee problems.

Often, visually intensive work requires the user to lean forward to clearly view or access the work area (e.g., for persons working at a microscope or performing industrial and electronic assembly and inspection, drafting and engineering, dentistry, or surgery). Sitting in a supported forward-inclined position can help relieve back and neck fatigue, especially for persons with issues related to the cervical spine. Two chairs in particular address this issue: the HÅG Capisco stool and the Neutral Posture AbStool or AbChair (Figure 12-5). In both of these chairs, the backrest, which in the former chair has a saddle-like design and in the latter is

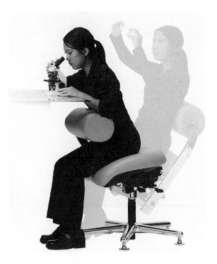

FIGURE **12-5** Neutral Posture's AbStool (or AbChair) can offer users support when the pillow backrest is in front or behind the torso as it swivels 360 degrees. (Courtesy Neutral Posture, Inc., Bryan, Tex.)

like a big cushioned roll, can be rotated 180 degrees so that the chair offers a front rest or abdominal support when the user leans over.

Jim required a chair that would allow him to get close to his work area, yet offer him support. Each dental work bench had its own design restrictions that could not be changed, so the chair became the primary adjustable feature. The HÅG Capisco chair was selected because it offered Jim the opportunity to lean forward with support or sit with the backrest in a more traditional posture and sit upright at both work benches. Jim is shown using his chair with both back support (Figure 12-6, *A*) and torso support (Figure 12-6, *B*), for different work applications. As this bench cannot be raised because of electrical power and other constraints, the work surface itself was raised.

New and innovative chair seating designs are continually entering the market. These include various reclining chairs integrated with special workstations that afford persons with special seated needs new options. Examples include but are not limited to the Stance Chair (Figure 12-7), which is considered a multiposture sit-to-stand shifting chair, and various models of the

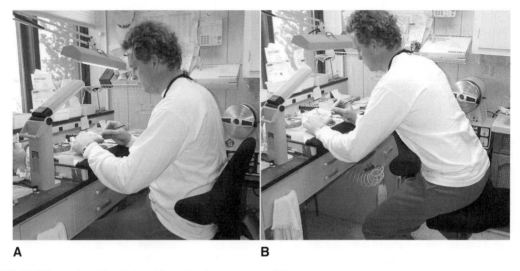

A   **B**

FIGURE **12-6** Jim using his chair with **A,** back support and **B,** torso support.

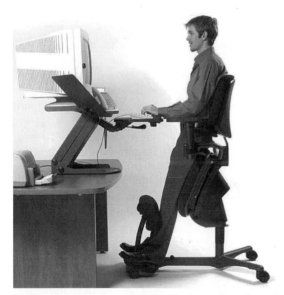

FIGURE **12-7** The Stance Angle Chair can be adapted to sitting, kneeling, and standing postures. This photograph illustrates a standing work posture, in conjunction with the TaskMate Height Adjustable Monitor and Keyboard Positioning Unit. (Courtesy HealthPostures, LLC, Glencoe, Minn.)

Ergoquest adjustable-height workstation, which can be used in supine, seated, or standing work positions. The use of wall-mounted large liquid crystal display (LCD) monitors and/or flat panel television screens is another option that allows people with severe back disabilities to work from bed or reclined chair postures.

SEATING STANDARDS

The original ANSI/HFES workstation guidelines, more commonly referred to as *ANSI-HFES 100-1988,* were published almost 20 years ago.[28] With significant technologic changes having occurred since that time, and along with the need for better guidelines, the *ANSI Standard for Human Factors Engineering of Visual Display Terminal Workstations* is nearing the end of its review period; a new version, to be known as the *Human Factors Engineering of Computer Workstations,* is expected in 2007. Because of variability in sitting and diversity of sitting preferences for different tasks, the *Human Factors Engineering of Computer Workstations canvass draft* refers to four reference postures for computer operators[27]:

- *Reclined sitting,* in which the user's torso and neck recline between 105 and 120 degrees to the horizontal

- *Upright sitting,* in which the user's torso and neck are approximately vertical and in line (between 90 and 105 degrees to the horizontal), the thighs are approximately horizontal, and the lower legs are vertical
- *Declined sitting,* in which the user's thighs are inclined below the horizontal, the torso is vertical or slightly reclined behind the vertical, and the angle between the thighs and torso is greater than 90 degrees
- *Standing,* in which the user's legs, torso, neck, and head are approximately in line and vertical

These four reference postures are intended only as guidelines from which variations can be expected (this is an important concept in ergonomics for which there are few absolutes, as comfort is intricately tied to individual preferences and variations). Because users require frequent movement and postural changes to achieve and maintain comfort and productivity, the specific workstation dimensional guidelines also relate to whether workplaces are designed for sit-only, stand-only, or sit-stand work postures.

Desired chair features in the ANSI standard follow well-established ergonomic design criteria. In addition to the basics of easy adjustability and good lumbar support, ANSI recommends the following:

- A backrest that reclines, that does not constrain the user's torso to a position forward of vertical or force a torso-thigh angle less than 90 degrees, and that allows for adjustments of the angle between the backrest and seat pan to an angle of 90 degrees or greater
- A seat pan that adjusts for height and tilt, that is wide enough to accommodate the clothed hip width of a 95th percentile female, and that is of sufficient depth to allow the user's back to be supported by the backrest yet allows clearance between the knee and seat edge
- The chair should provide support to the user's back and thighs in the chosen reference positions
- The chair should support at least one other seated reference posture in addition to the upright seated posture

The interested reader is referred to review the entire draft of this standard, which contains additional and very useful information, at the following website: www.hfes.org.

Ergonomists and health professionals rely mainly on the ANSI/HFES standards. The furniture industry has its own standard, *ANSI/BIFMA X5.1-2002 for General Purpose Office Chairs* (BIFMA). The Ergonomics Subcommittee of this organization has also developed an *Ergonomics Guideline for VDT (Video Display Terminal) Furniture used in Office Work Spaces,* which includes design requirements from the International Standards Organization, or the *ISO 9241.*

ERGONOMIC WORKSTATION CONSIDERATIONS

Workstation layout and design is intricately related to the seated person's comfort. Poorly designed workstations place workers at increased risk for musculoskeletal pain and injuries of the cervical and lumbar spines, the arms, and the legs and for eyestrain in computer or visually intensive jobs. Seated workers frequently complain of low back pain and overall discomfort, which can relate to the pure sustained nature of sitting in a fixed posture and resultant loads on the spine or to the chair itself. Perhaps of equal or more concern today are employee complaints of upper back and neck pain as related to sustained head postures for viewing full size or notebook screens and static sustained posturing of the entire arm while keying, using a mouse, or working on an assembly item.

As with any musculoskeletal condition, a person who has had an injury is more prone to reinjury or symptom exacerbation. In addressing workplace seating issues, ergonomists and therapists must apply their knowledge of biomechanical issues related to sitting to the conflicting demands on the body between the muscular and structural support systems (e.g., the spine and discs) and how these interface with individual postural needs and job requirements (see Chapter 6). Sitting is not the easy task that it appears to be when considering its demands on the body and the issues related to sustained static posturing.

Worker comfort is facilitated by whether the person can comfortably access needed work items and if a neutral body position can be assumed and/or maintained. This pertains to the height and vertical location of the work tool or object (e.g., the computer keyboard, input device, or assembly item). Ergonomic guidelines exist for preferred sitting and standing workstation heights, occasional and frequent reach distances, and loads handled in selected postures. Preferred reach distances or those within the work envelope that surrounds the employee have been established to help minimize muscle fatigue and pain. An easy rule to follow is for frequently used items to be within a forearm's length and occasionally used items within a full arm's reach.[2,18,41] Not surprisingly, greater reach distances and load weights handled are associated with shorter endurance times.

If the work surface is too high, the resultant elevated upper extremity places strain and fatigue on structures of the neck and shoulder. A common cause of this is the continued use of keyboard trays that are <20 inches wide and that can accommodate only the keyboard, resulting in elevated arm postures to access the input device that is atop the desk itself. Similarly, if the keyboard or input device is too far away, there can also be static loading on muscles of the shoulder and upper back. The recommended position for desk work involves shoulder abduction angles of less than 15 to 20 degrees and flexion of less than 25 degrees.[19] The elbows should be held comfortably at the user's sides and flexed 90 to 100 degrees, so that they are near the table or work level. Elbow flexion angles of at least 100 degrees have also been associated with a reduction in the static load of the trapezius muscle.[20] It is interesting to note that this open elbow posture correlates with that assumed when using a negative tilt keyboard tray. Keyboards that are too low should also be avoided, as this can result in wrist and forearm strain because of pressure on muscle, nerve, and tendon structures.

A commonly used guideline for establishing the correct hand and arm level is that a nearly straight line is formed among the elbow, wrist, and point of application of the work item. With respect to the point of application, it is the level of this item (which can range from <3 inches to >10 inches high) at which most work is being performed that is used as the reference point to which the user's hands and arms must comfortably reach. Ergonomic guidelines also recommend finetuning workstation heights by raising the elbow reference point or increasing the flexion angle while decreasing the viewing distance for work that requires high precision or visual acuity, and lowering them or reducing the flexion angle when strength exertions are required.[18]

In a small business the clinician or owner wears many hats. Jim did all the billing at his computer. Before his injury, the lack of a proper workstation setup had never presented issues for him. This included his use of a nonadjustable chair, rotation of the head to view a screen that was not in line with the keyboard, and extended hand and arm reaches to the mouse located beyond a fixed 24-inch high keyboard tray.

A built-up forearm rest was made (initially from two inverted screen risers and a keyboard tray with a built-in wrist rest) to provide hand and arm support and alleviate issues related to static, unsupported flexed shoulder postures of up to 40 degrees (Figure 12-8). After the therapist discussed how built-up gripping surfaces could minimize hand and arm strain from use of the dental tools, Jim became actively involved in the process and modified his tools using some of his dental epoxies.

When the workstation or desk height is fixed, the chair is the most flexible and usually the most critical piece of equipment to provide adjustability for a better worker-workstation fit. If the chair is elevated to a level where the person's feet dangle or cannot rest firmly on the floor, a footrest is indicated. More work height options are afforded users when the work surface is also adjustable. This can be via manual cranks or electric controls, adjustable keyboard trays, or various dual-level or sit-stand work units.

To minimize issues related to extended horizontal reaches, tables or desks with cutouts or curved edges that surround the worker may be considered to facilitate worker access to work

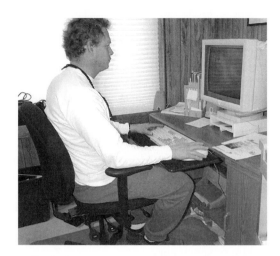

FIGURE **12-8** Modifications to the computer desk were required for this 6-foot, 1-inch tall man. These included a new chair, wider and adjustable-height keyboard tray, monitor risers, an antiglare screen, a larger mouse, and physically moving the desk away from the wall to create a preferred viewing distance to the screen.

items. Similarly, adding desk corner pieces to avoid the right angle juncture at L-shaped desks when the computer is located in this corner can minimize awkward hand-arm postures and provide additional forearm-arm support. Ergonomic devices that offer upper body support can also be added to facilitate worker access to the workstation; these include articulating arm supports or fixed position rests that extend out from the table or desk (e.g., the Morency Rest or Ergoport).

Keyboard and work heights must also be adjusted to allow a clearance of 1 to 2 inches between the undersurface and the seated person's thighs. A lack of clearance contributes to confined postures. Although the primary indication for negative tilt keyboard trays relates to the reduction of strain on the forearm extensor muscles, a practical secondary benefit of this angulation is increased clearance above the seated person's thighs. A crowded under-desk or workspace area is another factor that can contribute to confined sitting postures, thereby limiting freedom of lower body movement. This issue can be addressed by basic housekeeping and allocation of storage space.

It is easy to see that seating comfort in the workplace is not affected by any one ergonomic issue alone. Even adverse lighting conditions can affect how people assume awkward postures in efforts to better view their work areas, whether to obtain better lighting or to avoid glare. Similar compensatory postures can result from users who require visual correction. Numerous ergonomic equipment aides, including document holders and reading stands, headsets, monitor arms, antiglare screens, alternative keyboards, and input devices, also contribute to preferred sitting postures. Further benefits are afforded seated workers by integrating regular breaks into the work cycle and performing alternate job tasks that involve the dynamic use of different muscle groups. In a study by Dainoff and colleagues related to the use of an adjustable keyboard tray with sit-stand options,[15] the nonsitting or standing breaks were reported to be a beneficial postural change that was also associated with increased user productivity.

EMPLOYEE EDUCATION

Therapists may gain entry to the workplace by several routes, for example, as an extension of a return-to-work program or need to develop appropriate job accommodations or as industrial therapists who provide one-on-one or full ergonomic workplace assessments and wellness or ergonomic training. The therapist can influence industry practices not only by providing employee education, but by educating managers, supervisors, occupational medicine, safety and human resources personnel, and purchasing agents about the health and comfort needs of seated workers, proper chair selection, and general ergonomics. Therapists must emphasize to managers that although sitting appears to be low in its physical demands on the body, sustained sitting is not without its own health risks and prolonged sitting can be viewed as hazardous to a person's health. Therapists also need to encourage employers to involve their employees in the selection of new chairs, because a basic tenet of comprehensive ergonomic programs is employee participation.

Managers and purchasing agents often feel that once a new ergonomic chair has arrived on the workfloor, they have done all that is required with regard to that chair. However, receiving the chair is only the first step. Employee education and training are paramount to ensure that all users understand how their chairs work and how to finetune them in relation to the total workstation. An ergonomic chair, as with all ergonomic equipment, cannot be fully effective unless it fits workers properly and users are properly trained in its adjustment features. Although many chair vendors say they offer training, it is certainly not in the same context as that offered by therapists who understand how the body works and biomechanical issues related to seating and task and job analysis. The therapist's whole-person approach can help users fully make sense of why or how their ergonomic chairs can truly foster their seating comfort and well-being for one third of their daily hours.

Too often, employees who have used a chair for several months never realize several of its basic adjustment features, even if they are clearly described on the chair tag or illustrated directly on each control paddle or knob. This is evidenced by comments such as "I didn't know it could do this" or "I found it this way." This is why an essential part of an ergonomic assessment is to have employees demonstrate the various adjustment features on their chairs. Although this may sound obvious, this also provides further support to the need for employees to be present for their ergonomic workstation evaluation, as an ergonomist or therapist cannot make informed recommendations without seeing the user interfacing with his or her equipment or work area.

Ergonomics awareness seminars integrate the therapist's knowledge of anatomy, physiology, kinesiology, biomechanics, and task or job analysis. Therapists can also provide invaluable information related to the etiology of work-related musculoskeletal disorders, medical cost savings of purchasing the appropriate adjustable or ergonomic equipment, and educating users in its proper use. To emphasize the health benefits of good posture, therapists should actively engage their audience. Demonstrations with spine models help illustrate issues related to proper alignment and relative changes in disc pressure. Therapists should integrate a kinesthetic and tactile approach so that trainees are encouraged to palpate areas of increased or decreased muscle tension in different work postures and observe how people of varied sizes need different chair control adjustments. Trainees should be encouraged to assume preferred sitting postures: with approximate 90-degree angles at the hips, knees, and ankles; feet firmly on floor; shoulders aligned over the hips; and the head over the shoulders to help preserve the natural spinal curves.

After a classroom session, users should be encouraged to go back to their work areas to try to apply the didactic information. Therapists should also make themselves available for one-on-one assistance at the employee's workstation to address issues for which seminar attendees have a heightened awareness. This can include chair and workstation height adjustments, changes in the workstation layout, the use of various trial cushions or backrest options to achieve lumbosacral support, and/or information about the recommended equipment purchases. In addition to therapists providing their own handouts, several interactive programs are now available online. Figure 12-9 contains an excerpt from UCLA's *Computer Workstation Self-Evaluation.* An evaluation checklist developed by the U.S. Occupational Safety and Health Administration (OSHA) is shown in Figure 12-10.

Employee education needs to be ongoing. It should be provided for new hires, after periods of worker turnover and transfers, and after renovations. The latter is an ideal time to offer training, because the trainer has a captive audience with new equipment and furnishings, enabling the trainer to readily tie in the ergonomic benefits of new equipment with health and well-being issues. This is not the case, however, when ergonomists or therapists are asked to provide training as a substitute for new furnishings. Training in this context places the onus on the worker and his or her work methods and having to accommodate to

Computer Workstation
Self-Evaluation

Are your feet supported by the floor or by a footrest when seated?

Recommended Solutions
- Adjust the seat height so your feet can touch the floor with your knees equal to or slightly lower than your hips.
- If your chair is elevated for your keyboard or desk, use a footrest to support your feet.

Is there a small space (about 1") between the front edge of the chair and the back of your knee?

Recommended Solutions
- Adjust the seat depth if possible.
- If the seat does not adjust and is too long use a rolled up towel or lumbar cushion to push you forward in the seat.
- If the seat is short avoid using cushions or towels. They will push you forward and make it shorter.
- Try to adjust the backrest tilt to increase space.

Is the seat back adjusted so the inward curve of your lower back (lumbar) is supported?

Recommended Solutions
- Adjust the seat back height so the inward curve of your lower back is supported by the outward curve of the seat back.
- If the seat back does not adjust use a rolled up towel or lumbar cushion to support the curve of the lower back.

Are the armrests set so your shoulders are relaxed while your arms are supported?

Recommended Solutions
- Adjust the armrest height if possible.
- If available, adjust the armrest width to support your arms close to your body.
- If the armrests are too high and do not adjust, consider removing them.
- If the armrests are too low, pad them to make them higher.
- If the armrests get in the way, consider removing them.

FIGURE **12-9** Computer workstation self-evaluation. (Adapted from UCLA Ergonomics: Computer workstation self-evaluation. Retrieved October 2006, from www.ergonomics.ucla.edu/Seval_Chair.cfm.)

often less-than-ideal situations. Therapists should be wary of agreeing to this type of training.

Nelson and Silverstein[38] conducted a study of Washington State Department of Labor and Industries employees who were relocated to new office workspaces that included new modular units, height-adjustable keyboards, and fully adjustable chairs (seat-pan height and angle and seat-back tilt) that also came in three sizes. Initial study results reported improved worker satisfaction with the physical workstation and a reduction in the neck, shoulder, and back symptoms that were associated with improved chair comfort. Concurrent with the move, employees received 1 hour of ergonomic awareness training, instruction in chair

adjustments, and a personal workstation evaluation from a therapist, if requested.

In a study of garment workers by Herbert and co-workers,[26] new ergonomic chairs were introduced as part of an ergonomics program that also included an education program in the use of these chairs and issues related to work-related musculoskeletal disorders. The major finding of this study was a reduction in the percentage of the spoolers reporting upper extremity pain symptoms following introduction of new chairs and training. Similarly, this author was involved in a labor-management–sponsored textile workers' ergonomic training program that followed the introduction of new chairs and that led to the

WORKING POSTURES–The workstation is designed or arranged for doing computer tasks so it allows your	Y	N
1. **Head** and **neck** to be upright, or in-line with the torso (not bent down/back). If "no" refer to monitors, chairs, and work surfaces.		
2. **Head, neck,** and **trunk** to face forward (not twisted). If "no" refer to monitors or chairs.		
3. **Trunk** to be perpendicular to floor (may lean back into backrest but not forward). If "no" refer to chairs or monitors.		
4. **Shoulders** and **upper arms** to be in-line with the torso, generally about perpendicular to the floor and relaxed (not elevated or stretched forward). If "no" refer to chairs.		
5. **Upper arms** and **elbows** to be close to the body (not extended outward). If "no" refer to chairs, work surfaces, keyboards, and pointers.		
6. **Forearms, wrists,** and **hands** to be straight and in-line (forearm at about 90 degrees to the upper arm). If "no" refer to chairs, keyboards, and pointers.		
7. **Wrists** and **hands** to be straight (not bent up/down or sideways toward the little finger). If "no" refer to keyboards or pointers		
8. **Thighs** to be parallel to the floor and the **lower legs** to be perpendicular to the floor (thighs may be slightly elevated above knees). If "no" refer to chairs or work surfaces.		
9. **Feet** rest flat on the floor or are supported by a stable footrest. If "no" refer to chairs or work surfaces.		
Notes:		

SEATING–Consider these points when evaluating the chair:	Y	N
10. **Backrest** provides support for your lower back (lumbar area).		
11. **Seat width** and **depth** accommodate the specific user (seat pan not too big/small).		
12. **Seat front** does not press against the back of your knees and lower legs (seat pan not too long).		
13. **Seat** has cushioning and is rounded with a "waterfall" front (no sharp edge).		
14. **Armrests,** if used, support both forearms while you perform computer tasks and they do not interfere with movement.		
"No" answers to any of these questions should prompt a review of chairs.		
Notes:		

FIGURE **12-10** OSHA evaluation checklist. (From Occupational Safety and Health Administration: Evaluation checklist. Retrieved October 2006, from www.osha.gov/SLTC/etools/computerworkstations/pdffiles/checklist1.pdf.)

KEYBOARD/INPUT DEVICE–Consider these points when evaluating the keyboard or pointing device. The keyboard/input device is designed or arranged for doing computer tasks so the	Y	N
15. Keyboard/input device platform(s) is stable and large enough to hold a keyboard and an input device.		
16. Input device (mouse or trackball) is located right next to your keyboard so it can be operated without reaching.		
17. Input device is easy to activate and the shape/size fits your hand (not too big/small).		
18. Wrists and **hands** do not rest on sharp or hard edges.		
"No" answers to any of these questions should prompt a review of keyboards, pointers, or wrist rests.		
Notes:		

MONITOR–Consider these points when evaluating the monitor. The monitor is designed or arranged for computer tasks so the	Y	N
19. Top of the screen is at or below eye level so you can read it without bending your head or neck down/back.		
20. User with bifocals/trifocals can read the screen without bending the head or neck backward.		
21. Monitor distance allows you to read the screen without leaning your head, neck, or trunk forward/backward.		
22. Monitor position is directly in front of you so you do not have to twist your head or neck.		
23. Glare (for example, from windows, lights) is not reflected on your screen which can cause you to assume an awkward posture to clearly see information on your screen.		
"No" answers to any of these questions should prompt a review of monitors or workstation environment.		
Notes:		

WORK AREA–Consider these points when evaluating the desk and workstation. The work area is designed or arranged for doing computer tasks so the	Y	N
24. Thighs have sufficient clearance space between the top of the thighs and your computer table/keyboard platform (thighs are not trapped).		
25. Legs and **feet** have sufficient clearance space under the work surface so you are able to get close enough to the keyboard/input device.		
Notes:		

FIGURE **12-10**, cont'd   *Continued*

ACCESSORIES–Check to see if the	Y	N
26. Document holder, if provided, is stable and large enough to hold documents.		
27. Document holder, if provided, is placed at about the same height and distance as the monitor screen so there is little head movement or need to refocus when you look from the document to the screen.		
28. Wrist/palm rest, if provided, is padded and free of sharp or square edges that push on your wrists.		
29. Wrist/palm rest, if provided, allows you to keep your forearms, wrists, and hands straight and in-line when using the keyboard/input device.		
30. Telephone can be used with your head upright (not bent) and your shoulders relaxed (not elevated) if you do computer tasks at the same time.		
"No" answers to any of these questions should prompt a review of work surfaces, document holders, wrist rests, or telephones.		
Notes:		

GENERAL	Y	N
31. Workstation and equipment have sufficient adjustability so you are in a safe working posture and can make occasional changes in posture while performing computer tasks.		
32. Computer workstation, components, and accessories are maintained in serviceable condition and function properly.		
33. Computer tasks are organized in a way that allows you to vary tasks with other work activities, or to take microbreaks or recovery pauses while at the computer workstation.		
"No" answers to any of these questions should prompt a review of chairs, work surfaces, or work processes.		
Notes:		

FIGURE **12-10,** cont'd

development of an education booklet that was published in both English and Spanish.[3] Studies have also been conducted to assess productivity enhancements in relation to the introduction of ergonomic chairs, combined with ergonomics training. For example, Steelcase found that chair users who received training in conjunction with their new ergonomic chairs reported less pain and discomfort in their symptom surveys and had a productivity enhancement of almost 18%, in contrast to groups that received only ergonomic training or those that received training with their existing chairs.[50]

These training program examples illustrate the added and recommended benefits of training after new chair purchases. From a management perspective, training can be considered protecting an investment.

MANAGEMENT CONSIDERATIONS

In the office, management traditionally directs its attention to new technology—the hardware and software—with lesser attention paid to the furnishings used to support the computers or the user or the interactions between workers and various components of the total workstation or task. In the budgets of most companies, chairs are capital equipment. Employers should be encouraged to invest in better-quality, user-friendly, adjustable chairs as a first step toward improving the workplace. The employer should want to make wise and prudent decisions from the onset when investing in a large chair purchase. Managers need to be cognizant of the needs of their seated employees, as uncomfortable workers cannot be productive ones. Managers also need to be able to talk intelligently with vendors, purchasers, facility managers, and designers so that the proper chair for the intended user population is selected.[13]

When a company understands the needs of its users, it can intelligently select a chair or chairs from the myriad available and can allow this large investment to pay its dividends. As Bettendorf discusses, chair purchases are part of an ergonomic purchasing strategy that should also be integrated with a company's information systems strategy.[6] The chair and computer or work tool components need to mesh to ensure users' ergonomic compatibility. As ergonomists are aware, the successful implementation of an ergonomics program requires a systems approach, with the furnishings being only one component of the office system. Chair selection must consider the entire system and interrelationships among the component parts; otherwise, a misfit may occur, and new, unforeseen problems may be introduced at the workstation.[21] In Rice's discussion of an ergonomics systems approach, this approach is compared with and contrasted to the three-step process used in health care and rehabilitation (evaluation, intervention, and treatment).[42] Common to both approaches is the need to view the chair user or rehabilitation client as part of a larger system with multiple inputs and interacting performance factors.

The cost of an ergonomically correct office or industrial chair can vary from as low as $99 to several hundred dollars to over $1000. It is not possible for the cylinder of a $99 chair to sustain the test of time when used a minimum of 40 hours a week. When therapists are involved in helping to purchase a chair for an employee, they should not be concerned with only the cost factor. Rather, they should stress the needs of their client, especially if he or she has a medical condition. Furthermore, the price tag visible to the therapist, or the suggested retail price, differs greatly from the actual price a large company will pay for the chair. Chair costs are also affected by the total size of the order (with more costing less per unit), the number and type of adjustable features, and the fabric selected.

With any purchase that is intended for durability and when the total chair dollar cost is compared with total hours of usage over the life of the chair, the least expensive route is clearly not the route for the prudent employer to take. Many chair manufacturers have developed worksheets to help companies calculate the actual productivity enhancement value for each dollar spent on a chair. This can be very helpful in justifying the costs of this important investment. Similarly, the ability of an employee to sit comfortably or without additional breaks to relieve discomfort in and of itself increases the value of the chair from the perspective of productivity enhancement.

Companies, large or small, should never purchase chairs directly from a catalog without a trial usage period or simply at the recommendation of a salesperson. Several different styles of chairs should be assessed by users of different sizes, in different settings, and performing different job tasks, so that a good cross-section of the persons sampling the chairs can be established. A well-designed chair survey varies the order in which chairs are presented to users, to avoid the chance that people might feel either the first or last is best. Various comfort and discomfort questionnaires have been developed (Figure 12-11). Involving employees in the selection process also

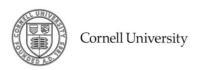

Cornell University

CORNELL ERGONOMIC SEATING EVALUATION ADMINISTRATION INSTRUCTIONS

Background

The seating evaluation is designed as a practical guide to help practitioners make comparative design decisions about different ergonomic chairs. The form started life as a >50-item list that was compiled based on published literature on seating evaluation research studies. Through iterative use and analysis the form was revised to a 25-item version that in turn was eventually refined to the current 15 items. This short evaluation form is designed to be quick and easy to use by nonergonomists as well as ergonomists.

The content of the evaluation form is based on those questions that most differentiate between chairs (or sitting experiences) and those that relate to ergonomic design considerations. The form does not evaluate design issues, such as color, style, etc., nor does it cover esthetic or economic considerations; it only addresses those features of greatest ergonomic importance.

How to score the evaluation form

The form is to be used to compare different chairs rather than as an absolute evaluation tool. Say that four chairs are being compared; each user would be allowed to sit in each chair for a specified period of time (it may be as brief as a few minutes, but this will limit some reactions [e.g., to seat pan comfort] and it is preferable that this is at least 90 minutes, unless the user really doesn't like the chair). At the end of this test period for each chair the user then rates the experience of sitting in that chair.

The use of the 11-point scale is based on a 10 cm linear rating scale design, but the defined intervals are given to speed scoring.

The use of 11 points gives a true midpoint value of 5 that represents a user rating that the experience is average for the chair, and the extremes are the scale bipolar anchors with a minimum of 0 defined as unacceptable and 10 as exceptional on the same acceptability scale so that responses to all items can be directly compared.

The rating responses are subjective but focus on factors such as the usability and comfort of the chair. The scale is organized into five separate sections (four component sections: chair adjustments, seat comfort, ease of use, and body support, and one overall comfort rating section). The scores for each section can either be totaled or averaged, and the same is true for all of the sections so that a total chair score is available.

In this way different chairs can be compared on individual items, on each of the four feature sections and on overall subjective performance, and then the total chair performance can be computed (an overall average score is the easiest summary).

FIGURE **12-11** Cornell ergonomic seating evaluation. (Copyright © Professor Alan Hedge, Cornell University, July 2003.)

CORNELL ERGONOMIC SEATING EVALUATION FORM

This form can help you to evaluate the ergonomic design of a chair. You should answer each question by giving a rating out of 10, with higher scores indicating better performance. This form can be used as part of your chair evaluation process and to compare the designs of different chairs. You can copy this form without permission for noncommercial and educational purposes. If you have any questions or comments please contact Professor Alan Hedge at the Department of Design & Environmental Analysis at Cornell University (ah29@cornell.edu).

Evaluator Name: _____   Date: _____

Chair Manufacturer _____   Model _____

Evaluation Criteria	Marks out of 10
A: Chair Adjustments (are these available and how usable are they?)	**Unacceptable(0) ----- Average(5) ---- Excellent(10)**
1. Usability of seat pan depth adjustment	0-1-2-3-4-5-6-7-8-9-10
2. Usability of back height adjustment while sitting	0-1-2-3-4-5-6-7-8-9-10
3. Adequacy of arm support width or width adjustment	0-1-2-3-4-5-6-7-8-9-10
	A: Chair Adjustments Score =
B: Seat Comfort	**Unacceptable(0) ----- Average(5) ---- Excellent(10)**
4. Seat cushion comfort (evaluate after at least 90 min. of sitting)	0-1-2-3-4-5-6-7-8-9-10
5. Backrest cushion comfort (at various recline positions)	0-1-2-3-4-5-6-7-8-9-10
6. Armrest comfort (when leaning on elbow)	0-1-2-3-4-5-6-7-8-9-10
	B: Comfort Score =
C: Ease of Use	**Unacceptable(0) ----- Average(5) ---- Excellent(10)**
7. Ease of chair height adjustment	0-1-2-3-4-5-6-7-8-9-10
8. Ease of armrest height adjustment	0-1-2-3-4-5-6-7-8-9-10
9. Ease of recline (without adjustments)	0-1-2-3-4-5-6-7-8-9-10
	C: Ease-of-Use Score =
D: Body Support	**Unacceptable(0) ----- Average(5) ---- Excellent(10)**
10. Back support at various recline positions (no forward push or fall back)	0-1-2-3-4-5-6-7-8-9-10
11. Lumbar support at various recline positions	0-1-2-3-4-5-6-7-8-9-10
12. Armrest height support range (below thigh level to above seated elbow height)	0-1-2-3-4-5-6-7-8-9-10
	D: Body Support Score =
E: Overall Chair Experience	**Unacceptable(0) ----- Average(5) ---- Excellent(10)**
13. Overall ease of use of the chair	0-1-2-3-4-5-6-7-8-9-10
14. Overall appearance of the chair	0-1-2-3-4-5-6-7-8-9-10
15. Overall comfort of the chair	0-1-2-3-4-5-6-7-8-9-10
	E: Overall Chair Experience Score =
TOTAL SCORE (A+B+C+D+E) =	

Comments:

FIGURE **12-11,** cont'd

Box 12-2	*Involving Chair Users in the Evaluation Process*

After purchasing selects chairs they feel are appropriate, users in the call center then test about five chairs in a real-work application. Users rate the chairs primarily on two of the five items in L.L. Bean's chair matrix: usability and comfort. The other factors addressed by the company are cost, warranty, and vendor reliability. Related to the importance for movement and a change in overall body postures that has been discussed in this chapter, a majority of the users in L.L. Bean's call centers (a near 24/7 operation) now use sit-stand chairs in conjunction with electronically adjustable stations. These sit-stand chairs are also used by all the company's support departments. For single-user applications, the work height is set at the individual's standing elbow height and a high footrest is used to provide these users with the necessary leg support when sitting in the adjustable high stools. In a study to assess comfort after ergonomic improvements (where modifications included additional upper extremity support, the addition of leg and back support, reductions in reach distances and neck movement), L.L. Bean used a simple 1 to 5 comfort rating scale, ranging from "no comfort" to "very comfortable." The comfort scores obtained 2 weeks after ergonomic modification found an 83.8% change in improvement, with scores increasing from 2.22 to 4.08.

Data from Morency RR, Roone EF, Forester DR: *A methodology to implement and validate ergonomic improvements to computer workstations at L.L. Bean,* International Industrial Ergonomics and Safety Conference, Copenhagen, Denmark, June 1993.

reaps a company benefit from the perspective of employee participation and buy-in, as it shows that their voice is important in influencing the equipment that they, and not the purchasing department, will be using. L.L. Bean is an example of one company that actively involves its chair users in the evaluation process (Box 12-2).

It cannot be emphasized enough that chairs must be tested in the context and the setting in which they will be used. Brief trial periods such as in a showroom do not suffice. Individuals trying out chairs in a showroom should be seated at a working desk and not simply sitting on a chair in isolation. Chairs for persons with medical issues, whom therapists are often called to see as part of the return-to-work plan, require an even more careful chair selection and trial usage period. People need time to get used to different chairs that promote correct posture, especially if they have been sitting with poor posture for a long time.

There are many ways to involve management in the chair-selection process. Perhaps one of the best is to have managers sit in the chairs that their production workers (on whom their company's ultimate profit depends) use. In ergonomics awareness seminars, managers should be afforded the opportunity to sit in chairs with good and poor ergonomic design, with and without adjustable features, and remain in these chairs for at least an hour, preferably while also working (this involves an extension of the training program outside the classroom itself). From this experience, it should not take management long to realize that the workforce can be more productive and comfortable in good ergonomic chairs, and that the investment in good chairs will surely reap the company dividends.

In contrast to the previously described situation in which managers were afforded the opportunity to sit in line-workers' chairs, chair selection for today's executives raises seating issues related to aesthetics and the perception of one's status in the company. The impressive-looking and often massive leather chair that has been associated with a management position is no longer the appropriate chair for every executive, as desktop or laptop computers are now a regular part of their desks and users cannot find the back support they need to perform productive desk work when seated in a chair of this style. Although these chairs are appropriate for allowing the executive to partially recline when having a meeting or on an extended phone call, they do not provide the necessary adjustability and support needed for desk work. Thus, we see another chair conflict related to the status symbol of selected chairs and their relative efficiency. When allocating chair dollar expenditures within a company, managers should resist the notion that it is acceptable to spend significantly more for their chairs and rather should be more willing to invest it in the high-end users whose productivity is key to the manager's success.[6]

CONCLUSION

Seated workers are exposed to musculoskeletal strain and circulatory issues when dynamic movement is limited and static postures are assumed for extended periods, particularly for the workforce of the twenty-first century that is not afforded diversity of movement or of job tasks. The use of easily adjustable ergonomic chairs can help alleviate many worker comfort issues, promote healthy postures, and in turn enhance productivity. Chair selection involves many considerations to address

the needs of diverse users. Training in the use of a new chair is equally important, so users can become informed as to its adjustable features and how this affects their interaction with their total workspace. The introduction of ergonomic chairs has often been viewed as a primary solution to office workplace problems. Although the chair is an integral part of an ergonomics program, the chair must be considered as only one of many interacting elements in the total work organization that affects seated workers' health and well-being.

Learning Exercise

Overview

This exercise is designed to help apply the principles of ergonomics in work settings.

Purpose

The purpose of this exercise is to evaluate your own work environment. You will determine if there are factors in your environment that may be enhancements to your work. You will also try to determine any characteristics of your work that could be altered using ergonomic principles.

Exercise

Collect anthropometric measures on yourself. Measure the parameters of your workstation. Identify potential risk factors (hazards). Prioritize controls. (Resource: Spaulding S: *Meaningful motion: biomechanics for occupational therapists,* London, 2005, Churchill Livingstone.)

Multiple Choice Review Questions

1. What is the *most* important feature to look for in the selection of an ergonomically appropriate chair?
   A. Backrest
   B. Adjustability
   C. Armrests
   D. Reasonable price

2. Research has shown that reduced disc pressure and reduced muscle strain occur in which of the following positions?
   A. Sitting forward slightly
   B. Sitting in an upright position
   C. Sitting back slightly

3. Radiographic studies show that the pelvis rotates backward and the lumbar spine _____ in sitting. This can cause disc herniation.
   A. rotates forward
   B. flattens
   C. is stretched
   D. is not affected

4. Which of the following should therapists consider when assisting in workstation design?
   A. Type of task being performed
   B. Body size and height of the worker
   C. Movement patterns of the work (workflow)
   D. All of the above

5. What workstation option should be considered when the worker must repetitively reach forward more than 16 inches or reach up more than 6 inches?
A. Higher work surface
B. Sit-stand position
C. Kneeling chair
D. Lower work surface

6. The benefits of sitting include:
A. relief of supporting muscles.
B. increased hand and arm support for fine motor activities.
C. increased demands on lower body circulation.
D. All of the above
E. Both A and B

7. Active movement is beneficial because it can:
A. decrease disc pressure and static muscle loading in seated workers.
B. increase blood flow throughout the body.
C. reduce the build-up of CO_2 and lactic acid.
D. All of the above

8. A full chair-user evaluation considers:
A. the user's knowledge of the adjustable features.
B. the task(s) being performed.
C. the overall work organization.
D. All of the above

9. Once a company invests in good ergonomic chairs, user training is not required, especially when the chair adjustability features have icons that indicate their proper use.
A. True
B. False

10. Chair selection should include attention to:
A. cost and durability factors.
B. the physical demands of the work being performed.
C. work flow and organization.
D. All of the above

REFERENCES

1. Åkerblom B: *Standing and sitting posture: with special reference to the construction of chairs,* Stockholm, 1948, Nordiska Bokhandeln.
2. Alexander D: *The practice and management of industrial ergonomics,* Princeton, NJ, 1986, Prentice-Hall.
3. Amalgamated Clothing & Textile Workers Union (ACTWU): *Stop the pain! A workers' guide to job design,* 1988, ACTWU.
4. Andersson GBJ, Murphy RW, Ortengren R et al: The influence of backrest inclination and lumbar support on the lumbar lordosis in sitting, *Spine* 4:52, 1979.
5. Andersson GBJ, Ortengren R: Lumbar disc pressure and myoelectric back muscle activity during sitting. 1. Studies on an experimental chair, *Scand J Rehabil Med* 3:104, 1974.
6. Bettendorf R: A low cost, effective approach to office design, *Occup Med State of the Art Reviews* 14(1):125, 1999.
7. Burandt U: Rontgenuntersuchung uber die Stellung von Becken und Wirbelsaule beim Sitzen auf vorgeneirten Flachen. In Grandjean E, editor: *Sitting posture,* London, 1969, Taylor & Francis.
8. Carlsoo S: *How man moves,* London, 1972, Heinemann.
9. Chaffin D, Andersson G: *Occupational biomechanics,* New York, 1984, Wiley & Sons.
10. Cornell P: *Dynamic and task seating: suiting the chair to the person, the machine, the task and the office environment,* Grand Rapids, Mich, 1989, Steelcase.
11. Cornell P: *The biomechanics of sitting,* ed 2, Grand Rapids, Mich, 1989, Steelcase.
12. Cortlett EN: *The evaluation of work: a practical ergonomic methodology,* London, 1990, Taylor & Francis.
13. Dainoff MJ: *People and productivity: a manager's guide to ergonomics in the electronic office,* Canada, 1986, Holt Reinhart & Winston of Canada.
14. Dainoff MJ: *The effect of ergonomic worktools on productivity in today's workstation design,* Oxford, Ohio, 1990, Center for Ergonomic Research, Miami University.

15. Dainoff MJ, Paasche J, Simons K et al: Periodic standing as a relief from fatigue in office work. In Alexander D, editor: *Applied ergonomics: case studies II,* Norcross, Ga, 1999, Institute of Industrial Engineers.

16. Eastman Kodak: *Ergonomic design for people at work,* vol 1, ed 1, New York, 1983, Van Nostrand Reinhold.

17. Eastman Kodak: *Ergonomic design for people at work,* vol 2, ed 1, New York, 1986, Van Nostrand Reinhold.

18. Eastman Kodak: *Ergonomic design for people at work,* ed 2, New York, 2004, John Wiley & Sons.

19. Engdahl S: Specification for office furniture. In Jonsson B, editor: *Sitting work postures,* No. 12, Solna, Sweden, 1978, National Board of Occupational Safety and Health.

20. Erdelyi A, Silhoven T, Helin P et al: Shoulder strain in keyboard workers and its alleviation by arm supports, *Int Arch Occup Environ Health* 60:119, 1988.

21. ErgoWeb: Is an "ergonomic chair" enough? *Ergon Today,* July 10, 2001.

22. Floyd WF, Roberts DF: Anatomical and physiological principles in chair and table design, *Ergonomics* 2(2):1, 1958.

23. Grandjean E: *Ergonomics in computerized offices,* Philadelphia, 1987, Taylor & Francis.

24. Grandjean E: *Fitting the task to the man,* ed 4, London, 1988, Taylor & Francis.

25. Hedge A: *Cornell University Ergonomics Page,* 2005, http://ergo.human.cornell.edu.

26. Herbert R, Dropkin J, Warren N et al: Impact of a joint labor-management ergonomics program on upper extremity musculoskeletal symptoms among garment workers, *Appl Ergon* 32(5):453, 2001.

27. Human Factors and Ergonomics Society (HFES): *HFES 100 human factors engineering standard for computer workstations,* Santa Monica, Calif, 2005, HFES.

28. Human Factors and Ergonomics Society (HFES): *HFES 100 human factors engineering standard for visual display workstations,* Santa Monica, Calif, 1998, HFES.

29. Keegan JJ: Alterations of the lumbar curve related to posture and seating, *J Bone Joint Surg Am* 35:589, 1953.

30. Krueger H: *Zur ergonomie von balans-sitzelementen im hinblick auf ihre verwendbarkeit als regulare arbeitsstuhle,* Report 8092, Zurich, 1984, Department of Ergonomics, Swiss Federal Institute of Technology.

31. Lundervold AJS: Electromyographic investigations during sedentary work especially typewriting, *Br J Phys Med* 14:31, 1951.

32. Lundervold AJS: Electromyographic investigations during typewriting, *Ergonomics* 1:226, 1958.

33. Lundervold AJS: Electromyographic investigations of position and manner of working in typewriting, *Acta Orthop Scand* (suppl 84), 1951.

34. Mandal A: Work-chair with tilting seat, *Ergonomics* 19(3):157, 1976.

35. McGrane S: Creating a generation of slouchers, *The New York Times,* January 4, 2001.

36. Nachemson A, Elfström G: Intravital dynamic pressure measurements in lumbar discs. A study of common movements, maneuvers and exercises, *Scand J Rehabil Med Suppl* 1:1, 1970.

37. Nachemson A, Morris JM: In vivo measurements of intradiscal pressure, *J Bone Joint Surg Am* 46:1077, 1964.

38. Nelson A, Silverstein B: Workplace changes with a reduction in musculoskeletal symptoms in office workers, *Hum Factors* 20:2:337, 1998.

39. Niebel B, Frievalds A: *Methods, standards, and work design,* ed 11, New York, 2003, McGraw-Hill.

40. Onishi N, Sakai K, Kogi K: Arm and shoulder muscle load in various keyboard operating jobs of women, *J Hum Ergol* 11:89, 1982.

41. Pulat BM, Alexander D: *Industrial ergonomics case studies,* Norcross, Ga, 1991, Industrial Engineering and Management Press.

42. Rice VB: *Ergonomics in health care and rehabilitation,* Boston, 1998, Butterworth- Heinemann.

43. Roberts S, Falkenburg S: *Biomechanics: problem solving for functional activity,* St Louis, 1992, Mosby.

44. Rodgers S: Recovery time needs for repetitive work, *Semin Occup Med* 2(1):19, 1987.

45. Rodgers S: *Working with backache,* New York, 1984, Perinton.

46. Roebuck J: *Anthropometric methods: designing to fit the human body,* Santa Monica, Calif, 1995, HFES.

47. Roebuck JA Jr, Kroemer KHE, Thomson WC: *Engineering anthropometry methods,* New York, 1975, Wiley.

48. Rosemeyer B: Eine methode zur beckenfixierung im arbeitssitz, *Z Orthop Ihre Grenzgeb* 110:514, 1972.

49. Schoberth H: *Sitzhaltung, sitzschaden, sitzmobel,* Berlin, 1962, Springer.

50. Steelcase: *Ergonomic study: leap productivity and health impact study,* Item @03-0003718, 2003, w w w . s t e e l c a s e . c o m / n a / f i l e s / d y n / 684f5dbc6c4e38f6331fb36d26104ad7/03-0003716. pdf#page=1.

51. Tichauer ER: *The biomechanical basis of ergonomics: anatomy applied to the design of workstations,* New York, 1978, Wiley & Sons.

52. Umezawa F: The study of comfortable sitting postures, *J Jpn Orthop Assoc* 45:1015, 1971.

53. Wells K, Luttgens K: *Kinesiology: a scientific basis of human motion,* Philadelphia, 1976, Saunders College Publishing.

54. Winkel J: Leg problems from long-lasting sitting. In Jonsson B, editor: *Sitting work postures,* No. 12, Solna, Sweden, 1978, National Board of Occupational Safety and Health.

55. Winkel J: Swelling of lower leg in sedentary work: a pilot study, *J Hum Ergol* 10:139, 1981.

56. Zacharkow D: *Posture: sitting, standing, chair design and exercise,* Springfield, Ill, 1988, Charles C Thomas.

SUGGESTED READING

Chaffin D, Andersson BJ, Marin B: *Occupational biomechanics,* ed 2, New York, 1997, John Wiley & Sons.

Karwowski W, Marras W, editors: *Occupational ergonomics: principles of work design,* Boca Raton, FL, 2003, CRC Press, LLC.

Kroemer K, Grandjean E: *Fitting the task to the human: a textbook of occupational ergonomics,* ed 5, Philadelphia, 1997, Taylor & Francis.

Linden P: *Comfort at your computer. Body awareness training for pain-free computer use,* Berkeley, Calif, 2000, North Atlantic Books.

Murphy DC: *Ergonomics and the dental care worker,* Washington, DC, 1998, American Public Health Association.

Oxenburgh M: *Increasing productivity and profit through health and safety,* Chicago, 1991, Commerce Clearing House/CCH International.

Pheasant S: *Bodyspace: anthropometry, ergonomics, and design,* London, 1986, Taylor & Francis.

Sanders MS, McCormick E: *Human factors in engineering and design,* ed 7, New York, 1993, McGraw-Hill.

Tadano P: A safety/prevention program for VDT operators: one company's approach, *J Hand Ther* 3:64, 1990.

Websites

www.bifma.org/standards/standards.html—BIFMA
www.cdc.gov/niosh/topics/ergonomics
www.ergonomics.ucla.edu/office_Chair.html
www.ergonomics.ucla.edu/Seval_ChairB.cfm
www.healthycomputing.com/office/buyersguides/chair_buyersguide.htm
www.healthycomputing.com/kids/computers.html
www.osha.gov/SLTC/etools/computerworkstations

13

Computers and Assistive Technology

Patrice L. (Tamar) Weiss, Chetwyn Che Hin Chan

Learning Objectives

After reading this chapter and completing the exercises, the reader should be able to do the following:

1. Understand the epidemiology of cumulative trauma disorder and apply the dose-response model to determine risk factors causing cumulative trauma disorder.
2. Identify different risk factors in using a video display terminal (VDT).
3. Apply ergonomic principles and recommendations to enhance workstation design for reducing the risks associated with prolonged use.

Cumulative trauma disorder (CTD). Injury from repeated stress placed on the tendons, muscles, or nerves, causing inflammation or damage.

Dose-response model. Model consisting of four interactive components—exposure, dose, capacity, and response—which are used to predict risk factors of CTDs.

Video display terminal (VDT). A combination of an electronic display screen, a keyboard, an input device, and furniture.

Workstation design. The organization of the VDTs in a work environment to minimize risk factors to VDT users.

CASE STUDY

Nancy is a 43-year-old woman who sustained bilateral hemiplegia (cerebrovascular accident [CVA]) as a result of cerebral aneurysms. The first CVA occurred when Nancy was 18 years old and resulted in a right-sided paresis. The second and more severe CVA occurred 20 years later and resulted in a complete left-sided paralysis of the upper extremity and moderate involvement of the lower extremity. Because of moderate balance problems and impaired judgment Nancy is able to ambulate only with assistance and under supervision. Her motor performance is impaired by a moderate nystagmus, psychomotor retardation, and a mild tremor. Her cognitive dysfunction is manifested primarily in difficulties related to motor planning, decision making, and following instructions.

Nancy is an artist who in the past used watercolors and oil paints to produce large landscape pictures. Since her second CVA, she has developed a method whereby she applies oil paints to her canvas with the aid of a broad knife. This method is slow and necessitates her reliance on unstable positions, which exacerbates her poor posture. Moreover it prevents Nancy from making use of the fine detail she had used in the past. Nancy was no longer participating in any active rehabilitation program and was referred by her family to an adapted computer access clinic in order to determine the possibility of augmenting her repertoire of artistic skills with the aid of computer graphics programs and to ensure that her posture does not deteriorate as a result of sustained awkward positions.

Nancy was scheduled for a series of 2-hour weekly evaluation-training sessions, which included assessment of her motor and cognitive functioning, introduction to basic computer skills, and instruction in the use of a computer graphics and painting program. This program enables the production of professional quality artwork even when using only the simplest tools. Nancy's data-entry problems were a result of her tremor, which prevented her from pressing the mouse buttons without changing the cursor's location. The tremor also made it difficult for her to release keys when using the alphanumeric keyboard; a single key press resulted in up to 10 repetitions of the same character.

These problems were solved with several accessibility and ergonomic adaptations. The mouse was replaced by a trackball, a device that permits the separation of cursor movement and icon selection. The Windows "Accessibility Options," a program supplied at no charge with all personal computers, enabled the removal of the key repeat function. Nancy was also provided with an office chair with an adjustable seat and back and arm support. Nancy continues to learn more computer graphics functions and is now working in this field professionally. This case study illustrates the ability of relatively simple computer access and ergonomic solutions to enable enhanced vocational opportunities.

1. What additional accessibility solutions could help Nancy advance in her use of computer graphics and painting programs?
2. What information about Nancy's posture and movements while using the computer graphics and painting program would help to determine whether she continues to face biomechanical risk factors?
3. What biomechanical accommodations can you suggest to enable Nancy to continue painting with watercolors and oil paints in addition to her computer-based art options?

The computer workstation has become common both at work and at home and is now used routinely for many purposes, including data entry, word processing, telecommunications, Web browsing, purchasing, inventory, designing, testing, and entertainment. Many computer operators type up to 60 words per minute (wpm) for more than 8 hours a day (i.e., more than 100,000 keystrokes per day).[86] Workers commonly spend long periods sitting in a static posture at computer workstations, with only minimal opportunities to reposition the trunk, neck, and arms.[149] Extensive evidence indicates that working with computer terminals and keyboards is associated with the development and exacerbation of a variety of work-related disorders involving the back, neck, and upper limbs.[10,86,116] Such conditions, known as *cumulative trauma disorders* (CTDs), are considered to be the "industrial injuries of the Information Age."[30] Other terms for CTD include *repetitive strain injury, muscle tendon syndrome,* and *occupational overuse syndrome.*[41] Medical problems commonly associated with CTD include tenosynovitis, wrist tendinitis, de Quervain's tenosynovitis, epicondylitis, carpal tunnel syndrome (CTS), and tension neck syndrome. More recently, there has been a greater awareness of the impact repetitive computer use has on the visual system.[20]

EPIDEMIOLOGY OF CUMULATIVE TRAUMA DISORDER

The Bureau of Labor Statistics has reported a rising incidence of musculoskeletal disorders of the upper extremity, which account for 70% of all occupational illnesses.[22] The National Institute for Occupational Safety and Health (NIOSH) estimates that 15% to 20% of the work force in the United States is at risk for developing a CTD. CTDs cost industries in the United States $27 billion in 1989,[84] and CTD claims made by workers in other developed countries, such as Australia and Canada, continue to escalate.[34,50] The number of computer keyboard workers with CTDs is as much as 12 times the number of nonkeyboard users with CTDs.[33,99] Among data processors the prevalence of musculoskeletal disorders is as high as 86%.[149] CTDs are reported to be more than twice as common in women as in men in workers between 30 and 50 years old.[15,47,54,79] Ekman and co-workers revealed that the odds ratio for women suffering from musculoskeletal symptoms was 11.9 times that for men.[32] CTDs can lead to a severe decline in worker performance with serious consequences to the employee, the employer, and medical and social service resources.[136]

A survey in Hong Kong examined musculoskeletal symptoms in office workers.[95] A total of 688 workers in 96 companies were interviewed, 65% of whom were female and 68% of whom operated a computer keyboard for more than 4 hours daily. Workers reported a high incidence of musculoskeletal symptoms, particularly in the shoulder (42%), lower back (39%), neck (39%), and upper back (36%). Lower rates of incidence were reported in the elbow (6%), forearm (9%), and fingers (13%). Similar findings were also reported by Sillanpaa and colleagues in 2003.[116] Approximately 60% of the workers felt that the onset of discomfort began after the commencement of their present employment. Among the workers who reported musculoskeletal discomfort, approximately 44% experienced reduced capacities in lifting more than a 10-pound load, 42% in sports, 37% in child care, and 32% in housework. Results of the study also indicated that workplace design (e.g., desktop, chair height, leg room), job design (e.g., workload and work hours), and hours of computer operation were the most important risk factors contributing to symptoms despite inconsistent results that were reported in later studies.[44,112]

The pathophysiology of CTDs is not completely known. Epidemiologic and clinical studies suggest that causes of CTDs consist of both intrinsic and extrinsic factors.[15,79] Studies have demonstrated that cumulative and repetitive force applied to the same muscle group, joint, or tendon causes soft-tissue microtears and trauma.[119] Barr, Barbe, and Clark revealed evidence on the causal effect of high-repetition negligible force on injury and inflammation of soft tissues.[17] This chronic soft-tissue condition is further aggravated by muscle exertion and excessive joint movements.[5,17] Several risk factors, including repetitive motion, excessive force, and awkward working posture, are closely associated with CTDs in keyboard operators.[18,69,140,154] The risk of CTDs is also associated with psychosocial factors such as personal characteristics, role conflict or ambiguity, excessive workload and work stress, and negative social interaction.[5,30,134,140,141]

DOSE-RESPONSE MODEL

Armstrong and colleagues proposed a dose-response model for determining risk factors of CTD.[10] The model has four interactive components: exposure, dose, capacity, and response. *Exposure* refers to the worker's external or work environment and includes physical characteristics of the job, including weight, size, and shape of tools, and psychologic factors such as job security. *Dose* refers to the internal environment of an individual's body and includes mechanical forces acting on the body tissues, physiologic consumption of metabolic substrates, and production of metabolites within the tissues, as well as psychologic disturbances, such as anxiety about work. These two factors are thought to act on every individual, in the workplace and at home.

Individuals react to these factors according to *capacity,* which is the physical and psychologic ability to resist destabilization caused by one or more doses.[10] An individual's reaction to exposure and dose, modified by his or her capacity, is a *response.* A vicious circle can occur in which responses elicit further disturbances within the body, often leading to severe tissue damage. CTDs are the consequences of these responses when the body's capacity (e.g., a particular muscle or tendon) is incapable of resisting deleterious changes induced by the exposure (i.e., body tissues cannot repair the damage as fast as it occurs).

The dose-response model predicts that an individual's capacity can be reduced by continued mechanical, physiologic, and psychologic events, such as muscle fatigue, minor injuries, and mental stress. CTDs occur when the exposure and doses exceed the capacity of an individual to respond in a healthy manner. The results of numerous experimental studies are consistent with the predictions of this model.[29,82,94,144,145]

The dose-response model is also useful in explaining interventions that may prevent or reduce CTDs. For example, interactions among an individual's capacity, dose, and response suggest that mobilization exercises, including stretching and strengthening of the body, can be beneficial in improving capacity by restoring weak and injured muscles.[17,128] Regular mobilization exercise of the involved body parts reduces the discrepancy between the dose and capacity of an individual, decreasing the effects of a deleterious response and the probability of developing a CTD.

RISK FACTORS OF CUMULATIVE TRAUMA DISORDER: EXACERBATION AND REDUCTION

Many investigators have identified risk factors that are closely associated with upper extremity CTDs, including repetitive motion, excessive force, maintenance of awkward or constrained postures for prolonged periods, mechanical stress via direct pressure, vibration, and extreme temperatures.[9,26,36,65,122,130] These factors are not equally relevant for all tasks, however.

According to the dose-response model, the probability of developing a CTD can be reduced by minimizing the exposure to the task and the

work environment and therefore to the dose. An effective job modification program reduces the frequency with which a worker is exposed to one or more risk factors.[15,65,144]

For most risk factors, exposure time is critical. Winkel and Westgaard recommended reducing exposure to less than 4 hours per day.[147] Nakazawa and colleagues found that increased mental and sleep-related symptoms were associated with daily video display terminal (VDT) operation that lasted longer than 5 hours.[93] Exposure time should be further reduced when the task is monotonous, the work environment is impoverished from a psychosocial viewpoint, an especially high demand is required for productivity, or rest breaks are infrequent. Varying the type of tasks in a work shift is advisable to ensure that the worker is not exposed to any single risk factor for an extended period. Taylor concluded that breaks or micropauses were effective for reducing muscle fatigue and musculoskeletal symptoms and improving performance.[127]

A number of studies suggest that keyboard tasks entail exposure to a number of risk factors and are prime factors in the development of CTDs.[28] Not only are keyboard tasks performed for extended periods, but the tasks also usually involve the simultaneous presence of two or more risk factors, further increasing the risk of developing a CTD.[106,108] The combined effect of excessive force and repetitive movement has been suggested to be considerably more injurious than either factor alone.* The relevance of working at a computer workstation to each of the major CTD risk factors is described in the following sections.

Repetitive Motion

Little doubt exists that high repetition is typical of the performance of many keyboard operators, who often type at rates of up to 100,000 keystrokes per day.[86,103,121] Pan and Schleifer observed that subjects with higher ratings of upper extremity discomfort during a data-entry task had lower keystroke rates.[100]

---

*References 17, 26, 108, 117, 121, 130.

Forceful Motion

Keyboard operators exert peak forces in the range of 2 to 3 N, approximately three to nine times more than the force actually required to activate the key.* The use of this amount of force means that keyboard keys are moved downward to their limit.[12,102] Not only does this result in greater travel than required to activate the keys, but the user may also encounter additional force by hitting down to the bottom of the key.

Whether the forces generated during each keystroke can be considered to be sufficiently high to be injurious is unclear, especially when their magnitude is compared with those generated during other manual jobs categorized as low (29 N) to high (125 N) force. Nevertheless, Feuerstein and colleagues[39] and Szeto and colleagues[126] found that office workers who reported upper extremity musculoskeletal symptoms with greater frequency and severity exerted higher levels of key force while typing than office workers who reported fewer and less severe symptoms. In contrast, Pan and Schleifer observed that subjects who had higher ratings of upper extremity discomfort during a data-entry task exerted *lower* key force.[100] The two studies differed in several respects, however, including the exact nature and duration of the tasks and whether the subjects reported previous symptoms. In tasks such as typing, which are performed for extended periods, the cumulative typing force, rather than the peak forces measured above, is highly likely to be more important.[42,121,126] Overall, the user's susceptibility to injury is affected by typing speed, the forces exerted on each key, total typing time, and the amount of time spent on each key.

With the surge in use of Windows-based software, menu-driven interfaces, and graphical user interfaces, manipulating a standard mouse now accounts for as much as 65% of the time spent at some computer tasks.[56] Certain mouse tasks, such as dragging, impose sustained loading on the finger flexor muscles. Andersen studied the use of the mouse and keyboard as related to develop-

ment of CTS.[7] The results indicated that participants spent more time using the mouse than the keyboard in a week—14.7 hours for the female subjects and 12.5 hours for the male subjects using the mouse versus 9.3 hours for the female subjects and 8 hours for the male subjects using the keyboard. The study also suggested elevated risks of CTS when using a mouse for more than 20 hours per week.

Awkward Postures and Constrained Positions

Typing is a composite task in which the arms, shoulders, and trunk provide a static support base while the digits engage primarily in dynamic work. In some cases, the same muscle alternately engages in both types of work. For example, the extensor digitorum communis provides both static wrist support and dynamic finger joint control.[121] In the classic typing position, elevated muscle activity has been found in the proximal musculature including the muscles responsible for shoulder elevation and abduction, forearm pronation, and ulnar deviation.[16,86,92,155] Pascarelli and Kella observed a number of postures used by keyboard operators who suffered from serious upper extremity symptoms.[101] These postures included the "alienated thumb" and the hyperextended fifth digit, both of which induce users to access the keyboard at potentially injurious joint angles and muscle lengths.[16]

Ulnar deviation of the wrist in excess of 20 degrees has frequently been observed[53,86,101] and has been associated with elevated pressure in the carpal tunnel.[16,86,109,142] Direct measurement of carpal tunnel pressure via a flexible catheter pressure transducer has shown that pressure is lowest when the wrist is slightly extended and slightly ulnar deviated.[16,142]

Sauter and co-workers[111] analyzed self-report data from several hundred computer users and found a number of posture-related factors associated with the presence of musculoskeletal discomfort.[140] In particular, low and soft seat surfaces were associated with leg discomfort, and keyboards placed above elbow level were associated with arm discomfort as well as high levels of neck and shoulder girdle discomfort. In one of the many studies that have documented the relation-

---

*References 12, 39, 42, 81, 103, 121, 140.

ship between user posture and CTD symptoms, Faucett and Rempel[35] showed that keyboard height was significantly related to severe pain and stiffness in the shoulders, neck, and upper back in a group of 150 computer operators working in a newsroom.[16,19,86]

Awkward and constrained postures also typify use of a standard mouse. Computer operators tend to maintain their shoulders in excessive external rotation and keep their wrists in extreme ulnar deviation for prolonged periods.[16,62,86] They also experience discomfort at the shoulder, elbow, and wrist. Significant increases in muscle activity levels and amount of perceived effort are related to the position of the arm and forearm during manipulation of the mouse and to users' anthropometric characteristics.[61,63] Less-than-optimal placement of the mouse was associated with a prevalence of upper-limb symptoms.[62] Aaras[1] concluded that the load on the trapezius muscle and pain intensity and duration were significantly reduced among computer operators when the workstation layout was adjusted by providing more work surface at the tabletop for operating the keyboard and mouse as well as an adjustable table and chair.[19,58,86,109,149]

Although awkward and constrained postures undoubtedly contribute to the development of CTDs, evidence exists that job design and work-style factors, such as task duration, are even more damaging.[88,126]

Mechanical Stress Caused by Direct Pressure

Mechanical stress caused by direct pressure, such as that exerted when objects press down on the base of the palm, can contribute to the development of CTDs. Feldman and co-workers[37] and Ruess and colleagues,[109] for example, suggested that cubital tunnel syndrome with subsequent ulnar neuropathy is commonly caused by a worker chronically leaning on his or her elbows on desks, armrests, or hard surfaces during working. Ruess and colleagues also suggested that sustaining the elbow in a position of prolonged flexion elevated the risk of ulna nerve compression and thus increased susceptibility to cubital tunnel syndrome.[109] This results in disturbed sensation in the fourth and fifth fingers and lateral side of the hand

and weakness of flexor carpi ulnaris, flexor digitorum profundus, and interossei.

Vibration

Exposure to excessive vibration at the work site can lead to sensory impairments such as paresthesia and diminished tactility, reducing the worker's ability to determine or gauge the amount of force necessary to hold and manipulate objects.[11,87] Affected individuals tend to exert too much force during repetitive manual tasks, causing soft-tissue damage. Although vibration is prevalent at many job sites, it rarely occurs during keyboard tasks.

Extreme Temperatures

Low temperature is another CTD risk factor. Low temperature (below 20° C) was found to reduce manual dexterity and performance[98] and to accentuate the symptoms of nerve impairment.[9,21]

EVALUATION OF THE IMPACT OF EXPOSURE

The dose-response model emphasizes that exposure is a crucial factor in the occurrence of CTDs. Methods commonly used to quantify the impact of exposure include self-report questionnaires, on-site observation, and electromyography (EMG). Self-report questionnaires are used to obtain information on workers' physical and psychologic symptoms and focus on perceived job demands, subjective analysis of the workstation, parts of the body in which symptoms occur, duration of symptoms over a particular period (e.g., the last 12 months, the previous 7 days), the effect of the symptoms on activities at work and during leisure time, and time off work. The standardized Nordic questionnaire is a well-known self-report form for the entire body.[74] Other questionnaires focus primarily on CTDs in the neck and upper extremities.[96] Self-report questionnaires, many of which have been shown to be reliable and valid, provide valuable information about workers, their behavior, and their environment without being overly invasive and time-consuming. Nevertheless, this method is inherently subjective and often not sufficiently accurate.

On-site observation and measurement can provide more detailed information on the interactions among workers, work tasks, and workstations. Information is commonly recorded on video, which can be reviewed with behavioral checklists to quantify the content and duration of the relevant aspects of task performance.[78] Metric measurement of the dimensions of the workstations and quantification of the job demands can be compared directly with the anthropometric database. The extent of the mismatch among workstation, task, and workers and its contribution to the occurrence of CTDs can be estimated. Validity of on-site observation methods can be compromised, however, when tasks are variable and not well defined. Furthermore, factors such as muscular load, angular velocity, and extent of fatigue cannot be addressed by observational methods.[57] The labor-intensive procedures of video analysis and the difficulty in applying the results to other jobs when tasks are heterogeneous and work environments are atypical are also drawbacks of this method.

EMG evaluation of the magnitude and duration of muscle activity is another method commonly used to analyze the muscular work pattern at workstations.[135] For example, EMG studies of the trapezius muscle under various load conditions revealed that workers who sat with the thoracolumbar spine slightly posteriorly inclined and with the cervical spine vertically aligned reported less strain on the muscle when compared with those who sat with the whole spine straight and vertical or with the whole spine flexed.[113] The occurrence of fatigue as shown by changes in the EMG spectral density can also be used to study the load on different muscles.[1] EMG evaluation is accurate in isolating and quantifying the effect of the exposure on the worker's musculoskeletal capacity and responses. However, EMG is perceived by the workers as more invasive than either the questionnaire or the on-site observation approaches. Care must be taken to avoid disturbances (e.g., excessive movement of wires) when using EMG in the work environment, to ensure that results are reliable.

EVALUATION OF WORK CAPACITY OF KEYBOARD USERS

A functional capacity evaluation (FCE) can determine whether a worker has the attributes neces-

sary for a specific job.[76,115] For the dose-response model, an FCE measures capacity in relation to the exposure imposed by the performance of tasks. An FCE can also help clinicians monitor the progress of workers with injury undergoing rehabilitation programs and identify any need for specific clinical interventions to meet work demands.

A number of commercial or custom-made evaluation packages and instruments have been designed to implement an FCE. The most common approach for evaluating work capacity is the use of work samples. A work sample is a set of activities involving tasks, materials, and tools that are identical or similar to those in an actual job or job clusters.[85] Because CTDs have many causes, a number of work samples and actual tasks are more useful than single examples for evaluating computer and keyboard operators. The activities that are important to computer workers are those involving the upper extremities (fingering, reaching, and using manual dexterity); those concerning the head, neck, and back (sustained erect posture, prolonged sitting, and eye-hand coordination); and those requiring sustained attention, concentration, and memory. The work samples selected should evaluate these job demands.

Unfortunately, appropriate work samples for computer workers are still uncommon. Valpar WorkSET components (available from Valpar International) include a few work sets that simulate the demands of sedentary work but are not specific to computer tasks. Other FCEs that simulate work tasks required in computer and keyboard operation include the BTE Primus (work simulator, available from Baltimore Therapeutic Equipment, Hanover, MD) and the LIDO Work Simulator (no longer available). The drawback of these computerized work simulators is that they involve the performance of isolated tasks in unnatural conditions, reducing the applicability of the results to real working environments. In addition to the work-sample approach, job-site evaluation, situational assessment, and psychometric instruments are used to address different clinical problems, leading to different strategies to improve work efficiency and minimize work-related injuries.

SOLUTIONS RELATED TO WORKSTATION SETUP

Modifying the work environment to suit the worker's anthropometric characteristics and performance requirements is important in CTD intervention. Recommendations, ideally based on analysis of the specific job site, include providing adjustable tables and chairs that permit a more relaxed shoulder position and desktop surfaces large enough to accommodate a keyboard, a mouse, and adjustable computer mounts.[1,25,43,88,104]

One of the greatest concerns in workstation design involves the need to accommodate varying task requirements and related postural requirements. For example, substantial differences exist between joint positions required when typing on a keyboard and those required when manipulating a pointing device. In some cases, the use of alternative devices, such as an ergonomic keyboard, requires support surfaces that are larger than the standard keyboard tray.[151] The larger size of some of the alternative "ergonomic" keyboards also forces users to make considerable changes in head, trunk, and upper extremity positions when switching between keyboard and mouse tasks such as reading, writing, and editing text.[151] Moreover, there is often a need to accommodate multiple users, each with his or her own anthropometric dimensions, at a single workstation.

Generally, users are advised to maintain their limbs in what is referred to as a neutral posture.[46,151] Neutral posture involves having the following:

- Head, neck, and trunk aligned at midline
- Head upright (not too far forward)
- Shoulders retracted and relaxed
- Upper arms relaxed at side of body
- Elbows flexed to approximately 90 degrees
- Forearms not completely pronated, preferably close to midline
- Wrists aligned with forearms with minimal ulnar or radial deviation and minimal flexion or extension

Adjustment of keyboard height and slope is one of the most frequently recommended changes in the computer workstation setup. Support for the importance of height adjustment comes from studies, such as that of Sauter and co-workers,[111] in which several hundred computer users reported that arm discomfort increased as keyboard height was raised above elbow level. Although most investigators agree that correct keyboard height is important in achieving comfortable, safe, and efficient use during prolonged data-entry tasks, the range in the values recommended for the general population is extremely wide.[90,92] This presumably reflects both a wide range of user preferences and significant variation in anthropometric characteristics.

Adjusting keyboard slope is another commonly recommended change. Almost all computer keyboards are constructed with a modest upward incline and have the option of achieving a small additional incline provided by two small pop-up support posts located beneath the keyboard. However, one study showed that subjects preferred typing on a keyboard that was declined by 12 degrees below the horizontal, essentially eliminating the built-in slope.[51] The subjects in this study chose to sit approximately 10 cm (4 in) farther from the computer screen when the keyboard angle was flattened. A more recent study showed that angles ranging from 0 to −30 degrees (i.e., a negative sloping keyboard) provided significant reductions in exposure to deviated wrist postures and muscle activity and comparable performance.[148] In another recent study, wrist extension decreased as the keyboard slope decreased, and there was a small decrease in muscle activity of the extensor carpi ulnaris (ECU).[118] The combined adjustment of slope and the proximity of the keyboard to the monitor did not have a significant effect on muscle activity of the upper trapezius.[129] Variations in a keyboard's pitch, roll, and yaw angles on finger motion, wrist motion, and tendon travel were examined; tendon travel was influenced by pitch, whereas wrist deviation was influenced by all three angles.[131]

Varying monitor height by 80 to 120 cm (31 to 47 in) has been shown to have a significant effect on neck angle, thoracic bending, and vertical eye position.[139] In contrast, Kietrys and colleagues[66] showed that raising the height of the computer monitor by approximately 13 cm (5 in), from an initial desktop height of 96.5 cm (38 in), had no significant effect on head and neck angle for a group of experienced computer users (at least not during the brief time they were monitored). A recent study of female bifocal wearers showed that although self-reported pain symptoms were correlated with hours of VDT work (with a threshold of about 5 hours for pain symptoms), there was no correlation for these users between pain and monitor placement.[83] Seghers and colleagues showed that lowering screen height resulted in a decreased ear-eye angle, an increased viewing angle, and increased muscle activity of the neck extensor muscles.[114] Based on EMG results, muscle fatigue was observed only rarely, although muscle activity did increase significantly in some muscles and for certain screen heights.

Hamilton found that source document position had a significant effect on muscle activity levels; the largest neck extensor and sternocleidomastoid EMGs were recorded when subjects read documents laid flat on a table.[48] Placement of documents farther from the user's midline in either vertical or horizontal directions also increased EMG activity. Ideally, source documents should be placed so that the head and body remain symmetrically aligned in a middle position.[48]

Note, however, that some recent studies[44] suggest that workstation dimensions are not as important as previously determined for computer workers (in particular for neck and upper extremity discomfort). Moreover, not all workstation characteristics affect posture, and many computer users do not work in neutral postures. Nevertheless, improvements in workstation characteristics were associated with an enhanced perception by users of ergonomic qualities, and they reported less upper back pain and greater satisfaction.[89]

ISSUES RELATED TO DESKTOP AND NOTEBOOK COMPUTERS

Compared with desktop computer users, notebook computer users are much more limited in their ability to adjust head and body posture to comfortable positions because the screen and keyboard of a notebook computer are joined. EMG and video studies have shown that notebook users have significantly more neck flexor activity and tilt their heads farther anteriorly than when they use a

desktop computer.[110,123] However, no other differences in body postures were observed, and users complained of more discomfort after their 20-minute session with the notebook than they experienced when using a desktop computer for the same amount of time. A more recent study has shown that more flexed postures were adopted when using smaller-sized computers, but there was greater neck movement when using desktop computers; the viewing distances decreased as the computer size decreased.[125] Whether and how much more habitual notebook users will suffer from CTD symptoms than desktop computer users remains to be determined. At the very least, users must be aware of the need to change their workstation support furniture when switching from a desktop to a notebook computer. Notebook design per se appears to have less impact on dose exposure than does the work position of the device (on the desk versus on the lap).[91] Particular caution should be taken when using very compact and lightweight portable personal computers, because it is tempting to use them while they are positioned in locations that lead to awkward postures.[138]

ISSUES RELATED TO KEYBOARD LAYOUT

Neither the layout nor the characteristics of individual keys in most standard computer keyboards take into account that fingers differ in strength, dexterity, and susceptibility to fatigue.[4,31,73] For example, although the thumb possesses the greatest strength and agility, it is generally allocated the least amount of work.[31,38]

Over the years the standard layout has been severely criticized. Ferguson and Duncan suggested that a more efficient layout would avoid the placement of commonly occurring letters in the front and back rows, unlike the standard QWERTY design, in which most of the typing is done on the back row.[38] A major objective of Dvorak's alphanumeric layout was to diminish digit and hand movement.[31] Indeed, this keyboard is considered by some to be an optimal layout because it permits the typing of an exceptionally large number of commonly used words exclusively with home row characters.[23] Despite the considerable interest in Dvorak's and other layouts over the years, the standard layout dominates the market. Although some studies have reported that the Dvorak layout is easier to learn and enables its users to achieve greater speed and accuracy,[31,135] others dispute these findings[68] and suggest that improvements of less than 5% to 10% are more realistic. Indeed, a critical examination of the evidence for and against the two keyboard layouts has shown that little, if any, advantage accompanies the Dvorak layout.[80] To date, no reliable evidence demonstrates that the Dvorak layout results in less fatiguing or injurious keyboard usage.

SOLUTIONS RELATED TO KEYBOARD STRUCTURE

Variations in keyboard structure have been the subject of fairly intensive study over the years, with the objective of providing faster, more accurate, less fatiguing, and more comfortable keyboard access.[73] Splitting the keyboard into symmetric half-keyboards provides the possibility of tremendous flexibility in hand and digit position. Each half-keyboard can be tilted laterally, enabling the typist to rotate the forearm from prone to a middle position. In some models, the angle between each half can also be enlarged, enabling greater flexibility of the wrist.

In an early study, lateral tilt appeared to increase key press rate and decrease errors but did not alter users' perceived fatigue.[24] In contrast, neither experienced nor inexperienced typists in Kroemer's[73] study of a split keyboard demonstrated any significant improvements in typing speed or accuracy, although they did claim to feel more comfortable with the split, tilted keyboard. Lateral tilts in the range of 10 to 30 degrees combined with a modest opening angle decreased muscle activity in the shoulder girdle and arm region, suggesting more comfortable keying.[92] The latter study also showed that, in comparison with a standard keyboard, the split, open-angled keyboard greatly decreased ulnar deviation.

A survey of more than 400 alternative keyboard users found that 81% were satisfied with their keyboards, noting improvements in posture and comfort and reduction in pain.[150] A more recent study, however, did not demonstrate any

significant difference in discomfort and fatigue reported by subjects who used both a standard and a split keyboard (over the 2-day period examined in the study).[124] Another study showed that the Comfort keyboard (adjusted to a lateral slope of 30 degrees and a horizontal split of 20 degrees) enabled subjects to type with less ulnar deviation and wrist extension.[107] In the same study, the Tru-Form keyboard also reduced ulnar deviation but caused subjects to type with wrist extension beyond accepted safe wrist-extension values (15 degrees). Long-term data examining the ability of split keyboards to reduce CTD incidence or to reduce symptoms in those who have been injured while using a traditional keyboard are unavailable, however.

Despite mixed evidence concerning their effectiveness in CTD reduction, a number of split keyboards that cater primarily to computer users who have an existing injury or wish to avoid a potential injury are available.[150] Given the relatively low cost of many of these alternatives, typists should consider trying one or more of these keyboards, making sure to monitor productivity and comfort. The trial period should be long enough to ensure that the new keyboard is used in an automatic and natural way.[151]

Fixed split keyboards, the most common and usually the least expensive of the alternative keyboards,[151] have a fixed lateral split angle and sometimes a slightly raised center. Some of the more popular brands are listed in Table 13-1. Some models are larger than the standard keyboard, forcing the user to reach an additional 5 to 7 cm (2 to 3 in) to operate the mouse.[151] With adjustable split keyboards, the lateral angle and, in some models, the vertical angle can be varied.

A recent metaanalysis examined the efficacy of three alternative keyboard designs, including adjustable slope, split fixed-angle, and adjustable open-tented keyboards, in reducing forearm pronation, wrist extension, and ulnar deviation.[16] Analyses of six studies indicated that the open-tented design had a large effect on pronation and ulnar deviation and that the split fixed-angle design had a large effect only on ulnar deviation. The adjustable slope design was found to have a large effect on wrist extension. None of the key-

TABLE 13-1   Example Keyboards with Characteristics Designed to Reduce Cumulative Trauma Disorders

Keyboard	Description	Manufacturer or Distributor	Estimated Cost (U.S. Dollars)
Acer Future	Fixed split keyboard with two keying fields that form a triangle; a touch pad is embedded in the center with four arrow keys surrounding it	Acer America Corporation www.dansdata.com/fkeyboard.htm	$100
Comfort keyboard	The comfort keyboard is the original three-piece folding keyboard with each section on a separate mount, permitting enormous adjustability; ErgoMagic and ErgoFlex are others also available	www.comfortkeyboard.com/keyboards_comfort.html	$150-$300
Ergomatic keyboard	Ergomatic keyboard is extended and expanded with redesigned "Malt" key structure and layout, which is easy to learn and ergonomically designed for the mind	www.ergo-comp.com/index.html	$175
Kinesis contoured ergonomic	Contoured keyboard with keys in curves suited to natural structure of hand and movement of the fingers; each hand has its own set of keys; thumb buttons handle many major functions	Kinesis Corporation www.kinesis-ergo.com	$289
Goldtouch keyboard	The Goldtouch adjustable keyboard allows for adjustment of the two alphanumeric sections; the separate sections allow for both horizontal and vertical movement	Keyovation www.keyovation.com	$199
Maltron	Contoured keyboard with split design and tilted keys and pads; thumb keys used for common function keys; palm resting pads	PCD Maltron Ltd. www.maltron.com	$295
MAXIM adjustable	Variable split keyboard with adjustable lateral tilt; removable palm supports	Kinesis Corporation www.kinesis-ergo.com	$149
MyKey	Fixed split keyboard with center peak and a V shape; built-in palm rests; front and rear elevators to customize hand and wrist position; circular function-key layout	Pelican Design www.pelic.com/MykeyPage.html	$275

Continued

TABLE 13-1 Example Keyboards with Characteristics Designed to Reduce Cumulative Trauma Disorders—cont'd

Keyboard	Description	Manufacturer or Distributor	Estimated Cost (U.S. Dollars)
Natural	Microsoft now has several alternate keyboards including a fixed split keyboard with built-in palm rest and adjustable wrist leveler; numeric keypad can be used to navigate pointer	Microsoft www.microsoft.com/products	$100
PACE adjustable	Two-section split; tented keyboard with easy adjustability	Pace Development www.ids2.com/pace	$245
PerfecTouch 101	PerfecTouch is a split angle adjustable that can be placed up to 14 inches apart and manipulated in various angles and positions for comfort	Ergostar www.ergostar.com/split2.shtml	$109
Safetype	Ergonomic-Interface Keyboard Systems, three-panel keyboard designed to eliminate harmful postures including extension, pronation, and deviation; it uses a handshake position with palms facing each other, and with the index fingers on the familiar "home"	SafeType www.safetype.com/	$179
SmartBoard	Fixed split keyboard with layout that fans the keys out slightly to match a typical relaxed hand; includes a comfortable palm rest and adjustable wrist leveler; keys are 20% smaller than on other split keyboards	Darwin Keyboards www.darwinkeyboards.com	$90
Truform	The Truform keyboard is a fixed split keyboard with a wave-shaped (similar to Microsoft's Natural keyboard); keyboard gently slopes to the sides to rotate the user's hands inward; Tru-Form is available with or without a built-in touchpad for both PC and Macintosh computers	www.sforh.com/keyboards/truform.html	$100

Data from Massachusetts Institute of Technology: *Access technology for information and computing*, http://web.mit.edu/afs/athena.mit.edu/project/atic/www/index.html; KS Wright, DS Wallach: *Alternative keyboard FAQ*, www.tifaq.com/keyboards.html; www.infogrip.com/category_view.asp?option = keyboard; www.alimed.com. These sources should be consulted before the purchase of keyboard to obtain further details and user feedback.

board designs was found to have a significant effect on all three postures. It is important to note that experienced 10-digit touch typists apparently adapt within about 10 minutes to many alternative keyboard structure features.[86] They are able to type with speed and accuracy similar to what they had with a conventional keyboard.

ISSUES RELATED TO KEY CHARACTERISTICS

Key activation forces should be kept low because the force exerted by typists increases by approximately 40% and finger flexor EMGs increase by approximately 20% when key activation force is increased from 0.47 to 1.02 N.[105] A reduction in key switch activation force levels to levels lower than those currently recommended by the American National Standard for Human Factors Engineering of Visual Display Terminal Workstations[6] would help decrease the biomechanical load on forearm tendons and muscles of keyboard users.

The most obvious method of reducing excessive force during keyboarding tasks is to decrease the magnitude of the force needed to activate keyboard keys. This solution is not easy to implement, however. Reducing key activation force could cause typists to inadvertently activate keys or require them to exert additional muscular effort to minimize accidental activations through contraction of proximal agonist-antagonist pairs.[102] Moreover, the results of several studies indicate that, in any case, users exert far more than the current key activation force, surpassing the activation value by as much as five times.[39] Thus, although the majority of manufactured keyboards comply with key switch standards published by organizations such as the American National Standards Institute, most typists continue to exert far more force than is actually needed.[143]

An alternative approach to reducing keyboard force has been proposed by Radwin.[102] Radwin had subjects tap repeatedly on a single key in a keyboard mock-up and found that the peak activation force could be lowered by approximately 24% simply by increasing the over travel (the displacement until a key hits bottom) from 0 to 3 mm. He suggested that the activation force was reduced because the additional over travel facili-tated finger deceleration. He further suggested that the increased over travel may provide increased proprioceptive feedback, possibly giving typists better control over the force they exert.

The effects of key switch characteristics on musculoskeletal tissue loading have been examined during tapping on computer key switches.[55] Joint torques and stiffness parameters differed across key switch designs and finger postures. Estimates of this type may help us reach a more in-depth understanding of specific injury mechanisms.

Some keyboards have sculpted keyboard and keys to facilitate natural postures and movement patterns of the fingers, hands, and arms. Examples of these contoured keyboards include the Kinesis and Maltron keyboards. Readers are advised to consult the Typing Injury Frequently Asked Questions website (www.tifaq.com) and the Massachusetts Institute of Technology's Access Technology for Information and Computing website (www.mit.edu/afs/athena.mit.edu/project/atic/www/index.html) for a frequently updated list of ergonomic alternative keyboards.

SOFTWARE SOLUTIONS

The ergonomic solutions described thus far exemplify the more traditional approach of attempting to reconfigure standard data-entry devices. An alternative approach is to use software solutions to improve the efficiency of the typist and decrease the workload. Examples of these techniques include automation of computer startup procedures, use of macros that store frequently used sequences of commands and phrases that can then be activated by one- or two-character commands, and command menus that minimize the number of key presses required to execute elaborate routines.

Another way to enhance the data-entry input-to-output ratio is word prediction. Often recommended for typists with severe motor disabilities,[8] this technique involves the use of software that presents a list of plausible completions to the initially typed characters from which the user selects the desired word. For example, subsequent to entering the initial characters *ex,* the words *exag-*

gerate, except, explore, and *extra* are listed. The appropriate word can then be selected by a single keystroke, reducing the total number of key-presses.[120,133] User performance with word-prediction software increases when more completions are presented[137] and when the choices are ordered by word length rather than alphabetically.[75] Research has focused on which systems and usage strategies are best for which types of users and tasks,[71] and considerable debate exists concerning the method's relative advantages and disadvantages. For words longer than three letters, word prediction can result in a considerable savings in keystrokes per word. Such savings may simply mean, however, that the users can complete a longer document in the same amount of time as a shorter one with no reduction of workload. As an additional asset, word prediction has been shown to have the potential to improve legibility and spelling of children with learning disabilities and handwriting difficulties.[49]

Austin and colleagues proposed that programmers consider ways to alleviate the stress placed on typists who use standard or alternative keyboard layouts when designing their software.[14] They recommend that, where possible, computer programs should be designed to avoid the use of keys that appear to be implicated in injurious typing and that frequently used commands should be allocated to keys that are more optimally placed.

SOLUTIONS RELATED TO ALTERNATE INPUT METHODS

Speech Recognition

Speech recognition is a computer input method in which the user's voice is used to enter all alphanumeric data and commands. Speech recognition has evolved from programs with a very limited vocabulary to those containing more than 100,000 words, and from programs that recognize only isolated letters to those that recognize free-flowing speech without pauses. Such systems allow for freer flow of thought and greater speed, theoretically as fast as natural speech rates (150 to 175 wpm).[72] Accuracy rates are also expected to improve, especially when systems become available that use context to recognize words and distinguish between homonyms.

Speech recognition has been intensely marketed as a way to avoid typing-induced CTDs of the neck, back, and upper extremities. Ironically, some users who use speech recognition as their primary typing method have subsequently developed CTDs in their vocal chords,[13,45,60] because some speech recognition systems require the user to speak in a monotonous tone and maintain a reasonably constant pitch and inflection. Such speech-recognition systems placed extended stress on the vocal cords, leading to swelling, hoarseness, and even complete loss of voice. Speech recognition can lead to increased activity in other muscles, namely the laryngeal muscles, leading to muscle tension dysphonia[97,146] as well as a decrease in productivity.[27]

The extent to which newer, continuous-speech systems may alleviate these problems has yet to be determined, although there is increasing evidence that speech recognition is associated with a reduction in the static muscle activity of the forearm, neck, and shoulder muscles during text entry and text editing.[59]

The continuous-speech systems offer the advantage of greater voice modulation but may strain the vocal apparatus even more by allowing the user to speak faster and more continuously. Although avoiding use of the speech-recognition system for extended periods is one way to reduce vocal fatigue and the risk of CTD, such a precaution could significantly mitigate the successful integration of its users into the vocational environment.

Mouse Pointing Devices and Mouse Alternatives

Ergonomics literature has begun to address ways to alleviate problems caused by the rapidly increasing use of the mouse and other pointing devices.[40,48,61,63] A number of variations in the design of the standard mouse have been proposed. Reductions in mouse size and modification of shape to fit the contours of a typical user's hand have frequently been advocated (Table 13-2). Even more interesting are devices that let the operator interact with graphical user interfaces by

TABLE 13-2	Example Mouse Pointing Devices with Characteristics Designed to Reduce Cumulative Trauma Disorders		
Pointing Device	**Description**	**Manufacturer or Distributor**	**Estimated Cost (U.S. Dollars)**
Anir	Designed like a pilot stick; promotes positioning of the supported forearm in midposition; switches activated by thumb	AnimaX International AS www.animax.no	$100
Perfit mouse	An optical tracking mouse that comes in several sizes for both left- and right-handed users, sculpted, elevated buttons, tilted palm support, elevated wrist support	Contour Design www.contourdesign.com/	$109
Evoluent vertical mouse	Hand supported in a completely relaxed handshake position	www.evoluent.com/vmouse2.html	$75
Goldtouch ergonomic mouse	Designed to support the hand in relaxed, neutral posture; has button-activated scrolling and panning capabilities and optical design	Goldtouch Technologies www.keyovation.com	$30
IntelliMouse Explorer	Optical mouse with four-way scrolling (including side-to-side)	Microsoft www.microsoft.com/products/hardware/inputdev.htm	$40
Natural wireless laser mouse 6000	Modeled to conform to hand in most relaxed posture	Microsoft www.microsoft.com/products/hardware/inputdev.htm	
Logitech MX Revolution	Contoured surface with conveniently located thumb and wheel buttons	Logitech www.logitech.com	$80-100
Thinking mouse whalemouse	Optical, contoured mouse with palm rest that encourages a neutral posture and promotes use of the large muscle of the arm	www.humanscale.com/products/whale_mouse.cfm	$90
Mouse in a box	Optical mouse with fast scroll wheel mechanisms	Kensington Microware www.kensington.com/products	$20

Data from Carroll D: *Ergonomic, adaptive and alternative pointing devices,* www.setbc.org/mouselist/ (Massachusetts Institute of Technology: *Access technology for information and computing,* http://web.mit.edu/afs/athena.mit.edu/project/atic/www/index.html; Mouse-Group Home Page, www.ami.dk/?lang = en, www.ami.dk/mousegroup; and KS Wright, DS Wallach: *Pointing device FAQ,* www.tifaq.com. These sources should be consulted before the purchase of any mouse pointing devices to obtain further detail and user feedback.

means quite different from those used to maneuver the standard mouse (Table 13-3). Users today can acquire pointing devices that incorporate different manipulation styles (e.g., push, roll, glide), control variables (e.g., position, force), and activation limbs (e.g., finger, hand, head, foot). The case study included at the beginning of this chapter illustrates how the use of a simple alternate pointing device (a trackball) can provide greater ease of access to computer graphics programs.

Different pointing devices must be evaluated for performance qualities, such as speed, accuracy, and endurance, and tendency to cause the user to develop CTDs. Not all pointing devices are equal in terms of speed and accuracy and thus are not equally suitable to the operation of all software. In an early study of pointing accuracy and speed, Albert compared the standard keyboard with five of the major cursor control methods.[3] The trackball was considerably more accurate than all other devices, whereas the touch screen was the least. However, the touch screen was the fastest control method, and the keyboard was the slowest. The trade-off between performance and safety should also be taken into consideration, as some devices provide excellent speed and accuracy but produce a significant load on the hand and forearm soft tissues.

Dennerlein and Johnson showed that frequent mouse use is associated with more constrained and nonneutral postures of the wrist and shoulder compared with keyboarding.[28] A variety of novel pointing device designs have been tested to determine their potential for decreasing exposure to CTD. For example, Ullman and colleagues examined a new mouse that is small and operated with a pivoting pen-shaped handle.[132] EMG activity was significantly less in the major shoulder muscles when computer users used the new mouse as compared with the traditional mouse. Some have studied efficiency, user satisfaction, and muscle activity of subjects using various pointing devices including an electromechanical force-feedback trackball,[64] a touch pen,[152] and a built-in touch pad.[77]

As for keyboard users, certain arm positions are more comfortable for mouse users. Karlqvist

and co-workers found that users preferred manipulating a standard mouse when they had arm support and were able to maintain the forearm in a middle position.[61] The user's body dimensions had a significant effect on preferred mouse location.

Certain mouse tasks, such as dragging, can be particularly taxing, causing sustained loading of the finger flexor muscles. Pointing-device manufacturers sometimes provide ways to carry out dragging without keeping the mouse button pressed. For example, the drag function can be locked by a third switch on some trackball devices or by some mouse driver programs. The user simply locks the cursor into drag mode then proceeds to move the mouse as in other mouse tasks. Releasing the switch returns the mouse to regular operation.

Researchers active in ergonomics continually explore innovative methods of cursor position manipulation. Devices should provide high performance but not expose the user to harmful positions or forces. The Anir mouse,[2] for example, allows users to manipulate cursor position by lightly gripping an upright stick. The mouse is operated with the forearm in a middle position instead of the usual pronated position, and the mouse buttons are activated by slight movements of the thumb. Subjects exhibited lower EMGs in the extensor digitorum communis, ECU, and trapezius muscle when using the Anir mouse than with a standard mouse, even when the standard mouse was accompanied by forearm support.[2] Another novel mouse alternative is based on a finger-motion recognition system in which finger position and shape are recorded and recognized.[70] This technique allows for direct manipulation of the cursor without exposure to potentially dangerous positions or external forces.

CONCLUSION

Various solutions to CTDs modify user comfort, increase efficiency, and reduce susceptibility. However, adjusting furniture, using alternative keyboards and pointing devices, and adopting various software solutions are only partial solutions to CTDs. Many computer workstation users,

TABLE 13-3 **Alternatives to Mouse Pointing Devices**

Pointing Device	Description	Manufacturer	Estimated Cost (U.S. Dollars)
Desktop 1.5-inch trackball	A compact, low-profile industrial trackball with a variety of button locations	Evergreen Systems International www.trackballs.com	N/A
Cirque Smart Cat Pro touchpad	Finger moves over small, touch-sensitive pad to control cursor position; one-touch hotlinks open up files quickly	Cirque Corporation www.cirque.com	$70
HeadMouse Extreme	Tracks a small reflective dot placed on user's forehead such that head movement is translated into cursor movement; button clicks are through an adaptive switch or by dwelling on an image	Origin Instruments www.orin.com	$995
Mouse Pen	This pen-shaped unit is a high-resolution optical mouse that can be used on almost any surface	www.ergo-items.com/mouse_pen.htm	$35-$80
Mouse-Trak	Large trackball with button on each side and a large button below; large padded base on which to rest hand	ITAC Systems www.mousetrak.com	$149
NoHands Mouse	Operated with the feet, one pedal moves the cursor, the other is used for clicking	Hunter Digital www.footmouse.com	$350
Orbit and Expert Mouse	Orbit is a trackball with optical features and large buttons on each side; Expert Mouse is a large programmable trackball with for large buttons on each side	Kensington http://ca.kensington.com	Orbit: $29 Expert: $99
Rollermouse Pro	Integrated in the center of a forearm support is a wide roller bar that controls the cursor and extends the length of the keyboard; has a scroll wheel and five buttons.	Contour Design www.contourdesign.com	$199
Logitech cordless Trackman wheel	Cordless device that allows the hand to rest over the programmable buttons while the thumb controls the trackball for cursor movement; includes a scroll wheel at the fingertips.	Logitech www.logitech.com	$50

Data from Carroll D: *The mouse list: adaptive and alternative pointing devices,* www.setbc.org/mouselist; Massachusetts Institute of Technology: *Access technology for information and computing,* http://web.mit.edu/afs/athena.mit.edu/project/atic/www/index.html; *Mouse-Group Home Page,* www.ami.dk/?lang=en; and KS Wright, DS Wallach: *Pointing device FAQ,* www.tifaq.com/mice.html. These sources should be consulted before the purchase of any pointing devices to obtain further details and user feedback.

particularly those who are highly motivated and who are working to meet one deadline after another, may need more than hardware and software solutions. Such users not only need to learn to use the equipment properly; they must learn to recognize the positions, postures, and working styles that place them at risk. Keeping workers aware of a taxonomy of injurious keyboard techniques serves to focus attention on technique errors that can be corrected with sufficient instruction.[101]

A number of studies have examined the efficacy of educating workers to recognize, report, and seek intervention for CTDs. Training programs of differing lengths and styles have aimed to teach workers to analyze their workstations, recognize hazards, and make appropriate changes.[67] Addressing specific habits that the worker has developed is often useful. For example, observing a typist for the amount of force exerted in keystrokes could lead to individual recommendations to correct injurious work styles.[39] A lack of synchrony between the internal physiologic rhythms of a worker and the rhythm set by the work has also been noted to be a potentially significant source of stress in tasks that are inherently repetitive, such as keyboarding.[52] Giving a worker greater control over his or her own work rhythm may help reduce this source of stress.

Learning Exercise

Overview

The learning exercises are designed to increase your practical understanding and application of some basic concepts and solutions to minimize or eliminate risk factors in prolonged use of a VDT at the workplace.

Purpose

The purpose of these learning exercises is to implement the dose-response model in a practical situation to predict the risk factors mentioned in the case study. You will also need to formulate a list of recommendations based on the principles learned in this chapter.

Exercise

Working with your peers, identify the possible risk factors of the workstation that a peer uses in his or her day-to-day work. You are encouraged to apply the dose-response model illustrated in the text. Once you have generated the risk factors, you can then proceed to work out a list of recommendations aimed at further improving the workstation. The recommendations should be justified by the ergonomic principles introduced in the text. More important, these recommendations should be suitable in terms of both their feasibility and their acceptability by your peers.

Multiple Choice Review Questions

1. Which of the following risk factors appear(s) to contribute to the pathophysiology of CTD?
   A. Repetitive motion
   B. Excessive force
   C. Awkward working posture
   D. Excessive vibration
   E. Answers A, B, and C

2. In the dose-response model of CTD, dose refers to:
   A. mechanical forces acting on the body tissues, physiologic consumption of metabolic substrates, and production of metabolites within the tissues, as well as psychologic disturbances such as anxiety about work.
   B. physical characteristics of the job, including the weight, size, and shape of tools, and psychologic factors such as job security.
   C. physical and psychologic ability to resist destabilization.
   D. an individual's reaction to exposure, modified by his or her capacity.
   E. None of the above

3. For most risk factors, exposure time is critical; thus:
   A. exposure should be reduced to less than 2 hours per day.
   B. exposure time should be reduced where the work environment is impoverished from a psychosocial viewpoint.
   C. varying the type of work tasks performed in a work shift such that the worker is not exposed to any single risk factor for an extended period is advisable.
   D. rest breaks are not always beneficial.
   E. Answers B, C, and D

4. EMG evaluation is used to analyze the muscular work pattern of workers at their workstations. This technique:
   A. reveals how a muscle responds to varying load conditions.
   B. shows when a muscle becomes fatigued.
   C. can identify which muscles are used to carry out specific tasks.
   D. is easy to use in all work environments.
   E. Answers A, B, and C

5. A keyboard user's susceptibility to injury will not be affected by:
   A. typing accuracy.
   B. force exerted on each key.
   C. total typing time.
   D. amount of time spent on each key.
   E. All of the above

6. Computer users are advised to maintain their limbs in a neutral posture, which includes:
   A. tilting the head anteriorly approximately 20 degrees.
   B. aligning the head, neck, and trunk midline.
   C. protracting the shoulders.
   D. pronating the forearms completely.
   E. All of the above

7. In comparison with desktop computers, notebook computers:
   A. limit the user's ability to adjust head and body posture to comfortable positions.
   B. cause users to generate significantly more neck flexor activity and tilt their heads anteriorly.
   C. cause greater discomfort to the user.
   D. Answers A and B
   E. Answers A, B, and C

8. Compared with the standard QWERTY keyboard layout, the Dvorak layout:
   A. is much easier to learn.
   B. enables its users to achieve greater speed and accuracy.
   C. is less fatiguing to use.
   D. is less injurious.
   E. None of the above

9. Word prediction:
   A. does not necessarily help the typist with CTD, because he or she is now able to complete a longer document in the same amount of time with no reduction of workload.
   B. was originally developed for users with severe motor disabilities to enhance their input and output efficiency.
   C. provides considerable savings in keystrokes per word only for words longer than six characters.
   D. Answers A and B
   E. Answers A, B, and C

10. Mouse and mouse-alternative pointing devices differ in:
    A. manipulation styles (e.g., push, roll, glide).
    B. control variables (e.g., position, force).
    C. activation limbs (e.g., finger, hand, head, foot).
    D. performance characteristics (e.g., speed, accuracy, endurance).
    E. All of the above

REFERENCES

1. Aaras A: Relationship between trapezius load and the incidence of musculoskeletal illness in the neck and shoulder, *Int J Ind Ergonomics* 14:341, 1994.
2. Aaras A, Westgaard RH, Stranden E et al: Postural load and the incidence of musculoskeletal illness. In *Proceedings from the NIOSH workshop: promoting health and productivity in the computerized office,* New York, 1997, Taylor & Francis.
3. Albert A: The effect of graphic input devices on performance in a cursor positioning task. In *Proceedings of the Human Factors Society 26th annual meeting,* Santa Monica, Calif, 1982, Human Factors Society.
4. Alden DA, Daniels RW, Kanarick AF: Keyboard design and operation: a review of the major issues, *Hum Factors* 14:275, 1972.
5. Alqattan MM, Bowen V: Cumulative trauma disorders of the hand and wrist, *Curr Opin Orthop* 4:68, 1993.
6. American National Standards Institute (ANSI): American national standard for human factors engineering of visual display terminal workstations, *ANSI HFS* 100, 1988.
7. Andersen JH, Thomsen JF, Overgaard E et al: Computer use and carpal tunnel syndrome: a 1-year follow-up study, JAMA 289:2963, 2003.
8. Anson D: The effect of word prediction on typing speed, *Am J Occup Ther* 47:1039, 1993.
9. Armstrong TJ: Ergonomics and cumulative trauma disorders of the hand and wrist. In Hunter JM, Schneider LH, Mackin EJ et al, editors: *Rehabilitation of the hand: surgery and therapy,* ed 3, St Louis, 1990, Mosby.
10. Armstrong TJ, Buckle P, Fine LJ et al: A conceptual model for work-related neck and upper-limb musculoskeletal disorders, *Scand J Work Environ Health* 19:73, 1993.
11. Armstrong TJ, Fine LJ, Radwin RG et al: Ergonomics and the effects of vibration in hand-intensive work, *Scand J Work Environ Health* 13:286, 1987.
12. Armstrong TJ, Foulke JA, Martin BJ et al: Investigation of applied forces in alphanumeric keyboard work, *Am Ind Hyg Assoc J* 55:30, 1994.
13. Arnaught G: Talking to computers has its hazards, *Globe and Mail,* September 15, 1995.
14. Austin H, Johnson M, Moras R: *Keyboard or software design?* Norcross, Ga, 1997, IIE Solutions.
15. Ballard J: Work related upper limb disorders, *Occup Health Rev* 46:9, 1993.
16. Baker NA, Cidboy EL: The effect of three alternative keyboard designs on forearm pronation, wrist extension, and ulnar deviation: a meta-analysis, *Am J Occup Ther* 60:40, 2006.
17. Barr AE, Barbe MF, Clark BD: Work-related musculoskeletal disorders of the hand and wrist: epidemiology, pathophysiology, and sensorimotor changes, *J Orthop Sports Phys Ther* 34(10):610, 2004.
18. Bartys S, Burton K, Main C: A prospective study of psychosocial risk factors and absence due to musculoskeletal disorders—implications for occupational screening, *Occup Med* 55(3):375, 2005.
19. Berkhout AL, Hendriksson-Larsen K, Bongers P: The effect of using a laptop station compared to using a standard laptop PC on the cervical spine torque, perceived strain and productivity, *Appl Ergon* 35:147, 2004.
20. Blehm C, Vishnu S, Khattak A et al: Computer vision syndrome: a review, *Surv Ophthalmol* 50:253, 2005.
21. Blomkvist AC, Bard G: Computer usage with cold hands; an experiment with pointing devices, *Int J Occup Saf Ergon* 6:429, 2000.
22. Bureau of Labor Statistics: Over half of workers used a computer in 2001, Washington DC, 2002, Bureau of Labor Statistics. Retrieved March 15, 2004, from www.bls.gov/opub/ted/2002/oct/wk3/art04.htm.
23. Cooper WE: *Cognitive aspects of skilled typewriting,* New York, 1983, Springer-Verlag.
24. Creamer LR, Trumbo DA: Multifinger tapping performance as a function of the direction of tapping movements, *J Appl Psychol* 44:376, 1960.
25. Dainoff MJ, Cohen BG, Dainoff MH: The effect of an ergonomic intervention on musculoskeletal, psychosocial, and visual strain of VDT data entry work: the United States part of the international study, *Int J Occup Safety Ergon* 11:49, 2005.
26. Davis L, Wellman H, Punnett L: Surveillance of work related carpal tunnel syndrome in Massachusetts, 1992-1997: a report from the Massachusetts Sentinel Event Notification System for Occupational Risks (SENSOR), *Am J Ind Med* 39:58, 2001.
27. de Korte EM, van Lingen P: The effect of speech recognition on working postures, productivity and the perception of user friendliness, *Appl Ergon* 37:341, 2006.
28. Dennerlein JT, Johnson PW: Different computer tasks affect the exposure of the upper extremity to biomechanical risk factors, *Ergonomics* 49:45, 2006.
29. Dobyns JH: Balancing psyche, soma and society in overuse syndromes. In Vastasmaki M, editor: *Current trends in hand surgery,* Amsterdam, 1995, Elsevier.

30. Doheny M, Linden P, Sedlak C: Reducing orthopaedic hazards of the computer work environment, *Orthop Nurs* 14:7, 1995.

31. Dvorak A: There is a better typewriter keyboard, *Natl Business Educ Q* 12:51, 1943.

32. Ekman A, Andersson A, Hagberg M et al: Gender differences in musculoskeletal health of computer and mouse users in the Swedish workforce, *Occup Med* 50:608, 2000.

33. Fahrback PA, Chapman LJ: VDT work duration and musculoskeletal discomfort, *Am Assoc Occup Health Nurses J* 38:32, 1990.

34. Fast C: Repetitive strain injury: an overview of the condition and its implications for occupational therapy practice, *Can J Occup Ther* 62:119, 1995.

35. Faucett J, Rempel DM: VDT-related musculoskeletal symptoms: interactions between work posture and psychosocial work factors, *Am J Ind Med* 26:597, 1994.

36. Feely CA, Seaton MK, Arfken CL et al: Effects of work and rest on upper extremity signs and symptoms of workers performing repetitive tasks, *J Occup Rehabil* 5:145, 1995.

37. Feldman RG, Goldman R, Keyserling WM: Peripheral nerve entrapment syndromes and ergonomic factors, *Am J Ind Med* 4:661, 1983.

38. Ferguson D, Duncan J: Keyboard design and operating postures, *Ergonomics* 17:731, 1974.

39. Feuerstein M, Armstrong T, Hickey P et al: Computer keyboard force and upper extremity symptoms, *J Occup Environ Med* 12:1144, 1997.

40. Fogelman M, Brogmas G: Computer mouse use and cumulative trauma disorders of the upper extremities, *Ergonomics* 38:2465, 1995.

41. Frederick L: Cumulative trauma disorders, *Am Assoc Occup Health Nurses J* 40:113, 1992.

42. Gerard MJ, Armstrong TJ, Rempel DA et al: Short term and long term effects of enhanced auditory feedback on typing force, EMG and comfort while typing, *Appl Ergon* 33:129, 2002.

43. Gerr F, Marcus M, Monteilh C et al: A randomised controlled trial of postural interventions for prevention of musculoskeletal symptoms among computer users, *Occup Environment Med* 6:478, 2005.

44. Gerr F, Marcus M, Ortiz D et al: Computer users' postures and associations with workstation characteristics, *Am Ind Hyg Assoc J* 61:223, 2000.

45. Gooderham M: High-tech RSI aid creates new problem, *Globe and Mail,* September 4, 1995.

46. Grandjean E: *Fitting the task to the man. A textbook of occupational ergonomics,* ed 4, London, 1988, Taylor & Francis.

47. Gun RT: The incidence and distribution of RSI in South Australia 1980-1981 and 1986-1987, *Med J Aust* 153:376, 1990.

48. Hamilton N: Source document position as it affects head position and neck muscle tension, *Ergonomics* 39:593, 1996.

49. Handley-More D, Deitz J, Billingsley FF et al: Facilitating written work using computer word processing and word prediction, *Am J Occup Ther* 57:139, 2003.

50. Hashemi L, Webster BS, Clancy EA et al: Length of disability and cost of work-related musculoskeletal disorders of the upper extremity, *J Occup Environ Med* 40:261, 1998.

51. Hedge A, Powers JR: Wrist postures while keyboarding: effects of a negative slope keyboard system and full motion forearm supports, *Ergonomics* 38:508, 1995.

52. Henning RA, Sauter SL, Krieg EF: Work rhythm and physiological rhythms in repetitive computer work: effects of synchronization on well-being, *Int J Hum Comput Interact* 4:233, 1992.

53. Hunting W, Laubli T, Grandjean E: Postural and visual loads at VDT workplaces. I. Constrained postures, *Ergonomics* 24:917, 1981.

54. Islam SS, Velilla AM, Doyle EJ, Ducatman AM: Gender differences in work-related injury/illness: analysis of workers compensation claims, *Am J Ind Med* 39:84, 2001.

55. Jindrich DL, Balakrishnan AD, Dennerlein JT: Effects of keyswitch design and finger posture on finger joint kinematics and dynamics during tapping on computer keyswitches, *Clin Biomech* 19:600, 2004.

56. Johnson P, Dropkin J, Hewes J et al: Office ergonomics: motion analysis of computer mouse usage. In *Proceedings of the American Industrial Hygiene Conference and Exposition,* Fairfax, Va, 1993, American Industrial Hygiene Association.

57. Juul-Kristensen B, Fallentin N, Ekdahl C: Criteria for classification of posture in repetitive work by observation methods: a review, *Int J Indust Ergonomics* 19:397, 1997.

58. Juul-Kristensen B, Jensen C: Self-reported workplace related ergonomics conditions as prognostic factors for musculoskeletal symptoms: the "BIT" follow up study on office workers, *Occup Environ Med* 62:188, 2005.

59. Juul-Kristensen B, Laursen B, Pilegaard M et al: Physical workload during use of speech recognition and traditional computer input devices, *Ergonomics* 47:119, 2004.

60. Kambeyanda D, Singer L, Cronk S: Potential problems associated with use of speech recognition products, *Assist Technol* 9:95, 1997.

61. Karlqvist LK, Bernmark E, Ekenvall L et al: Computer mouse position as a determinant of posture, muscular load and perceived exertion, *Scand J Work Environ Health* 24:62, 1998.

62. Karlqvist LK, Hagberg M: Musculoskeletal symptoms among computer-assisted design (CAD) operators and evaluation of a self-assessment questionnaire, *Int J Occup Environ Health* 2:185, 1996.

63. Karlqvist LK, Hagberg M, Selin K: Variation in upper limb posture and movement during word processing with and without mouse use, *Ergonomics* 37:1261, 1994.

64. Keuning H, Monne TK, IJsselsteijn WA et al: The form of augmented force-feedback fields and the efficiency and satisfaction in computer-aided pointing tasks, *Hum Factors* 47:418, 2005.

65. Kierklo E, Jones S: Stop repetitive injuries before they start, *Safety Health* 150:68, 1994.

66. Kietrys DM, McClure PW, Fitzgerald GK: The relationship between head and neck posture and VDT screen height in keyboard operators, *Phys Ther* 78:395, 1998.

67. King PM, Fisher JC, Garg A: Evaluation of the impact of employee ergonomics training in industry, *Appl Ergon* 28:249, 1997.

68. Kinkead R: Typing speed, keying rates, and optimal keyboard layout. In *Proceedings of the Human Factors Society Nineteenth Annual Meeting*, Dallas, 1975, Human Factors Society.

69. Knardahl S: Psychophysiological mechanisms of pain in computer work: the blood vessel–nociceptor interaction hypotheses, *Work Stress* 16:179, 2002.

70. Ko BK, Yang HS: Finger mouse and gesture recognition system as a new human computer interface, *Comput Graphics* 21:555, 1997.

71. Koester HH, Levine SP: Model simulations of user performance with word prediction, *Augment Altern Commun* 14:25, 1998.

72. Kraat A: *Communication interaction between aided and natural speakers*, Madison, Wis, 1987, Trace Research and Development Center.

73. Kroemer KH: Human engineering the keyboard, *Hum Factors* 14:51, 1972.

74. Kuorinka I, Johnsson B, Kilbom A et al: Standardized Nordic questionnaire for the analysis of musculoskeletal symptoms, *Appl Ergon* 18:233, 1987.

75. Lanspa A, Wood LA, Beukelman DR: Efficiency with which disabled and nondisabled students locate words in cue windows: study of three organizational strategies—frequency of word use, word length and alphabetic order, *Augment Altern Commun* 13:117, 1997.

76. Lechner D, Roth D, Straaton X: Functional capacity evaluation in work disability, *Work* 1:37, 1991.

77. Lee TH: Ergonomic comparison of operating a built-in touch-pad pointing device and a trackball mouse on posture and muscle activity, *Percept Mot Skills* 101:730, 2005.

78. Leinonen T, Kisko K: A new method for work analysis, *Int J Indust Ergon* 21:361, 1998.

79. Leung PC, Wong SKM: Extensor origin tendinitis around the elbow: its relationship with occupation. In Vastasmaki M, editor: *Current trends in hand surgery*, Amsterdam, 1995, Elsevier.

80. Liebowitz SJ, Margolis SE: The fable of the keys, *J Law Econ* 33:1, 1990.

81. Loeb KM: Membrane keyboards and human performance, *Bell Syst Tech J* 62:1773, 1983.

82. Lundborg G, Dahlin LB: Vibration-induced hand problems. In Vastasmaki M, editor: *Current trends in hand surgery*, Amsterdam, 1995, Elsevier.

83. Lyon JL Jr, Lillquist DR, Alder S et al: An analysis of VDT monitor placement and daily hours of use for female bifocal users, *Work* 20:77, 2003.

84. Mallory M, Bradford H: An invisible work place hazard gets harder to ignore, *Business Week* January 30, 1989, p 92.

85. Malzahn DE, Fernandez JE, Kattel BP: Design-oriented functional capacity evaluation: the available motion inventory—a review, *Disabil Rehabil* 18:382, 1996.

86. Marklin RW, Simoneau GG: Design features of alternative computer keyboards: a review of experimental data, *J Orthop Sport Phys Ther* 34:638, 2004.

87. Mason HJ, Poole K, Elms J: Upper limb disability in HAVS cases—how does it relate to the neurosensory or vascular elements of HAVS? *Occup Med* 55:389, 2005.

88. Matias AC, Salvendy G, Kuczek T: Predictive models of carpal tunnel syndrome causation among VDT operators, *Ergonomics* 41:213, 1998.

89. May DR, Reed K, Schwoerer CE et al: Ergonomic office design and aging: a quasi-experimental field study of employee reactions to an ergonomics intervention program, *J Occup Health Psychol* 9:123, 2004.

90. Miller W, Suther TW: Display station and anthropometrics: preferred height and angle settings of CRT and keyboard, *Hum Factors* 25:401, 1983.

91. Moffet H, Hagberg M, Hansson-Risberg E et al: Influence of laptop computer design and working position on physical exposure variables, *Clin Biomech* 17:368, 2002.

92. Nakaseko E, Grandjean E, Hunting W et al: Studies on ergonomically designed alphanumeric keyboards, *Hum Factors* 27:175, 1985.

93. Nakazawa T, Okubo Y, Suwazono Y et al: Association between duration of daily VDT use and subjective symptoms, *Am J Ind Med* 42:421, 2002.

94. Nathan PA, Meadows KD, Doyle LS: Occupation as a risk factor for impaired sensory conduction of the median nerve at the carpal tunnel, *J Hand Surg* 13:167, 1988.

95. Occupational Safety and Health Council: *Report on survey of office environment and the occupational health of visual display terminals (VDT) users,* Hong Kong, 1997, Occupational Safety and Health Council.

96. Ohlsson K, Attewell RG, Johnsson B et al: An assessment of neck and upper extremity disorders by questionnaire and clinical evaluation, *Ergonomics* 37:891, 1994.

97. Olson DE, Cruz RM, Izdebski K et al: Muscle tension dysphonia in patients who use computerized speech recognition systems, *Ear Nose Throat J* 83:195, 2004.

98. Oksa J: Neuromuscular performance limitations in cold, *Int J Circumpolar Health,* 61:154, 2002.

99. Oxenburgh M: Musculoskeletal injuries occurring in word processor operators. In Adams A, Stevenson M, editors: *Ergonomics and technological change: proceedings of the 21st Annual Conference of the Ergonomics Society of Australia and New Zealand,* Sydney, Victoria, Australia, November 28-30, 1984, Ergonomics Society of Australia and New Zealand.

100. Pan CS, Schleifer LM: An exploratory study of the relationship between biomechanical factors and right-arm musculoskeletal discomfort and fatigue in a VDT data entry task, *Appl Ergon* 26:195, 1996.

101. Pascarelli EF, Kella JJ: Soft-tissue injuries related to use of the computer keyboard, *J Occup Med* 35:522, 1993.

102. Radwin RG: Activation force and travel effects on overexertion in repetitive key tapping, *Hum Factors* 39:130, 1997.

103. Rempel DM, Harrison RJ, Barnhart S: Work-related cumulative trauma disorders of the upper extremity, *JAMA* 267:838, 1991.

104. Rempel DM, Krause N, Goldberg R et al: A randomised controlled trial evaluating the effects of two workstation interventions on upper body pain and incident musculoskeletal disorders among computer operators, *Occup Environ Med* 63:297, 2006.

105. Rempel DM, Serina E, Kinenberg E et al: The effect of keyboard keyswitch make force on applied force and finger flexor muscle activity, *Ergonomics* 40:800, 1997.

106. Rizzo TH, Pelletier KR, Serxner S et al: Reducing risk factors for cumulative trauma disorders (CTDs): the impact of preventive ergonomic training on knowledge, intentions, and practices related to computer use, *Am J Health Promot* 11(4):250, 1997.

107. Ro J, Jacobs K: Wrist postures in video display terminal operators (VDT) using different keyboards, *Work* 9:155, 1997.

108. Rossignol M, Patry L, Sacks S: Carpal tunnel syndrome: validation of an interview questionnaire on occupational exposure, *Am J Ind Med* 33:224, 1998.

109. Ruess L, O'Connor SC, Cho KH et al: Carpal tunnel syndrome and cubital tunnel syndrome: work-related musculoskeletal disorders in four symptomatic radiologists, Am J Roentgenol 181:37, 2003.

110. Saito S, Miyao M, Kondo T et al: Ergonomic evaluation of working posture of VDT operation using personal computer with flat panel display, *Ind Health* 35:264, 1997.

111. Sauter SL, Schleifer LM, Knutson SJ: Work posture, workstation design, and musculoskeletal discomfort in a VDT data entry task, *Hum Factors* 33:151, 1991.

112. Schreuer N, Lifshitz Y, Weiss PL: The effect of typing frequency and speed on the incidence of upper extremity cumulative trauma disorder, *Work* 6:87, 1996.

113. Schuldt K, Ekholm J, Harms-Ringdahl K et al: Effects of changes in sitting work posture on static neck and shoulder muscle activity, *Ergonomics* 12:1525, 1986.

114. Seghers J, Jochem A, Spaepen A: Posture, muscle activity and muscle fatigue in prolonged VDT work at different screen height settings, *Ergonomics* 10:714, 2003.

115. Shaw WS, Feuerstein M, Miller VI et al: Clinical tools to facilitate workplace accommodation after treatment for an upper extremity disorder, *Assist Technol* 3:94, 2001.

116. Sillanpaa J, Huikko S, Nyberg M et al: Effect of work with visual display units on musculo-skeletal disorders in the office environment, *Occup Med* 53(7):443, 2003.

117. Silverstein B, Armstrong TJ, Fine LJ Hand wrist cumulative trauma disorders in industry, *J Ind Med* 43:779, 1986.

118. Simoneau GG, Marklin RW, Berman JE: Effect of computer keyboard slope on wrist position and forearm electromyography of typists without musculoskeletal disorders, *Phys Ther* 83:816, 2003.

119. Sjogaard J: Work induced muscle fatigue and its relation to muscle pain. In *Conference Proceedings: Occupational Disorders of the Upper Extremity*, Ann Arbor, Mich, March 29-30, 1990, University of Michigan.

120. Smith RO, Christiaasen R, Borden B et al: Effectiveness of a writing system using a computerized long-range optical pointer 10-branch abbreviation expansion, *J Rehabil Res Dev* 26:51, 1989.

121. Sommerich CM, Marras WS, Parnianpour M: Activity of index finger muscles during typing. In *Proceeding of the Human Factors and Ergonomics Society 39th Annual Meeting*, Philadelphia 1996.

122. Stetson DS, Keyserling WM, Silverstein BA et al: Observational analysis of the hand and wrist: a pilot study, *J Appl Occup Environ Hyg* 6:927, 1991.

123. Straker L, Jones KJ, Miller J: A comparison of the postures assumed when using laptop computers and desktop computers, *Appl Ergon* 28:263, 1997.

124. Swanson NG, Galinsky TL, Cole LL et al: The impact of keyboard design on comfort and productivity in a text-entry task, *Appl Ergon* 28:9, 1997.

125. Szeto GPY, Lee R: An ergonomic evaluation comparing desktop, notebook, and subnotebook computers, *Arch Phys Med Rehabil* 83:527, 2002.

126. Szeto GPY, Straker LM, O'Sullivan PB: The effects of typing speed and force on motor control in symptomatic and asymptomatic office workers, *Ind Ergon* 35:779, 2005.

127. Taylor K: Research paper on repetitive strain injury (RSI) and breaks, 2002, Niche Software.

128. Taylor PM, Braun KA: Stretching exercise. In Taylor PM, Taylor DK, editors: *Conquering athletic injuries*, Champaign, Ill, 1988, Leisure Press.

129. Tepper M, Vollenbroek-Hutten MM, Hermens HJ et al: The effect of an ergonomic computer device on muscle activity of the upper trapezius muscle during typing, *Appl Ergon* 34:125, 2003.

130. Thomsen JF, Hansson GA, Mikkelsen S et al: Carpal tunnel syndrome in repetitive work: a follow-up study, *Am J Ind Med* 42:344, 2002.

131. Treaster DE, Marras WS: An assessment of alternate keyboards using finger motion, wrist motion and tendon travel, *Clin Biomech* 15:499, 2000.

132. Ullman J, Kangas N, Ullman P et al: A new approach to the mouse arm syndrome, *Int J Occup Saf Ergon* 9:463, 2003.

133. Vanderheiden GC: The practical use of microcomputers in rehabilitation, *Rehabil Lit* 44:66, 1981.

134. van Eijsden-Besseling MDF, Peeters FPML, Reijnen JAW et al: Perfectionism and coping strategies as risk factors for the development of non-specific work-related upper limb disorders, *Occup Med* 54:122, 2004.

135. Veiersted KB, Westgaard RH, Andersen P: Electromyographic evaluation of muscular work pattern as a predictor of trapezius myalgia, *Scand J Work Environ Health* 19:284, 1993.

136. Vender MI, Kasdan ML, Truppa KL: Upper extremity disorders: a literature review to determine work-relatedness, *J Hand Surg* 20:534, 1995.

137. Venkatagiri HS: Effect of window size on rate of communication in a lexical prediction AAC system, *Augment Altern Comm* 10:105, 1994.

138. Villanueva MB, Jonai H, Saito S: Ergonomic aspects of portable personal computers with flat panel displays (PC-FPDs): evaluation of posture, muscle activities, discomfort and performance, *Ind Health* 36:282, 1998.

139. Villanueva MB, Sotoyama M, Jonai H et al: Adjustments of posture and viewing parameters of the eye to changes in the screen height of the visual display terminal, *Ergonomics* 39:933, 1996.

140. Wahlstrom J: Ergonomics, musculoskeletal disorders and computer work, *Occup Med* 55:168, 2005.

141. Wahlstrom J, Hagberg M, Toomingas A et al: Perceived muscular tension, job strain, physical exposure, and associations with neck pain among VDU users; a prospective cohort study, *Occup Environ Med* 61:523, 2004.

142. Weiss ND, Gordon L, Bloom T et al: Position of the wrist associated with the lowest carpal-tunnel pressure: implications for splint design, *J Bone Joint Surg Am* 77:1695, 1995.

143. Weiss PL: Mechanical characteristics of microswitches adapted for the physically disabled, *J Biomed Eng* 12:398, 1990.

144. Wells R: Job modification—check out challenge, *Occup Health Safety Can* 9:62, 1993.

145. Wieslander G, Norback D, Gothe CJ et al: Carpal tunnel syndrome (CTS) and exposure to vibration, repetitive wrist movements, and heavy manual work: a case-referent study, *Br J Ind Med* 46:43, 1989.

146. Williams NR: Voice recognition products—an occupational risk for users with ULDs? *Occup Med* 53:452, 2003.

147. Winkel J, Westgaard R: Occupational and individual risk factors for shoulder-neck complaints. Part I—guidelines for the practitioner, *Int J Ind Ergon* 10:79, 1992.

148. Woods M, Babski-Reeves K: Effects of negatively sloped keyboard wedges on risk factors for upper extremity work-related musculoskeletal disorders and user performance, *Ergonomics* 48:1793, 2005.

149. Woods V: Musculoskeletal disorders and visual strain in intensive data processing workers, *Occup Med* 55(3):121, 2005.

150. Wright KS, Andre AD: Alternative keyboard characteristics: a survey study. In *Conference Proceedings: ErgoCon*, San Jose, Calif, 1996, Silicon Valley Ergonomics Institute.

151. Wright KS, Wallach DS: *CTD Resource Network* (www.tifaq.com), 1998.

152. Wu FG, Luo S: Performance study on touch-pens size in three screen tasks, *Appl Ergon* 37:149, 2006.

153. Yamada H: A historical study of typewriters and typing methods: from the position of planning Japanese parallels, *J Inform Process* 2:177, 1980.

154. Yassi A: Repetitive strain injuries, *Lancet* 349:943, 1997.

155. Zipp P, Haider E, Halpern N et al: Keyboard design through physiological strain measurements, *Appl Ergon* 14:117 1981.

14

Ergonomics for Children and Youth in the Educational Environment

Asnat Bar-Haim Erez, Orit Shenkar, Karen Jacobs, Robin Mary Gillespie

Learning Objectives

After reading this chapter and completing the exercises, the reader should be able to do the following:

1. Increase awareness concerning ergonomic factors affecting children and youth.
2. Increase knowledge about ergonomic factors in learning environments and in carrying schoolbags.
3. Develop basic ergonomics tools for analysis of learning environments and carrying schoolbags.

Classroom design. The organization of furniture, materials, equipment, and activity space in the classroom.

Learning environments. Places where organized teaching and learning occur.

Anthropometrics. The study of body dimensions.

CASE STUDY

Vera is a 12-year-old seventh grader who attends middle school. Vera is a healthy girl with no known learning disabilities; however, she is short for her age and weighs about 40 kg (88 pounds). Vera lives 1.5 km from school (1 mile), about 10 to 15 minutes walking distance, and usually walks to school.

Vera uses a school backpack on a regular basis (Figure 14-1). The bag weight varies with her school schedule. On average, her schoolbag and contents weighs 8 kg (about 17 pounds), or 20% of her body weight.

Vera's school class is organized in rows facing the teacher. During the last summer vacation, the school administration purchased new school furniture. The chairs are fixed to the table and the table to the floor. The furniture does not allow for any adjustments and modifications, such as changing the distance of the chair from the table. The furniture purchased was the same size for all the students. This school serves students from seventh to twelfth grades.

There is a large computer laboratory used by all the students. Each workstation is designed for use by two students at a time. The chairs are designed for computer use and are adjustable. Vera uses the computers only in the 2 hours per week of computer laboratory class. Most of her computer use, about 3 hours daily, occurs at home, doing homework, surfing the Internet, and playing video games.

Other than school, Vera loves soccer and plays both in the neighborhood with friends and in a local youth league.

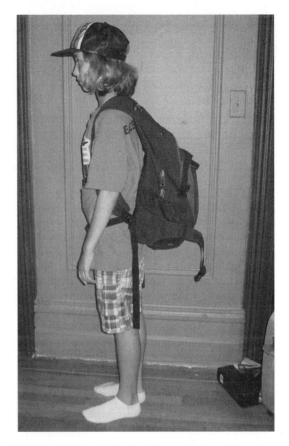

FIGURE **14-1** Vera's backpack can get very heavy.

Children's learning environments are an emerging area in ergonomics. The effect of musculoskeletal risk factors on the health of adults in various work environments is widely researched, and the public has become familiar with the concept of computer ergonomics at work. However, what happens to the musculoskeletal system of children who sit for hours in front of the computer or at a desk in the classroom is still being investigated. Table 14-1 provides an overview of research concerning children's learning environments.

Children encounter learning environments at school, home, and the library, usually sitting at a desk or in front of the computer. Besides the learning stations, children carry the environment with them in school backpacks and bags. This chapter will concentrate on these two issues.

THE LEARNING ENVIRONMENTS

Computer Environment

Electronic media use by children has increased over the past 15 years. The Longitudinal Study of American Youth found that in 1990 only one in 50 kids used a computer outside of class for 10 or more hours during a school year,[46] with significant classroom computer use defined as more than 10

Text continued on p. 252.

TABLE 14-1	Current Research in the Area of Ergonomics and Children in the School Environment

Year	Title	First Author
Anthropometrics		
1998	An anthropometric and postural risk assessment of children's school computer work environments	Oates, S.
1990	Sex differences in anthropometry for school furniture design	Jeong, B.Y.
1969	Anthropometric and physiological considerations in school, office, and factory seating	Floyd, W.F.
1969	Anthropometric data for educational chairs	Oxford, H.W.
Computer Use		
2006	Navigation in children's educational software: the influence of multimedia elements	Carusi, A.
2006	ITKids: does computer use reduce postural variation in children?	Ciccarelli, M.
2006	Effect of computer-based instruction on students' functional task performance	Chiang, H.
2006	Size, strength and physical exposure differences between adult and child computer users	Blackstone, J.M.
2006	Survey of ergonomics issues in computer classrooms of Latvian and Lithuanian schools	Gedrovic, J.
2006	Musculoskeletal complaints by middle school students with computer use	Jacobs, K.
2006	ITKids: is a high computer display more physically demanding for children?	Straker, L.
2006	ITKids: exposure to computers and adolescents' neck posture and pain	Straker, L.
2006	Musculoskeletal impact of computer and electronic game use on children and adolescents	Gillespie, R.M.
2006	Computer-related posture and musculoskeletal discomfort in schoolchildren	Dockrell, S.
2006	Children and instant messaging	Crenzel, S.R.
2006	CAKE (computers and kids' ergonomics): the musculoskeletal impact of computer and electronic game use on children and adolescents	Gillespie, R.M.
2003	The research and design of more legible and readable key legends for school children while operating Chinese computer keyboard	Chen, J-C
2003	Psycho-physiological reactions in children using computer games	Horie, Y.
2003	Delivering the power of computers to children, without harming their health	Straker, L.
2003	ITKids: reading from computers creates different biomechanical and physiological stresses for children?	Straker, L.
2003	Potential health problems faced by an Asian youth population with increasing trends for computer use	Szeto, G.
2002	A healthy approach to classroom computers: preventing a generation of students from developing repetitive strain injuries	Bradley Royster, L.
2002	Ergonomics for grade school students using laptop computers	Fraser, M.
2002	Legislating computer use in the classroom: is it possible?	Hainsworth, A.
2002	Middle school children and their use of interactive media	Jacobs, K.

TABLE 14-1	Current Research in the Area of Ergonomics and Children in the School Environment—cont'd

Year	Title	First Author
2001	Are children at more risk of developing musculoskeletal disorders from working with computers or with paper?	Straker, L.
2001	Physical and psychosocial aspects of the learning environment in information technology rich classrooms	Zandvliet, D.B.
2001	Ergonomics programs for schools: challenges and opportunities	Hedge, A.
2001	The physical impact of IT use on children	Straker, L.
2001	Making sure technology works for kids: the role of research	Atkinson, N.L.
2001	Computers and children's physical fitness: a reason for concern?	Gabbard, C.P.
2001	Computer associated upper extremity symptoms and disability in college students: prevalence, risk factors, impact and strategies for prevention.	Katz, J.N.
2001	Ergonomic aspects of introduction of information technology into schools in Japan	Saito, S.
2001	Vision issues: children in a high tech world	Sheedy, J.
2001	Growing up with interactive media: what we know and what we don't about the impact of new media on children.	Wartella, E.
2001	Is computer ergonomics for elementary and middle school students important?	Williams, I.M.
2000	Survey of physical ergonomics issues associated with school children's use of laptop computers	Harris, C.
2000	Scarring a generation of school children through poor introduction of information technology in schools	Straker, L.
2000	Children, computers and classrooms	Bennett, C.
2000	Ergonomic issues for classroom computing	Hedge, A.
2000	Research activities on the ergonomics of computers in schools in Japan	Saito, S.
2000	Computer ergonomics for teachers and students	Williams, I.M.
1999	A computer in every classroom—are school children at risk for repetitive stress injuries (RSIs)?	Royster, L.
1998	Information technology in the New Zealand curriculum and occupational overuse syndrome	Grant, A.
1998	Ergonomics in schools: some issues	McMillan, N.
1997	Computers in schools—an international project under planning	Bergvist, U.
1997	Aspects on the Swedish provisions on work with VDUs in telework and at school	Jonsson, C.
1997	Computer operation by primary school children in Japan—present condition and issues	Noro, K.

Computers and Vision

2003	A case report of ophthalmologic problems associated with the use of information technology among young students in Japan	Marumoto, T.

Continued

TABLE 14-1   Current Research in the Area of Ergonomics and Children in the School Environment—cont'd

Year	Title	First Author
2002	Students' musculoskeletal and visual concerns	Williams, I.M.
2002	Physician perspectives on children's musculoskeletal and vision disorders in Geneva, Switzerland	Gierlach, P.

School Furniture Design

Year	Title	First Author
2006	Development of a furniture system to match student needs in New Zealand schools	Kane, P.J.
2006	Evaluation of three types of school furniture according to prEN 1729	Motmans, R.R.E.E.
2006	Development and testing of school furniture for disabled pupils	Huwiler, H.
2003	Adjustable tables and chairs correct posture and lower muscle tension and pain in high school students	Hänninen, O.
2002	Juvenile computer seating design recommendations and analogs	Herring, D.
1998	The effect of computer workstation design on student posture	Laeser, K.
1998	A preliminary ergonomic and postural assessment of computer work settings in American elementary schools	Oates, S.
1997	Changing standards for school furniture	Mandal, A.C.
1996	The potential use and measurement of alternative work stations in UK schools	Taylour, J.A.
1995	A comparative study of three different kinds of school furniture	Aagaard-Hansen, J.
1995	Effect of workstation design on sitting posture in young children	Marschall, M.
1994	The working position of school children	Storr-Paulsen, A.
1993	Evaluation of working position of school children	Mandal, A.C.
1993	CEN/207/WGS/TG1 1993, European standards for chairs and tables for school furniture	CEN/TC
1992	Is school furniture responsible for student seating discomfort?	Evans, O.
1991	Why ergonomic designs and school?	Kayis, B.
1990	School seating arrangements—an example of school based research in ergonomics	Oates, E.
1983	Postural fault in school children	Johnsson, B.
1982	The correct height of school furniture	Mandal, A.C.
1980	An ergonomic appraisal of educational desks	Hira, D.S.
1976	School furniture: standing and sitting postures	Dillon, J.
1962	Preliminary report on the sitting postures of school children	Karvonen, M.J.

TABLE 14-1	**Current Research in the Area of Ergonomics and Children in the School Environment—cont'd**

Year	Title	First Author
School Furniture Design and Behavior		
1999	Children's behaviour and the design of school furniture	Knight, G.
1994	The effects of ergonomically designed school furniture on pupils' attitudes, symptoms and behaviour	Linton, S.J.
1992	Seating arrangements and classroom behaviour	Wheldall, K.
Backpacks and Carrying Cases		
2006	Schoolbag weight and the effects of schoolbag carriage on secondary school students	Dockrell, S.
2006	Effects of a two-school-year multi-factorial back education program in elementary schoolchildren	Geldhof, E.
2002	Are backpacks making our children beasts of burden?	Jacobs, K.
1996	A pilot study of the weight of schoolbags carried by 10-year-old children	Casey, G.
Issues for Teachers		
2003	An investigation of primary school teachers education on computer related ergonomics	Dockrell, S.
2001	Elementary school teachers' working comfort while using computers in school and at home	Williams, I.M.
2000	Health risks with computer use in New Zealand schools	Lai, K-W.
2000	Teachers' tools for the 21st century: a report on teachers' use of technology NCES 2000-102	U.S. Department of Education
1999	Will new teachers be prepared to teach in a digital age?	Moursund, D.
Ergonomics Curriculum		
2006	Developing hands-on ergonomic lessons for youth	Bennett, C.L.
2006	Buildings for schools—a case study	Newman, M.
2006	Ergonomic programs in the school curriculum: attitudes of teachers' college students	Heyman, E.
2006	Ergonomics for children: an educational program for physical education students	Heyman, E.
2002	Ergonomics in secondary school curriculum	Woodcock, A.
General Children and Ergonomics Issues		
2006	Sleepiness in working teens attending evening classes	Teixeiraf, L.R.
2003	ErgoKids: How will future generations deal with current exposures?	Schultz, L.J.H.
2003	Ergonomics for children and educational environments—around the world	Bennett, C.

Adapted from International Ergonomics Association: *Summary of research and applied work papers and references,* www.iea.cc/ergonomics4children/sumtab.html.

times per subject in the school year.[45] The most recent statistics in the United States are provided through the Current Population Survey of 56,000 households, representing 29,000 children aged 3 to 18. These telephone interview data, reported by adult household members, indicate that 80% of kindergartners (5 years old) use computers; by sixth grade (11 years old) almost all U.S. students use computers at home, school, or work.[38] In these survey results, girls and boys used computers with similar frequency, but race and socioeconomic status affected use.

Daily use time has not been characterized consistently yet. According to the Media in the Home annual telephone survey in 2000, based on parent reports, the average U.S. child used a computer for 34 minutes a day, the Internet for 14 minutes, and a video game for 33 minutes.[55] In one Australian study of notebook use, average daily use in the past month was 3.2 hours; the highest total daily use reported was 15 hours, with a mean longest single period of use of 102 minutes.[21] Among the students surveyed by Gillespie,[16] frequent computer users reported a mean of 2.2 hours on weekdays and 2.9 hours on the weekend, whereas less frequent users reported 1.3 hours and 1.7 hours, respectively. Among the 376 sixth and seventh graders surveyed by Jacobs, Hudak, and McGiffert,[26] 90% reported spending 0 to 6 hours per day using the computer, with 10% reporting using the computer for 4 to 6 hours per day.

Electronic or video game use is also frequent and common. However, unlike video games, computers and the Internet are considered by parents to be a resource for their children's education and enrichment as well as entertainment, with 92% of mothers believing that the Web is a great tool for their children and 53% saying that the Web has brought their family closer together.[1] According to this America Online/Digital Marketing Services, Inc. non-random online survey of more than 2,000 kids aged 7 to 12 years and their parents, 46% go online at least four times a week and nearly 20% go online every day.[1] The question is whether the extensive time children spend on computers affects their health. If it does, can the furniture and equipment they use be adjusted to their needs, or should access or other activity be adjusted to keep them safer?

Research in adults points to the relationship between extensive computer use and the development of musculoskeletal disorders (MSDs).[4,39] This has not been definitively established for children; however, it is being investigated in light of the potential risks to young users.[2,25,50,54]

A few studies that have examined the effect of computer use on children's health suggest possible adverse health effects. Researchers have described children working with computers in awkward postures that are considered risk factors for the musculoskeletal system.[30,43,54] Harris and Straker,[21] in a survey of 314 notebook computer users aged 10 to 17 years in Western Australia, found that on average students used a notebook computer for 3.2 hours daily (Figure 14-2). The students reported that at home they are mostly sitting on the floor, lying prone, or sitting in a beanbag chair. At school the postures were mostly sitting at a desk or lying on the floor. These postures probably place the children in awkward postures, and 60% of those surveyed reported discomfort from using or carrying their notebook computer.

Jacobs and Baker,[25] looking at the association between musculoskeletal discomfort and computer use in 152 sixth-grade children, reported that more than 40% reported some musculoskel-

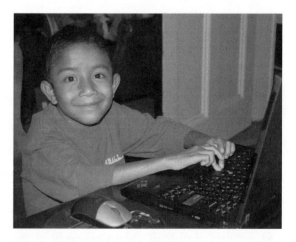

FIGURE **14-2** On average, students use a notebook computer for 3.2 hours per day.

etal discomfort within the last year and that the pain could be made worse by computer use. There was a small unadjusted correlation between hours of computer use and a composite musculoskeletal discomfort score (Pearson's r = 0.19, p = 0.05).[25] A student's ability to touch type was suggested as a protective factor against developing musculoskeletal aches and pains with computer use. In a survey of high school business classes, 28% of 382 respondents reported hand discomfort.[27] The unadjusted odds of reporting neck or back pain were significantly higher in those reporting more than 2 hours of daily computer use. When 212 children (grades 1 to 12, mean age 12 years), interviewed by college-aged siblings, were asked about symptoms occurring "following, during or immediately after your computer/computer game use," back discomfort was significantly higher in children in the highest category of game use time.[7]

More recently Jacobs and colleagues[26] reported that 41% of the 352 sixth- and seventh-grade students who participated in their study complained of having musculoskeletal discomfort or pain after working on a computer. In a cross-sectional survey of 476 U.S. students aged 12 to 18, Gillespie reported significantly increased neck and upper extremity symptoms among children who used a computer daily or almost daily, compared with those who used a computer less or not at all (OR = 1.7, adjusted for age, race, and gender).[16] The relationship between use and symptoms may not be linear; in a study of 884 adolescents, Straker and co-workers found increased odds of neck and shoulder pain among "never" and among frequent computer users (OR = 1.8 and 2.5, respectively).[51]

Another concern about computer use is the environmental setting, and the way the workstation is arranged and fits the user. A comfortable and relatively safe workstation allows the user to sit with back, feet, and arms supported, shoulders relaxed, and neck and wrists neutral. From the limited published research it appears that the typical computer station at school is not well adjusted for most children.[6,42,43,50,56] Young children also use adult-sized equipment differently than they use smaller equipment, with more force and awkward postures.[5]

Recent intervention studies have investigated the effect of education and changes in the school setting on musculoskeletal complaints. Jacobs and co-workers conducted a 3-year study with 376 middle-school students.[26] They administered a yearly questionnaire concerning musculoskeletal symptoms and computing behavior and carried out computer workstation analysis and education on healthy computing. The study design included intervention and control groups. Results indicated that overall complaints of musculoskeletal discomfort decreased among the students who received education concerning changes in computing behavior and the computer workstation. The researchers concluded that increased awareness of proper positioning, proper computer workstation arrangement, and changes in work habits such as taking stretch breaks may assist in decreasing the degree and frequency of reported musculoskeletal discomfort and pain in children. More such research is needed to measure and understand how working with computers influences children's health.

Taken as a whole, this research base can guide us, as clinicians, to take a proactive approach with Vera, the case study student. She does not complain about MSD symptoms. This might be because of her high physical activity levels (playing soccer several times a week and doing fitness activities), as exercise has been suggested as a protective factor against MSDs.[16] It might be that we did not ask her how she feels after spending a long time at the computer and thus are missing her most symptomatic times. Given her frequent computer use and the likelihood of increased use as she gets older, it would be good to assess her computer setting at home and provide her with education concerning the best way for her to configure the computer station.[54] It will also be important to teach her appropriate and healthy posture at the computer and work habits that include breaks. Such education will help to prevent MSDs as well as provide her with future healthy work habits.

Classroom Environment

Schoolchildren are one group of workers who appear to be particularly at risk for musculoskeletal strain related to sitting because of their wide range of body size leading to furniture mismatch, combined with prolonged seated posture.[14] In the classroom, students do much of their work while sitting—listening to the teacher, looking at the blackboard, copying from the blackboard or free writing, doing group work, and more. Performance of these activities affects how children sit (e.g., writing vs. copying from the board). The amount of sitting changes throughout the student's years at school. For example, preschool children are expected to be physically active 73% of the time, whereas children in the ninth grade move only 19% of the time they are in school.[49] Most of the time (57%) seated was spent leaning forward (for activities such as writing and reading), and rest leaning (such as watching the teacher or the board). In a recent study of 8-year-olds in Germany it was observed that children spent an average of 97% of the lesson time sitting statically, one third of the time with the trunk bent forward more than 45 degrees.[8]

Because children vary so greatly in size, over the years and within the same ages, much of the ergonomic research on children in learning environments has focused on the potential mismatch between children and their classroom furniture. A growing body of evidence implicates school furniture size and design in back pain and other symptoms in children.* Evans and colleagues[14] reported variation in anthropometric measurements in schoolchildren ages 6 to 18 and suggested that furniture should be organized according to size not age. Evans and co-workers[13] also examined the relations between reported discomfort and the mismatch between individual anthropometry and related chair and table dimensions. The findings from 224 students from four schools, aged 12 to 16, suggest that the high incidence of reported pain and discomfort (55%) was mainly related to a mismatch between thigh length and seat depth (associated with seated discomfort) and mismatch between seated elbow height and desk height (associated with pain in the shoulder and neck). Another study of 74 sixth- to eighth-grade students reported a substantial mismatch between

students' body dimensions and classroom furniture; only 20% could find a suitable table and chair for their needs.[44]

Think about our case study: what are the odds that the chair and table in Vera's class do not fit her anthropometric measurements? Can she adjust the setup to suit his needs? Contrary to expectations, in a study of 1269 Australian children aged approximately 14 to 18, the smallest quartile of students had the best fit with the furniture, based on seat size and height and working surface height.[37] The tallest quartile had higher odds of reporting back pain, even within age groups.

It has long been asserted that good posture in sitting is important in the prevention of back strain in children and adults,[53] but this is hard to achieve without the support of adjusted chairs and tables. Furniture design aside, notable classroom seating problems have been described, such as children sitting with their backs or their sides to the teacher, which requires twisting during lessons.[31]

Some studies report specifications for schoolchildren's furniture. Mandal recommended that a chair be at least one third the height of the person using it and the desk at least one half the height of the person using it.[33,35] In his study, he reported that the participants (ages 7 to 50 years) preferred to sit higher with the seat pan sloping forward 10 to 15 degrees. Despite studies separated by 15 years, Storr-Paulsen and Aagaard-Hensen[49] and Hira[23] reported similar results. They recommended adjustable tabletops and emphasized the importance of proper chair backrests. Yeats[56] stated that it is assumed that chairs and desks in the classroom fit all children; however, adjustability and variability of furniture are still needed to satisfy the child's postural and educational needs.

Yeats, reviewing the literature to determine the effect of school furniture design on the postural health of schoolchildren, proposed that the adjustability of school furniture is an important factor in the health of children.[56] One study compared muscular activities using electromyography (EMG) in 10 children who were performing a tracing task while seated in traditional vs. ergonomically designed workstations.[36] Researchers found that when the children were seated at the ergonomic workstations, there was a preferable postural

---

*References 31, 32, 34, 44, 56.

alignment, and activities in lower and middle trunk muscles were decreased compared with children using the traditional workstations. The children favored the ergonomic workstations over the traditional ones. The researchers hypothesized that decreased muscle activities will result in less fatigue and stress on the spine. Troussier and Tesnier[52] asked 263 students ages 8 to 11 to compare furniture with a forward tilted seat and a slanted desk, based on Mandal's recommendations[35] and available in various sizes, to standard International Organization of Standardization (ISO) issue, single-size furniture. After 4 to 5 years of use, the children using the ergonomically designed furniture rated it higher than the others rated the standard furniture, but they did not report less back pain as predicted.

Linton and co-workers evaluated the effect of ergonomically designed school furniture on the attitudes, symptoms, and behavior of tenth-grade students.[32] This study followed government laws in Sweden that called for applying safe work regulations to schoolchildren. Although the students who used the ergonomic furniture reported being more comfortable and experiencing less physical discomfort, no change in what we think of as healthier sitting behavior was recorded. It has also been reported that the preferred furniture may lead to more active, out-of-seat behavior.[29] Although this may appeal to supporters of the "Moving School,"[8] teachers with more traditional expectations may find the change disruptive.

In any case, letting students select furniture solely based on their perception or expectation of comfort may not be enough to achieve a good match. When typical students select furniture, they choose a chair that is one size bigger and a table that is too high for their anthropometric measurements.[2] This suggests that continued effort to educate children as to how to arrange and adjust their sitting postures and furniture needs to address anthropometry and a consideration of tasks they do (working at the computer, writing, reading, and so on).

Our case study describes an apparently extreme but, in fact, realistic situation. The school furniture design has two faults. First, there is one size for students in the seventh through ninth grades,

both boys and girls, despite the wide variation in height and weight within this age range. One size of table and chair will not fit all. Second, both desks and chairs are fixed to the floor, so even the simplest adjustment is not possible. Vera is smaller than average and thus must reach farther than larger students, relative to her size. In Vera's case the parents' council is very involved; they quickly understood the problem and hired an ergonomic consultant to provide recommendations. These included detaching the chairs and tables, providing several sizes of desks and chairs, and assessing the fit and comfort of the children twice a year. Regular stretch and activity breaks were also recommended.

QUESTIONS TO ASK ABOUT THE SEATED LEARNING ENVIRONMENT

Questions for the Clinician

Computer work is associated with upper back and shoulder pain related to raising the arms to reach a keyboard or mouse, to back pain because of extended sitting, to hand, wrist, and forearm disorders because of use of the hand while rotated, and to neck pain because of sustained tilted postures. One approach to assessing ergonomics risks is to ask whether and where the individual has pain, discomfort, or numbness. The type and location of the symptoms can indicate which aspect of the environment is causing the problem. If a child has neck symptoms, monitor height must be assessed, as well as seated demands, such as twisting to see the board. If shoulder or upper back symptoms are reported, the height of the writing surface or keyboard placement could be the cause. In addition, shoulder symptoms, along with those in the forearm, wrist, or hand, could indicate a problem with the distance or angle of the surface or computer control devices. How far the mouse is from the side of the user and how far forward it is, the angle in which the keyboard or mouse places the hands, and how strongly the child holds the mouse or hits the keys will need to be assessed. Handwriting demands including grip angle and force can also contribute to symptoms in the hands and forearms. Back pain could

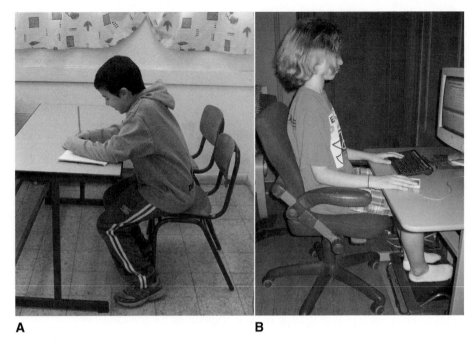

A   **B**

FIGURE **14-3** Comfortable workstation setup. **A,** School. **B,** Home.

be related to chair and table mismatch, to inadequate back or foot support, and to excessive carrying as described later.

Parents, teachers, and school districts will want to know exactly how the computer or workstation should be set up. Unfortunately the physical therapist will not be able to provide one answer. A good workstation is one that allows all users of that station to sit with the neck fairly straight, looking slightly down at the work, with the shoulders relaxed and the arms close to the body and supported for extended work (Figure 14-3, *A*). The forearms should not be rotated or the wrists deviated. The feet should be supported on the ground or a footrest, and the back supported by a rest that allows the person to lean back or stretch as desired. This means that in a shared workstation, heights and distances should be adjustable for the range of sizes in the group. For home and dedicated school workstations, the furniture should be selected and adjusted to the child and changed as he or she grows (Figure 14-3, *B*).

Perhaps the most important question to ask if symptoms appear (after other health problems are ruled out, of course) is, "What else is this child doing?" A healthy amount of physical activity and a varied set of activities throughout the day are important for all aspects of health—physical, psychologic, and cognitive.[47] The "Moving School" described by Cardon and colleagues[8] is based on this premise.

Questions for the Researcher

The literature asks whether the known ergonomic risk factors that are important to the working adult are relevant to the child and youth studying at school or home and using the computer. Researchers and clinicians involved in ergonomics with children and youth have suggested the following[2,25]:

- Collect thorough updated anthropometric data, and apply them to furniture for children and youth at school and home.

- Conduct epidemiologic studies to investigate the effect of various learning environments and workstations on children's health.
- Systematically explore ergonomic issues and identify possible risk factors for MSDs in children.
- Provide guidelines for children's furniture design.
- Provide education for school staff and parents in ergonomic principles and their relevance to furniture and work habits.
- Influence school, national, and international guidelines for matching furniture to children not on the basis of age alone, but according to gender, ethnic background, and other contributors to size and task differences.
- Examine the best way to integrate ergonomic intervention programs at school.
- Develop physical education programs to reduce the impact of the learning environment.

It appears that even if there is not yet clear evidence for adverse effects of specific learning environments and technologies on schoolchildren's health, it is important to provide preventive work habit education. This can include how to set up a good workstation for writing, reading, and computer use, how to select and arrange the chair relative to the working surface, and how to maintain musculoskeletal health while studying and working. Geldhof and co-workers conducted a 2-year back education program for 9- to 11-year-old students with 193 students in the intervention group and 172 serving as controls.[15] The education program included six back education sessions to teach principles of biomechanically favorable postures during various activities. The program also rehearsed dynamic sitting while preventing prolonged static sitting, including teaching short movement breaks between lessons, and teachers were instructed to carry over the principles into their regular day. A follow-up measure of postural behavior and pain complaints was measured after 2 school years. The researchers reported that the intervention appeared to result in increased back posture knowledge and behavior in the class, as well as decreased trunk flexion and neck torsion during classes. Boys reported decreased back or neck pain, but girls did not.

In-depth ergonomics training that can be integrated into the science curriculum is being developed that will allow teachers to provide training without taking up extra time.[3] Another avenue has been to teach ergonomics and movement concepts to physical education student teachers, so that they can spread this awareness to their students.[22]

CARRYING SCHOOLBAGS

Students don't just sit, they also carry. Parents, students, teachers, and clinicians have expressed concerns about schoolbags. Problems related to schoolbags include the weight of the bag, how it is packed, and how it is carried. In this section we explore the risk factors associated with schoolbag use and provide recommendations to reduce these factors. Kistner recently reviewed the potential musculoskeletal and physiologic health effects and summarized the research literature.[28]

Musculoskeletal Symptoms and Complaints

References to children's schoolbags on the websites of the American Academy of Pediatrics (AAP), the American Occupational Therapy Association (AOTA), and the American Physical Therapy Association (APTA) revealed a wide range of symptoms and complaints associated with backpacks. Children report discomfort, aches, and pain in their neck, shoulders, and back associated with carrying a heavy schoolbag. Muscle weakness, tingling in the arms, stooped posture, and headaches have also been reported as associated with carrying a heavy schoolbag. The children are not alone in this problematic situation: parents and teachers are concerned and describe signs of pressures. Those signs are reported at the shoulder girdle, caused by the bag's straps, or at the palms in cases of carrying a trolley.

Main Concerns and Causes for the Complaints

Although earlier recommendations for backpack use by adults were to limit the weight to 10% to 15% of body weight,[28] measured loads carried by children are frequently higher. Negrini,

Carabalona, and Sibilla found that students carried an average of 22% of their body weight.[41] Casey and Dockrell[9] reported an average weight of 15% of primary school students' body weight in their study of 10-year-old children; in 2006 the mean load was 12% in students aged 13.[12]

What is so wrong with those overweight bags? How do they harm our children? The main areas of concern are fatigue, both to specific muscles, causing irritation or injury, and to the whole system; postural constraint leading to stressful accommodation affecting the musculoskeletal system in the short run; and long-term or developmental impacts on the spine. The following studies illustrate these concerns.

Several studies suggest that heavier backpacks are associated with increased pain and discomfort symptoms. Negrini and Carabalona reported that back pain was associated with fatigue during carrying of a bag.[40] Guyer compared students ages 9 to 20 years old from India and Houston and reported that almost 60% of the students, from both countries, felt chronic back pain.[19] However, Haig and colleagues did not find a significant association between backpack use and pain when correcting for age.[20] This could suggest that the heavy bags do not cause strain, or more likely that the strain is not linearly related to weight or is not experienced identically by all students.

Carrying affects posture and balance. The effect of backpack weight on standing posture and balance was examined by Chow and co-workers.[11] The standing posture of 26 schoolgirls (mean age 13) with adolescent idiopathic scoliosis (AIS) and 20 age-matched normal schoolgirls was recorded while the subjects were without a backpack and while they carried a standard dual-strap school backpack loaded at 7.5%, 10%, 12.5%, and 15% of the subject's weight. Kinematics of the pelvis, trunk, and head were recorded using a motion analysis system, and center of pressure (COP) data were recorded using a force platform. Increasing backpack load caused significantly increased flexion of the trunk in relation to the pelvis and extension of the head in relation to the trunk, as well as increased anteroposterior range of COP motion. Although backpack load appeared to affect balance predominantly in the anteroposte-

rior direction, differences between groups were more evident in the mediolateral direction, with AIS subjects showing poor balance in this direction. Overall, carrying a backpack caused similar sagittal plane changes in posture and balance in both the normal and the AIS groups. Load size or subject group did not influence balance, but the additive effect of backpack carrying and AIS on postural control increases the risk of falling in this population.

Grimmer and colleagues focused on the way the backpack is worn and its impact on posture.[18] Findings reported from a study of 250 Australian students demonstrated a correlation between positioning of the bag and the posture. Positioning of the bag higher has the largest negative effect on posture, which may affect the development of the spine. Positioning the bag on the lower spine, close to the body's center of gravity, has the least effect on posture.

The impact on posture of the way the bag is carried was examined by Chansirinukor and co-workers.[10] They examined the posture of high school students and found that carrying the bag on both shoulders has the least potential for harm. However, carrying a heavy bag causes students to lean forward in order to balance the body against the bag's weight. This compensation had a greater effect when the subjects carried a bag that weighed 15% of the body weight.

Based on these and similar findings, some organizations have recommended limiting the bag's weight to 15% of the child's body weight.[48] However, debate continues in this area as no specific level of load has been shown to be safe for every age and size of child. A set percentage may not be possible to establish. For an average U.S. girl of age 7 weighing 24 kg (53 pounds), 15% means carrying only 3.6 kg (8 pounds). This is very different from a 90-kg (200-pound) 16-year-old; should he be allowed to carry 14 kg (30 pounds) of books every day?

What do you think about Vera's bag's weight? Does carrying the bag affect her? In what ways?

Controls

Reducing weight and postural demands are the main issues when dealing with schoolbags and children and adolescents. The most common recommendations to reduce the harm caused by carrying schoolbags can be found on websites of physicians and health care professions. Israel has a federal standard for schoolbags as determined by the Standards Institution of Israel (SIL) and as accepted by the Occupational Safety and Health Agency in Israel (OSH). Those recommendations are described according to the classic distribution of controls: engineering, administrative, and work practice controls.

Engineering controls, as described by Jacobs, are "changes to the workstation, equipment or tools" (p. 11).[24] Engineering controls are the preferred method of control, as their modification eliminates hazards at the source. In the case of schoolbags, the design, size, and weight of the bags themselves are engineering controls. Achieving engineering controls may require educating manufacturers.

On examination of the schoolbag design, we should have a look at three components: the back of the bag, the straps, and the handles. The back of the bag should be firm and padded. It should prevent or adequately reduce the pressure on the child's back. The level of the bag should be adjusted to the child's back. The straps should be padded and adjustable. The bag handles should be smooth and comfortable for handling, without any rough edges or sharp angles.

The bag size is another element of the engineering controls. According to SIL the size of the bag should be as follows: height: 40 ± 2 cm ($16 \pm \frac{3}{4}$ in), width 29 ± 1 cm ($11 \pm \frac{1}{2}$ in). If there is a waist or hip belt, it should be at least 50 mm (2 in) wide. The straps should be 30 mm ($1\frac{1}{4}$ in) wide or more. Lightweight materials are preferred. However, as with all standards-based recommendations, these suit only a segment of the population. The actual size, age, and body linkage dimensions of each child must be considered.

Administrative controls are "decisions made by management to reduce the duration, frequency, and severity of exposure to existing hazards. It leaves the hazards at the workplace, but attempts to diminish the effects on the worker" (p. 40).[24] Applying this method of control requires collaboration between teachers and students. Controlling

the weight of the bag's contents is the most obvious administrative control. Rather than carrying large books every day, it is recommended that books and files be organized not as one unit but in subunits. Using this approach, children will carry only what they need for that particular day. Homework should be given in separate sheets, so students will bring only the papers they need. Having books and assignments on computer disks or using websites and e-mail can reduce excess weight.

Other solutions can be tailored to each school, such as using drawers and lockers that will allow students to leave part of their school books, equipment, or tools at school. Another attempt to diminish the effect of schoolbag weight on children is having two sets of books: one for home use and another at school. This requires financial resources that might not be applicable to every setting and school system.

Work practice controls are (1) safe and proper work techniques and (2) fitness and flexibility.[24] Work techniques, in term of schoolbags, relate to packing and carrying the bag. Educating parents and their children is essential in reducing risk factors associated with carrying schoolbags. We should instruct the students about right packing, to pack only what is needed for that particular day, to place heavy contents at the back of the bag, and to keep the contents in balance.

Carrying the bag is the next issue to address. Appropriate schoolbag carrying means keeping both straps on both shoulders (Figure 14-4). It is essential to adjust the straps in a way that will make the bag sit properly on the child's back, meaning the lower part of the bag will be located around the lumbar curve of the spine. Straps should be short enough to keep the bag close to the back, but not so short or tight as to discourage using both straps. Hip and chest straps help distribute the weight and maintain stability.

Work practice controls can also include making sure students don't carry bags when they don't need them. Adequate physical activity to maintain cardiovascular and musculoskeletal strength is also important. A child carrying 20 pounds is less likely to run home—or even to want to walk—than those carrying the minimum necessary.

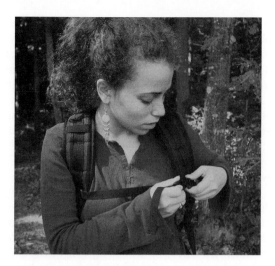

FIGURE 14-4 Carrying a backpack properly can help distribute the weight and maintain stability.

Finally, educating parents, school administrators, and teachers is essential in reducing overuse syndrome caused by carrying schoolbags. The administrative and work practice controls depend on their awareness and knowledge.

What will you recommend in order to minimize Vera's exposure to risk factors associated with the schoolbag?

CONCLUSION

Schoolchildren are affected by physical demands. Although they may recover more quickly and do not typically spend long hours doing one thing as adults do, they are effectively workers in training. Strain they experience now may compound with the strain they encounter in working life. Perhaps more important, what they learn about their bodies, about movement, and about work habits now will affect them throughout their lives. Computer use, sitting at school, and carrying schoolbags pose challenges to teachers, parents, and physical therapists. Of course, sports, playing instruments, using hand-held devices, and other hobbies and activities are also important. Using the model of controls (engineering, administrative and work practice) and paying attention to size,

posture, and physical activity, the adults responsible for children's health can reduce the strains encountered in learning environments and build health habits and knowledge. By sharing knowledge and engaging involvement, you can help children protect themselves in the future.

Learning Exercise

Overview

This exercise applies the principles of ergonomics for children in the two main areas covered in this chapter: learning environments and carrying schoolbags.

Purpose

The purpose of this exercise is to identify musculoskeletal and related risk factors that might affect the children during their learning activities, both at school and home, and to suggest ways to reduce those factors.

Exercises

1. Choose several different learning activities, such as doing homework at home, working with computers at school, sitting in the classroom, or carrying a schoolbag. Observe the child's posture while he or she sits in front of the computer or in front of a table doing various learning activities. You can also choose to observe a child who is either carrying a backpack or pulling a trolley. Assess the match between the child and the furniture he or she is using, both at home and at school. Do the same for the schoolbag, in terms of size, weight, and carrying practices.
2. Apply the controls principles (engineering, administrative, and work practice) used in the section on backpacks to the computer workstation. Give an example of each type of control. Prioritize controls that might be applicable to the child you observed. What role do children, teachers, and parents play?
3. Appraise whether the child himself and others in his environment are aware of ergonomics issues. Suggest education interventions that are appropriate for this setting.

Multiple Choice Review Questions

1. A study by Harris and Straker[22] on students' notebook computer use in Western Australia found that:
   A. 10% of the students reported discomfort from using or carrying their notebook computers.
   B. 20% of the students reported discomfort from using or carrying their notebook computers.
   C. 40% of the students reported discomfort from using or carrying their notebook computers.
   D. 60% of the students reported discomfort from using or carrying their notebook computers.

2. A study by Jacobs and co-workers[26] on students' computer use determined that:
   A. approximately 10% of the students reported discomfort from using their notebook computers.
   B. approximately 20% of the students reported discomfort from using their notebook computers.
   C. approximately 30% of the students reported discomfort from using their notebook computers.
   D. approximately 40% of the students reported discomfort from using their notebook computers.

3. Evans and co-workers[14] reported variation in anthropometric measurements in schoolchildren ages 6 to 18 and suggested that furniture should be organized according to:
   A. size not age.
   B. age not size.
   C. seat depth.
   D. thigh length.

4. In the case of schoolbags, you should refer to the design, size, and weight of the bag as a(n) _____ control.

A. work practice
B. administrative
C. engineering
D. ergonomic

5. Girls reach 95% of their stature at what age?
   A. 11 years
   B. 13 years
   C. 15 years
   D. 17 years

6. Boys reach 95% of their stature at what age?
   A. 11 years
   B. 13 years
   C. 15 years
   D. 17 years

7. Among the students surveyed by Gillespie,[16] frequent computer users reported a mean of _____ hours on weekdays and _____ hours on weekends.
   A. 2.2 and 2.9
   B. 3.2 and 3.9
   C. 4.2 and 4.9
   D. 5.2 and 5.9

8. For home and dedicated school workstations, the furniture should be selected and adjusted to the child and changed _____.
   A. as he or she grows
   B. every year
   C. at age 13
   D. at age 15

9. A healthy amount of _____ and a varied set of activities throughout the day is important for all aspects of a child's health—physical, psychologic, and cognitive.
   A. sitting
   B. standing
   C. physical activity
   D. computing

10. Researchers and clinicians involved in ergonomics with children and youth have suggested the following:
    A. Collect thorough updated anthropometric data and apply it to furniture for children and youth at school and home.
    B. Conduct epidemiologic studies to investigate the effect of various learning environments and workstations on children's health.
    C. Influence school, national, and international guidelines for matching furniture to children not on the basis of age alone, but according to gender, ethnic background, and other contributors to size and task differences.
    D. All of the above

REFERENCES

1. America Online Press Center: *America Online "youth wired" survey*, www.aol.com, 2003, (retrieved 2/9/06).
2. Barrero M Hedge A: *School ergonomics program: guidelines for parents*, 2000, http://ergo.human.cornell.edu/MBergo/intro.html, accessed April 12, 2007.
3. Bennett CL, Alexandre MM, Jacobs K: Developing hands-on ergonomics lessons for youth. In Koningsveld E, editor: *Proceedings of the 16th World Congress of the International Ergonomics Association (IEA)*, CD-ROM, Maastricht, Netherlands, 2006, Elsevier.
4. Bernard B, editor: *Musculoskeletal disorders in the workplace*, Washington DC, 1997, National Institutes for Occupational Safety and Health.
5. Blackstone JM, Johnson PW: Size, strength and physical exposure differences between adult and child computer users. In Koningsveld E, editor: *Proceedings of the 16th World Congress of the International Ergonomics Association (IEA)*, CD-ROM, Maastricht, Netherlands, 2006, Elsevier.
6. Brown MR: *Hardware ergonomic considerations in middle school classroom computer and video display terminal installations*, Denton, Tex, 1992, University of North Texas.
7. Burke A, Peper E: Cumulative trauma disorder risk for children using computer products: results of a pilot investigation with a student convenient sample, *Public Health Rep* 117:350, 2002.
8. Cardon G, De Clercq D, De Bourdeaudhuij I et al: Sitting habits in elementary schoolchildren: a traditional versus a moving school, *Patient Educ Couns* 54(2):133, 2004.
9. Casey G, Dockrell S: A pilot study of the weight of schoolbags carried by 10-year old children, *Physiother Ireland* 17(2):1, 1996.
10. Chansirinukor W, Wilson D, Grimmer K et al: Effects of backpacks on students: measurement of cervical and shoulder posture, *Austr J Physiol* 47:110, 2001.
11. Chow DHK, Kwok MLY, Cheng JCY et al: The effect of backpack weight on the standing posture and balance of schoolgirls with adolescent idiopathic scoliosis and normal controls, *Gait Posture* 24:173, 2006.
12. Dockrell S, Kane C, O'Keefe E: Schoolbag weight and the effects of schoolbag carriage on secondary school students. In Koningsveld E, editor: *Proceedings of the 16th World Congress of the International Ergonomics Association (IEA)*, CD-ROM, Maastricht, Netherlands, 2006, Elsevier.
13. Evans O, Collins B, Stewart A: Is school furniture responsible for student sitting discomfort? In *Proceedings of 2nd Pan-Pacific Conference on Occupational Ergonomics*, Wuhan, 1992.
14. Evans WA, Courtney AJ, Fox KF: The design of school furniture of Hong Kong schoolchildren, *Appl Ergon* 19:122, 1988.
15. Geldhof E, Cardon G, De Bourdeaudhuij I et al: Effects of a two-school-year multi-factorial back education program in elementary schoolchildren. In Koningsveld E, editor: *Proceedings of the 16th World Congress of the International Ergonomics Association (IEA)*, CD-ROM, Maastricht, Netherlands, 2006, Elsevier.
16. Gillespie RM: CAKE (computers and kids' ergonomics): the musculoskeletal impact of computer and electronic game use on children and adolescents, Unpublished dissertation, 2006, New York University.
17. Gillespie RM: The physical impact of computers and electronic game use on children and adolescents, a review of current literature, *Work* 18:249, 2002.
18. Grimmer K, Dansie B, Milanese S et al: Adolescent standing postural response to backpack loads: a randomized controlled experimental study, *BMC Musculoskelet Disord* 3:10, 2002.
19. Guyer RL: Backpack = back pain, *Am J Public Health* 91(1):16, 2001.
20. Young IA, Haig AJ, Yamakawa KS: The association between backpack weight and low back pain in children, *Journal of back and musculoskeletal rehabilitation*, 19:25, 2006.

21. Harris C, Straker L: Survey of physical ergonomics issues associated with school children's use of laptop computers, *Int J Ind Ergon* 26:337, 2000.

22. Heyman E, Dekel H: Ergonomics for children: an educational program for physical education students. In Koningsveld E, editor: *Proceedings of the 16th World Congress of the International Ergonomics Association (IEA)*, CD-ROM, Maastricht, Netherlands, 2006, Elsevier.

23. Hira DS: An ergonomic appraisal of education desks, *Ergonomics* 23:213, 1980.

24. Jacobs K: *Ergonomics for therapists*, Handouts from workshop given at Tel-Aviv University, Israel, 1997.

25. Jacobs K, Baker NA: The association between children's computer use and musculoskeletal discomfort, *Work* 18:221, 2002.

26. Jacobs K, Hudak S, McGiffert J: Musculoskeletal complaints by middle school students with computer use. In Koningsveld E, editor: *Proceedings of the 16th World Congress of the International Ergonomics Association (IEA)*, CD-ROM, Maastricht, Netherlands, 2006, Elsevier.

27. Jones C, Orr B: Computer-related musculoskeletal pain and discomfort among high school students, *Am J Health Studies* 14(1):26, 1998.

28. Kistner FE: Backpacks as a risk factor for musculoskeletal disorders. In Koningsveld E, editor: *Proceedings of the 16th World Congress of the International Ergonomics Association (IEA)*, CD-ROM, Maastricht, Netherlands, 2006, Elsevier.

29. Knight G, Noyes J: Children's behaviour and the design of school furniture, *Ergonomics* 42(5):747, 1999.

30. Laeser KL, Maxwell LE, Hedge A: The effects of computer workstation design on students' posture, *J Res Comput Educ* 31:173, 1998.

31. Limon S, Valinsky LJ, Ben-Shalom Y: Children at risk: risk factors for low back pain in the elementary school environment, *Spine* 29(6):697, 2004.

32. Linton SJ, Hellsing AL, Halme T et al: The effects of ergonomically designed school furniture on pupils' attitudes, symptoms, and behavior, *Appl Ergon* 25:299, 1994.

33. Mandal AC: *Balanced sitting posture on forward sloping seat*, 2005, Copenhagen. Retrieved from www.acmandal.com, accessed 2/9/06.

34. Mandal AC: The prevention of back pain in school children. In Lueder R, Noro K, editors: *Hard facts about soft machines*, Bristol, Penna, 1994, Taylor & Francis.

35. Mandal AC: The seated man, the seated work position. Theory and practice, *Appl Ergon* 12:19, 1981.

36. Marschall M, Harrington AC, Steele JR: Effect of workstation design on sitting posture in young children, *Ergonomics* 9:1932, 1995.

37. Milanese S, Grimmer K: School furniture and the user population: an anthropometric perspective, *Ergonomics* 47(4):416, 2004.

38. National Center for Education Statistics: *Rates of computer and Internet use by children in nursery school and students in kindergarten through 12th grade: 2003*, Washington DC, 2005, U.S. Department of Education.

39. National Research Council and Institute of Medicine: *Musculoskeletal disorders and the workplace: low back and upper extremities*, Washington DC, 2001, National Academies Press.

40. Negrini S, Carabalona R: Backpacks on! Schoolchildren's perceptions of load, associations with back pain and factors determining the load, *Spine* 27(2):187, 2002.

41. Negrini S, Carabalona R, Sibilla P: Backpack as a daily load for schoolchildren, *Lancet* 354:1974, 1999.

42. Noro K, Okamoto T, Kojima M: Computer operation by primary school children in Japan—present condition and issues, International Conference on Work with Display Units (WWDU), 1997, Tokyo.

43. Oates S, Evans G, Hedge A: A preliminary ergonomic and postural assessment of computer work setting in American elementary schools, *Comput Sch* 14:55, 1998.

44. Parcells C, Stommel M, Hubbard RP: Mismatch of classroom furniture and student body dimensions, *J Adolesc Health* 24:265, 1999.

45. Pelgrum W: Information technology and children from a global perspective. In Collins BA, Knezek GA, Lai KW et al, editors: *Children and computers in school*, Mahweh, NJ, 1996, Lawrence Erlbaum Associates.

46. Rocheleau B: Computer use by school-age children: trends, patterns and predictors, *J Educ Comput Res* 12(1):1, 1995.

47. Salminen JJ, Oksanen A, Maki P et al: Leisure time physical activity in the young. Correlation with low-back pain, spinal mobility and trunk muscle strength in 15-year-old school children, *Int J Sports Med* 14(7):406, 1993.

48. Standards Institution of Israel (SIL): *SI 873*, 2006. Retrieved August 13, 2006, from www.sil.org.

49. Storr-Paulsen A, Aagaard-Hensen J: The working positions of schoolchildren, *Appl Ergon* 25:63, 1994.

50. Straker L, Briggs A, Greig A: The effect of individually adjusted workstations on upper quadrant posture and muscle activity in school children, *Work* 18(3):239, 2002.

51. Straker L, O'Sullivan P, Kendall G et al: IT kids: exposure to computers and adolescents' neck

posture and pain. In Koningsveld E, editor: *Proceedings of the 16th World Congress of the International Ergonomics Association (IEA),* CD-ROM, Maastricht, Netherlands, 2006, Elsevier.

52. Troussier B, Tesnier C: Comparative study of two different kinds of school furniture among children, *Ergonomics* 42:516, 1999.

53. Wheatley GM, Hallock GT: *Health observation of school children,* New York, 1951, McGraw-Hill.

54. Williams CD, Jacobs K: The effectiveness of a home-based ergonomics intervention on the proper use of computers by middle school children, *Work* 18:261, 2002.

55. Woodard EH, Gridina N: *Media in the home,* Survey Series, 2000, Annenberg Public Policy Center.

56. Yeats B: Factors that may influence the postural health of schoolchildren (K-12), *Work* 9(1):45, 1997.

15

Ergonomics of Aging*

E. Kent Gillin, Alan Salmoni, Lynn Shaw

Learning Objectives

After reading this chapter and completing the exercises, the reader should be able to do the following:

1. Understand how physiologic, biologic, psychologic, and sociologic theories of aging combine to explain the aging process.
2. Understand how theories of aging can inform ergonomic practice in workplace design and in interactions with workers, co-workers, and employers.
3. Apply knowledge of aging processes to address ergonomic concerns of older workers.

Theories of aging. Theories of aging offer explanations of the factors or issues that affect the aging process. Aging theories in this chapter focus on biologic, physiologic, psychologic, and sociologic processes.

Productive work. Work for which older workers receive monetary compensation to produce a high-quality product in a safe and timely manner.

Older workers. Older workers include persons who are 50 years of age and older who are engaged in productive work.

---

*Portions of this chapter © 2006 E. Kent Gillin.

CASE STUDY

Garment workers from a factory located in Montreal participated in a study to understand issues associated with aging and productive work. Garment workers (76 women and 3 men) from diverse ethnic backgrounds were interviewed during focus groups. Key findings revealed that, in response to a cost-reduction initiative and because of a strong bias against older workers (ageism), many older workers were forced to retire or quit early. Many of those who retired were 50 to 60 years of age. In addition, managers did not organize work routines to accommodate an aging workforce. For example, physically easier jobs were subcontracted, rather than offering them to older workers. Managers admitted to wanting to be rid of the older workers and to replace them with younger workers who would work for less pay.

This case overview is based on the study of garment workers in Montreal, Canada by McMullin and Marshall,[20] who examined the complexities of aging and work.

In the past, many countries imposed mandatory retirement and forced early retirement onto workers. Thus, the knowledge base on preparing aging-friendly workplace environments is not extensive. However, more recently, mandatory retirement policies are being removed and the age of retirement is moving beyond age 65. This societal change underscores the need for a better understanding of how organizations and therapists can assist in applying ergonomics to the new age of workers—older workers. This chapter introduces the prominent physiologic, biologic, psychologic, and sociologic theories of aging to demonstrate the need for a more holistic consideration of factors and ergonomic interventions that will influence optimal health and productivity of older workers. Aging theories can guide therapists in planning ergonomic interventions and in creating workplaces congruent with the needs of older workers.

The World Health Organization considers the age of 65 years to be the beginning of old age in developed countries and 60 years in developing countries.[2] In Canada and most developed countries, chronologically defined age categories often used are *young-old* (ages 65 to 74 years), *old* (75 to 84 years), and *very-old* (85 years and older). These three categories define old age and place labels on the process of senescence.[26] However, to define aging chronologically is more a convenience for political governance[25] than it is an accurate prediction of functional ability to participate in productive work. There are many very-old people who engage in productive work. Indeed, many of them would be classified as much younger than their chronologic age if they were assessed from a physiologic, psychologic, or sociologic standpoint.[15]

As a group, the population of older adults is increasing at a much faster rate than the rest of the population. The population aged 65 years or older in the early twenty-first century totals nearly 4 million (Figure 15-1). In the year 2020 the Baby Boom generation, those born between 1946 and 1964, will enter the ranks of those over 65 years of age. In the next 45 years the older adult population in North America is expected to triple in size.[24] The aging population of the world is also stepping into uncharted territory, as can be seen in Figure 15-1.

In addition to experiencing a rapidly aging workforce, mandatory retirement regulations in North America are quickly disappearing. Consequently, health care professionals, researchers, politicians, employers, and the public at large must become more cognizant of the effect this trend will have on society and use all available knowledge to enhance the ability of older adults to maintain an injury-free, productive work environment.

BIOLOGIC AND PHYSIOLOGIC THEORIES OF AGING

There are over 70 biologic and physiologic theories of aging. Figure 15-2 summarizes the predominant physiologic and biologic aging theories. Many of these theories can be categorized into major factors responsible for decline during the aging process, such as genetic mutation or decline in cellular function through wear and tear and/or accumulation of waste. These processes manifest

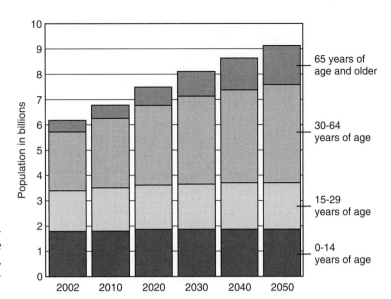

FIGURE **15-1** Predicted world population 2002-2050 by specific age groups. (From U.S. Census Bureau, International Programs Center, International Data Base.)

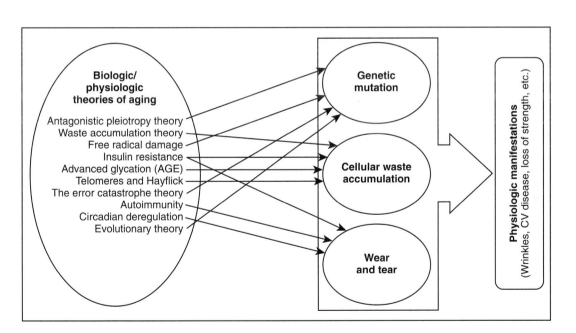

FIGURE **15-2** This summary of prominent biologic and physiologic theories of aging identifies three main categories of biologic theories (genetic mutation, cellular waste accumulation, and wear and tear) of physiologic manifestations of age.

at the biologic and physiologic levels, resulting in age-related changes (e.g., osteoarthritis, chondromalacia, graying of hair, reduced elasticity of skin, rigidity of the arteries, decline in kidney function, opacification of the lens of the eye, and decline in oxygen uptake and delivery of oxygen throughout the body, among others).

Biologic theories are linked with physiologic theories of aging through physical signs of aging. For instance, wrinkles are the manifestation of collagen cross-linkage, decreased endurance is the partial result of decreased oxygen uptake, and cellular changes in metabolism, joint stiffness, and arthritis are thought to be partially a result of insulin and autoimmunity disorders. Physiologic theory, when combined with biologic theory, contributes somewhat more to our understanding of functional ability and aging in relation to the performance of productive work. The functional implications of these changes are numerous. Several important functional changes associated with age include decreased strength, decline in timed respiratory measures, increased brittleness of bones, increased stiffness of tendons, ligaments, and muscles, reduced vision, and reduced hearing. It is, however, important to note that there is great variability in functional ability and decline as one ages.[27] Yet many of these functional changes have implications for older workers that can be addressed through ergonomic interventions. For instance, changes in workstation design, use of workplace modifications, and use of assistive technologies can offer the older worker opportunities to remain at work and to maintain optimal performance. Many functional problems such as inability to see or hear can be ameliorated through assistive technologies such as electronic magnifiers or computer magnification software. Hearing technologies such as hearing aids, adapted headsets and telephones, and frequency modulation (FM) field sound systems can be installed in the workplace to assist older workers in interacting with team members, servicing customers, and participating in meetings. Other opportunities also exist in workstation setup and design such as adjusting color contrast of computer screens to optimize vision, using lighting, enlarging numbers on phones, and increasing grip sizes on tools.

Other strategies could focus on changes to work processes. As older workers experience stiffness and decreased flexibility as a natural aging process, efforts are needed to redesign work processes and procedures to support opportunities for movement and mobility and to reduce periods of stationary work.

Although older workers will be increasingly more common in the workplace, customers are also aging. Many ergonomic concepts are being used in the redesign of workspaces to support older workers and older customers. One example of this change is appearing in many financial institutions such as banks. Customer service and support employees in banks have traditionally serviced customers in standing positions. Now banks are redesigning service carrels with sit-stand chairs, adjustable height counters, and adjustable keyboards that enable the bank employees and the customer to sit or stand while banking.

Consider the biologic and physiologic changes that will affect productivity of older workers such as repetitive work (lifting, cutting, sewing, folding, and packing) in the garment industry. The ergonomist needs to identify types of workplace modifications, workstation redesign, or assistive technologies that would support older workers staying beyond the age of 50.

How would you go about relaying the need for these changes to the employer? The employer and employee will require education about aging and the changes that will occur. Identify the physiologic challenges that you know will occur. Next, the employer and employee need to prepare for these changes related to the effects of aging. Table 15-1 examines some of the changes related to vision, hearing, skin, muscle, endocrine, and immune systems that might be necessary. What justification would you use to implement some or all of the recommendations? The physiologic effects of aging are happening inevitably to the employee and consequently the employer is affected. If the employer is to ensure that the employees, with their experience and the training that has been invested in them, remain viable and healthy, the employer must provide opportunities such as those mentioned to capitalize on this investment.

TABLE 15-1	**Preparing for Changes Related to the Effects of Aging**
Changes	**What Can the Ergonomist Do?**
Vision changes	Brighter lighting Reduce or eliminate glare with indirect lighting Use special-purpose lighting Use high-contrast materials
Hearing changes	Avoid high-frequency noise Reduce background noise Use equipment with adjustable noise levels Combine noise-based systems with visual and perceptual features
Skin changes	Improve hydration opportunities Avoid work in extreme hot or cold temperatures or improve work rest schedules Avoid work with chemicals with defatting properties
Muscle changes	Reduce work with static muscle effort (e.g., sustained positions) Increase use of mechanical lifts or automation Keep work in "neutral zone" Eliminate twisting Stretch upper body throughout the day Encourage regular work exercise programs
Endocrine changes	Encourage liquid nutrition intake at work Take breaks each hour to stretch and walk Avoid work in hot or cold environments Encourage regulation through medical or natural means available
Immune system changes	Avoid repetitive-motion work that could fatigue the employee Take precautions to avoid infection such as increased hand washing, flu shots Encourage exercise to enhance the autoimmune system Encourage stable shifts when working

PSYCHOLOGIC THEORIES OF AGING

Functional ability and participation in productive work are directly affected by psychologic factors. To date, psychologic theories of aging have focused mainly on postretirement ages. Thus, in general, little is known about preretirement aging, with the possible exception of personality development. Some researchers suggest that individuals who are motivated and active are more likely to be able to adapt and continue to participate in productive work and consequently are less likely to retire prematurely.[1,4,16]

The most prominent psychologic theories of aging include longevity, productivity, adaptive capacity, disengagement, activity, and continuity theories. Figure 15-3 groups these theories into three distinct themes (i.e., genetic, adaptive, and static). These theories and themes contribute to how older workers perceive, as well as believe in, their ability and capacity to function as they age.

A psychologic theory of aging that aids in understanding functional ability and productive work is the activity theory.[12] This theory suggests that the more psychologically active and resourceful an adult becomes in gathering and linking islands of information[3] to allow himself or herself to continue productive activity at work, the more likely it is that he or she will remain healthy and productive. In addition, it is believed that in-

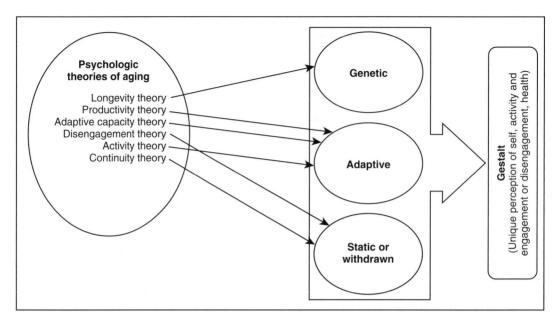

FIGURE 15-3 This is a summary of the prominent psychologic theories of aging that are categorized into three areas (genetic, adaptive, and static or withdrawn). The figure illustrates the unique gestalt that emerges as the life course progresses.

dividuals who are motivated and active are more likely to be able to adapt and therefore to continue to participate in productive work. Consequently they are less likely to retire prematurely.[11,13] Activity theory is believed to be an important contributor to older adult health and older worker productivity.[12]

Psychologic theories of aging direct ergonomists and therapists to consider the older worker's self-efficacy and personal views relevant to his or her level of activity and engagement in safe and productive work. Older workers who lack or begin to lose confidence in their ability to continue to be physically active at work may be at risk for an injury. In contrast, some older workers may be somewhat overenthusiastic in taking on new job demands and tasks, inadvertently placing them at risk for injury. Strategies that focus on the older worker could be structured to reduce these risks. As they age, older workers need opportunities to become more self-aware of abilities and learn how to self-monitor their capacities to adapt and

adjust to work demands. Access to information on working safely as a person ages is a new area for therapists to consider in ergonomic practice. Provision of information and education sessions that engage older workers in knowledge exchange about their own physical and mental health will increase self-awareness. In addition, education sessions on how older workers can monitor personal readiness for work to maintain health and safety will also benefit workers. Therapists can draw on the growing body of evidence on the older worker and information on websites that offer older worker–to–older worker knowledge transfer (Box 15-1).

The workers at the garment factory indicated that the employer encouraged departure from work before age 65. Drawing on the psychologic theories of aging, what might an ergonomist provide by way of education or information as these workers are making decisions about continuing to work? You know from psychologic theories of aging that activity theory is the most

<table>
<tr><td>

Box 15-1 *Websites on the Older Worker*

American Association of Retired People—Lists
  organizations with an older worker focus
www.aarp.org
Society of Human Resource Professionals—
  Offers information on hiring older workers
www.wishrm.org
NIOSH—Site on issues for older miners
www.cdc.gov/niosh/mining/topics/
  humanfactors/olderworkers.htm
International Labour Organization—Lists many
  websites with information on older workers
www.ilo.org/public/english/employment/skills/
  older/link.htm

</td></tr>
</table>

positive approach to encouraging long-term
healthy aging. You consider this important, and
develop educational materials that outline what to
expect physically and psychologically while aging.
You also provide information pamphlets that
outline the importance of remaining actively
involved with work and peers. What information
would you give people about health and safety
and future engagement in other work occupations? You could offer alternative methods to
safely work by introducing concepts of work rotation or suggesting ways of reducing awkward postures, forces, or static loading that could be contributing to increasing the risk of injury. If the
garment industry changed its views of older
workers, what types of education sessions might
you provide for older workers in this factory? An
example would be as follows:

- Session 1: Aging-myths and facts
- Session 2: Safe work strategies for an aging
  employee
- Session 3: Coping with injury
- Session 4: Injury prevention strategies

How would you convince the employer to support these sessions? You could first educate the
employer about the facts and myths regarding the
aging workforce. Outline benefits and expectations of an older worker, especially the prospect
of higher productivity through proper ergonomics
assessment and remediation. Also highlight that

older workers are absent less often than younger
workers if they are working in a positive, supportive environment.

SOCIOLOGIC THEORIES OF AGING

Sociologists have approached the study of aging
and work performance through investigations of
social structures such as gender, race and ethnicity,[19] life course research,[6,9] and reexamination of
the concepts of ambivalence.[7,18] The prominent
theories of aging include age stratification, aging
and society paradigm, political economy of aging,
and ambivalence. The underlying themes within
these theories can be grouped into social expectations and social policy as indicated in Figure 15-4.
Sociologic aging theories and related themes can
help therapists understand the older worker's
ability to participate in the environment and remain active in productive work. For instance,
societal expectations can influence the acceptance
of older workers. If an older worker is valued in
the work role and for his or her wisdom and
experience, he or she can contribute longer and
more productively.[5,8,10,21] Organizational support
for older workers at the corporate level within
a workplace can create opportunities for older
workers.[17] In addition, co-workers and peers can
also influence an older worker's ability to engage
and remain employed in productive work. Conversely, there are many examples of ageism (social
expectation and beliefs that older people are
unable to work) that are a major cause for early
retirement. One example discussed in the case
study at the beginning of this chapter was the
finding that garment workers were encouraged to
leave or retire because of age and perceived lower
productivity issues. Less-demanding jobs were
contracted out, leaving only difficult positions for
the older employees, thereby forcing the older
workers to retire.[20]

Social policies such as mandatory retirement
also shape and reflect national perspectives on
ageism and the stereotyping of older persons as
not having the physical or cognitive capacity to
be economically productive and to contribute to
society. With removal of mandatory retirement,
new views and perceptions about the capacity of

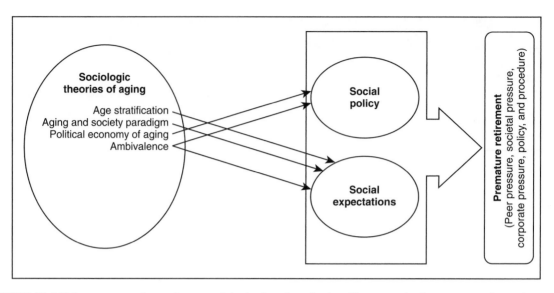

FIGURE **15-4** This summary of prominent sociologic theories of aging illustrates the importance of two themes (social policy and social expectations) in socially constructing an atmosphere that can lead to premature retirement.

older workers will emerge over time. These insights from the sociologic theories provide therapists with information that might influence future ergonomic planning and interventions to address the needs of the older worker in the workplace context. Therapists in work practice must understand the social context in the workplace and the degree of acceptance and support for employing and retaining older workers. If older workers are going to succeed in maintaining their health and optimizing their productivity, they need environments that provide instrumental and social supports as well as employers who embrace their contribution. Not every workplace will be receptive to older workers, nor will they know how best to support older workers. Therapists can work with employers to help identify the strengths and potential of older workers and create older-worker–friendly workplaces. This can be achieved through appropriate changes in physical workspace and equipment, but also by shaping a workplace context that supports older worker participation. To work toward this goal, the therapist can provide education and evidence about the capacity and potential of older workers to employ-

ers, co-workers, and older workers. Other efforts may include therapist participation in health and safety committees, in development of policies that support older workers (e.g., the need for flexible breaks), as well as in advocating for the redesign of workplace environments to support older workers (e.g., changes in lighting or health and safety signage to include increased color contrast and larger letters).

If the mandatory retirement policy changes, employees at the garment factory may begin to exert pressure through union agreements or on their own to try to stay at work longer. Consider the impact of the change in mandatory retirement and older workers deciding to remain at work in the garment factory. As a therapist you are being asked to come to a health and safety meeting and advise the employer on how to create an ergonomically older-worker–friendly workplace. You identify the following issues and recommend steps to develop a plan to assist this workplace:

Issue 1: Employer Ambivalence

The employer wishes to remain productive and profitable. The employer feels that older workers will lose the company profits and take more sick time because they cannot do the essential duties of the job. This may result in plant downsizing or closure.

Therapist Recommendations

1. Conduct a task analysis to identify essential duties of each job.
2. Determine the areas of productivity that place the company most at risk.

Issue 2: Employee Ambivalence

The employee enjoys the work and peer support. The employee feels that he or she is constantly at risk for replacement by younger workers.

Therapist Recommendations

Use the information obtained from task analysis and productivity determination from issue 1 and identify through workstation and employee assessment how to improve productivity without increasing risk to the worker.

Issue 3: Workplace Readiness for Change

Some workplaces do not have policies and procedures in place that can be used as a platform on which to return an employee to work or accommodate an aging workforce.

Therapist Recommendations

The workplace should have an accommodation policy in place to remain in compliance with human rights legislation. Suggest that you work with the health and safety committee to develop a joint policy with management and union input.

Issue 4: Physical Job Demands That Are Occasionally Untenable for Older Employees

Therapist Recommendations

Use the information gleaned from the task analysis in issue 1 to develop a risk reduction plan for employees. Conduct a physical demands analysis to highlight job severity indices. Such items can be proposed using simple ergonomic principles such as moving a load closer to the employee, tilting a table, or providing work rotation.

CONCLUSION

Aging theories provide a platform to guide therapists in holistically addressing ergonomic interventions relevant to older workers in the workplace. Biologic and physiologic theories of aging primarily assist the therapist in understanding the areas of body structure and function by classifying the ability of bodily systems to function with or without limitations. Psychologic theories primarily inform us about older workers' personal views of activity and participation. Sociologic theories can assist the therapist in understanding the contextual factors affecting older worker success on the job. However, given the relatively young age of "older" workers, the influence of biologic and physiologic factors in determining whether or not individuals can engage in productive work will likely play a smaller role than psychologic and sociologic factors. The effect of physiologic decline over time and its relevance to the therapist in understanding the productivity of older adults should not be overlooked; however, it should be put into perspective. It has been shown that physical function declines about 0.5% per year after the age of 30 years.[27] Therefore even the average 65-year-old employee will have retained a majority of his or her physical function. In addition, jobs can be modified to overcome much of this physical decline by reducing postural demands and the amount of lifting, force, and repetition, along with making other accommodations.[14,15,22,23] An elevated importance should be given to the sociologic findings because of the enormous influence (usually negative) that society, policy makers, employers, and peers have on an older worker's ability to participate in productive work.

Change in government and employer policies, increase in employer productivity demand, physical inability to work productively, or lack of appreciation by employers and co-workers for older employees can lead to an early exit from the workforce, often not by the worker's choice.[20] Employers and therapists are encouraged to establish and follow improved policies that will assist in enhancing universal access to workplaces, provide flexible time schedules, offer care-giving allowances, and give fair and equitable accom-

Purpose

The purpose of this exercise is to encourage therapists to consider the application of these theories in creating older-worker–friendly workplaces.

Exercises

1. You should work in two groups. On a flip chart the first group will create a list of all of the functional problems related to physical changes of aging and the commonly understood reasons why older workers may be at risk for occupational injury. The second group will create a similar list on a flip chart. However, group two will identify and list all of the functional problems related to cognitive changes of aging and the commonly understood reasons why older workers may be at risk for occupational injury. Groups will then exchange the lists and identify ergonomic enablers and

interventions for each item on the list that might be used to address the functional problems of older workers in the workplace. The groups will then share strategies using a group discussion format.

2. Develop a list of topics and health education sessions that could be offered to older workers to help them maintain their health, monitor their performance at work, and evaluate their readiness for considering alternative work occupations. Create an advertisement inviting older workers to attend an education session; include the goals and objectives as well as the benefits to workers.

3. Create an outline for an education session that could be delivered to employers about the benefits of older workers and strategies needed to support older workers in the workplace.

modation considerations. Particular attention should be given to the ambivalence faced by older workers as they negotiate to remain productive in increasingly hostile environments filled with employer pressure, peer pressure, social forces, and political policies to leave the workforce as soon as functional ability is questioned. In most cases older workers can be accommodated and can continue to work productively, given a caring social and psychologic climate.

Multiple Choice Review Questions

1. Older workers will become more common in the workplace because:
   A. employers typically embrace older workers.
   B. policies on mandatory retirement are changing.
   C. more people are getting older.
   D. more jobs are being designed for the older worker.

2. Social supports can contribute to older worker success in the workplace. This concept is linked to:
   A. biologic theories of aging.
   B. activity theory.
   C. psychologic theories of aging.
   D. sociologic theories of aging.

3. Biologic theories of aging can assist therapists in understanding:
   A. older workers' reluctance to leave work.
   B. functional problems of older workers.
   C. employers' reluctance to hire older workers.
   D. co-workers' attitudes toward older workers.

4. Older workers include workers who are:
   A. 50 to 65 years of age.
   B. 65 to 70 years of age.
   C. 60 to 65 years of age.
   D. 50 years of age and older.

5. Aging theories can assist the therapist in:
   A. planning ergonomic interventions for all workers.
   B. planning ergonomic interventions for older workers.
   C. deciding when a worker is too old to work.
   D. deciding if an older worker has the motivation to work.

6. Sociologic theories of aging suggest that the therapist focus interventions on:
   A. the older worker.
   B. the workplace context.
   C. assistive technologies.
   D. modifications to the tools older workers use.

7. Psychologic theories of aging suggest that the therapist needs to focus interventions on:
   A. co-workers' attitudes toward older workers.
   B. employers' attitudes toward older workers.
   C. older workers' confidence.
   D. older workers' decisions to retire.

8. Workers in the garment factory indicated that they were encouraged to leave work around the age of 50 because:
   A. the employer did not value older workers.
   B. younger workers could perform the work better.
   C. the mandatory retirement policy supported early exit from work.
   D. the work was physically and emotionally challenging.

9. Aging theories can inform a more:
   A. simplistic approach to address older worker issues.
   B. collaborative approach to address older worker issues.
   C. legislative approach to address older worker issues.
   D. holistic approach to address older worker issues.

10. Therapists can help create a workplace context that embraces older workers by:
    A. changing workstations.
    B. advocating for social policy change.
    C. advocating for older workers to remain at work.
    D. educating workers, co-workers, and employers.

REFERENCES

1. Achenbaum WA, Bengtson VL: Re-engaging the disengagement theory of aging: on the history and assessment of theory development in gerontology, *Gerontologist* 34(6):756, 1994.
2. Beaglehole R, Irwin A: *The world health report 2003: shaping the future,* London, 2003, Thomson Prentice.
3. Birren JE, Bengtson VL: A contribution to the theory of the psychology of aging: as a counterpart of development. In Birren JE: *Emergent theories of aging,* New York, 1998, Springer.
4. Burbank PM: Psychosocial theories of aging: a critical evaluation, *ANS Adv Nurs Sci* 9(1):73, 1986.
5. Chou KL, Chi I: Social support exchange among elderly Chinese people and their family members in Hong Kong: a longitudinal study, *Int J Aging Hum Dev* 53(4):329, 2001.
6. Connidis IA: *Speaking to ourselves: who is listening? Aging and the life course,* Chicago, 2002, American Sociological Association.
7. Connidis IA, McMullin JA: Ambivalence and family ties: a critical perspective, *J Marriage Fam* 63(3):558, 2002.
8. Dudley KC, Goins RT: Guardianship capacity evaluations of older adults: comparing current practice to legal standards in two states, *J Aging Soc Policy* 15(1):97, 2003.
9. Elder GHJ: Theoretical advances in life course research. In Heinz W, editor: *Theoretical advances in life course research,* Weinham, 1991, Deutscher Studies Verlag.
10. Fone S, Lundgren-Lindquist B: Health status and functional capacity in a group of successfully ageing 65-85-year-olds, *Disabil Rehabil* 25(18):1044, 2003.
11. Franche RL, Krause N: Readiness for return to work following injury or illness: conceptualizing the interpersonal impact of health care, workplace, and insurance factors, *J Occup Rehabil* 12(4):233, 2002.
12. Goldberg E: A healthy retirement, *Aorn J* 76(5):873, 2002.

13. Hansson RO, Robson SM, Limas MJ: Stress and coping among older workers, *Work* 17(3):247, 2001.

14. Ilmarinen J: Aging workers, *Occup Environ Med* 58(8):546, 2001.

15. Ilmarinen J: Physical requirements associated with the work of aging workers in the European Union, *Exp Aging Res* 28(1):7, 2002.

16. Karp DA: A decade of reminders: changing age consciousness between fifty and sixty years old. In Gubrium JF, Holstein JA, editors: *Ageing and everyday life,* Oxford, 2000, Blackwell.

17. Liang J, Shaw BA, Drause NM et al: Changes in functional status among older adults in Japan: successful and usual aging, *Psychol Aging* 18(4):684, 2003.

18. Luscher K: Intergenerational ambivalence: further steps in theory and research, *J Marriage Fam* 64(3):564, 2002.

19. Marshall VW, Matthews SH, Rosenthal CJ: Elusiveness of family life: a challenge for the sociology of aging. In Maddox GL, Lawton MP: *Annual review of gerontology and geriatrics,* vol 13, New York, 1993, Springer.

20. McMullin JA, Marshall VW: Ageism, age relations, and garment industry work in Montreal, *Gerontologist* 41(1):111, 2001.

21. Mulvey J: Retirement behavior and retirement plan designs: strategies to retain an aging workforce, *Benefits Q* 19(4):25, 2003.

22. Savinainen M, Nygard CH, Korhonen O et al: Changes in physical capacity among middle-aged municipal employees over 16 years, *Exp Aging Res* 30(1):1, 2004.

23. Tuomi K, Huuhtanen P, Nykyri E et al: Promotion of work ability, the quality of work and retirement, *Occup Med (Lond)* 51(5):318, 2001.

24. United Nations: *World population ageing: 1950-2050,* World Assembly on Ageing, Geneva, 2002, United Nations.

25. Vincent J: *Old age,* New York, 2003, Routledge.

26. Volkert D, Kreuel K, Heseker H et al: Energy and nutrient intake of young-old, old-old and very-old elderly in Germany, *Eur J Clin Nutr* 58(8):1190, 2004.

27. Yates FE: Complexity of a human being, *Neurobiol Aging* 23(1):17, 2002.

16

Ergonomics in Disability Management

Susan A. Domanski, Nancy J. Gowan, Rhysa Tagen Leyshon, Melanie Weller*

Learning Objectives

After reading this chapter and doing the exercises, the reader should be able to do the following:

1. Define the participatory ergonomics process.
2. List the return-to-work process.
3. Describe a process of reflective analysis when implementing ergonomics in disability management.

Participatory ergonomics. The implementation of ergonomic solutions involving participation of the worker and other workplace staff, such as the supervisor.

Primary prevention. Intervention that is undertaken before members of the population at risk have acquired a condition of concern.

Secondary prevention. Intervention that is undertaken after individuals have experienced a condition of concern.

Tertiary prevention. Intervention designed for individuals with chronically disabling musculoskeletal disorders with the goal of achieving maximal functional capacity.[27]

---

*Although the authors of this chapter have been listed alphabetically, each contributed their time and expertise equally in its development.

Accident prevention and disability management (DM) in the workplace are everyone's responsibility and succeed only when there is continuous support, commitment, and a willingness to change from the employer and employees. Creating and nurturing a culture of safety requires the employer and upper management to understand and provide the necessary financial, human, and time resources for processes to succeed.[14,17] This commitment is essential if frontline workers are expected to follow through and benefit from ergonomic programs. Such support and commitment to safety and ergonomic programs have been shown to lead to increased profits through reduced insurance claim costs, increased productivity, and reduced DM costs, and to healthier workforces because of reduced injuries, less strenuous work tasks, reduced worker turnover, and increased employee satisfaction and morale.[14,29,34,38]

Because therapists are not typically trained in business and management, topics such as cost justification and cost-benefit analysis are not familiar to us. Instead of presenting ergonomic projects to management from a business perspective, we do so in the language of health, engineering design, and quality of work life. When we are not able to "sell" our product to management in these terms, we complain that we are not appreciated.[14] Hendrick offers explanations for why employers are not always open and accepting of ergonomics solutions.[15] First, many have been exposed to "bad" ergonomics, in which the product or work environment fails because of incompetence and lack of training by a person representing himself or herself as an ergonomic professional. Second, many ergonomic solutions appear to be common sense, and everyone is capable of coming up with the correct solution. As we know, this is not always the case. Third, employers are often expected to support ergonomics because it is the "right thing to do," but management has a need to be able to justify any investment as a benefit to the organization. The fourth explanation offered by Hendrick is that professionals working in the ergonomic community have done a poor job of documenting and advertising the cost benefits of good

ergonomics—that good ergonomics is good economics.[15]

In order to gain the necessary organizational support from the employer, therapists must learn to present ergonomic proposals in business terms. Management needs to be able to justify any funds necessary for the ergonomic intervention from an economic perspective. In determining the cost of the project it is necessary to consider four major areas: (1) personnel, (2) equipment and materials, (3) reduced productivity or sales, and (4) overhead. Chapter 20 provides information on the economics and marketing of ergonomic services. For further details on determining the cost benefit of the ergonomic intervention, refer directly to Hendrick.[14]

Of particular relevance to ergonomics is the fact that most work injuries fall into the musculoskeletal disorder (MSD) category. Other terms used to describe these injuries include *cumulative trauma disorder* (CTD), *soft tissue injury* (STI), and *repetitive strain injury* (RSI). MSDs not only are the result of the physical components of a job but also are attributed to the psychosocial aspects of the work environment.[13] The consequences of MSDs are far-reaching, potentially affecting every aspect of a worker's life. These injuries are also costly for employers. MSDs are the number one reason for lost-time claims reported in most industrialized nations, constituting 30% to 60% of all work-related injuries,[2,3,5,8] yet most are believed to be preventable.[29] These injuries result in billions of dollars in direct and indirect costs to employers worldwide.[8,27] In addition to the direct costs of insurance and rehabilitation, employers' indirect costs include overtime, equipment modifications, administration, retraining, and lost productivity.[27]

In addition to MSDs, other work-related illnesses and traumatic injuries are preventable through ergonomic solutions. Ergonomic strategies not only prevent illness and injury, but also assist in returning workers with an illness or injury to meaningful and productive employment.

Throughout the chapter, we will use the case of Compufone to assist in describing ergonomics in DM.

CASE STUDY

Compufone is a small call center in a rural town, with 120 full-time and 20 part-time employees. The employees have a limited employee-paid health plan with short-term disability and long-term disability. They work rotating 8-hour shifts and share 60 workstations. The employees start at minimum wage in this nonunionized environment where the jobs are considered either entry-level or exit-level positions. The employees are primarily in the age ranges of 20 to 35 years and over 50 years. The role of the company is to perform market research and fundraising for local charities.

Compufone's chief financial officer (CFO) has contacted the therapist, as the latest company financial review indicates high turnover rates, high worker's compensation rates, and high absenteeism. There have been fluctuations in productivity over the past 6 months. A recent employee survey noted low morale and low employee empowerment. Employee comments were related to workstation conditions (e.g., desk chairs broken or uncomfortable, headsets that do not fit properly, desks too high or low).

The therapist begins by meeting with the CFO and the senior management team to educate them on ergonomic principles and to ensure that there is senior management commitment to undertake a participatory approach to finding a solution. During the meeting, it is determined that Compufone recently formed an ergonomics team, but the team lacks direction and knowledge. It is also determined that compensation claims for telephone operators have gradually been increasing over the past 2 years and are overwhelmingly related to neck, arm, and low back MSDs. As a priority, Compufone would like to see decreased compensation claims resulting from MSDs. The therapist approaches this request by examining the ergonomics of the telephone operators and reviewing the company's return-to-work (RTW) policy and program.

DISABILITY MANAGEMENT

Typically, DM is associated with the handling of workers with an injury, once an injury has been reported. DM has been defined as the process of minimizing the impact of an impairment (resulting from work-related and non–work-related injury, illness, or disease) on a worker's ability and capacity to engage in competitive employment.[26] However, part of managing injuries is preventing them. Rather than separating injury prevention strategies from DM, we have chosen to consider DM as part of the whole process. Within a DM program, the use of both macroergonomics and microergonomics is essential.

MACROERGONOMICS

Often the most challenging task for therapists is not to identify the ergonomic problem or solution, but to overcome the cultural barriers and lack of trust between workers and management.[19] Management blames the workers for lack of safe work practices, and workers blame management for failure to supply the necessary resources to allow safe work practices. Macroergonomics are solutions that are implemented to overcome these cultural barriers (see Chapter 3).

Macroergonomics refers to employer- and upper management–directed, global, large-scale organizational solutions to ergonomic problems that, when successful, result in the existence of an effective culture of health and safety throughout the organization.[11,24,32] Workplaces that demonstrate concern for employees, involve employees in decision making, show evidence of effective accident prevention programs, and provide early and supportive DM programs to workers with illnesses or injuries demonstrate lower compensation claim rates.[11,20,32]

Macroergonomics should be thought of as a process, implying continuity, rather than a program, which implies an end point. Workers need to know that the employer and management are committed to ensuring the health and well-being of each and every worker, and this message must be relayed through a system of cooperation, open communication, and continual learning and advancement.[7] Within this large-scale process are smaller programs aimed at specific problems but that generally benefit all workers and are not specific to any one job or task. One basic example would be the use of an ergonomics team, referred to as *participatory ergonomics* (PE).[17,24]

PARTICIPATORY ERGONOMICS

From a preventative perspective, PE appears to be the most effective method of applying ergonomics in the workplace.* Evidence also exists regarding the benefit for PE in returning workers with injuries to work.[4,21] The success of PE can be attributed to the involvement of workers in the entire process—from identifying the risks and hazards, to recommending solutions, to implementing the solutions and evaluating the outcomes.[24] PE has been defined as "the involvement of people in the planning and controlling of a significant amount of their own work activities, with sufficient knowledge and power to influence both processes and outcomes to achieve desirable goals."[37] PE recognizes that all members of the team are capable of identifying and solving the problem through reflection of past and present experiences.[39]

The therapist, as an ergonomic consultant, is not seen as the expert but rather acts as a reflective facilitator or advisor, once the team is educated on the basics of ergonomics[24] with the employees taking the role of expert.[37,39] The therapist can provide ergonomic training in the following areas: structure of the human body, energy expenditures of movement, healthy versus harmful body mechanics and postures, the importance of rest and fatigue prevention, ergonomic relations among human, equipment, and work process, psychologic implications of job satisfaction, cognitive aspects of work activity, and ergonomic techniques for analyzing the workplace.[28] Generally, a PE team may consist of representatives from management, occupational health, maintenance, engineering, union, and front-line workers, supervisors, and a therapist or ergonomist.[24,33]

The aim of the PE program is to generate enthusiasm for the change and process, allow identification, exploration, and evaluation of alternatives for redesign, contribute to development of criteria and methods of evaluation, and provide a basis for future participation and implementation, including acceptance of the current change. Numerous models for implementing PE programs have been described in the literature and are briefly reviewed in this chapter. The advantages of using PE have been shown to include an overall sense of community among workers, decreased injury rates, increased investment and motivation of workers, increased all-around safety awareness, increased confidence of workers, and an increased sense of power for workers to make change.[24,31,37]

Using Participatory Ergonomics in the Workplace

It is less expensive for employers to prevent an injury than it is to make changes and corrections after an injury has occurred. Often, making straightforward and basic ergonomic changes can reduce MSD risks significantly.[28] This proactive ergonomic approach has proven effective when PE is implemented.[25,30] *Proactive ergonomics* refers to the process of applying ergonomics in the early stages of developing work processes and tasks to avoid injuries and potentially expensive retrofitting of lines or equipment. This forms an essential primary prevention strategy. Proactive ergonomics may include such activities as having an ergonomics team assess a production line before a company purchases certain equipment or ordering ergonomic office chairs and desks right from the start of a new business venture. In other words, proactive ergonomics eliminates or reduces the chance that workers will be put at risk for developing injuries in the first place and is an example of a macroergonomic process.

Primary prevention ergonomics is undertaken when a risk for injury has been identified but before workers acquire an injury or when injuries have been reported but the goal is to reduce the chance of injuries to additional workers.[25] For example, a manufacturing plant may introduce back care education to reduce the number of low back pain claims. Other examples of primary preventative ergonomics include regularly scheduled stretch breaks and job or task rotation.[16,18]

Generally, PE teams undertake risk assessments of various jobs to identify where risk of injury is present. This would include examining incidences of reported MSDs over the past few years, the amount of lost time resulting from the MSD, and the cost of treating the worker and re-

---

*References 6, 21, 24, 33, 35, 38.

turning him or her to work.[38] The goal of the PE team is to identify what part of the job or task causes the MSD. This can be done by observing workers performing the job, interviewing healthy workers and workers with injuries, and having workers and the PE team complete questionnaires.[28,38] The PE team deals only with risk factors that have an ergonomic solution.[28] Having a checklist to identify risk factors for each job is beneficial. Various checklists exist and can be customized according to the needs of the team. Typically MSD risk factors are related to awkward postures or positions, forceful exertions, highly repetitive movements, or sustained static positioning. Some of the checklists also include perception of exertion as well as using objective measurements of the risk factors. Examples of checklists include the Rapid Upper Limb Assessment (Figure 16-1), the Washington Hazards Checklist (Figure 16-2), and the Activity Risk Checklist (Figure 16-3).

Models of Participatory Ergonomics

There is no one model of PE that is suitable in all situations, so the most appropriate model should be chosen for each project.[38] Regardless of the exact model that is used to implement a preventative PE program, it is essential that the process be seen as one of reflection. Without evaluating outcomes to ensure that solutions have in fact solved the problem, the PE intervention will not succeed. Taken from the business literature, the Deming cycle of Plan-Do-Check-Act (PDCA) is a simple and basic systemic approach to problem solving[7] that works well within the participatory ergonomic framework. The "plan" stage identifies the actual problem (ergonomic risk factor or hazard) and the root cause. The "do" stage represents the implementation of the solution to the ergonomic risk factor. The "check" stage evaluates the results of the solution and compares it with the original method, identifying benefits and any gaps between the two. The "act" stage engages the participant in reflection of the change process and encourages participants to act on the new learning gained through the change process. Each of the following PE programs can be evaluated using the PDCA system.

Once the ergonomic team has identified the potential risks and hazards, a process for implementing change to reduce risks must be undertaken. Numerous models or frameworks have been identified in the literature for implementing a PE process. Five will be briefly described here, but you are strongly encouraged to complete further reading before attempting to use any of the models.

Design Decision Group

The Design Decision Group (DDG) method reported by Wilson[38] includes the following stages: (1) familiarization with tasks, jobs, workplace, and team, (2) field visits to similar sites, (3) DDG problem solving (brainstorming, visualization techniques, wordmaps, round-robin questionnaires, drawings, discussing and critiquing problems, and suggesting improvements), (4) implementation simulation, (5) sourcing and costing of solutions, (6) implementation of solutions, and (7) continual improvements. The focus of this method is on group-based problem solving. The workers are the experts and the therapist or ergonomist acts as a facilitator. No idea is rejected unless it is deemed unsafe by the therapist. The goal is to implement not necessarily the best solution from an ergonomic perspective, but the solution that the workers are most likely to feel confident about and motivated to use. Workers are expected to build mockup simulations of their suggestions in order to identify potential problems before purchasing new equipment or resources. The workers are also involved in the sourcing and costing of solutions, which ensures that they are completely vested in the process and understand how the solutions may affect the employer overall. The expectation is that the therapist will gradually remove himself or herself from the picture and another team member will ensure ongoing evaluation of the process.

The DDG method was determined to be an appropriate approach to the problems in Compufone. The following are the steps that were taken with Compufone.

1. The therapist became familiar with the ergonomics team.

Text continued on p. 291.

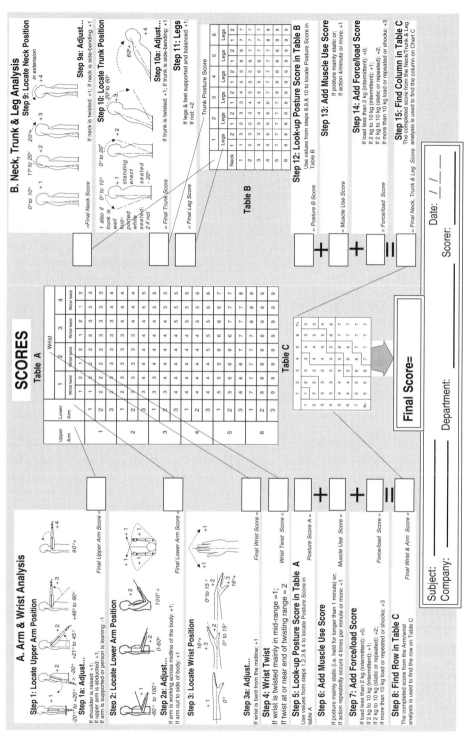

FIGURE 16-1 Rapid Upper Limb Assessment (RULA). (Copyright © Professor Alan Hedge, Cornell University, February 2000.)

Job		Date / /
Notes		Analyst(s)

Reading across the page, determine if any of the conditions are present in the work activities. For many of the risk factors, two conditions are presented, which are the indicators for Caution (a lower level of risk) and Hazard (a higher level of risk). Most of the conditions are based on duration. If the lower threshold condition is not met, no box is checked. If the lower condition is met but the higher is not, then Caution is checked. If the higher condition is met (generally a longer period of time), then Hazard is checked.

If only Caution boxes are checked, the risk is present but immediate action (further analysis or interventions) are not recommended. It is worthwhile to continue to monitor Caution level jobs for changes that might increase the risk and for injuries or symptoms that may occur.

If one or more Hazard boxes are checked, a work-related musculoskeletal disorder (WMSD) hazard exists, and further action is recommended.

Awkward Posture				Check (✓) as applicable
Body Part	**Physical Risk Factor**	**Duration**	**Visual Aid**	
Shoulders	Working with the hand(s) above the head or the elbow(s) above the shoulder(s)	More than 2 hours total per day		Caution ☐
		More than 4 hours total per day		Hazard ☐
	Repetitively raising the hand(s) above the head or the elbow(s) above the shoulder(s) more than once per minute	More than 2 hours total per day		Caution ☐
		More than 4 hours total per day		Hazard ☐
Neck	Working with the neck bent more than 45° (without support or the ability to vary posture)	More than 2 hours total per day	45°	Caution ☐
		More than 4 hours total per day		Hazard ☐

FIGURE **16-2** Washington Hazards Checklist. (Adapted from State of Washington Department of Labor and Industries Ergonomic Rule.)   *Continued*

Awkward Posture (continued)				Check (✓) as applicable
Body Part	**Physical Risk Factor**	**Duration**	**Visual Aid**	
Back	Working with the back bent forward more than 30° (without support, or the ability to vary posture)	More than 2 hours total per day More than 4 hours total per day	30°	Caution ☐ Hazard ☐
	Working with the back bent forward more than 45° (without support or the ability to vary posture)	More than 2 hours total per day	45°	Hazard ☐
Knees	Squatting	More than 2 hours total per day More than 4 hours total per day		Caution ☐ Hazard ☐
	Kneeling	More than 2 hours total per day More than 4 hours total per day		Caution ☐ Hazard ☐

FIGURE **16-2**, cont'd

High Hand Force—Pinch					Check (✓) as applicable
Body Part	**Physical Risk Factor**	**Combined with**	**Duration**	**Visual Aid**	
Arms, wrists, hands	Pinching an unsupported object(s) weighing 2 or more pounds per hand, or pinching with a force of 4 or more pounds per hand (comparable to pinching half a ream of paper)	Highly repetitive motion	More than 3 hours total per day		Hazard ❏
		Wrists bent in flexion 30° or more, or in extension 45° or more, or in ulnar deviation 30° or more	More than 3 hours total per day	Flexion / Extension / Ulnar deviation	Hazard ❏
		No other risk factors	More than 2 hours total per day		Caution ❏
			More than 4 hours total per day		Hazard ❏

FIGURE **16-2, cont'd**   *Continued*

High Hand Force—Grasp					Check (✓) as applicable
Body Part	**Physical Risk Factor**	**Combined with**	**Duration**	**Visual Aid**	
Arms, wrists, hands	Gripping an unsupported object(s) weighing 10 or more pounds per hand, or gripping with a force of 10 pounds or more per hand (comparable to clamping light-duty automotive jumper cables onto a battery)	Highly repetitive motion	More than 3 hours total per day		Hazard ☐
		Wrists bent in flexion 30° or more, or in extension 45° or more, or in ulnar deviation 30° or more	More than 3 hours total per day	Flexion Extension Ulnar deviation	Hazard ☐
		No other risk factors	More than 2 hours total per day		Caution ☐
			More than 4 hours total per day		Hazard ☐

FIGURE **16-2,** cont'd

Highly Repetitive Motion

Body Part	Physical Risk Factor	Combined with	Duration	Check (✓) as applicable
Neck, shoulders, elbows, wrists, hands	Using the same motion with little or no variation every few seconds (excluding keying activities)	No other risk factors	More than 2 hours total per day	Caution ☐
			More than 6 hours total per day	Hazard ☐
	Using the same motion with little or no variation every few seconds (excluding keying activities)	Wrists bent in flexion 30° or more, or in extension 45° or more, or in ulnar deviation 30° or more **AND** High, forceful exertions with the hand(s)	More than 2 hours total per day	Hazard ☐
	Intensive keying	Awkward posture, including wrists bent in flexion 30° or more, or in extension 45° or more, or in ulnar deviation 30° or more	More than 4 hours total per day	Hazard ☐
		No other risk factors	More than 4 hours total per day	Caution ☐
			More than 7 hours total per day	Hazard ☐

Repeated Impact

Body Part	Physical Risk Factor	Duration	Visual Aid	Check (✓) as applicable
Hands	Using the hand (heel/base of palm) as a hammer more than 10 times per hr	More than 2 hours total per day		Caution ☐
	Using the hand (heel/base of palm) as a hammer more than 60 times per hr			Hazard ☐
Knees	Using the knee as a hammer more than 10 times per hour	More than 2 hours total per day		Caution ☐
	Using the knee as a hammer more than 60 times per hour			Hazard ☐

FIGURE **16-2, cont'd**

Continued

Heavy, Frequent, or Awkward Lifting				Check (✓) as applicable
Body Part	**Physical Risk Factor**	**Combined with**	**Duration**	
Back and shoulders	Lifting 75 or more pounds	No other risk factors	One or more times per day	Caution ☐
	Lifting 55 or more pounds	No other risk factors	More than 10 times per day	Caution ☐
	Lifting more than 10 pounds	More than 2 times per minute	More than 2 hours total per day	Caution ☐
	Lifting more than 25 pounds	Above the shoulders Below the knees At arm's length	More than 25 times per day	Caution ☐
	WISHA Lifting Analysis – Perform if any Caution condition exists. Actual weight is greater than the Weight Limit (See separate work sheet)			Hazard ☐

Moderate to High Hand-Arm Vibration			Check (✓) as applicable
Body Part	**Physical Risk Factor**	**Duration**	
Hands, wrists, and elbows	Using impact wrenches, carpet strippers, chain saws, percussive tools (jack hammers, scalers, riveting or chipping hammers) or other hand tools that typically have high vibration levels	More than 30 minutes total per day	Caution ☐
	Using grinders, sanders, jig saws or other hand tools that typically have moderate vibration levels	More than 2 hours total per day	Caution ☐
	WISHA HAV Analysis – Perform if any Caution condition exists. Actual exposure time is greater than the Hazard Level Exposure Time (See separate work sheet)		Hazard ☐

FIGURE **16-2**, cont'd

ACGIH® TLV® for Hand Activity

Job	Analyst	Date / /
	Left	Right
Hand Activity Level (HAL) (See scale below)		
Normalized Peak Force (NPF) (See table below)		
Ratio = NPF/(10-HAL)		
Determine result TLV = 0.78 AL = 0.56	>TLV ☐ AL to TLV ☐ <AL ☐	>TLV ☐ AL to TLV ☐ <AL ☐

Hand Activity Level Rating

0	2	4	6	8	10
Hands idle most of the time; no regular exertions	Consistent conspicuous long pauses; or very slow motions	Slow steady motion/exertions; frequent brief pauses	Steady motion/ exertion; infrequent pauses	Rapid steady motion/exertions; no regular pauses	Rapid steady motion/ difficulty keeping up or continuous exertion

Estimation of Normalized Peak Force for Hand Forces

% MVC	Borg scale		Moore-Garg Observation (Alternative method)	NPF
	Score	Verbal Anchor		
0	0	Nothing at all		0
5	0.5	Extremely weak (just noticeable)	Barely noticeable or relaxed effort	0.5
10	1	Very weak		1
20	2	Weak (light)	Noticeable or definite effort	2
30	3	Moderate		3
40	4		Obvious effort, but unchanged facial expression	4
50	5	Strong (heavy)		5
60	6		Substantial effort with changed facial expression	6
70	7	Very strong		7
80	8			8
90	9		Uses shoulder or truck for force	9
100	10	Extremely strong (almost maximum)		10

FIGURE **16-3** Activity Risk Checklist. (Copyright © 2002 Thomas E. Bernard.)

Continued

ACGIH® TLV® for Hand Activity

The American Conference of Governmental Industrial Hygienists (ACGIH®) Threshold Limit Value® (TLV®) for Hand Activity (2001) is offered for the evaluation of job risk factors associated with musculoskeletal disorders of the hand and wrist. The evaluation is based an assessment of hand activity and the level of effort for a typical posture while performing a short cycle task.

The data collection form on the previous page is an adaptation that guides the gathering of information on job risk. The first step is to identify the level of hand activity on a scale of 0 to 10, where zero is virtually no activity to a level of 10 (highest imaginable hand activity). Hand activity accounts for the combined influences of effort repetition and effort duration in a qualitative assessment. The second step characterizes the effort level by noting the effort associated with a typically high force within the cycle of work. The normalized peak force (NPF) is the relative level of effort on a scale of 0 to 10 that a person of average strength would exert in the same posture required by the task. Three methods are suggested for assessing NPF: Noting the measured % of maximum voluntary contraction and a subjective report of perceived exertion (Borg Scale) as well as an observational method borrowed from the Moore-Garg Strain Index. The third step is to locate the combination of HAL and NPF on the following TLV graph. For more information see the TLV and associated documentation.

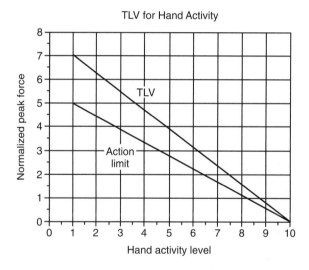

American Conference of Governmental Industrial Hygienists (ACGIH). Threshold limit values and biological exposure indices for 2001. Cincinnati: ACGIH, 2001. See www.acgih.org for more information.

FIGURE **16-3,** cont'd

2. The ergonomic team and therapist reviewed the tasks, jobs, and workplace environment of the call-center operators. This helped all of the team members to assess what the problems were and what they felt were the causes.

3. During this stage, team members had opportunities to interview workers, observe workers, and take measurements of workstations. A problem list was generated by the team and included the following:

   Office chairs lack adjustability and comfort, and many are broken.

   Telephone headsets are shared, which results in some being stretched and not fitting other workers' heads.

   Mouse and keyboards are located on the desktop, and this is too high for many workers.

   No adjustability in monitor height—too high or too low for some workers.

   Workers complain of generalized stiffness, especially on calls that last for extended periods.

4. Once the actual problems had been identified, arrangements were made to visit another call center where a PE team had been operating for some time. This allowed team members to see possible solutions to situations similar to their own.

5. Following the visit to the other call center, the PE team met to problem solve and come up with recommendations for how they would try to resolve the problems identified previously. (Subsequent to the visit to the other call center, the PE team identified countermeasures to resolve the problems.) This was accomplished using flip charts and having each team member write a suggestion down and continuing one by one until no further suggestions were made. Then each suggestion was discussed by the group and either accepted or rejected. The team was left with the following suggestions:

   Have each employee assigned his or her own personal chair. Chairs would be chosen from a sampling of three or four ergonomically sound chairs, then ordered specifically for each employee.

   Find an ergonomically sound chair that has maximal adjustability in seat height, depth, back height and angle, armrest height, and tilt. Order one for each workstation, but attempt to assign workers of similar size and body type to the same workstations. Educate workers on how to adjust and operate the chairs for maximal comfort and correct positioning.

   Allow workers to choose their own style of headset from an appointed vendor, and have that headset assigned to only one worker.

   Attach height- and angle-adjustable keyboard and mouse trays to the underside of each desk.

   Provide education to each worker regarding correct monitor height at his or her workstation. (Educate workers on correct height of monitor for them.) As old monitors are replaced, new ones should be liquid crystal display (LCD) flat screens with adjustability built into the stand.

   Workers will be instructed and educated on stretches that can be performed at their desks to minimize complaints of stiffness. Workers will also be given an option of taking six 5-minute breaks during their shift instead of two 15-minute breaks. Finally, workers should be allowed to stand at their desks if not on a call or if still able to handle calls from the standing position.

6. A simulation was undertaken for each solution to determine which was most feasible and/or to determine if other problems arose as a result of the proposed solution.

7. The team then voted on which solutions would be implemented for each problem.

8. Samples of each equipment suggestion were borrowed from vendors and installed in sample workstations. Other suggestions not involving equipment were tried at two or three workstations for a period of 1

week. This resulted in a choice for desk chairs.

9. Team members were then assigned to sourcing and costing of the solutions.
10. Once this information was compiled, the team approached management for permission to proceed, which was granted.
11. During this time the therapist began to gradually withdraw from the process and allowed natural leaders to take on more of a leadership role. The therapist was contacted for information as needed.
12. Over a period of 8 months the solutions were implemented and the PE team continued to assess and monitor the situation. Minor changes were made as needed and based on input from all workers.

Participatory Ergonomics Program

Maciel described the Participatory Ergonomics Program (PEP).[22] PEP is basically an ergonomic team that meets on a regular basis to discuss ergonomic issues and is made up of workers, supervisors, and medical and engineering staff. Extensive ergonomic training is provided in an informal manner. Once a working knowledge of ergonomics is attained, the group plans the major changes that are needed to improve working conditions. Teams made up of front-line workers are selected to test possible solutions for an appropriate length of time. The work team is responsible for meeting and arriving at a consensus regarding their opinions and concerns about the solution. The health and quality of work of the work team is monitored and compared with that of those workers not taking part in the new solution.

Advanced Knowledge and Design Acquisition Methodology

The main focus of Advanced Knowledge and Design Acquisition Methodology (AKADAM)[23] is for the therapist (knowledge elicitor) to gain knowledge from the worker (domain expert). The worker (user) is considered the most knowledgeable regarding the work tasks and work environment and therefore is the expert. The reason the therapist (designer) requires knowledge from

the worker is that the designer often misjudges the impact of designs on the user. In order to succeed with ergonomic interventions, there needs to be an exchange of knowledge between the user and designer (worker and therapist). The authors of AKADAM argue that the ergonomist cannot rely solely on observation of the user but must incorporate direct interaction to understand the contextual interdependencies of the user and work.

Work Analysis

Work analysis[10] has been defined as a global approach in which activity analysis takes place in relation to an analysis of the work determinants (employer financial constraints, workforce characteristics, production organization and technical processes, and time and quality constraints). Many workers unconsciously develop strategies to reduce injury risk. The role of the therapist in the work analysis model of PE is to modify the representation of work involved in the process. In other words, the work analysis must identify the worker activity (postures, efforts, decision making, communication) as a personal response to either a set of work determinants (e.g., time constraints, production speed, workstation organization) or operator-related determinants (e.g., age, size, strength, experience). Work analysis reveals aspects of work that are not usually readily apparent, such as strategies to cope with incidents and communication networks. Work analysis emphasizes differences between performance reached at the workplace and decreased cost of performance to the worker (e.g., fatigue, health problems, mental processes).

Ergonomic Coordinator Program

The Ergonomic Coordinator (EC) Program[12] begins with an external expert in ergonomics coming to assist the organization with a PE program and ends with internal regulation of the program. The expert provides extensive ergonomic training to volunteer employees. These employees become the ECs. The ECs develop a mission and purpose statement, then proceed with an evaluation of work environments. The final stages of the program focus on improving working conditions and confirming the program's future. The EC members decide how the worksite will be evaluated and prioritize identified problems. It is during these last stages that the ECs begin moving away from the external agent.

RETURN TO WORK

Successful return to work depends on (1) early injury reporting, (2) injury intervention, (3) continuous contact and communication among the worker, employer, and health care providers, and (4) a management team and workforce educated in the importance of early and safe return to work, provision of ergonomic modifications to worksites, and specific and meaningful DM policies and procedures.[9,36] Using ergonomic strategies in the return to work process provides for sustainable ways for workers with limitations to return earlier to the workforce and remain in the workplace longer.

The role of the therapist in the return-to-work process is significant, as the therapist is often the only direct link between the workplace and the health care system. The therapist can provide insight into how to match the worker to the workplace without causing reinjury or impeding the employer's work activities. In all organizations there is a legal and financial responsibility to assist workers in the return-to-work or accommodation process, but many organizations are unaware of how to effectively adjust the workplace and work duties to meet the needs of an employee with a disability. The therapist has the opportunity to demonstrate effective methods by applying the knowledge of the mechanism of injury, the impact on the individual, and residual capabilities, while understanding the corporate cultures that affect work.

When reviewing Compufone's compensation records the therapist noted the following: Compufone had an average of 15 lost-time days per employee per year; a number of employees never returned to work; and long-term disability premiums for the coming year were doubling. In order to demonstrate legal due diligence, financial improvements, and workplace culture improvements the therapist recommended the development of a company return-to-work program.

The therapist worked with the management team and representatives from the union to develop a return-to-work policy that met the workplace cultural needs and ensured a return-to-work process aimed at early and safe return to work. A successful return-to-work program requires a combination of several elements.

A Written Return-to-Work Policy

The policy should outline the company's philosophy on and dedication to returning employees to productive employment. It should spell out how the program works, such as what benefits are available, how to report an injury, and roles and responsibilities of all workplace parties. The RTW policy should include the role of the consulting therapist as a RTW coordinator or consultant to the RTW team, depending on the company internal resources.

Maintaining "Occupational Bond"

Before an injury, an employee typically has personal and professional relationships at work that give him or her a sense of self-worth and identity. When an individual is injured, these relationships and feelings of self-worth begin to erode. It is a downward spiral that often causes employees to lose their drive to return to work. Employers must counter these negative "psychosocial" factors by maintaining early and appropriate communication with the employee. This can be accomplished by communication with the employee to inform them of new developments at work. In short, keep them in the loop.

Job Descriptions and Physical Demands Analysis

The purpose of detailed job descriptions is to give the employee's treatment team an idea of whether the employee is able to safely return to work within his or her medical restrictions. It can also help the physician write specific medical restrictions that apply directly to the employee's work. The job tasks should be separated into "essential" and "nonessential" duties for purposes of the Americans with Disabilities Act (ADA), workers' compensation, or human rights requirements. Some employers complement the written descriptions with digital photographs or videotape to ensure accuracy and complete understanding.

Completing a physical demands analysis (PDA) of a job is one way of identifying risks. PDAs include basic job descriptions, level of work (sedentary, light, medium, heavy), a description of the workstation and environment, hours of work and break times, physical demands (walking, lifting, reaching, etc.), and sensory and/or cognitive demands (vision, hearing, memory, writing, reading, etc.). The frequency and duration required for each demand are recorded, as is any other information that would allow replication or simulation of the demand. For example, standing may be done on a frequent basis over the course of the day (5 hours) and up to 20 minutes continuously, on a wet cement floor, while working at a counter 42 inches high, with a rail 10 inches high. PDAs are job specific, not worker specific, and any measurement should be related to the workstation and not to the individual worker (e.g., counter is 36 inches high, not counter is waist high). Clarity of the PDA is important so that the treatment team has an understanding of the workplace demands and can support the RTW process through thorough assessment and RTW recommendations. PDAs are important when using functional assessments as part of the RTW process. A sample PDA is shown in Figure 16-4.

Early Communication Between the Health Care Team and the Workplace

The therapist can be a conduit between the treatment team and the workplace. It is important to ensure that the therapist understands not only the job components but also the functional capabilities of the individual and how to communicate this match to the workplace in a meaningful way. It is important that the therapist has the informed consent of the worker and does not share diagnosis, but only functional and work-based capabilities and limitations with the employer.

Creating a Return-to-Work Team

An RTW coordinator (which may be the therapist) should oversee the program. The RTW coordinator should be supported by all members of the RTW team, which may include the treating physician, the supervisor, the employee with an injury, the union representative, the human resources contact, and the safety specialist. The coordinator's responsibilities may include early communication with the worker and healthcare team, communicating with the insurance claims person, overseeing all RTW activities, obtaining job descriptions for the treatment team, developing an RTW plan with all stakeholders, and conducting progress reviews to ensure the success of the program. The supervisor would be involved in individual cases when one of his or her employees is involved. Among other things, he or she might participate in the accident investigation and suggest a worksite modification to ease the transition back to work.

Training of the Supervisors and Employees

The program should be communicated to all employees and supervisors so everyone knows what to expect when an injury occurs. A systematic review of the literature demonstrated that education of supervisors about ergonomics and health and safety improved disability durations and RTW success.[9]

Offering Accommodation and Transitional Duty

The employer should offer an accommodation and transitional duty program aimed at returning the worker to productive work as soon as he or she is able to perform such work. The therapist can provide input into appropriate offers of transitional work. *Transitional work* is defined as work that has been modified temporarily to be able to accommodate an individual's reduced capabilities because of an illness or injury during an RTW process to allow for safe and timely transition into the workplace duties. Generally, three types of transitional duty may be offered. First, the worker's regular job may be modified to meet medical restrictions. Modifications may include the provision of ergonomic equipment, removal of nonessential work duties, or providing a work buddy to complete tasks that do not meet the restrictions. The second type of transitional duty is modified work. Modified work is not the worker's regular

Text continued on p. 305.

Job Demands Analysis – <Job Classification>

Date:

Job title:

Union:

Location:

Description: Narrative overview of the job analyzed

Form completed by: _____

Nancy J. Gowan, BHSc(OT), OT Reg(Ont), CDMP

Reviewed by:

I have reviewed the physical demands analysis for the xxx position within the xxx and I agree with the stated demands of the position as noted.

_____   _____
Client name   *Date*

I have reviewed the physical demands analysis for the xxx position within the xxx and I agree with the stated demands of the position as noted.

_____   _____
Contact name, title   *Date*

Essential Duties and Tasks

0) Duty 1
) Task 1
     (0) Sub-task
     (0) Sub-task
) Task 2
     (0)
     (0)
     (0)
) Task 3
     (0)

0) Duty 2
) Task 1
     (0) Sub-task 1
     (0) Etc.

0) Duty 3
) Task 1
     (0) Sub-task 1
     (0) Etc.

Time for tasks observed <Start/finish>

FIGURE **16-4** A sample physical demands analysis.   *Continued*

	Summary	
Critical Physical Demands	**Details** (force, distance, range of motion)	**Frequency** **(see scale)**
Maximum lift	•	
Maximum carry	•	
Maximum push/pull	•	
Range of motion	•	
Extended reach	•	
Standing/sitting	•	

Ergonomic concerns/comments (if ANY box is checked, inform Safety Dept.)

☐ **Contact stress** (hand or knee as a hammer >10 × hr/ >2 hr total/day)	☐ **Repetition (same motion** with neck, shoulders, elbows, wrists, or hands every few seconds with little or no variation >2 hr total/day)	☐ **Intensive keying** (>4 hrs/day)	☐ **Grip force (pinch grip** unsupported object >1 kg or with force of more than 4 kg >2 hrs/day)
☐ **Grip force (power grip** unsupported object >5 kg or with force of >5 kg/>2 hrs/day)	☐ **Lift Lower Force (lifting >35 kg** >once/ day)	☐ **Lift Lower Force (lifting >25 kg/**>10 × hr/>2 hrs/day)	☐ **Lift Lower Force (lifting >5 kg**>2 × minute/>2 hrs/day)
☐ **Lift Lower Force (lift >11 kg**>25 × day AND - above shoulders or - below knees or - at arm's length)	☐ **Awkward Posture** (working with **neck or back bent** more than 30° >2 hrs/day)	☐ **Awkward Posture** (working with **hand above head or elbow above shoulder** >2 hrs/day)	☐ **Awkward Posture (kneeling** >2 hrs/day)
☐ **Vibration** (use of **high-vibration tools**— chain saw, jack hammer, etc.->30 min/day)	☐ **Vibration** (use of **moderate vibration tools**—grinders, sanders, jig saw->2 hrs/day)	**Frequency Scale** 5–Constantly, more than 75% of shift 4–Frequently, 50-75% of shift 3–Occasionally, 25-50% of shift 2–Seldom, less than 25% of shift 1–Never	

Comments:

FIGURE **16-4,** cont'd

Work schedule:

Avg. hrs. per shift: _____   Week: _____

Shift rotation: _____

Voluntary overtime: _____

Work pace:

☐ Unpaced

☐ Deadline

☐ Machine paced

Tools, equipment, and machines	**Special clothes and personal protective equipment**

Tools, equipment, and machines

- Banding cutters
- Small sledge hammer

Special clothes and personal protective equipment

☐ Hard hat

☐ Safety shoes/boots

☐ Hearing protection

☐ Respiratory protection

☐ Safety glasses

Vehicles and mobile equipment

- Equipment 1
   Sub-types
- Equipment 2

Others: _____

FIGURE **16-4, cont'd**

Continued

Physical Demands

For each item, show the corresponding amount of time the movement is made per shift:

5–Constantly, more than 75% of shift
4–Frequently, 50-75% of shift
3–Occasionally, 25-50% of shift
2–Seldom, less than 25% of shift
1–Never

Physical demands (whole body)	Task description	Frequency (1-5)
Sitting/driving	•	
Standing	•	
Walking (level, rough ground, slopes)	•	
Low level work (Crouching/squatting/ kneeling/crawling) Squat Kneel	•	
Going up or down stairs or steps	•	
Climbing ladders	•	
Climbing on or over equipment	•	
Balancing (when on narrow or slippery surfaces)	•	

FIGURE **16-4**, cont'd

Physical Demands (cont.)

For each item, show the corresponding amount of time the movement is made per shift:

5–Constantly, more than 75% of shift
4–Frequently, 50-75% of shift
3–Occasionally, 25-50% of shift
2–Seldom, less than 25% of shift
1–Never

Posture/ movement	Task description	Frequency (1-5)
Bending from waist	•	
Bending laterally	•	
Twisting	•	
Sitting unsupported	•	
Neck flexion	•	
Neck extension	•	
Neck lateral flexion	•	
Neck rotation	•	

FIGURE **16-4, cont'd**   *Continued*

Physical Demands (cont.)

For each item, show the corresponding amount of time the movement is made per shift:

5–Constantly, more than 75% of shift
4–Frequently, 50-75% of shift
3–Occasionally, 25-50% of shift
2–Seldom, less than 25% of shift
1–Never

Movements	One hand/ arm use	Both hands/ arms used together	Task description	Frequency (1-5)
Shoulder extension	☐	☐	•	
Shoulder flexion	☐	☐	•	
Shoulder abduction	☐	☐	•	
Elbow flexion	☐	☐	•	
Elbow pronate/supinate Pronation Supination	☐	☐	•	
Hand (power grip)	☐	☐	•	
Hand (pinch grip)	☐	☐	•	

FIGURE **16-4,** cont'd

Physical Demands (cont.)

For each item, show the corresponding amount of time the movement is made per shift:

5–Constantly, more than 75% of shift
4–Frequently, 50-75% of shift
3–Occasionally, 25-50% of shift
2–Seldom, less than 25% of shift
1–Never

Movements	One hand/ arm use	Both hands/ arms used together	Task description	Frequency (1-5)
Hand (side-side deviation) Ulnar deviation Radial deviation	☐	☐	•	
Flexion Wrist flexion	☐	☐	•	
Extension Wrist extension	☐	☐	•	
Leg extension	☐	☐	•	
Ankle flexion/extension/ use of pedals	☐	☐	•	

FIGURE **16-4, cont'd**

Continued

Lift/Carry/Push/Pull

Manual lifting	Rating (1-5)	Object(s) handled (dimensions)	Lowest point (floor, waist, chest)	Highest point (waist, chest, overhead)
1-10 lbs.		•		
11-25 lbs.		•		
26-50 lbs.		•		
50+ lbs.		•		

Carrying	Rating		Average distance moved	
			Min.	Max.
1-10 lbs.				
11-25 lbs.				
26-50 lbs.				
50+ lbs.				

Pushing/pulling	Rating	Rough smooth wheels Flat slope	Min.	Max.
1-10 lbs.				
11-25 lbs.				
26-50 lbs.		•		
50+ lbs.				

Comments:

FIGURE **16-4, cont'd**

Working Conditions

Check ✓ **"Yes"** or **"No"** for each item to show whether or not a person would be exposed to it while doing the job.

Description	Exposure		Comments/explanations
	Yes	No	
Slippery or uneven surfaces (rough ground, steps, slopes, etc.)			•
Work around moving machinery or mobile equipment			•
On and off moving equipment			•
Moving objects/parts			•
High workplaces (>10 ft.)			•
Confined spaces (tanks, pits, etc.)			•
Noise levels (give dB levels)			•
Low levels of lighting			•
Vibration or jarring (from mobile equipment, power tools, etc.)			•
Contact with chemicals			•
Breathing chemicals or dust			•
Electrical hazards			•
>20 mins. from advanced medical aid			•
Welding, cutting, plasma torches			•
Other (please specify)			•

Percentage of time spent indoors	Percentage of time spent outdoors
Approximate temperature range	**Humidity range of work area**

FIGURE **16-4, cont'd**

Continued

Visual/Communication

Description	Required		Comments/explanations
	Yes	No	
• Near vision			•
• Far vision			•
• Depth perception			•
• Side vision			•
• Color discrimination			•
• Reading			•
• Hearing			•

Cognitive/Psychological Demands

5–Constantly, more than 75% of shift
4–Frequently, 50-75% of shift
3–Occasionally, 25-50% of shift
2–Seldom, less than 25% of shift
1–Never

Description	Rating (1-5)	Comments/explanations
• Self-supervision		•
• Supervision exercised over others		•
• Deadline pressures		•
• Attention to detail		•
• Performance of multiple tasks		•
• Reading		•
• Writing		•
• Mathematics		•
• Speaking		•
• Memory		•
• Listening		•

FIGURE **16-4**, cont'd

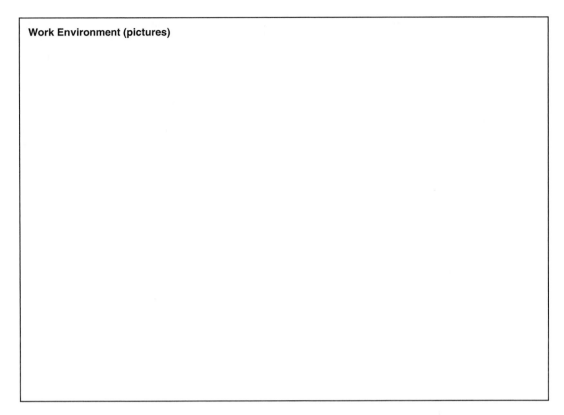

Work Environment (pictures)

FIGURE **16-4, cont'd**

job, but rather an alternate job that meets the worker's medical restrictions. The third type of transitional duty is work hardening. Work hardening involves the worker performing his or her regular work for fewer hours, and gradually building up to the required hours. The transitional duty, in whichever form, should have a timeline, be goal oriented, and involve meaningful and productive work. The work should focus on the employee's abilities and have a goal of returning the worker to regular duties.

Performing Ergonomic Visits (Job Coaching)

Moderate evidence exists that onsite ergonomic visits by the therapist and the involvement of the therapist with responsibility for the RTW coordination reduces work disability duration and costs.[9] The onsite visit should include a worksite assessment or job analysis specific to the worker with an injury. Typically, these types of assessments are more in-depth than a PDA and are worker specific. The therapist also provides coaching to the employee on strategies to safely perform the work, manage symptoms at work, and improve productivity through the work program.

Coaching involves an interactive education and support process at the workplace. When coaching a worker with an injury the therapist provides regular onsite instruction on a one-on-one basis. Coaching allows the therapist and worker to problem solve together on ways to allow a worker to complete the job tasks within the confines of the work requirements without risk of reinjury. As a coach in the workplace, the therapist helps the worker with an injury develop mastery over the job duties through integration of all of the strategies developed during the rehabilitation period in the real workplace environment.

Applying Secondary and Tertiary Prevention Strategies

Microergonomics refers to ergonomic solutions that are applied to a specific job for a specific individual's need. RTW processes must employ a microergonomic strategy that is specific to the needs of the worker with an illness or injury while ensuring that the changes made for that worker do not affect the safety and productivity of other workers. Knowing the worker's injury and any limitations or restrictions will enable the therapist to identify worker-specific risk factors. Making modifications or adaptations to any aspect of the job will often allow early return to work without risk of reinjury or exacerbation of the injury. These changes could be applied to the worker (change the way the worker physically performs the job, such as eliminating forward trunk bending by training the worker to squat or flex at the hip), the workplace equipment (e.g., customized, fully adjustable office chair in place of old, nonadjustable oversized chair used preinjury), or the work processes (e.g., rotate job tasks to avoid prolonged static positioning, or begin with reduced work hours and gradually increase as worker tolerates).

Secondary prevention is an ergonomic solution applied to jobs in which injuries have been reported.[25] These types of ergonomic solutions are geared to a specific worker and job and are not usually generalizable to the entire workforce. An example may be a telephone headset for a receptionist complaining of neck pain.

Tertiary prevention would also be considered a form of microergonomics, whereby solutions are found for individuals with chronic, disabling MSD limitations in order for them to achieve maximal functioning at work.[25] The therapist applies the principles of ergonomics to find strategies that will allow individuals with impairments to perform the work without further risk of injury. Some of the strategies may apply to the larger workforce but generally need to consider the specific needs of the worker with a disability.

Evaluating the Results of the Program

Once an employee completes the RTW program, the therapist should sit down with the employee and supervisor and evaluate the RTW process and the program outcome. Areas for improvement should be noted. The employer should also track certain program indicators, such as days away from work, medical costs of disability, length of transitional duty, and so on. These benchmarks will help the employer measure the success of the program.

Throughout the RTW process, it is paramount that the therapist understand that early return to work must be appropriate to the worker's capabilities and restrictions and must take into consideration that both the employee and employer only benefit from sustainable RTW solutions. Taking time to properly assess all of the workplace barriers from a physical, cognitive, and psychosocial point of view will ensure that any strategy implemented will have increased likelihood of success. For example, rushing return to work without fully understanding the productivity demands of the workplace or the workplace culture may lead to reinjury or lack of buy-in from the supervisor with regard to the RTW plan.

The therapist's role in the RTW process may vary depending on the relationship with the workplace and the workplace's resources. The therapist may be the RTW coordinator, work in a supporting clinic, or consult on ergonomic adjustments for accommodation of workers with illnesses or injuries. No matter which role the therapist is involved in, use of evidence-based ergonomic strategies and treatment or intervention recommendations should focus on matching the worker to the workplace early to avoid the additional issues that are associated with delayed return to work.

RETURN-TO-WORK MODEL

Berthelette and Baril have developed an explanatory model for implementation of early RTW programs considering stakeholder interactions.[1] The focus of the model is on RTW intervention, but it considers the influences of the RTW processes, organizational factors, and socioenvironmental factors. For example, company size and sector affect how the RTW interventions are implemented and how resources are allocated. A large organization may have access to resources internally and have the flexibility to offer many options for returning to work (including bundling and unbundling tasks to modify the work), but a smaller organization may require outside resources and be unable to financially afford some of the ergonomic strategies that may be most beneficial to an employee returning to work (e.g., having only a few job options that may be similar in job demands). Senior management commitment to a safety-oriented culture is also important, because RTW outcomes are improved in such a culture. Organizational cultures affect the relationships among the internal and external stakeholders. A culture of safety ensures that all stakeholders understand their roles and responsibilities in the process. People and safety-oriented organizational cultures are associated with improved RTW outcomes. Management can influence all aspects of the RTW process; therefore, commitment of senior management to a safety-oriented culture is important. Ensuring that all stakeholders understand their roles and responsibilities in the process will facilitate RTW success.

In order to better understand the RTW process we will return to Compufone and the case of Ms. Jones. The therapist was asked to assist Ms. Jones in an RTW process. Ms. Jones is a call-center employee with less than 3 years of service. She has been off work for 3 weeks under the care of her family physician. A recent electromyogram (EMG) indicated moderate symptoms of carpal tunnel syndrome (CTS). Her physician has asked Ms. Jones to remain off work while attending physiotherapy and wearing night splints. The physician is unsure if Ms. Jones will be able to return to her job at the call center.

The therapist met with Ms. Jones the following day to obtain information about her current capabilities and discuss Compufone's new RTW plan. In the interview the therapist is informed by Ms. Jones that she has made improvements in the physiotherapy program and that she is concerned that a return to work would affect her CTS. She indicated that she does not wish to have surgery. She also cares for three small children at home, aged 6, 4, and 2.

The therapist performs a complete PDA of the work demands in order to analyze the essential work duties and risks for CTS. Ms. Jones and her supervisor participate in the PDA.

Through this analysis it is determined that the work requires repetitive keyboarding activities. The therapist communicates with the treatment team after gaining consent from Ms. Jones. Once the therapist has an understanding of Ms. Jones' current capabilities, the therapist, worker, and supervisor examine whether the job requires adjustments. These adjustments may include the following:

- Ergonomic changes at the workplace (provision of an adjustable chair with adjustable forearm rests, a natural keyboard, and a footrest)
- Adjustment in hours (gradual return to work starting at 4 hours per day)
- Workflow (alternating phone and keyboarding activities)
- Productivity amounts (starting with reduced productivity of 25% and gradually increasing to 100% at the end of the program)
- Work and rest breaks (scheduled stretches at each hour)
- Bundling or unbundling of various jobs (reassignment of data entry tasks)
- Trials of tools (large-grip pens, chair, thumb paper turners)
- Education on proper body mechanics
- Coaching on managing symptoms at work

The therapist provides Ms. Jones with education on work, home, and leisure activities in order to ensure that all 24-hour body care is addressed.

The therapist sets up an RTW meeting with Ms. Jones, the supervisor, and the union representative. The purpose of the meeting is to develop an RTW plan in collaboration with the employee and the treatment team. A written plan is created that includes specific roles and responsibilities for each stakeholder, details of the week-to-week duties, and progression of duties (Figure 16-5).

Before the commencement of the RTW plan the therapist ensures that appropriate ergonomic equipment is in place and that on-site orientation and training is provided to Ms. Jones on return to work.

Name:	Ms. Jones	Phone number:
Employer:	Compufone	Phone number:
Therapist:	Ms. Ideas	Phone number:
Job title:	Call Center Attendant	
Date of plan:		

Return to work restrictions: Limit repetitive keyboarding, gripping and awkward postures of the wrist, implement rest breaks every hour

Return to work goal: Gradual return to work to call center attendant activities

Return to work schedule:

Week dates	Hours	Duties
Week 1-2	4 hours (rest break every hour for stretches; 15-minute break)	Answering calls, inputting basic data only, using tape recorder for documenting calls (25% productivity week 1; 40% productivity week 2)
Week 3-4	6 hours (rest break for stretches each hour; 15-minute break and 30-minute lunch)	Answering calls, inputting screen 2 and 3 only, using tape recorder for documenting calls (50% productivity week 3; 65% productivity week 4)
Week 5-6	7.5 hours (rest break every hour for stretches; 30-minute lunch, two 15-minute breaks)	Answering calls, inputting all screens 1-4, using tape recorder when fatigued (75% productivity week 5 and 100% productivity week 6)

Review schedule:
- Therapist to review with employee weekly
- Concerns regarding the workplace should be directed to the employer or the therapist

Approved by:

_____   _____

Employee (Ms. Jones)   Supervisor (John Doe)

_____   _____

Therapist (Ms. Ideas)   Physician (Dr. Smith)

Parameters of the Return to Work Program:

The Employee is responsible for:
❑ Reporting any concerns to the supervisor and therapist as the concerns arise
❑ Being on time
❑ Performing all duties as assigned
❑ Contacting the therapist as outlined
❑ Reporting directly to therapist and supervisor any absences prior to shift start times

The supervisor is responsible for:
❑ Ensuring job duties meet employee's capabilities as outlined
❑ Reporting any concerns to the employee and therapist as they arise
❑ Monitoring job performance
❑ Providing feedback to the employee on job performance

The therapist is responsible for:
❑ Ensuring job duties are appropriate for employee's capabilities
❑ Monitoring any concerns brought forth by supervisor or employee
❑ Reviewing return-to-work plan at scheduled intervals
❑ Providing education to employee on proper body mechanics and work pacing

FIGURE **16-5** A return-to-work outline for Ms. Jones.

As the RTW plan is implemented the therapist provides on-site job coaching and evaluation in order to ensure that all the strategies are implemented well. The job coaching is gradually reduced throughout the program as Ms. Jones becomes confident in the RTW process. The therapist must listen effectively to all the stakeholders to identify barriers and to adjust and modify as the plan continues.

As barriers are identified early in the process, the therapist adjusts and modifies the plan in collaboration with the employee and the supervisor on site.

Once the therapist has had the opportunity to evaluate the outcome of RTW plans for various workers, the company's RTW program should be revised accordingly to meet identified needs and reduce gaps. The evaluation process should also identify any training and education needs required to standardize the program and thus ensure consistency within Compufone. Within 1 year of implementing the RTW program, Compufone is provided with an evaluation report that notes a

Learning Exercise One

Overview

This exercise helps in understanding return-to-work roles and responsibilities.

Purpose

The purpose of this exercise is to help the reader become familiar with what roles the therapist can have in the RTW process.

Exercise

Contact a local company to request a copy of their RTW policies and procedures. Review the policies and procedures. Provide recommendations on how to incorporate ergonomic principles and models into the company's RTW policies and procedures. Determine what evaluation processes they may wish to include in the RTW program to reduce risks for all employees. What recommendations would you make to improve the role of the therapist in the RTW programs of this company?

Learning Exercise Two

Overview

This exercise is designed to emphasize reflective facilitation within a team setting.

Purpose

The purpose of this exercise is to investigate your understanding of the reflective facilitation approach as an ergonomic consultant.

Exercise

Discuss the tools that the therapist could use to facilitate the PE team members in identifying their individual skills and knowledge for use in the ergonomic process.

Learning Exercise Three

Overview

This exercise involves applying problem-solving techniques in a team setting.

Purpose

The purpose of this exercise is to approach problem solving in a systematic manner.

Exercise

Review and discuss the suggested Design Decision Group problem-solving tools.

Learning Exercise Four

Overview

This exercise involves promoting ergonomics and DM within the business and management environment.

Purpose

The purpose of this exercise is to become familiar with the business and management justifications for ergonomics within a DM program.

Exercise

Identify some of the components of a business proposal to provide ergonomic services to a manufacturing employer.

reduction of 30% in lost-time injuries and accidents and 90% effective RTW plans. This allows Compufone to reinvest in the program once again toward health promotion and DM strategies.

What are the barriers within Compufone that may affect Ms. Jones' RTW success? How would you use ergonomic principles to address the issues observed at Compufone? What checklists would be appropriate to consider, and how would you use these with the Compufone ergonomic team?

Multiple Choice Review Questions

1. What is disability management?
   A. The study of matching the workplace to the worker
   B. The return-to-work process for workers with work-related injuries
   C. The process of minimizing the impact of an impairment (resulting from work-related and non–work-related injury, illness, or disease) on a worker's ability and capacity to engage in competitive employment
   D. The process of implementing injury-prevention strategies in the workplace

2. Primary prevention is intervention provided to reduce risk:
   A. before a condition exists.
   B. once a condition exists, to reduce further risk.
   C. to maximize function for a chronic condition.
   D. to make ergonomic changes in a team.

3. An example of macroergonomics is:
   A. intervention aimed at one group of workers.
   B. intervention aimed at a worker with a condition.
   C. company policies and procedures.
   D. back education for injured employees.

4. Which of the following is not an ergonomic model?
   A. Design, deliver, delight
   B. Plan, do, check, act
   C. Participatory Ergonomic Program
   D. Advanced Knowledge and Design Acquisition Methodology

5. An example of a strategy to maintain occupational bond is:
   A. applying glue to the desk to prevent keyboard slippage.
   B. calling a worker when he or she is off work to offer modified work.
   C. providing an ergonomic chair.
   D. providing the physician with a copy of the PDA.

6. Key components of return to work include:
   A. job descriptions, communication with treatment team, return-to-work plan.
   B. worksite visits, investigations, surveillance.
   C. union meetings, employee luncheons, ergonomic changes.
   D. early reporting, investigations, long-term disability benefits.

7. Coaching is a strategy to provide the ergonomics team with suggestions on how to implement ergonomics in the workplace during alternate shifts.
   A. True
   B. False

8. In the model of return to work designed by Berthelette and Baril, organizational structure does not affect return to work for employees.
   A. True
   B. False

9. When implementing an ergonomic committee in the workplace, it is important that all workers understand how to use the checklists for identifying hazards and for the company to approve

all ergonomic suggestions provided by the committee.
A. True
B. False

10. In determining the cost of the project it is necessary to consider these major areas:
    A. Personnel, equipment and materials, reduced productivity or sales, and overhead
    B. Current organizational structure and salary grades
    C. Ergonomic equipment sale prices, maintenance fees, lost-time costs
    D. Number of illnesses and injuries in the workplace over the last 3 years

REFERENCES

1. Berthelette D, Baril R: A theoretical model of the implementation of early return to work measures. Conference proceedings. In *Back pain and disability—unraveling the puzzle,* New York, 2000, CIRPD International Conference.
2. Bureau of Labor Statistics: *Lost work-time injuries and illnesses: characteristics and resulting time away from work,* 2005. Retrieved June 3, 2006, from www.bls.gov/news.release/osh2.nr0.htm.
3. Canadian Centre for Occupational Health and Safety: *Work related musculoskeletal disorders,* 2005. Retrieved June 3, 2006, from http://www.ccohs.ca/oshanswers/diseases/rmirsi.html
4. Carrivick PJ, Lee AH, Yau KK et al: Evaluating the effectiveness of a participatory ergonomics approach in reducing the risk and severity of injuries from manual handling, *Ergonomics* 48(8):907, 2005.
5. Chao E: *The need to reduce musculoskeletal disorders in America's workforce.* Speech to the Subcommittee on Labor, Health and Human Services, and Education of the Senate Appropriations Committee, April 26, 2001. Retrieved June 3, 2006, from www.osha.gov/pls/oshaweb/owadisp.show_document?p_table=TESTIMONIES&p_id-245.
6. deJong AM, Vink P: Participatory ergonomics applied in installation work, *Appl Ergon* 33(5):439, 2002.
7. Deming WE: *The new economics for industry, government, education,* ed 2, Cambridge, MA, 1994, Massachusetts Institute of Technology Center for Advanced Educational Services.
8. European Agency for Safety and Health at Work: *Occupational accidents and work related diseases in Sweden,* 2000. Retrieved June 20, 2006, http://www.av.se/dokument/inenglish/reports/2000_15.pdf.
9. Franche RL, Baril R, Shaw W et al: Workplace-based return-to-work interventions: optimizing the role of stakeholders in implementations and research, *J Occup Rehabil* 15(4):525, 2005.
10. Garrigou A, Daniellou F, Caraballeda G et al: Activity analysis in participatory design and analysis of participatory design activity, *Int J Ind Ergon* 15(5):311, 1995.
11. Habeck R, Leahy M, Hunt H et al: Employer factors related to workers' compensation claims and disability management, *Rehabil Couns Bull* 34(3):210, 1991.
12. Haims MC, Carayon P: Theory and practice for the implementation of 'in-house,' continuous improvement participatory ergonomic programs, *Appl Ergon* 29(6):461, 1998.
13. Hanse JJ, Forsman M: Identification and analysis of unsatisfactory psychosocial work situations: a participatory approach employing video-computer interaction, *Appl Ergon* 32(1):23, 2001.
14. Hendrick HW: Determining the cost-benefits of ergonomics projects and factors that lead to their success, *Appl Ergon* 34(5):419, 2003.
15. Hendrick HW: *Good ergonomics is good economics,* 1996. Retrieved June 10, 2006, from www.hfesorg//Web/PubPages/goodergo.pdf.
16. Holmstrom E, Ahlborg B: Morning warm-up exercises on musculoskeletal fitness in construction workers, *Appl Ergon* 36(4):513, 2005.
17. Imada AS, Nagamachi M: Introduction to participatory ergonomics, *Int J Ind Ergon* 15(5):309, 1995.
18. Koningsveld EAP, Dul J, Rhijn GW et al: Enhancing the impact of ergonomics interventions, *Ergonomics* 48(5):559, 2005.
19. Laitenen H, Saari J, Kuusela J: Initiating an innovative change process for improved working conditions and ergonomics with participation and performance feedback: a case study in an engineering workshop, *Int J Ind Ergon* 19(4):299, 1997.
20. Lewin D, Shecter SM: Four factors lower disability rates, *Pers J* 70(5):99, 1991.
21. Loisel P, Gosselin L, Durand P et al: Implementation of a participatory ergonomics program in the rehabilitation of workers suffering from subacute back pain, *Appl Ergon* 32(1):53, 2001.
22. Maciel R: Participatory ergonomics and organizational change, *Int J Ind Ergon* 22(4-5):319, 1998.
23. McNeese MD, Zaff BS, Citera M et al: AKADAM: eliciting user knowledge to support participatory ergonomics, *Int J Ind Ergon* 15(5):345, 1995.

24. Nagamachi M: Requisites and practices of participatory ergonomics, *Int J Ind Ergon* 15(5):329, 1995.

25. National Academy of Sciences: *Musculoskeletal disorders and the workplace: low back and upper extremities,* 2001. Retrieved May 13, 2006, from http://books.nap.edu/openbook.php?isbn = 0309072840&page = 301.

26. National Institute of Disability Management and Research: *Occupational standards for disability management professionals and return to work coordinators,* 2005, Vancouver British Columbia, NIDMAR.

27. National Research Council and Institute of Medicine: *Musculoskeletal disorders and the workplace: low back and upper extremities,* 2001, Panel on Musculoskeletal Disorders and the Workplace, Commission on Behavioral and Social Sciences and Education. Retrieved June 3, 2006, from http://fermat.nap.edu/catalog/10032.html#toc.

28. Occupational Health and Safety Agency for Healthcare in BC: Participatory ergonomics literature review. Retrieved on May 18, 2006, from www.ohsah.bc.ca/index.php?section_id = 1350&section_copy_id = 5416.

29. Ontario Ministry of Labour: Prevent workplace pains and strains. Retrieved May 19, 2006, from www.labour.gov.on.ca/english/hs/pdf/is_ergonomics.pdf.

30. Rempel DM, Krause N, Goldberg R et al: A randomized control trial evaluating the effects of two workstation interventions on upper body pain and incident musculoskeletal disorders among computer operators, *Occup Environ Med* 63:300, 2006.

31. Sankaran S: Notes from the field: action research conversations, *Action Res* 3(4):341, 2005.

32. Shannon HS, Walters V, Lewchuk W et al: Workplace organizational correlates of lost-time accident rates in manufacturing, *Am J Ind Med* 29(3):258, 1996.

33. Theberge N, Granzow K, Cole D et al: Negotiating participation: understanding the "how" in an ergonomic change team, *Appl Ergon* 37(2):239, 2006.

34. U.S. General Accounting Office: *Worker protection: private sector ergonomics programs yield positive results* (GAO/HEHS-97-163), Washington DC, 1997, U.S. General Accounting Office.

35. Vink P, Kompier MAJ: Improving office work: a participatory ergonomic experiment in a naturalistic setting, *Ergonomics* 40(4):435, 1997.

36. Westmorland MG, Williams RM, Amick BC et al: Disability management practices in Ontario workplaces: employees' perceptions, *Disabil Rehabil* 27(14):825, 20005.

37. Wilson JR: Ergonomics and participation. In Wilson JR, Corlett EN, editors: *Evaluation of human work,* ed 2, London, 1995, Taylor & Francis.

38. Wilson JR: Solution ownership in participative work redesign: the case of a crane control room, *Ind Ergon* 15:329, 1995.

39. Zuber-Skerritt O: Action learning and action research: paradigm, praxis and program. In *Effective change management using action learning and action research,* Australia, 2001, Southern Cross University Press.

SUGGESTED RESOURCES

Accommodations
www.abledata.com
www.ccrw.com
www.disabilityresources.org
www.ncddr.org/rpp/techaf/techdfdw/rerc/index.html
www.jan.wvu.edu
www.resna.org
http://trace.wisc.edu
www.dmec.org

Disability Management Resources
www.psychdismgmt.com
www.nidmar.ca
www.equalopportunity.on.ca
www.dm-edge.com
www.WORKink.com
www.gowanhealth.com

Health and Safety Resources
www.ccohs.ca
www.cdc.gov/niosh/homepage.html
www.whsc.on.ca
www.wsib.on.ca
www.iwh.on.ca
http://www.iea.cc/index.cfm

17

Ergonomics of Play and Leisure

Mary Frances Baxter

Learning Objectives

After reading this chapter and completing the exercises, the reader should be able to do the following:

1. The learner will understand how ergonomic principles apply to activities of leisure and sport.
2. The learner will identify risk factors for quilting, golf, and gardening and apply the same concepts to other leisure activities.
3. The learner will identify strategies to improve effort and efficiency in leisure tasks using ergonomic principles.

Crafts. A variety of activities and hobbies that are related to making things with one's own hands and skill.

Sports. Activities requiring physical ability, physical fitness, or physical skill which usually, but not always, involve competition between two or more people.

Tools. Pieces of equipment that most commonly provide a mechanical advantage in accomplishing a physical task.

Positions. Arrangement or posture of one human body; in this context, body positions used when participating in crafts and sports and when using tools to accomplish tasks.

CASE STUDY

Betty is a 55-year-old woman currently working in a mid-level management job. She began quilting 20 years ago and quilts an average of 2 to 4 hours each evening, sometimes more if she can fit it into her schedule. Betty has a defined space for her quilting, which is a 12-foot by 12-foot room that is also used for other craft projects and storage as well as her computer. However, she also uses other parts of the house, such as the kitchen table for cutting fabric and the living room floor for laying out large sections of the project she is working on. Betty enjoys quilting so much that she reports that she occasionally loses track of time while involved in a project. Her favorite part of the quilting process is piecing the tops of the quilts using her sewing machine.

During the warmer weather, Betty also likes to garden, doing the raking, weeding, pruning, planting, and other tasks with minimal help. In addition, Betty has decided to play golf again, which she has not done since she was in her 30s. She is currently taking lessons at the local golf course.

Typically, ergonomics focuses on work. In this chapter we will apply the principles and foundations of ergonomics to leisure, recreation, and activities of choice.

Issues related to the use of computers in the workplace are well represented in the literature and in this text. However, the burgeoning use of home computers for leisure activities compounds the effects of the musculoskeletal strains and injuries experienced in the work environment. For instance, quilters may use computer-based programs to design templates, choose colors, and determine size, shape, and placement of quilt blocks. Golfers and other athletes use computers to play virtual golf, monitor player statistics, or track their own game statistics. Gardeners use computers to design garden layouts and choose plants for placement in a garden design. Practitioners of a number of leisure and sports activities visit chat rooms and Internet sites that support their interests.

The field of kinesiology provides extensive research and information about a number of sports and activities. The main goal of studying athletes is to improve performance in the selected sport. By studying and analyzing performance in a sport, kinesiologists have helped athletes such as swimmers, runners, skiers, and rowers improve competition performance through faster times of completion.[*] Studying the work and movement involved in a sport has also helped increase distance and accuracy obtained. Athletes involved in track and field events achieve longer jumps or higher pole vaults. Other benefits of performance analysis are found in athletic competition.[†] Accuracy of actions such as in putting a golf ball, throwing a basketball, and shooting skeet is improved.[49,51,66,96] Kinesiology combined with sports medicine also provides valuable information about the number and types of injuries associated with a variety of sports[‡] to facilitate injury prevention measures and improved treatment.

BACKGROUND

To illustrate the application of principles of ergonomics to leisure and sports, three activities were selected: gardening, quilting, and golf. These activities were selected because of their popularity and the variety of tasks involved in each activity. In addition, each of these activities has a wide range of participants, from casual engagement to intense involvement and even to professional involvement by which a person engages in the activity as a means of employment.

Quilting was chosen to represent a generally sedentary activity involving a creative process. Similar activities include scrapbooking, bead or leather work, some types of ceramics such as mosaics, and most crafts. Gardening also involves a creative process but is more physically demanding. Similar activities might include woodworking, home repair, and pottery. Golf is defined as

---

*References 1, 5, 13, 14, 16, 78, 79, 88.
† References 6, 11, 15, 25, 26, 39, 43, 45, 56, 71.
‡References 5, 13, 22, 31, 41, 42, 44, 72, 75, 99.

a sport and can be physically demanding, but includes a competitive factor. Each of these activities involves an assortment of tools to accomplish different tasks within the activity as well as a variety of positions for different tasks embedded in the activity.

RISK FACTORS FOR LEISURE OCCUPATIONS

Risk factors are associated with many leisure activities, and much of the information about the risks comes from the study of persons who engage in the performance, arts, or sports industries as professionals. Persons such as professional golfers, athletes, musicians, and dancers generated interest in risk factors and injuries related to their professions.* As a result of the study of professionals, interest expanded to include persons who engage in a myriad of activities or occupations for leisure or during uncommitted time. Ergonomic analysis and injury rate prediction have been gathered for boaters, gardeners, golfers, swimmers, and runners, as well as for contact sports participants and even children (see Chapter 14).† In addition, with the aging of baby boomers (see Chapter 15) and the increase in health awareness in the general public, there is an increase in knowledge related to ergonomics as well as an increase in the number of ergonomic products available to the general public.[48,60,92]

Injuries of the back and the effects of cumulative trauma and repetitive strain are most typically reported in the work environment. There are, however, several risk factors not typically encountered in the office and work environment that may be seen in sports and leisure activities. In addition to unique and challenging musculoskeletal injuries, some leisure-time activities such as hunting, backpacking, biking, paintball, rock climbing, boating, bungee-cord jumping, and other challenging leisure time pursuits can generate outcomes such as ocular injuries, head injuries,

injuries from lightning strikes, and even death.* Gardening, photography, ceramics, and other creative outlets have resulted in health conditions and illnesses related to environmental toxins.[19,58,69,82]

The case study of Betty will be used to discuss the information and apply the principles presented in this chapter. The intent is that the reader will be able to apply the same principles and process to persons engaged in other leisure, play, or sport activities.

PARTICIPATION AND DEMOGRAPHICS

Much of the information about the demographics of participants in activities comes from marketing research, especially when the activity involves purchase or rental of equipment or space. Marketing research is an integral part of business in the United States. Some limited data from other countries are available, depending on the particular market.

Quilting

The largest quilt show in the world is held yearly in Houston, Texas, with reports of 53,000 attendees from all over the world. Every 3 years Quilts, Inc. produces a survey for the retail quilt community identifying the demographics of American quilters. According to the National Survey of Quilting in America, 16.27 million households (15% of the population) have someone who participates in quilting as a hobby or a profession.[77] The average quilter is female and 55 to 65 years of age. Quilters report an average of 11.5 hours per week of involvement in a quilting-related task. Machine piecing is the most commonly reported of the array of tasks associated with quilting.[77] Some quilters report spending as much as 40 to 60 hours per week.[4,77] Although there are quilters throughout the world, there is limited information on the demographics of any particular country. Japan hosts several large quilt exhibits and competitions each year, bringing approximately 32,000 visitors to the larger shows, indicating a strong

---

*References 13, 14, 17, 42, 48, 55, 57, 68, 75, 89, 91, 95, 97, 99, 100.
†References 12, 27, 30, 37, 47, 59, 65, 73, 74, 86.

*References 3, 10, 21, 38, 40, 47, 52, 53.

popularity of quilting in Japan. In addition, the European Quilt Association shows a membership of 48,215 members from 14 European countries. The largest member organization in Europe is in the Netherlands, with 14,000 members. Not all quilters join organizations and quilt guilds, but these numbers give an indication of the popularity of quilting worldwide.

Gardening

Gardening continues to be a popular activity for pleasure and leisure. The European Commission reports 107 million gardens or garden allotments across the European Union, which includes 10 European countries.[24] The report further indicates that Europeans spend an average of 10 minutes per day in gardening tasks. Statistics Canada indicates that 80% of Canadians participate in some form of gardening, but limited detail is found about gardeners or their participation.[90] In the United States the National Gardening Association indicates that approximately 91 million or 83% of American households participate in one or more types of do-it-yourself indoor and outdoor lawn and garden activities.[67] The same survey identifies several categories of people who garden, including master gardeners, garden enthusiasts, casual gardeners, reluctant gardeners, and "just cut the grass" gardeners, indicating that there is a wide variety of participation levels in gardening.[20,67] Demographic information for the Pacific-Asian countries as well as Australia is not readily available.

Golfing

The invention of golf is generally attributed to the Scots; however, there is debate among historians that the origins of golf may be Chinese, French, or Dutch. There is evidence that the oldest playing golf course in the world is the Old Links at Musselburgh, Scotland, where Mary, Queen of Scots reputedly played in 1567. Today, golf is more popular than ever, with 32,000 golf courses in the world, approximately half of them in the United States.

There are approximately 27 million golfers in the United States.[18] Of those 27 million golfers, 73% are male and 27% are female. The average

golfer is a 39-year-old married man who plays more than 20 rounds per year. An avid or devoted golfer is defined as someone who plays 25 or more rounds per year. The category of avid golfer includes 6.1 million people. Considering that a round of golf is typically 18 holes and can take as little as 2.5 hours but as long as 6 hours, it is easy to see that a large amount of time per week can be spent on golf.

Marketing reports from other countries indicate similar demographics of golfers. Australia has 1.28 million golfers, and golf is identified as the second most popular physical activity among Australian men.[2,32] The Royal Canadian Golf Association reports 25.2 million golfers across Canada,[84] marketing reports indicate 11 million golfers in Japan,[83] and the London Golf Show reports 6.1 million golfers across the United Kingdom.[54] In all these countries, the average golfer is a young adult male.

According to the demographics presented, Betty fits the model of the average quilter and gardener but not necessarily the average golfer.

COMMON INJURIES

It may be difficult to think of a task that is identified as a leisure pursuit as an activity that is prone to cause injuries. Nevertheless, quilting, gardening, and golf injuries can be common and concomitant with the positions, movements, and forces associated with the tasks. It is important for therapists to be aware of the patterns of musculoskeletal injuries associated with various leisure activities so problems can be avoided or corrected. In addition, it is important to understand the relationship between the work activities and the leisure activities. For example, a woman who quilts may also have a job that requires extensive computer work. Both contexts can be contributing to the musculoskeletal problems a person is experiencing.

Quilting

Several studies on garment industry workers have shown that extensive time spent sewing or using poor positioning leaning forward over the sewing machine leads to musculoskeletal disorders, especially in the neck, shoulders, elbows, and hands.[46,87] Comparable problems are seen in quilters. Quilters report discomfort and pain in the neck, shoulders, and back.[4,74] It should be easy to see that participation in activities that require the same forward-leaning position with concentrated engagement of the upper extremities, such as woodworking, ceramics, scrapbooking, and other crafts, could cause similar discomforts, pain, or musculoskeletal injuries.

From the National Survey of Quilting in America, 59% of the respondents indicated that they would increase their weekly amount of time in making quilts in the next 3 years. Quilting time may approach 20 to 40 hours a week and would likely increase musculoskeletal complaints. In the same survey a number of people indicated that they would spend less time quilting (2%). Of those who indicated that they would spend less time quilting, health reasons (48%) was the primary reason for the decline in participation.[74]

Several authors suggest that the repetitive tasks in quilting can put quilters at risk for other musculoskeletal injuries including repetitive stress disorders, specifically carpal tunnel syndrome, tendonitis, de Quervain's syndrome, and epicondylitis,[50,63,98] especially when awkward positions of the body and extremities are used in the tasks (Figure 17-1). Although there is little research to substantiate these claims in quilters and other crafters, repetitive stress disorders are well documented in professional musicians and performers as well as in workers who perform repetitive fine motor tasks.*

In addition, eyestrain can occur when vision is needed for a prolonged period of time in an unsuitably lighted working environment. Many quilters rely on household lighting that is not effective enough for intense fine motor work to complete the tasks of quilting. Conversely, quilters may have adequate lighting such as high spectrum lighting but have poor positioning of the light relative to the task, resulting in glare. Lighting should be bright and directed toward the work surface or the task and not toward the eyes. Quilters report

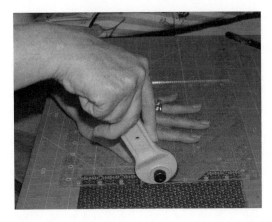

FIGURE **17-1** Weight-bearing on the left hand to hold the ruler and excessive flexion of the right wrist while using a nonergonomic rotary cutter can lead to repetitive strain injuries and other musculoskeletal injuries during a cutting task.

symptoms such as eye soreness or fatigue, headache, blurred vision, double vision, and dry, itching, burning, or irritated eyes.[50,63,98]

Gardening

Surprisingly, there is very little information about injury rates among gardeners. Powell and colleagues describe a self-reported injury rate among gardeners of 2.1 million in the 30-day period before their interview.[76] They also suggest that younger gardeners (ages 18 to 44 years) were more likely to be injured during gardening than older gardeners (ages 45+ years) and that men and women were equally likely to be injured. Unfortunately, the researchers do not have data that show what types of injuries occurred and what effect the injuries had on participation in daily activities. It is suggested that there is a relatively low risk of injury in gardening and other low- to moderate-intensity activities such as home repair, hunting and fishing, swimming, and walking. However, because of the high participation rate, the absolute number of injuries is high.[72,76]

Golfing

The golf swing is a multiphase coordinated movement that uses the whole body and includes ro-

---

*References 17, 64, 70, 80, 81, 85.

tation or twisting of the legs and back in a forceful manner. Injuries also occur as a result of the action of the fast-moving golf club combined with the twisting action of the torso to generate power.

Common injuries seen in golfers can result from repetitive overuse, poor body mechanics, or trauma.[28,34,36,61,62] Because of the amount of time spent in practice or play, professional golfers tend to acquire overuse injuries. Conversely, amateur golfers tend to have musculoskeletal injuries from incorrect movements and general deconditioning.[62] Common injuries in the amateur golf population include low back, hand and wrist, elbow, and shoulder injuries, as well as injuries of the knee.[62]

These injuries are often the result of an explosive or ballistic-type twisting motion, with the lower back and shoulders as the axes of the motion paired with lack of warmup or conditioning. It is interesting to note that men and women have different types of injuries, which may be related to body morphology as well as technique (Table 17-1). Men show injuries of the back and hand and wrist at 36% and 32% respectively, whereas women show an injury rate of 51% at the elbow and 25% at the shoulder.

Betty reports that her lower back hurts when she cuts fabric at the kitchen table even after cutting for only a short amount of time. She also complains of a persistent ache in her shoulders and neck, especially after a long period of working at the sewing machine. Betty was hoping that the use of her recently purchased ergonomic chair would reduce or eliminate her persistent pains. Betty also sought medical attention for her neck, shoulder, and upper arm pain and a new complaint of tingling and numbness in her fingers. She was referred by her primary physician to occupational therapy for evaluation and treatment of her upper extremity discomforts.

Betty does not currently have any complaints of discomfort related to gardening or golf. Taking golf lessons will teach Betty proper technique and positioning and will help reduce her chances for injury or musculoskeletal discomfort.

POSTURES AND POSITIONING

Consideration of positioning and postures is important in leisure pursuits just as it is in the work environment. The difficulty with considering the ergonomics of postures and positions is the tremendous variability of the body mechanics needed for different activities and the forces generated, especially in sports and the environmental factors that affect positioning.

Quilting

In quilting, there are three basic positions that can be considered: sitting at a sewing machine, standing at a cutting table or ironing board, and sitting to quilt by hand. With each of these tasks, variables affect the postures. For example, the amount of arm excursion and trunk rotation during pressing is related to whether a person is pressing multiple small pieces of fabric to make a 12-inch quilt block or pressing the seams of a 90-inch by 70-inch quilt top. Kaergaard[46] and Chan,[9] in separate studies, reported that the musculoskeletal strain on the neck and shoulders of workers in the garment industry could be reduced by modifying the angle of the sewing machine and the needle on the machine. Several authors recommend that quilters tilt the sewing machine forward by approximately 15 degrees to put the shoulders and neck in a more neutral position and thereby allevi-

TABLE 17-1   Injury Rate Among Amateur Golfers

Injuries	Men	Women
Back	36%	12%
Shoulder	4%	25%
Elbow	8%	51%
Hand and wrist	32%	12%
Knee	8%	NR
Ankle	8%	NR
Other	6%	NR

Shamus E, Shamus, J: (2001). *Sports injury prevention and rehabilitation*, New York, 2001, MacGraw-Hill.
NR, Not reported.

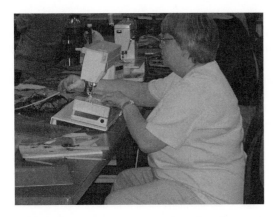

FIGURE **17-2** A wedge positioned under the sewing machine tilts the machine approximately 15 degrees and reduces neck and shoulder strain.

ate musculoskeletal discomfort in the shoulders and neck (Figure 17-2).[50,63,98]

Modifying the relationship between the worker and the surface that is used for cutting or ironing can alleviate back, shoulder, and neck discomforts. By raising the work surface or lowering the worker, the task can be brought into the easy reach area, and a more effective and efficient work area can be created. Tables can be raised using blocks of wood, risers used to raise the height of a bed (Figure 17-3, *A*), or homemade risers created using polyvinyl chloride (PVC) pipe (Figure 17-3, *B*). A person can also sit to position herself in the easy reach areas of the work area. In addition, cushioned floor padding has been found to reduce the strain on the legs, feet, and back during long periods of standing, as seen in the cutting or pressing stages during quilting. These same principles can be applied to other leisure activities such as woodworking, ceramics, painting, and other crafts.

Gardening

Gardeners use a wide range of postures and positions in the multiple and varied tasks involved in gardening. A gardener may be pruning a tree with an overhead reach or weeding a garden, requiring a lot of bending and grip strength. To decrease the amount of overhead reach, ladders and stepstools are available to raise a person closer to the working

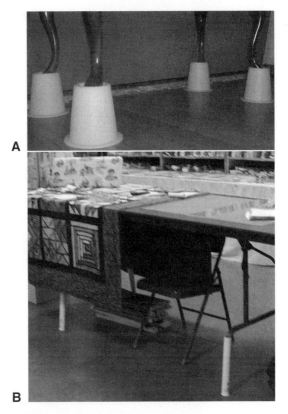

FIGURE **17-3 A,** Risers or elevators typically used for beds are used to increase the height of a table. **B,** Home-made table elevators or risers have been made of PVC pipe and used to increase the height of a folding table.

area, and long-handled cutting tools are available to permit access to higher branches (Figure 17-4).

To reduce the amount of bending, small stools are recommended so the gardener sits to dig in the dirt rather than bending or kneeling. Cushioned pads can be used for gardening tasks involving kneeling. When raking, hoeing, or sweeping, a common technique used is to lean forward from the hips and pull back using the back and arms. This technique can lead to aches in the shoulders, upper arms, and back. A better technique would be to place one leg forward of the other, then use a rocking motion to alternate weight on the front leg then the back leg, thereby using the stronger leg muscles more effectively to accomplish the task with less discomfort (Figure 17-5).

Golfing

Body positioning, posture, and body mechanics are especially important in athletics because body position can directly affect performance as measured by accuracy, speed, or distance and there-

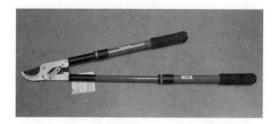

FIGURE **17-4** Bypass pruners used for cutting branches. On this model the grip is padded for comfort and the handles are adjustable. In this picture the lower handle has been extended.

fore affect the outcome of the athletic event. Poor body position or technique in athletics such as running, swimming, golf, baseball, and so on, can hinder performance, directly affect the outcome, and lead to injuries. In golf, during the set-up phase, the preferred position is to have 50% to 60% of the body weight on the back foot. The knees are flexed approximately 20 to 25 degrees, the trunk is flexed forward at the hips 40 to 50 degrees, and the back is straight in a neutral position (Figure 17-6). This position creates an axis of rotation at the hips. If the back is rounded there is less rotation from the hips and more rotation from the lower back, resulting in back injuries. This is the basic position for golf swings, whether a drive or a putt.[7,29,35,43,94] However, golfers adjust their body position, sometimes very subtly, relative to the ball to produce a particular angle and distance they want the ball to go.

In athletic activities, measures of accuracy, speed, or distance provide a rate of performance as well as an indication of winning or losing. To

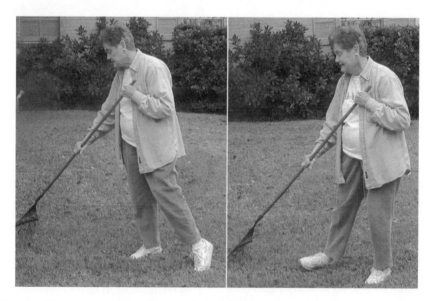

FIGURE **17-5** When raking, use a stance with one foot forward and the other foot back. Then rock back and forth from the front foot *(left image)* to the back foot *(right image)*. This technique uses the stronger leg muscles and reduces the strain on the back and shoulders. This technique can be used for similar tasks such as sweeping.

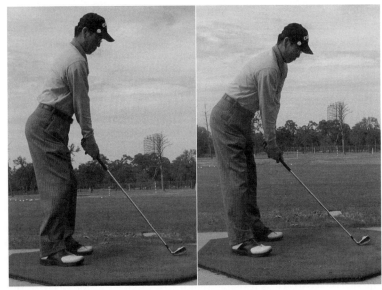

FIGURE **17-6 A,** The proper setup for the golf swing includes approximately 40 degrees of flexion at the hip and a straight back. **B,** Improper setup increases the rotation at the lower back and increases the risk of injury.   **A**   **B**

improve performance in their sport, athletes are more likely to take lessons or hire a professional to evaluate and train their skill and improve the outcome of their sport than other leisure participants. Conversely, people who engage in nonathletic leisure activity such as quilting, gardening, fishing, crafting, woodworking, and so on may not be aware of their posture during the activity, and the positions used are not critical to the outcome but do influence the comfort of the person and the effectiveness of the tasks. Poor or awkward positions in leisure activities may compound any musculoskeletal discomforts that occur from work, especially if the tasks for leisure and work are similar, such as quilting and computer work.

Although Betty has a dedicated quilting space (12-foot by 12-foot room), it is also used for other craft projects and storage as well as her computer. In addition, she also uses other space in the house such as the 29-inch–high kitchen table for cutting fabric and the living room floor for laying out large sections of the project she is working on.

Both of Betty's musculoskeletal complaints noted earlier (low back pain when cutting fabric at the kitchen table and persistent ache in her shoul-

ders and neck after a long period at the sewing machine) could be related to the postures she is using during her quilting tasks. Specifically, the 29-inch table is probably too low for cutting fabric, leading to the back pain. The typical position used at the sewing machine, especially when used for 2 to 4 hours, is likely contributing to the neck and shoulder discomfort Betty is experiencing.

A site evaluation of her sewing and craft room can identify ergonomic concerns in the setup of her space and work surfaces. Raising the height of the current cutting surface (kitchen table) or providing a cutting surface that is within her easy reach area will help alleviate the back pain she is experiencing. Identifying other awkward postures or positions can be accomplished through a site evaluation and clinical observations. Betty appears to have some knowledge and concerns about ergonomic factors as evidenced by the recent purchase of a sewing chair labeled "ergonomic." An additional concern is the amount of focused and uninterrupted time that Betty spends in quilting. She reports that she occasionally loses track of time when involved in a project. Education in frequent stretch breaks and time management strategies will help alleviate some of Betty's musculoskeletal complaints.

TOOL USE

Many leisure activities and sports require the use of specialized tools and equipment. As seen in the work environment, proper fitting and use of tools can make the difference between comfort and discomfort or injury in leisure pursuits.

Quilters and other crafters have available a wide range of tools that can make a particular task easier and more efficient. Examples of tools that have been modified in the quilting arena to improve comfort and skill in quilting include the invention of such things as the rotary cutter for cutting multiple pieces quickly and easily, spring-loaded scissors that open with a spring, making the use of scissors less resistive (Figure 17-7), and quilting gloves that are soft and breathable and have a slip-resistant grip on the palm used when machine quilting to control the quilt with increased ease. Examples of common quilting tools that have been modified to increase comfort and ease of use include thimbles modified to change the position of the hand during hand quilting, quilting hoops that have a swivel base to reduce poten-

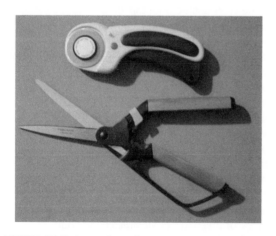

FIGURE 17-7 Examples of ergonomic cutting tools used in sewing and other crafts. *Top,* An ergonomic rotary cutter with an automatic closing safety feature. *Bottom,* Soft-handled scissors with a spring-loaded automatic opening feature.

tially awkward angles of the motion of the quilting stitch, and rotary cutters modified to increase the size of the blade and create an angle of the handle, thus creating an ergonomic rotary cutter. In quilting and craft, these types of objects are labeled "ergonomic," and many users find they improve comfort in the tasks they do.[50,63,98] These tools and others are well promoted, but there is limited, if any, research to determine their effectiveness and support the marketing claims.

Several authors offer guidelines for choosing and using hand tools, including those used for gardening.[8,74,93] They suggest that tools should be lightweight, have a nonslip handle, and fit the user's hand. They further suggest that cutting tools such as garden pruners and clippers be kept sharp and free of rust or corrosion.

It should be noted that the National Institute for Occupational Safety and Health (NIOSH) suggests that the use of the term "ergonomic" in defining tools can be misleading. Padding the grip and curving a handle is not enough to make a tool ergonomic. NIOSH recommends that for a tool to be ergonomic it needs to fit both the user and the task being performed without creating awkward postures, harmful contact pressures, or other safety and health risks.[8] In a study comparing gardening trowels labeled "ergonomic" with regular gardening trowels, Tebben and Thomas reported that the ergonomic gardening trowels did not differ from standard trowels in the extremes of wrist movements.[92] In addition, the participants in their study rated both types of trowels similarly for comfort and ease of use. They suggest that the correct gardening trowel addresses the effects of the tool not only on hand and wrist positioning, but also on the individual perceptions of comfort and ease of use (Figure 17-8).[92]

Equipment or tools used for any sport are most effective when fitted to the individual. Sport equipment companies and kinesiologists support the concept that equipment used in sports should be matched to the individual based on the human factors that affect that particular sport. In golf those factors are the person's height, arm length, hand size, and swing speed. In addition, Ellis indicates that the use and maintenance of well-fitting, high-quality, athletic protective equipment

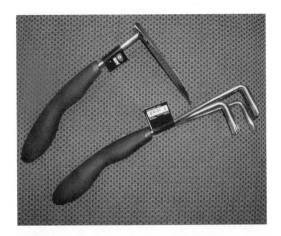

FIGURE **17-8** Samples of gardening tools identified as "ergonomic." These have large handles and are heavy, which may not be the best option for someone with smaller hands.

is one of the variables in the prevention of injury in sports.[22] Using the example of golf, golf shops and golf professionals can help an individual find equipment to match his or her anthropometric and skill characteristics. Shops that specialize in other sports can provide a similar service, such as finding the right running shoes or ski equipment, fitting a bicycle, or determining the right protective gear for team sports.[33]

During many leisure activities, especially crafts, sewing, quilting, and gardening, tools are an integral part of the participation. Betty has a pair of scissors dedicated to her sewing and quilting and she keeps them sharp. She uses an ergonomic rotary cutter with a cutting mat for cutting multiple pieces of cloth quickly. If Betty develops pain in her hands, the therapist should evaluate the current tools to determine if they are contributing to the pain.

Betty also gardens. She recently bought an ergonomic trowel but found that the handle was too large and it was too heavy for her to use comfortably. She now uses a smaller, lighter, plastic model that works well for her. Betty also uses gardening gloves with a nonslip coating on the palm. This helps her maintain her grip on the gardening tools, as well as protecting her hands

from thorns, prickles, and rough substances. Of further note, Betty gave the ergonomic trowel to her grown son, who also gardens. She reports that he finds the trowel quite comfortable.

EVALUATION

Information about the assessment or evaluation of the ergonomic concerns of persons engaged in leisure activities is limited. Assessment should include three components: physical performance measures, interview, and observation. Formal testing of physical performance, such as tests of strength and range of motion, may be useful but does not address the concerns of the person in the context of the activity. Furthermore, it is important to consider the person's participation in other daily activities and routines. A thorough interview that includes the client's daily routine and habits helps identify problem areas. Clinical observation of the person engaged in the leisure activity provides the best information for the individual. If possible, an on-site assessment using the principles from work-site assessments also provides valuable information about the factors leading to the injuries or discomforts experienced by the participant.

Betty works at a computer all day and then continues in a similar posture at her sewing machine at night. Each activity therefore contributes to the musculoskeletal problems in her neck and shoulders. This information can be obtained from a thorough interview to identify routines and habits. Betty may also be able to identify some of the factors that contribute to her discomforts but needs help in identifying the combinations of activities that contribute to her pain. Observing Betty in her leisure tasks provides valuable information regarding the ergonomic factors of her postures, the positions she uses for various tasks, and her skill and techniques with the tools.

What are of the some environmental factors contributing to Betty's musculoskeletal discomforts? What components of the quilting tasks could be compared with tasks in the work environment? Can the evaluations or assessments that are used in the work environment be applied to leisure tasks? What strategies or suggestions would you give to Betty to modify the environment or tasks to decrease her musculoskeletal discomforts?

CONCLUSION

Leisure activities are an important part of people's lives. People today have a myriad of crafts, sports, and leisure activities from which to choose. In addition, participation in leisure activities ranges from sedentary to very physically active, from casual engagement to intense involvement. The Ergonomic Society indicates that people involved in leisure activities have a very wide range of capabilities and limitations (including people with disabilities and the elderly); therefore, human variability is greatest in leisure activities. A further confounding variable is that leisure participants seldom train for the tasks in which they engage.[23] Based on these factors, the Ergonomics Society suggests that a key ingredient in ergonomics is the understanding of the participant.

Learning Exercises

Overview

This exercise applies the principles of ergonomics to a leisure activity or sport.

Purpose

The purpose of this exercise is to observe and analyze a person while he or she is engaged in a leisure activity. You will determine the factors in the environment in which the task is performed that may be enhancements or hindrances to engagement in the leisure activity. You will also determine any characteristics of the activity that could be altered using ergonomic principles.

Exercise

Find a person who regularly engages in a leisure activity (choosing a person doing a craft will be more straightforward). Collect anthropometric measures on the person. Measure the parameters of the workstations. Identify potential risk factors (hazards).

Participation in any activity that is done for prolonged periods of time, done with poor or awkward body mechanics, or with a competitive nature can contribute to musculoskeletal difficulties. Although there is limited information about the ergonomics of leisure activities, the principles of ergonomics for work situations can be applied to activities that are done for pleasure during uncommitted time. Considering and understanding the individual's engagement in leisure activities should be part of the evaluation and treatment of ergonomic concerns.

Multiple Choice Review Questions

1. Where on the body do seamstresses and quilters more frequently experience musculoskeletal discomfort?
   A. Hands, from manipulating the fabric
   B. Lower leg, from using the control foot of the sewing machine
   C. Shoulders, from leaning over the sewing machine
   D. Lower back, from sitting forward toward the machine

2. Men who are amateur golfers experience a high rate of injury at which body site?
   A. The lower back
   B. The shoulder
   C. The elbow
   D. The knee

3. The ideal angle of the hip when addressing the ball to begin the golf swing is:
   A. 20-degree hip flexion.
   B. 30-degree hip flexion.
   C. 40-degree hip flexion.
   D. 50-degree hip flexion.

4. To decrease musculoskeletal discomforts during sewing and similar tasks, adjust the angle of the sewing machine or work surface to:
   A. 5 degrees toward the worker.
   B. 15 degrees toward the worker.

C. 25 degrees toward the worker.

D. 35 degrees toward the worker.

5. Information about participation and success rate in sports comes from which field of study?
   A. Ergonomics
   B. Occupational therapy
   C. Sports medicine
   D. Kinesiology

6. According to available demographic information the most common quilting task is:
   A. hand quilting.
   B. machine quilting.
   C. hand piecing.
   D. machine piecing.

7. Which of the following is most likely to lead to back injury in golf?
   A. Rounding of the back during the setup phase
   B. Too much force used to "drive" or hit the ball
   C. Weakness of the shoulders causing excessive force on the back
   D. Missing the ball during the drive

8. To decrease the risk of musculoskeletal problems, the ideal tool should:
   A. have an ergonomic grip.
   B. fit the user.
   C. be lightweight.
   D. be adjustable for multiple use.

9. The evaluation of the person experiencing discomfort from leisure activities should include:
   A. electromyography tests for muscle performance in that particular leisure activity.
   B. thorough knowledge of the particular leisure task.
   C. observation of performance of the individual in the leisure activity.
   D. manual muscle and range-of-motion testing for physical performance.

10. Evaluation of individuals participating in leisure activities is difficult because of:
    A. greater human variability in leisure participants.
    B. therapists' limited knowledge of leisure activities.
    C. lack of formalized tests for leisure activity participation.
    D. limited ergonomic information related to leisure activities.

REFERENCES

1. Annet J: The learning of motor skills: sports science and ergonomics perspectives, *Ergonomics* 37(1):5, 1994.
2. Australian Bureau of Statistics: http://www.abs.gov.au/AUSSTATS/, Accessed 11/20/06.
3. Avery JG, Harper P, Ackroyd S: Do we pay too dearly for our sport and leisure activities? An investigation into fatalities as a result of sporting and leisure activities in England and Wales, 1982-1988, *Public Health* 104(6): 417, 1990.
4. Baxter MF: *Quilter's health and lifestyle survey,* Houston, Tex, 2005, Texas Woman's University:
5. Bernstein IA, Webber O, Woledge R: An ergonomic comparison of rowing machine designs: possible implications for safety, *Br J Sports Med* 36(2):108, 2002.
6. Breed RV, Young WB: The effect of a resistance training programme on the grab, track and swing starts in swimming, *J Sports Sci* 21(3):213, 2003.
7. Burdorf A, Van Der Steenhoven GA, Tromp-Klaren EG: A one-year prospective study on back pain among novice golfers, *Am J Sports Med* 24(5):659, 1996.
8. California Occupational Safety and Health Administration (Cal/OSHA), The National Institute for Occupational Safety and Health (NIOSH), C.f.D.C.a.P. (CDC): *Easy ergonomics: a guide to selecting non-powered hand tools,* California, 2004, California Department of Industrial Relations and NIOSH.
9. Chan J, Janowitz I, Lashuay N et al: Preventing musculoskeletal disorders in garment workers: preliminary results regarding ergonomics risk factors and proposed interventions among sewing machine operators in the San Francisco Bay Area, *Appl Occup Environ Hyg* 17(4):247, 2002.
10. Cherington M: Lightning injuries in sports: situations to avoid, *Sports Med* 31(4):301, 2001.

11. Cheuvront SN, Carter R, Deruisseau KC et al: Running performance differences between men and women: an update, *Sports Med* 35(12):1017, 2005.

12. Ciraulo DL, Smith P, Ciraulo SC: A trauma systems assessment of boating safety: a comparison of commercial and recreational boating practices, *Am Surg* 66(6):604, 2000.

13. Ciullo JV, Stevens GG: The prevention and treatment of injuries to the shoulder in swimming, *Sports Med* 7(3):182, 1989.

14. Clarys JP, Publie J, Zinzen E: Ergonomic analyses of downhill skiing, *J Sports Sci* 12(3):243, 1994.

15. Cronin J, McNair PJ, Marshall RN: The effects of bungy weight training on muscle function and functional performance, *J Sports Sci* 21(1):59, 2003.

16. Cross R, Bower R: Effects of swing-weight on swing speed and racket power, *J Sports Sci* 24(1):23, 2006.

17. Davies C: Musculoskeletal pain from repetitive strain in musicians: insights into an alternative approach, *Med Probl Performing Artists* 17(1):42, 2002.

18. *Demographics overview,* 2001, Golfserv. Retrieved from http://handicap.golf.com/corporate/media/demographics.asp, 8/26/06.

19. Dorevitch S, Babin A: Health hazards of ceramic artists, *Occup Med* 16(4):iii, 563, 2001.

20. Dortch S: *American demographics,* 1996, Advertising Age.

21. Driscoll TR, Mitchell RJ, Hendrie AL et al: Unintentional fatal injuries arising from unpaid work at home, *Inj Prev* 9(1):15, 2003.

22. Ellis TH: Sports protective equipment, *Prim Care* 18(4):889, 1991.

23. Ergonomic Society: *What is ergonomics?* Retrieved from http://www.ergonomics.org.uk/, 10/07/06.

24. European Commission: *Comparable time use statistics; national tables from 10 European countries,* Luxembourg, 2005, Office for Official Publications of the European Communities.

25. Fattorini L, Ferraresi A, Rodio A et al: Motor performance changes induced by muscle vibration, *Eur J Appl Physiol* 98(1):79, 2006.

26. Fletcher IM, Hartwell M: Effect of an 8-week combined weights and plyometrics training program on golf drive performance, *J Strength Cond Res* 18(1):59, 2004.

27. Flynn JM, Lou JE, Ganley TJ: Prevention of sports injuries in children, *Curr Opin Pediatr* 14(6):719, 2002.

28. Fradkin AJ, Cameron PA, Gabbe BJ: Golf injuries—common and potentially avoidable, *J Sci Med Sport* 8(2):63, 2005.

29. Fradkin AJ, Cameron PA, Gabbe BJ: Opportunities for prevention of golfing injuries, *Int J Inj Contr Saf Promot* 13(1):46, 2006.

30. Gillespie RM: The physical impact of computers and electronic game use on children and adolescents, a review of current literature, *Work* 18(3):249, 2002.

31. Giza E, Fuller C, Junge A et al: Mechanisms of foot and ankle injuries in soccer, *Am J Sports Med* 31(4): 550, 2003.

32. *Golf advisory,* 2003, Ernst & Young. Retrieved from http://www.ey.com/GLOBAL/content.nsf/Australia/Golf_Advisory-FAQ, 11/23/06.

33. Golfsmith International: *Custom club fitting,* 2006, Golfsmith International.

34. Gosheger G, Liem D, Ludwig K et al: Injuries and overuse syndromes in golf, *Am J Sports Med* 31(3):438, 2003.

35. Grimshaw PN, Burden AM: Case report: reduction of low back pain in a professional golfer, *Med Sci Sports Exerc* 32(10):1667, 2000.

36. Grimshaw P, Giles A, Tong R et al: Lower back and elbow injuries in golf, *Sports Med* 32(10):655, 2002.

37. Haapasalo H, Parkkari J, Kannus P et al: Knee injuries in leisure-time physical activities: a prospective one-year follow-up of a Finnish population cohort, *Int J Sports Med* 2006.

38. Haas JC, Meyers MC: Rock climbing injuries, *Sports Med* 20(3):199, 1995.

39. Hoffman JR, Cooper J, Wendell M et al: Comparison of Olympic vs. traditional power lifting training programs in football players, *J Strength Cond Res* 18(1):129, 2004.

40. Hollander DA, Aldave AJ: Ocular bungee cord injuries, *Curr Opin Ophthalmol* 13(3):167, 2002.

41. Holtzhausen LM, Noakes TD: Elbow, forearm, wrist, and hand injuries among sport rock climbers, *Clin J Sport Med* 6(3):196, 1996.

42. Hulstyn MJ, Fadale PD: Shoulder injuries in the athlete, *Clin Sports Med* 16(4):663, 1997.

43. Hume PA, Keogh J, Reid D: The role of biomechanics in maximising distance and accuracy of golf shots, *Sports Med* 35(5):429, 2005.

44. Jacobson JA, Miller BS, Morag Y: Golf and racquet sports injuries, *Semin Musculoskelet Radiol* 9(4):346, 2005.

45. Jung AP: The impact of resistance training on distance running performance, *Sports Med* 33(7):539, 2003.

46. Kaergaard A, Andersen JH: Musculoskeletal disorders of the neck and shoulders in female sewing machine operators: prevalence, incidence, and prognosis, *Occup Environ Med,* 57(8):528, 2000.

47. Kim PT, Jangra D, Ritchie AH et al: Mountain biking injuries requiring trauma center admission: a 10-year regional trauma system experience, *J Trauma* 60(2):312, 2006.

48. Lake MJ: Determining the protective function of sports footwear, *Ergonomics* 43(10):1610, 2000.

49. Lamirand M, Rainey D: Mental imagery, relaxation, and accuracy of basketball foul shooting, *Percept Mot Skills* 78(3 Pt 2):1229, 1994.

50. LeRoy C: *Pain-free quilting,* Appleton, Wis, 2002, Pain-Free Quilting.

51. Libkuman TM, Otani H, Steger N: Training in timing improves accuracy in golf, *J Gen Psychol* 129(1):77, 2002.

52. Listman DA: Paintball injuries in children: more than meets the eye, *Pediatrics* 113(1 Pt 1):e15, 2004.

53. Logan AJ, Mason G, Dias J et al: Can rock climbing lead to Dupuytren's disease? *Br J Sports Med* 39(9):639, 2005.

54. London Golf Show: *Facts and figures,* 2006. Retrieved from http://www.londongolfshow.com/facts and figures.cfm, 11/23/06.

55. Marmaras N, Zarboutis N: Ergonomic redesign of the electric guitar, *Appl Ergon* 28(1):59, 1997.

56. Martel GF, Harmer ML, Logan JM et al: Aquatic plyometric training increases vertical jump in female volleyball players, *Med Sci Sports Exerc* 37(10):1814, 2005.

57. Masters B: Sport as a health risk, *Educ Health* 21(3):43, 2003.

58. McCunney RJ, Russo PK, Doyle JR: Occupational illness in the arts, *Am Fam Physician* 36(5):145, 1987.

59. McDermott C, Quinlan JF, Kelly IP: Trampoline injuries in children, *J Bone Joint Surg Br* 88(6):796, 2006.

60. McGorry RW, Dempsey PG, Casey JS: The effect of force distribution and magnitude at the hand-tool interface on the accuracy of grip force estimates, *J Occup Rehabil* 14(4):255, 2004.

61. McHardy AJ, Pollard HP: Golf and upper limb injuries: a summary and review of the literature, *Chiropr Osteopath* 13:7, 2005.

62. McHardy A, Pollard H, Luo K: Golf injuries: a review of the literature, *Sports Med* 36(2):171, 2006.

63. Mech SD: *Rx for quilters; stitcher-friendly advice for every body,* Lafayette, 2000, C & T Publishers.

64. Mohamed OJ: *Testing and assessing the postural stresses associated with sedentary work,* Cincinnati, 1997, University of Cincinnati.

65. Moody-Jones WD, Jenkins IS: Water slides—are safety standards sliding? *Arch Emerg Med* 6(3):231, 1989.

66. Muller H, Sternad D: Decomposition of variability in the execution of goal-oriented tasks: three components of skill improvement, *J Exp Psychol Hum Percept Perform* 30(1):212, 2004.

67. National Gardening Association: *Garden market research,* 2006. Retrieved from http://www.gardenresearch.com/index.php?q = show&id = 2602, 08/24/06.

68. Norris RN: Applied ergonomics: adaptive equipment and instrument modification for musicians, *Md Med J* 42(3):271, 1993.

69. O'Connor BA, Carman J, Eckert K et al: Does using potting mix make you sick? Results from a *Legionella longbeachae* case-control study in South Australia, *Epidemiol Infect* 135(1):34, 2006.

70. Ohara H, Aoyama H, Itani T: Health hazard among cash register operators and the effect of improved working conditions, *J Hum Ergol* (Tokyo), 5(1):31, 1976.

71. Ostwald PF, Baron BC, Byl NM et al: Performing arts medicine, *West J Med* 160(1):48, 1994.

72. Parkkari J, Kannus P, Natri A et al: Active living and injury risk, *Int J Sports Med* 25(3):209, 2004.

73. Pelletier RL, Anderson G, Stark RM: Profile of sport/leisure injuries treated at emergency rooms of urban hospitals, *Can J Sport Sci* 16(2):99, 1991.

74. Pitt-Nairn EJ, Relf PD, McDaniel AR: Analysis of factors which can affect the preferences of older individuals for hand pruners, *Phys Occup Ther Geriatr* 10(4):77, 1992.

75. Pluim BM, Staal JB, Windler GE et al: Tennis injuries: occurrence, aetiology, and prevention, *Br J Sports Med* 40(5):415, 2006.

76. Powell KE, Heath GW, Kresnow MJ et al: Injury rates from walking, gardening, weightlifting, outdoor bicycling, and aerobics, *Med Sci Sports Exerc* 30(8):1246, 1998.

77. Promedia, Quilts Inc: *The national survey of quilting in America, 2003,* Golden, Colo, 2004, Promedia Consumer Media & Magazine Group.

78. Reilly T: Ergonomic aspects of sport and recreation, *Can J Appl Sport Sci* 6(1):1, 1981.

79. Renstrom P, Johnson RJ: Cross-country skiing injuries and biomechanics, *Sports Med* 8(6):346, 1989.

80. Rettig AC: Wrist and hand overuse syndromes, *Clin Sports Med* 20(3):591, 2001.

81. Ro JI: *Risk factors for musculoskeletal disorders among performing musicians,* Lowell, Mass, 2006, University of Massachusetts.

82. Rosenthal J, Forst L: Health hazards of photography, *Occup Med* 16(4):iv, 577, 2001.

83. Rowley I: Japan: cashing in on golf's comeback, *Business Week,* 2006.

84. Royal Canadian Golf Association: *Golf participation in Canada quick facts,* 1999. Retrieved from http://www.rcga.org/english/Membership/research-1999-summary.asp, 11/22/06.

85. Rozmaryn LM: Upper extremity disorders in performing artists, *Md Med J* 42(3):255, 1993.

86. Salmon J, Owen N, Bauman A et al: Leisure-time, occupational, and household physical activity among professional, skilled, and less-skilled workers and homemakers, *Prev Med* 30(3): 191, 2000.

87. Schibye B, Skov T, Ekner D et al: Musculoskeletal symptoms among sewing machine operators, *Scand J Work Environ Health* 21(6):427, 1995.

88. Shan G: Comparison of repetitive movements between ballet dancers and martial artists: risk assessment of muscle overuse injuries and prevention strategies, *Res Sports Med* 13(1):63, 2005.

89. Shan G, Westerhoff P: Full-body kinematic characteristics of the maximal instep soccer kick by male soccer players and parameters related to kick quality, *Sports Biomech* 4(1):59, 2005.

90. Statistics Canada: Ottowa, 2006. Retrieved from http://www.statcan.ca/, 11/20/06.

91. Taunton JE, Ryan MB, Clement DB et al: A retrospective case-control analysis of 2002 running injuries, *Br J Sports Med* 36(2):95, 2002.

92. Tebben AB, Thomas JJ: Trowels labeled ergonomic versus standard design: preferences and effects on wrist range of motion during a gardening occupation, *Am J Occup Ther* 58(3):317, 2004.

93. Tichauer ER, Gage H: Ergonomic principles basic to hand tool design, *Am Ind Hyg Assoc J* 38(11):622, 1977.

94. Vad VB, Bhat AL, Basrai D et al: Low back pain in professional golfers: the role of associated hip and low back range-of-motion deficits, *Am J Sports Med* 32(2):494, 2004.

95. Vanlandewijck Y, Theisen D, Daly D: Wheelchair propulsion biomechanics: implications for wheelchair sports, *Sports Med* 31(5):339, 2001.

96. Van Wieringen PC, Emmen HH, Bootsma RJ et al: The effect of video-feedback on the learning of the tennis service by intermediate players, *J Sports Sci* 7(2):153, 1989.

97. Wang Q: Baseball and softball injuries, *Curr Sports Med Rep* 5(3):115, 2006.

98. Watts C: *The hidden hazards of quilting,* Saskatoon, 1996, Physio-Diversity.

99. Wilk BR, Fisher KL, Rangelli D: The incidence of musculoskeletal injuries in an amateur triathlete racing club, *J Orthop Sports Phys Ther* 22(3):108, 1995.

100. Winspur I: Controversies surrounding "misuse," "overuse," and "repetition" in musicians, *Hand Clin* 19(2):325, 2003.

SUGGESTED RESOURCES

Quilting and Crafts Resources

Ergonomic sewing tools: www.ergonomicadvantage.com

Ergonomic tips for beaders: http://beadwork.about.com/od/tipstricksandtems/ss/Hand_Care.htm

Ergonomic tips for crafters: www.handhelpers.com/docs/crafttips.htm

Ergonomics for the craft professional: www.createforless.com/advice/biz_ergonomics.asp

European Quilt Association: http://eqa.homepage.dk

Quilts Inc.: www.quilts.com

Studio Safety: www.craftsreport.com/june00/studiosafety.html

U.S. Department of Labor Occupational Safety and Health Administration: www.osha.gov/SLTC/etools/sewing/index.html

Gardening Resources

Ergonomic Gardening Tips: www.indianahandcenter.com/erg_garden.html

Source for ergonomic garden tools: www.lifewithease.com/garden.html

Sports Resources

Canadian track and field: www.ergoweb.com/news/detail.cfm?id = 1142

Ergonomic Sports: www.ergonomics.org.uk/page.php?s = 15&p = 115

Motion analysis system for sports: www.sports-motion.com/aw2.htm

Working Well: www.working-well.org/sports_guideln.html

18

Evidence-Based Practice

Chetwyn Che Hin Chan, Connie Y.Y. Sung, Tatia M.C. Lee,
Cecilia W.P. Li-Tsang, Paul C.W. Lam

Learning Objectives

After reading this chapter and completing the exercises, the reader should be able to do the following:

1. Outline methods to access systematic reviews for establishing scientific evidence to guide the practice.
2. Describe relevance and relationships among evidence-based practice, clinical research, and practice guidelines.
3. Appreciate the importance of incorporating evidence-based practice in research and clinical practices.

Evidence-based practice. An approach to a profession informed by the review of evidence gathered in systematic ways. It uses research results, reasoning, and best practices to inform the improvement of whatever professional task is at hand.

Randomized control trial. A form of clinical trial or scientific procedure used in the testing of the efficacy of medicines or medical procedures. It is widely considered the most reliable form of scientific evidence because it is the best-known design for eliminating the variety of biases that regularly compromise the validity of medical research.

Work rehabilitation. Refers to rehabilitation services for providing a transition between acute care and return to work while addressing the issues of safety, physical tolerances, work behaviors, and functional abilities. It helps the client in regaining his or her earning capacity and employment in the open labor market.

CASE STUDY

James had worked as a welder in a ship construction factory for 15 years before his injury. His job required him to carry and lift equipment and metal materials weighing over 50 pounds. He was also required to assume a prolonged crouching position during his work.

James felt severe pain in the right forearm when he was transporting the equipment to and from two welding sites. He was admitted to the accident and emergency department in a nearby hospital and was diagnosed with tendonitis in the extensor tendons of the right forearm. Despite repeated rehabilitative interventions, the pain remained in his right elbow and at times radiated down to the right forearm and wrist. On assessment, James was able to perform household chores but was not ready to return to work. He was under the workers' compensation system, receiving partial salary and subsidy for medical and rehabilitation expenses.

Tendinitis in the forearm is a common type of injury at the workplace. It leads to disability among the workers, which is undesirable in the work force. More important, injury at the workplace results in billions of dollars spent on benefit payments, lost productivity, replacement workers, and increased workers' compensation premiums. There have been plenty of clinical studies supporting different return-to-work strategies and outcomes for workers who have back pain. If you were James' case therapist, it would be your responsibility to get a good grasp of the evidence at hand and provide the best intervention for enhancing his return-to-work process. But how can this be done? This chapter will lead you through the process of evidence-based practice.

Evidence-based practice (EBP) began in the early 1980s and has since been adopted by many health care professionals, including occupational and physical therapists and nurses.[5,14] EBP contributes significantly to improved clinical effectiveness, increased ability to provide clients access to information about services received, and increased success meeting administrators' target costs.[25,62,93] This chapter discusses methods for establishing scientific evidence in ergonomics, including work-related rehabilitation, and explains relationships among EBP, clinical research, and practice guidelines. It also discusses difficulties that clinicians and researchers encounter in pursuing EBP in work rehabilitation.

Evidence-based medicine (EBM) was introduced in the 1980s at McMaster University in Canada for training medical practitioners.[24,29,65] In contrast to conventional curriculums, EBM introduced practitioners to problem-based learning and less structured tutorial groups. The EBM program helped McMaster graduates develop self-directed learning skills that enabled them to attain high levels of clinical competence for years after their graduation. In comparison, the clinical competence of non-McMaster graduates tended to deteriorate progressively. The positive effect of self-directed learning among medical practitioners provided the impetus for the development of EBP. EBM is primarily associated with the practice of medicine, whereas EBP is used in many professional services.[24]

Evidence-based clinical practice (EBP) is an approach to decision making in which clinicians use the best evidence available, in consultation with the client, to decide on the option that suits that client best.[6,61,68,69] EBP incorporates not only the clinician's knowledge of scientific evidence and clinical judgment, but also the values and beliefs of the client.[11,18] EBP involves the use of the best available evidence, preferably generated scientifically, to guide decisions on clinical diagnosis, treatment, and intervention.[6,67] At the operational level, EBP circumscribes different systems of reviewing and integrating clinical evidence through organizations such as the Cochrane Collaboration[32,34,42,44] and the Journal Club.[15,60,62] Reviewed evidence is disseminated through CD-ROMs and the Internet.[36,39,74] The American Occupational Therapy Association (AOTA) also published the Evidence-Based Literature Review Project together with the practice guidelines and use of OTseeker.[7,55,80]

The process of EBP is complicated and multidimensional.[37,38,41,76] EBP begins with the identification of a problem and systematically reviews, analyzes, evaluates, and synthesizes existing published and unpublished evidence. According to Holm,[45] EBP should provide research on what each intervention consists of and how each is to be implemented for yielding the best outcomes for particular client populations. Results of the review are then used to determine the most efficient and cost-effective interventions. Various methods, such as critical reviews, database building, and instructional workshops, are used to disseminate the results to clinicians, researchers, managers, and clients.[21] Clinical experts use the reviewed evidence to develop practice guidelines. Different review groups update existing systems and establish new databases. Because results of EBP directly influence clinicians' decisions in practice, stringent and bias-free criteria are used to ensure the best-quality information is gathered and disseminated.[16,18]

Although discussion of EBP is abundant, information on EBP applied to ergonomics and work rehabilitation is scarce. Issues identified in rehabilitation-related literature include advantages versus disadvantages of EBM in the clinical practice,[46,54,83,92] methods of establishing evidence,[42,86] and integration of evidence into clinical practice.[18,29,47,79,84] Various questions are raised concerning whether EBP can be equally applied to ergonomics and work rehabilitation: What is the best evidence? Can the evidence be pooled? Is the evidence available? Can research evidence be realistically generalized to be incorporated in daily clinical practice?

DETERMINING THE CLINICAL QUESTION

The process of gathering evidence in EBP requires a well-defined question relevant to day-to-day clinical practice rather than to theoretic or philosophic propositions.[79,82] Compared with clinical research, EBP involves several factors, such as theoretic work, empiric findings, and clinical applications.[51] In contrast to a general question such as "What is the best intervention for clients with cumulative trauma disorder?" a typical EBP clinical question is "Is the combined mobilization and work hardening program increasing work endurance of workers with tennis elbow?" However, a question such as "Is Armstrong's dose-and-response model sufficient to explain the phenomenon of cumulative trauma disorders?" is too theoretic.

In James' case, the case therapist should identify the information needs—for example, whether there is any evidence to support a return-to-work program for people with work-related injuries. Then the therapist should formulate clinical questions based on the information needs. The clinical questions can be "Does the return-to-work program facilitate return to work for temporarily and permanently disabled workers?" or "Does the return-to-work program improve the return-to-work rate of workers with work-related injuries in the intermediate to long term?"

SOURCES OF INFORMATION AND EVIDENCE

After a clinical question is defined, the next step is to gather information and evidence relevant to the question. Assembling a group of practitioners and researchers is an efficient way to form a review group that can identify a number of sources for information before the search. In addition to being found in CD-ROMs, citation indices, and Internet searches, information can be requested from authors and relevant national and international agencies, foundations, associations, and content experts and can be found through bibliographic screening of all articles. The Cochrane Collaboration (www.cochrane.org/) has developed a system to coordinate activities and provide technical support for journal searches through a methods working group.[17,77] Examples of search strategies are available in the abstracts of review of the Cochrane Library at the Cochrane Collaboration Internet site. The site contains two search fields called "Cochrane Rehabilitation and Related Therapies" and "Occupational Health Field," which are the closest search field for rehabilitation disciplines at this time. No search field on ergonomic and work rehabilitation was available.

For James' case, the case therapist should conduct a literature search including a review of electronic specialist databases, journals, websites of preappraised research related to work-related injuries and workers' compensation, government websites, and various Internet sites such as Cochrane Library, PubMed, and OTseeker. In this case, the following "key words" can be used for

TABLE 18-1	Rating of Evidence
Category	Criteria from Which Evidence Is Derived
I	Systematic review of all relevant randomized controlled trials
II	At least one properly designed randomized controlled trial
III-1	Well-designed controlled trial without randomization
III-2	Well-designed cohort or case-control analytic studies
III-3	Multiple time series with or without the intervention; dramatic results in uncontrolled experiments
IV	Opinions of respected authorities, based on clinical experience, or reports of expert committees

From Wallace MC, Shorten A, Russell KG: Paving the way: stepping stones to evidence-based nursing, *Int J Nurs Pract* 3:147, 1997.

TABLE 18-2	Levels of Scientific Evidence, Based on the Quality and the Outcome of the Studies
Level	Characteristics
Level 1—Strong research-based evidence	Generally consistent findings in multiple high-quality randomized controlled trials (RCTs)
Level 2— Moderate research-based evidence	Generally consistent findings in one high-quality RCT plus one or more low-quality RCTs, or generally consistent findings in multiple low-quality RCTs
Level 3—Limited research-based evidence	One RCT (either high- or low-quality) or inconsistent or contradictory findings in multiple RCTs
Level 4—No research-based evidence	No RCTs

From rating system with levels of evidence proposed by Heymans MW, van Tulder MW, Esmail R et al: Back schools for nonspecific low back pain: a systematic review within the framework of the Cochrane Collaboration Back Review Group, *Spine* 30:2153, 2005; and van Tulder MW, Assendelft WJ, Koes BW et al: Method guidelines for systematic reviews in the Cochrane Collaboration Back Review Group for Spinal Disorders, *Spine* 22:2323, 1997.

searching: *return to work, work placement accommodation, modified work, light duties,* and *disability management.* Among all the articles listed, those related to the effectiveness of return-to-work interventions including the benefits of a return-to-work program and the barriers to implementing a successful return-to-work program should be chosen for reviews.

RANDOMIZED CLINICAL TRIALS

The quality of the evidence reviewed on a clinical question plays a significant role in EBP. Various organizations have established different criteria for evaluating to what extent the evidence established is free of bias.[27,63,86] The Quality of Evidence Ratings used by the National Health and Medical Research Council (NHMRC) classify evidence into four categories; category I indicates the best evidence and category IV indicates less reliable evidence (Table 18-1).[92] Category I identifies evidence completely generated by randomized controlled trials (RCTs), and category II includes evidence

based primarily but not exclusively on RCTs. Evidence obtained from stringent study designs such as controlled trials without randomization, cohort or case-control analytic design, and multibaseline and time series is identified as category III. Category IV includes evidence generated from descriptive studies, respected authorities, and clinical experience. Table 18-2 gives another example of rating the levels of evidence.[44,85]

The most commonly used method for evaluating the level of evidence is the Cochrane Collaboration system adopted by the Oxford Centre

```
                              ----------------------------------------
                              O₁e        X_I        O₂e     Experimental group (e)
                    R         ----------------------------------------
                              O₁p                   O₂p     Placebo group (p)
                              ----------------------------------------
```

```
                              ----------------------------------------
                              O₁e        X_I        O₂e     Experimental group
                    R         ----------------------------------------
                              O₁c        X_II       O₂c     Standard treatment group
                              ----------------------------------------
```

FIGURE **18-1** Typical randomized controlled trial. O_1, pretreatment observations; O_2, posttreatment observations; X_I, intervention used in experimental group; X_{II}, intervention used in comparison group; R, randomization.

for Evidence Based Medicine.[2,51] The American Academy of Neurology's system has been widely used by the American Congress of Rehabilitation Medicine's Clinical Practice Committee for evaluating clinical studies relevant to practice in rehabilitation. This system adopts a four-tiered rating for assessing the risk of biases; Class I indicates the lowest risk, and Class IV indicates the highest (Table 18-3).[27,51]

The NHMRC ratings identify evidence gathered from RCTs as the best, based on internal validity and reliability of the research design.[94] Another system, used by Raphael and Marbach,[63] also considers RCTs the best source of reliable data, primarily because of randomization. Clinical trials that are uncontrolled or nonrandomized have an intermediate strength of inference. Case series or case studies involving prospective follow-up of clients have the weakest strength of inference.

Why do RCTs produce the best evidence? The answer is random assignment and control for testing the efficacy of a therapy or treatment (Figure 18-1).[2] RCTs require participants to be assigned randomly to two or more intervention groups. Randomization can eliminate potential biases attributable to differences (e.g., age, gender, ethnic backgrounds, severity of disability, and prior clinical interventions) that create nonequivalent baselines between the experiment and control groups. Randomization helps achieve a condition of equivalence for intervention and control groups.[66,73]

The control in an RCT can be a placebo or a standard treatment group (see Figure 18-1). A controlled placebo group helps ensure that performance is solely caused by the intervention provided. Problems with natural changes in clients (maturation effect) or other environmental factors (history effect) (O2e – O2p = effect due to XI; where O2e and O2p are posttreatment observations of experimental and placebo groups, respectively) can be eliminated. In contrast, treatment comparison groups are less desirable because net gain in the experimental group can be caused by differences in the strength of interventions (O2e – O2c = effect due to XI – XII; where O2e and O2c are posttreatment observations of experimental and standard treatment groups, respectively). Effects of the experimental intervention XI therefore cannot be interpreted directly. The clinical trials most able to provide strong data are, in descending order, randomized placebo-controlled, randomized comparison-controlled, nonrandomized placebo, nonrandomized comparison, and uncontrolled single-group trials.

Results obtained by clinical trials are also evaluated for methodologic quality. EBP differentiates results generated by studies with higher internal validity from those produced from studies with lower standards. An excellent example is the review study conducted by van Tulder and co-workers[86] in which a maximum of 100 points were assigned to trials according to a set of criteria on study population, interventions, effect, and data

TABLE 18-3 American Academy of Neurology Criteria for Grading Diagnostic and Therapeutic Studies

Class	Rating of Prognostic Article	Rating of Therapeutic Article
I	Evidence provided by a prospective study of a broad spectrum of persons who may be at risk for developing the outcome (e.g., target disease, work status). The study measures the predictive ability using an independent gold standard for case definition. The predictor is measured in an evaluation that is masked to clinical presentation, and the outcome is measured in an evaluation that is masked to the presence of the predictor. All patients have the predictor and outcome variables measured.	Prospective, randomized, controlled clinical trial with masked outcome assessment, in a representative population. The following are required: a. Primary outcome(s) are clearly defined. b. Exclusion and inclusion criteria are clearly defined. c. There is adequate accounting for dropouts and cross-overs, with numbers sufficiently low to have minimal potential for bias. d. Relevant baseline characteristics are presented and substantially equivalent among treatment groups, or there is appropriate statistical adjustment for differences.
II	Evidence provided by a prospective study of a narrow spectrum of persons at risk for having the condition, or by a retrospective study of a broad spectrum of persons with the condition compared with a broad spectrum of controls. The study measures the prognostic accuracy of the risk factor using an acceptable independent gold standard for case definition measured in an evaluation that is masked to the outcome.	Prospective matched group cohort study in a representative population with masked outcome assessment that meets a-d above or a randomized controlled study in a representative population that lacks one criterion of a-d.
III	Evidence provided by a retrospective study in which either the persons with the condition or the controls are of a narrow spectrum. The study measures the predictive ability using an acceptable independent gold standard for case definition. The outcome, if not objective, is determined by someone other than the person who measured the predictor.	All other controlled trials (including well-defined natural history controls or patients serving as own controls) in a representative population, where outcome is independently assessed or independently derived by objective outcome measurement.
IV	Any design in which the predictor is not applied in an independent evaluation or evidence provided by expert opinion or case series without controls.	Evidence from uncontrolled studies, case series, case reports, or expert opinion.

From Edlund W, Gronseth G, So Y et al: *American Academy of Neurology clinical practice guideline process manual,* St. Paul, Minn, 2004, American Academy of Neurology.

presentation and analysis. Studies were classified by high (≥50) or low (50) qualities. Other useful criteria can also be found in the writings of Alderson and colleagues,[2] Edlund and co-workers,[27] Raphael and Marbach,[63] Wallace and co-workers,[92] and West and colleagues.[94] For instance, clearly defined outcome measure and intervention, confidence intervals (CIs) or magnitude-of-effect sizes, use of statistical analysis methods, possible measurement biases and treatment contamination, and number of consistent studies can influence the quality of the data collected and hence the conclusion drawn from the studies.

A review of the literature in rehabilitation for low back pain and cumulative trauma disorders revealed that RCTs are not commonly used. Furthermore, the quality of results presented in the studies that were available ranged from moderately high to poor. In a review of studies on treatment of acute and chronic low back pain, only 34.6% of 150 articles that studied acute low back pain and 25% that studied chronic low back pain were graded as high-quality RCTs.[86] Another study, conducted by Gross and colleagues,[40] examining the effect of education on clients with mechanical neck disorders, reported that the two RCTs related to the topic were rated moderately strong in terms of methodologic quality. In a review of studies on the effectiveness of a physical conditioning program (work conditioning, work hardening, and functional restoration) for workers with back and neck pain,[71] the mean internal validity methodologic quality score was 4.7 out of 8 (58%, range between 3 and 8). The results of this review suggest variations in the quality of the studies conducted in this field. Verhagen and co-workers[90] examined the effect of ergonomic and physiotherapeutic interventions for upper extremity work-related disorders. They found that only three of 15 studies gained an overall quality score of 50% or above. None of these studies, however, was considered to be of high quality in terms of "having a concealed randomization procedure and a form of blinding." Similarly, the study conducted by Karjalainen and colleagues[52] on the effect of a multidisciplinary rehabilitation program for workers with neck and shoulder pain was regarded as low on its methodologic quality, as

only one of the two trials reported in the paper was randomized. Both of these trials involved lack of blinding of therapist and observers, and similarity of the baseline characteristics and co-interventions.

AMALGAMATION OF RESULTS

After the review and evaluation of methodologic quality, evidence is compared. This process involves pooling results of studies with similar characteristics, such as methodologic quality, demographics, diagnoses, and treatment interventions. The purpose of amalgamation is to increase the strength of the inference by increasing the total sample size and the number of observations contributed from individual studies, enabling conclusions drawn from reviews to be more objective and powerful compared with those based on single studies.

Different methods can be used to amalgamate results of various studies, ranging from simple frequency counts of studies for positive or negative effects to sophisticated metaanalytic procedures that consider mean differences, effect sizes (ESs), and sample sizes. The selection of a particular method is determined by the methodologic quality of studies reviewed and whether placebo groups and similar measures were used in the studies.

Metaanalysis is a statistical procedure that combines the ES of different studies. ES is a scale-free index of effect magnitude, or the mean difference between experimental and control groups divided by the group's standard deviation.[35] ESs are estimated for each study in terms of either a d or g index.[35,43] The g index is a biased ES estimate that overestimates the population ES when sample size is small (Figure 18-2). The d index is an unbiased ES estimate derived for studies with small sample sizes. The mathematic expression of ES indicates that studies with a placebo group design obtain the most information on the effects of the clinical intervention under investigation because the difference between experimental interventions (Me) and control interventions (Mc) yields the treatment effect. This conclusion is substantially weakened if a comparison group is used.

$$g = \frac{(M_e - M_c)}{S_p}$$ where

Me = Posttest mean score of experimental group

Mc = Posttest mean score of control group

Sp = Pooled standard deviation

$$d = g\{1 - [3/(4N - 9)]\}$$ where

N = Ne + Nc

Ne = sample size of experimental group

Nc = sample size of control group

FIGURE **18-2** Mathematical expression of indices g and d. The g index is a biased ES estimate that overestimates the population ES when sample size is small. The d index is an unbiased ES estimate derived for studies with small sample sizes.

Pooling results becomes even less meaningful if the interventions used in control groups differ among studies. The estimated ESs are pooled by weighted integration methods that consider the sample size of each study. A mean ES and its 95% CI are calculated. Positive effect of a particular intervention is indicated if the 95% CI of the ES is not 0. An overlap of the 95% CI of mean ES and 0 indicates that clinical intervention has no effect. Validity of the pooled ESs is tested by homogeneity statistics, which determine whether all ESs belong to the same population.[43]

An example of a descriptive method that integrates the results of review is found in the study conducted by van Tulder and colleagues.[86] Of 81 RCTs relevant to treatment for chronic low back pain clients, 10 studies employed back schools as the clinical intervention. For the two studies that were regarded as having high methodologic quality, the effectiveness of back schools was positive in both studies when compared with no actual treatment. In the other four studies with low quality, three reported positive and one reported negative results. The conclusion of van Tulder and co-workers was as follows: "There is strong evidence (level 1) that an intensive back school program in an occupational setting is more effective than no actual treatment for chronic low back pain. There is limited evidence (level 3) that a back school is more effective than other conservative types of treatment for chronic low back pain" (p. 2135).[86]

Another example of a descriptive method that integrates the results of review is by Verhagen and colleagues.[90] Of the 15 RCTs relevant to ergonomic and physiotherapeutic interventions for upper extremity work-related disorders, three studies employed ergonomic intervention; two high-quality studies were on evaluating the efficacy of six different keyboards in reducing complaints made from the workers. One study reported significant positive results in reducing workers' pain in 12 weeks after use of a particular type of keyboard, but another study did not reveal significant treatment effects across different type of keyboards. The conclusion reached by Verhagen and co-workers was that there is "limited evidence of the efficacy of some keyboards in people with a carpal tunnel syndrome compared with other keyboards."[90] Review of the EBP materials in the field of ergonomics and work rehabilitation emphasizes the field's underdevelopment.

In James' case, throughout the literature review and critique process the case therapist started to think about some critical issues. First, is the evidence valid? This is determined by whether the methodology adopted, sampling strategy, subject selection, means of eliminating biases and confounding factors, and methods used for data analysis are appropriate. Second, is the evidence important? This is determined by whether the study outcomes have clinical significance and large effect. Third, is the evidence good enough? This is determined by the size of the effect, the level of confidence of the observed effect, and the number of studies confirming the result.

RESULTS INTEGRATION AND DISSEMINATION

EBP is highly dependent on the dissemination of evidence to clinical communities. In the past the flow of information relied heavily on professional journals, conferences (e.g., the International Conference on Evidence-Based Practice[21]), symposiums, seminars, workshops, professional meetings, electronic bulletin boards, and continuing education.[91] To further enhance the dissemination of the results of evidence-based research, Cameron and colleagues[14] suggested the professional associations take up the responsibility for putting the evidence into practices for their members. In fact, therapists in some countries (e.g., Canada) have constructed websites that have served as the platform for information exchange for its users.[28]

The Cochrane Collaboration was founded in 1993 to help health care professionals "make well informed decisions about health care by preparing, maintaining and ensuring the accessibility of systematic reviews of the effects of health care interventions." It produces and disseminates systematic reviews of health care interventions and promotes the search for evidence in the form of clinical trials and other studies of interventions.[19] Core activities are carried out by the collaborative review groups. In 2006, approximately 50 groups covered most of the important areas of health care. These groups consisted of researchers, health care professionals,

consumers, and others who shared an interest in generating reliable, up-to-date evidence for clinical interventions. Globally, more than 13,000 consumers, clinicians, policymakers, and researchers are involved with the Cochrane Collaboration and have to date produced more than 2500 systematic reviews that can be used to inform knowledge-translation activities.[39] A full list of all review groups is available at the Cochrane Collaboration website (Table 18-4). Activities of the review groups are enhanced by the Cochrane Library, which includes Cochrane review groups (CRGs), Cochrane fields, Cochrane centers, and Cochrane methods groups (see details at www.cochrane.org/reviews/clibintro.htm), which were established to coordinate the interests and review activities of the groups by fostering international and interdisciplinary collaboration, organizing workshops, and initiating and participating in exploratory discussions and meetings.

The Cochrane fields most closely associated with work rehabilitation are the following (see Table 18-4 for websites):
- Back Review Group
- Bone, Joint and Muscle Trauma Group
- Injuries Group
- Musculoskeletal Group
- Occupational Health Field
- Rehabilitation and Related Therapies Field

Back Review Group

The Back Review Group has an international editorial board with members from the United States, the United Kingdom, the Netherlands, France, Canada, and Sweden.[50] The scope of the group is to cover RCTs and controlled clinical trials (CCTs) of primary and secondary prevention and treatment of neck pain, back pain, and other spinal disorders, excluding inflammatory diseases and fractures. Approximately 40 members actively engage in conducting systematic reviews of interventions for back and neck pain (around 43 reviews and protocols, 1751 RCT references). In-terventions reviewed and under review include transcutaneous electrical nerve stimulation (TENS), acupuncture-like TENS, spinal manipulation, client education, exercise therapy, back school, behavioral therapy, herbal medicine, superficial

TABLE 18-4 Cochrane Internet Sites, Centers, and Review Groups Relevant to Work Rehabilitation

Center	Web Address
The Cochrane Collaboration	www.cochrane.org
Cochrane Brochure	www.cochrane.org/resources/brochure.htm
Information Management System	www.cc-ims.net
ISI Web of Science	www.isiknowledge.com Cochrane reviews (new or substantively updated) published from Issue 1, 2005, now appear on the website for the ISI Web of Science
Update software	www.update-software.com/publications/cochrane/
Update abstract	www.update-software.com/ABSTRACTS/MainIndex.htm
Cochrane Centers	
Australian Cochrane Centre	www.cochrane.org.au
Canadian Cochrane Network and Centre	www.cochrane.uottawa.ca
Nordic (Denmark) Cochrane Centre	www.cochrane.dk
U.K. Cochrane Centre	www.cochrane.co.uk
U.S. Cochrane Center	www.cochrane.us
Cochrane Libraries	
The Cochrane Library	www.thecochranelibrary.com
Cochrane Library Gateway (National Electronic Library for Health)	www.nelh.nhs.uk/cochrane.asp
Cochrane Library Gateway (Australia)	www.nicsl.com.au/cochrane
Cochrane Library Gateway (New Zealand)	www.moh.govt.nz/cochranelibrary
Cochrane Library Gateway (Scotland)	www.nes.scot.nhs.uk
Cochrane Review Groups (CRGs)	
Cochrane Review Index	www.cochrane.org/reviews/en
Back Review Group	www.cochrane.iwh.on.ca Covers the areas of primary and secondary prevention and treatment of neck and back pain and other spinal disorders, excluding inflammatory diseases and fractures
Bone, Joint and Muscle Trauma Group	http://cmsig.tees.ac.uk Covers areas of fractures.

TABLE 18-4	**Cochrane Internet Sites, Centers, and Review Groups Relevant to Work Rehabilitation—cont'd**

Center	Web Address
Injuries Group	www.cochrane-injuries.lshtm.ac.uk (lindsey.shaw@manchester.ac.uk) Covers areas of traumatic injuries
Musculoskeletal Group	www.cochranemsk.org Covers areas of musculoskeletal conditions, including: gout, lupus erythematosus, osteoarthritis, osteoporosis, pediatric rheumatology, rheumatoid arthritis, soft tissue conditions, spondyloarthropathy, systemic sclerosis and vasculitis
Fields/Networks	
Occupational Health Field	www.cohf.fi
Rehabilitation and Related Therapies Field	www.fdg.unimaas.nl/epid/cochrane/field.htm Occupational therapy: www.otseeker.com Physical therapy: https://www.cebp.nl
Method Groups	
Applicability and Recommendations Methods Group	Email: hjs@buffalo.edu
Campbell and Cochrane Economics Methods Group	www.med.uea.ac.uk/research/research_econ/cochrane/cochrane_home.htm
Individual Patient Data Metaanalysis Methods Group	Email: lhr@ctu.mrc.ac.uk
Information Retrieval Methods Group	www.cochrane.org/docs/irmg.htm
Patient Reported Outcomes Methods Group	www.cochrane-hrqol-mg.org
Prospective Metaanalysis Methods Group	www.cochrane.org/docs/pma.htm
Qualitative Research Methods Group	www.joannabriggs.edu.au/cqrmg
Reporting Bias Methods Group	www.chalmersresearch.com/rbmg
Screening and Diagnostic Tests Methods Group	Email: gatsonis@stat.brown.edu
Statistical Methods Group	Email: doug.altman@cancer.org.uk

heat and cold, traction, multidisciplinary biopsychosocial rehabilitation, work conditioning, work hardening, functional restoration, worksite interventions, advices, and assistive devices.

Bone, Joint and Muscle Trauma Group

The Cochrane Bone, Joint and Muscle Trauma Group, formerly called the Musculoskeletal Injuries Group, provides work on the prevention, treatment, and rehabilitation of traumatic injury, especially orthopedic trauma.[75]

Injuries Group

The Injuries Group also has an international editorial board with members from the United States, the United Kingdom, Switzerland, Australia, and Italy.[56] The scope of the group is to prepare, maintain, and promote the accessibility of systematic reviews in the prevention, treatment, and rehabilitation of traumatic injury (e.g., occupational injuries). Approximately 12 members actively engage in conducting systematic reviews of interventions for traumatic injuries excluding orthopedic trauma and burn wounds (approximately 68 reviews).

Musculoskeletal Group

The Cochrane Musculoskeletal Group (CMSG) editorial base is located at the Institute for Population Health of the University of Ottawa, Canada, and supported by the Canadian Cochrane Centre.[49] The group has 20 members who are health care professionals, researchers, and consumers from around the world. Reviews produced by the CMSG cover many areas of musculoskeletal conditions, such as gout, lupus, fibromyalgia, osteoarthritis, osteoporosis, rheumatoid arthritis, pediatric rheumatology, soft-tissue conditions, spondyloarthropathy, systemic sclerosis, and vasculitis. Interventions reviewed and under review include treatment of pain in the shoulder, elbow, wrist, hand, hip, knee, ankle, and so on, caused by, for instance, rotator cuff tendonitis, epicondylitis, extensor tenosynovitis and de Quervain's tenosynovitis, and flexor tenosynovitis.

Occupational Health Field

Cochrane Occupational Health Field (COHF) was established in 2003 by Verbeek and colleagues of the Department of Research and Development in Occupational Health Services of the Finnish Institute of Occupational Health in Finland.[31,89] COHF aims to gather evidence on the effectiveness of occupational health interventions and stimulate the completion of systematic reviews on these interventions. The scope of the occupational health field covers all interventions related to the prevention or treatment of occupational or work-related diseases, injuries, and disorders. There are approximately 40 reviews and protocols related to work rehabilitation. The role of COHF mainly is to maintain two databases of occupational interventions and systematic reviews; develop a search strategy for PubMed; organize hand searches of occupational health journals; communicate by email with those interested in the field; maintain a list of desirable systematic reviews; organize funding for systematic reviews; and develop methodologic support for occupational health reviews.

Rehabilitation and Related Therapies Field

The Rehabilitation and Related Therapies Field (PTRF) was established in 1996 by de Vet and de Bie of the Department of Epidemiology of the University of Maastricht in the Netherlands.[23] The PTRF hosted a number of specialties (Rehabilitation Medicine, Speech and Language Therapies, Occupational Therapies, Manual and Physical Therapies) and has collaborated with two new partners, the Knowledge Centre for Professions Allied to Health (NPI) and PeDro (the Physiotherapy Evidence Database). Until now, the field altogether has reviewed nearly 5600 articles related to rehabilitation and physical therapy, of which approximately 3700 address RCTs, 500 CCTs, 400 cross-over trials, 900 reviews, and 80 guidelines. All articles are available in the form of electronic copies that have been converted from the hard copies of the paper and CD-ROM versions for members of PTRF and Cochrane Collaboration reviewers, and PTRF issues newsletters that are available for all interested individuals. A large number of journals related to work rehabilitation are also surveyed for information, including the *British Journal of Occupational Therapy,* the *American Journal of Occupational Therapy, Physiotherapy Theory and Practice, Physiotherapy,* the *European Journal of Physical Medicine and Rehabilitation,* and the *Austrian Journal of Physical Medicine.* In 2003, apart from PeDro for the physical therapy area, OTseeker websites have been developed particularly for the occupational therapy area.[81]

To disseminate results of various review groups, the Cochrane Collaboration has established a formal channel called the *Cochrane Library* that assembles reviews in electronic formats. Several databases are included in the Cochrane Library (Table 18-5). Hayes and McGrath detail the purpose and format of each database.[42] The Cochrane Library can be accessed by subscription through Wiley InterScience (email: emrw@wiley.com or cs–cochrane@wiley.co.uk). Residents in the following countries can access the Cochrane Library for free through a national provision: Australia, Denmark, Finland, Ireland and the Island of Ireland, New Zealand, Norway, Scotland, Sweden, and Wales. Access is also possible through special schemes for the following: Higher Education & Further Education Institutions in the Caribbean, the United Kingdom, Latin America, and Low-Income Countries. The Cochrane Library is also available in CD-ROM and online versions, which are reviewed and updated quarterly.

In 2005 the Cochrane Collaboration introduced a new Information Management System (IMS) (www.cc-ims.net). The main purpose of the new IMS is to support more efficient preparation, maintenance, and publication of high-quality Cochrane reviews. The new IMS also integrated the software currently used by Review Groups (RevMan, ModMan) into one streamlined Internet-based system. Using a standard Internet browser, accurate and up-to-date resources such as contact details, protocols, reviews, studies, review group topic lists, and other information are easily accessible to all Cochrane entities (with the appropriate access rights). Additional advantages of the new IMS include the avoidance of duplication of data; centralized backup and archiving of reviews and other documents; a check-in/check-out system that ensures that authors, editors, and CRG staff are always working with the latest version of a RevMan file; the ability to track reviews during their preparation and maintenance; and the automation of some administrative and editorial tasks.

After critical appraisal of the evidence, James' case therapist was able to provide a synthesis of relevant information such as previous work and research on and discussion of the topic of a return-to-work program. The case therapist was able to find out the way to design and implement the return-to-work program and its benefits, including substantial reductions in disability and therefore a significant reduction in the number of lost workdays as well as workers' compensation costs. The therapist was also able to find the major barriers to the implementation of an effective return-to-work program: (1) lack of knowledge and understanding of the impact of the program and lack of social support in the workplace, (2) lack of possibilities for work task modification, (3) lack of involvement of workers and supervisors in the design and content, and (4) negative attitudes toward a return-to-work program. It is proposed that a successful return-to-work program should be characterized by employer-employee participation, a multidisciplinary approach, worksite-based rehabilitation, and necessary follow-up and monitoring.

The therapist started to think of other key issues. First, could the results or findings apply to James? Second, do the findings fit in with James' context? Third, are there resources available to implement the return-to-work program for James? With all these considerations, advice was sought from other disciplines for James' readiness to return to work, and a meeting was held with James and his family for a briefing about the arrangements for returning to work and to discuss the expectations of different parties. After that, James' case therapist conducted a job site visit and arranged a meeting with James' supervisor and co-workers on issues related to James' return to work and light job duties to develop an encour-

TABLE 18-5	Databases Associated with the Cochrane Library

Database	Function
Cochrane Database of Systematic Reviews (CDSR) (Total records: 4320)	Contains protocols and reviews prepared and maintained by Cochrane Review Groups. It is available via the Internet and on CD-ROM, which includes a feedback system to enable users to help improve the quality of Cochrane Reviews.
Database of Abstracts of Reviews of Effects (DARE) (Total records: 6019)	Contains critical assessments, structured abstracts, and bibliographic references of systematic reviews of the effects of healthcare intervention assembled and maintained by the Centre for Reviews and Dissemination in York, England.
Cochrane Central Register of Controlled Trials (CENTRAL) (Total records: 473442)	Contains bibliographic information on tens of thousands of controlled trials, including reports published in conference proceedings and many other sources not currently listed in other bibliographic databases.
Cochrane Database of Methodology Review (CDMR) (Total records: 22)	Contains two types of documents: Cochrane methods reviews and protocols in which methods reviews are full-text systematic reviews of methodological studies; and protocols that provide place-markers for reviews that are currently being written. (Methods Reviews are included in the browse lists for Cochrane Reviews.)
Cochrane Methodology Register (CMR) (Total records: 8255)	Contains bibliography of articles and books about methodologic issues relevant to summarizing evidence of the effects of health care.
Health Technology Assessment Database (HTA) (Total records: 5648)	Contains structured records describing health technology assessment projects.
NHS Economic Evaluation Database (NHS EED) (Total records: 17639)	Contains structured abstracts of articles describing the economic evaluation of health care interventions.
Software Review Manager (RevMan)	Used for preparing and maintaining reviews (www.cc-ims.net/RevMan).
Software Module Manager (ModMan)	Used by editorial team to assemble protocols and complete reviews (www.cc-ims.net/ModMan).

aging environment for welcoming James' return. Discussions on the return-to-work plan were also held with human resource personnel to assess the possibility of redeploying James to a new position or giving him other jobs that involved handling of lighter equipment and materials and less job responsibility. Finally, regular phone and job site visit follow-ups were conducted to monitor James' progress.

EVIDENCE-BASED PRACTICE, ERGONOMICS, AND WORK REHABILITATION

Review of existing systems indicates that EBP is still underdeveloped in the areas of ergonomics and work rehabilitation. The Back Review Group and Rehabilitation and Related Therapies Field are the two established groups closest to the subject of ergonomics and work rehabilitation. However, the abstracts published by these two groups do not seem to cover this aspect of rehabilitation. Research has already been conducted on barriers to evidence-based occupational therapy[8,59] and preferred strategies for disseminating research to occupational therapists in Australia.[8]

Lack of Theoretic Background

Well-established theoretic backgrounds supporting the effectiveness of different rehabilitation interventions, such as ergonomics, are scarce. According to Brandt and Pope,[10] little formal theory exists in rehabilitation to guide research and clinical decisions.[48,91] Schiller[70] also commented that the diffusion of research findings into practice is slow and that practice-based research was scarce. In addition, as cited by Law and Baum,[54] the practitioner may lack the skills, familiarity, and time necessary to search for and interpret the evidence, as well as to integrate the research knowledge into daily practice. Similar concern was also found in other studies investigating the perceptions of therapists in using research evidence for EBP.[13,26,30,33] The practice of clinicians is often based on experience (the lowest level of clinical evidence). Alsop[3] also commented that occupational therapy practice had primarily used opinion-based decisions that originated from values and resources rather than evidence to guide decision making and intervention planning processes. The majority of evidence is accumulated for studying causes of impairments rather than their consequences or resulting disabilities, and advances in ergonomics and work rehabilitation are over-studied causes of the problems. For example, the study of cumulative trauma disorders has been dominated by exploring the effects of repetitive tasks,[87,88] predicting the model of carpal tunnel syndrome,[58] and establishing relationships between trapezius load and incidence of musculoskeletal illness.[1] Other important areas of focus are the development of instruments for objective and accurate measurement and the establishment of the validity and consistency of functional capacity evaluations, such as the Baltimore Therapeutic Equipment (BTE) Work Simulator evaluation[9] and the available motions inventory.[57] The ErgoScience FCE System is also another example that has compre-

hensive reliability and validity research publication in a peer-reviewed journal. It can be used as an objective research-based, accurate assessment tool on rehabilitation and prevention of work-related injuries in order to minimize clinical guesswork (see details at www.ergoscience.com).

Outcomes of Ergonomic Interventions

Outcomes of ergonomic interventions are difficult to define, partly because they are multifaceted. Most studies emphasize the physical outcomes of different work health improvement programs, such as those that examine the incidence of trapezius myalgia[84] and those that involve statometric measurements obtained from inclinometer through subjective acceptability.[4] In contrast, data with higher ecologic validity, such as those regarding long-term health, work style, and quality of life, are rather uncommon.

Method of Investigation

RCTs are seldom used as the primary method of investigation. Instead, most studies use quasi-experimental designs with or without comparison groups. A good example is the study by Schuldt and colleagues that adopted single-group pretest and posttest design and used electromyelography as the outcome parameter.[72] Another example is from a study by Westgaard and Aaras[95] in which the effectiveness of ergonomic factors for improving the health of workers was studied through single-group pretest and posttest design. The difficulties of using RCTs to test the effectiveness of ergonomic interventions are largely due to labor law protection and objections from employers and labor unions. It is not ethical to randomly assign clients to a less-than-optimal treatment or no treatment when it is known (presumably based on clinical experience) that the treatment is the best option. Even if an ethical, well-designed trial could be developed, the human and financial resources that would be required to actually conduct an RCT with an adequate number of participants would be prohibitive.[18]

Technology

Technology is not transferred from research institutions to clinical practitioners, particularly in rehabilitation. According to Brandt and Pope,[10] some of the reasons for the failure of such information transfer are that clinical rehabilitation research lacks funds; little formal theory has emerged across the disciplines in rehabilitation; formal mechanisms for transferring knowledge are limited; and a market link that ties the products of research to the market economy, such as employers and workers' associations, is absent.

Conflict of Values

Even when they are familiar with the evidence, clinicians are less likely to follow practice guidelines that require new skills or skills that are inconsistent with their clinical experience, norms, and values.[12,13] A study conducted by Dubouloz and colleagues[26] on the perceptions of EBP by occupational therapists indicated that practitioners perceived EBP as a process of understanding and associating research and as a potential threat to their clinical reasoning and experience. Some researchers revealed that some practitioners might even perceive EBP as an attempt to subvert the knowledge and autonomy of individual clinicians.[20] Such perceived threats to professional competency and individual clinical judgment may result in therapists being less likely to engage in and use EBP.[26,30,48,64]

EBP in ergonomics and work rehabilitation should establish a theoretic framework for explaining the phenomenon of how tasks, the physical and psychologic environment, and the worker's capacity affect work performance. Instead of solely focusing on the impact of a particular factor, studies should strive to be multidimensional to facilitate better understanding of an ergonomic intervention's impact on long-term occupational health. More studies that use RCTs should be conducted to test the effectiveness of particular ergonomics and work interventions. The benefits of EBP to rehabilitation should be explained to clients, employers, and unions. More channels should be established to facilitate the transfer of knowledge, methodology, and results of clinical trials from researchers to clinicians. Both researchers and clinicians should be active in collaboration and sharing of knowledge.

EVIDENCE-BASED PRACTICE AND CLINICAL GUIDELINES

The development of clinical guidelines based on evidence is the goal of EBP. Systematic methods linking evidence to daily clinical practice are still in their infancy. Formulating clinical pathways using Clinical Pathway Constructor (CPC) computer software[36] demonstrates the potential of EBP. CPC computer software is equipped with a database that contains a large number of review abstracts on different clinical conditions and categories of care for acute medical and surgical conditions, such as total hip replacement and stroke. A typical clinical pathway is constructed as a computer grid consisting of standardized categories of care (e.g., diagnostic procedures and discharge planning) and a timeline (in terms of postadmission days or phases) in which the care should be carried out. Clinicians should review all available evidence and determine guidelines to be encoded in different clinical pathways. These pathways can be printed, disseminated to all team members, and used as guidelines for service provision. The guidelines can also be submitted to quality-assurance offices as targets for clinical audit. It is also suggested that continuing professional development, higher education, and work-based activities can help in the development of clinical guidelines[22] as well as identify ways to validate the experience and clinical reasoning skills of the practitioner with EBP information.[26]

In James' case, the development of clear guidelines for the return-to-work process outlining the roles and responsibilities of each key player may actually improve the implementation of the return-to-work program. Procedures developed may also create a more comprehensive guideline for injured workers and other stakeholders to follow.

Greengold and Weingarten's clinical pathway is inpatient acute care–oriented, however. Clinicians working in different settings and dealing with different clinical populations should be more innovative in designing their own systems using information (and evidence) resulting from the systematic reviews in EBP. More interinstitutional and multidisciplinary collaborations should also be developed to make this process an effective and efficient effort.

As rehabilitation education has advanced to postgraduate level, there is much room to integrate scientific basis and research findings into the originally clinical-based curriculum.[53] On one hand, this can further promote the concept of EBP in the training of student clinicians, and on other hand it can bridge the "theory versus practice" gap commonly found in entry-level programs.[78]

CONCLUSION

EBP is both an old and a new concept in health care. The preference for RCTs, detailed review and evaluation of literature, collation, and amalgamation of evidence is not new in scientific and critical inquiry circles. However, the quality of evidence reviewed, the comprehensiveness of methods used, and collaboration between researchers and clinicians has distinguished EBP by improving the quality of clinical decision-making, clinical practices, professional accountability, and client choice. Although EBP has not been widely developed to facilitate clinical practices in ergonomics and work rehabilitation, the benefits and potential for its development are well recognized.

Learning Exercise

Overview

This exercise applies the principle of EBP in daily practice. It is used to collect evidence from published research literature and from one's own practice to answer questions that arise in everyday practice.

Purpose

The purpose of this exercise is to understand and become familiar with the sequential steps in practicing EPB: (1) how to write answerable occupational therapy questions, (2) how to understand the ethics of research and practice collaboration with clients, (3) how to search for evidence on the Internet and in the library, and (4) how to summarize study information in an outline format.

Exercise

1. Write a clinical question related to the intervention for upper limb work-related musculoskeletal disorder.
2. Gather four or five current published articles via an Internet and library search that might answer the question.
3. Evaluate the gathered evidence to determine what is the "best" evidence for answering the question.
4. Interpret the evidence to determine a possible answer to the question.
5. Communicate with classmates or colleagues about the evidence as evaluation and intervention decisions are being made during therapy.
6. Use research procedure to document implementation of clinical decisions and to record assessments, progress, revisions, and outcomes.

Multiple Choice Review Questions

1. The concept of EBP is not based on which one of the following statements?
   A. Individuals are life-long learners.
   B. Professionals should choose the best interventions.
   C. Clients have the right to know what is best for them.
   D. Health services are operated as a business that imposes quality control.

2. Which of the following should be less likely to be involved in the clinical reasoning of EBP?
   A. Therapists' clinical experience and expertise
   B. Clients' preferences and goals
   C. Cost-effectiveness of the intervention
   D. High-quality evidence available (both quantitative and qualitative)

3. What is the relationship between EBP and RCTs?
   A. EBP considers all results other than those obtained from RCTs.
   B. EBP accepts the results obtained only from RCTs.
   C. EBP prefers to gather the results obtained from RCTs.
   D. EBP has no relationship to RCTs.

4. In a randomized controlled trial, which of the following types of biases can be reduced by randomization?
   A. Measurement bias
   B. Selection bias
   C. Intervention bias
   D. Bias in handling dropouts

5. Methodologic quality of studies reviewed in EBP cannot be assessed for the:
   A. presence of control or placebo groups.
   B. equivalence among different comparison groups.
   C. factors related to internal validity.
   D. differences in scores on the outcome measures before and after the intervention.

6. Which of the following methods is not relevant to the process of amalgamating the results in EBP?
   A. Determination of sample sizes
   B. Combination of ES
   C. Estimation of CI
   D. Computation of standardized differences

7. The conclusions of a metaanalysis may be rendered invalid if:
   A. the primary trials are statistically compatible with one another.
   B. the research participants differ significantly from one another.
   C. the selection of primary studies is complete and bias-free.
   D. the sample size of each primary study is different.

8. Which of the following is not a reason for the underdevelopment of EBP in work rehabilitation?
   A. Lack of well-defined outcome variables
   B. More emphasis on workers' impairment than on disability and handicap
   C. Lack of studies with high methodologic quality
   D. Weak technologic support from companies

9. Which of the following is less likely to enhance the evidence-based practice in work rehabilitation?
   A. Put more emphasis on the impact of a particular factor in affecting workers' work performance
   B. Conduct more RCTs to test the effectiveness of particular ergonomics and work interventions
   C. Establish more channels to facilitate transfer and sharing of knowledge among researchers and clinicians
   D. Construct a theoretic framework for explaining ergonomic phenomena and promoting occupational health

10. Throughout the development process of clinical guidelines based on evidence, which of the following should be avoided?
   A. Clinicians review available evidence and determine guidelines to be encoded in clinical pathways.
   B. Clinicians adopt a universal set of guidelines for different clinical conditions.
   C. Clinicians disseminate and use the guidelines for service provision.
   D. Clinicians submit the guidelines to quality-assurance offices for clinical audit.

REFERENCES

1. Aaras A: Relationship between trapezius load and the incidence of musculoskeletal illness in the neck and shoulder, *Int J Ind Ergon* 14:341, 1994.
2. Alderson P, Green S, Higgins JPT: *Cochrane reviewers' handbook 4.2.2,* Chichester, United Kingdom, 2004, John Wiley & Sons.
3. Alsop A: Evidence-based practice and continuing professional development, *Br J Occup Ther* 60:503, 1997.
4. Bendix T: Seated trunk posture at various seat inclinations, seat heights, and table heights, *Hum Factors* 26:695, 1984.
5. Bennett JW, Sackett DL, Haynes RB et al: A controlled trial of teaching critical appraisal of the clinical literature to medical students, *JAMA* 257:2451, 1987.
6. Bennett S, Bennett JW: The process of evidence-based practice in occupational therapy: informing clinical decisions, *Aust Occup Ther J* 47:171, 2000.
7. Bennett S, Hoffman T, McCluskey A et al: Introducing OTseeker (Occupational Therapy Systematic Evaluation of Evidence): a new evidence database for occupational therapists, *Am J Occup Ther* 57:635, 2003.
8. Bennett S, Tooth L, McKenna K et al: Perceptions of evidence based practice: a survey of occupational therapists, *Aust Occup Ther J* 50:13, 2003.
9. Bhambhani Y, Esmail S, Brintnell S: The Baltimore Therapeutic Equipment work simulator: biomechanical and physiological norms for three attachments in healthy men, *Am J Occup Ther* 48:19, 1994.
10. Brandt EN, Pope AM, editors: *Enabling America. Assessing the role of rehabilitation science and engineering,* Washington, DC, 1997, National Academies Press.
11. Brown M, Gordon WA: Empowerment in measurement: "muscle," "voice," and subjective quality of life as a gold standard, *Arch Phys Med Rehabil* 85:13, 2004.
12. Burgers JS, Grol RP, Zaat JO et al: Characteristics of effective clinical guidelines for general practice, *Br J Gen Pract* 53:15, 2003.
13. Cabana MD, Rand CS, Powe NR et al: Why don't physicians follow clinical practice guidelines? A framework for improvement, *JAMA* 282:1458, 1999.
14. Cameron KAV, Ballantyne KA, Margolis-Gal M et al: Utilization of evidence-based practice by registered occupational therapists, *Occup Ther Int* 12:123, 2005.
15. Carter AO, Griffin GH, Carter TP: A survey identified publication bias in the secondary literature, *J Clin Epidemiol* 59:241, 2006.
16. Cassell EJ: *Doctoring: the nature of primary care medicine,* New York, 1997, Oxford University Press.
17. Chalmers I: The prehistory of the UK Cochrane Centre. In Bosch FX, Molas R, editors: *Archie Cochrane: back to the front,* Barcelona, 2003, Thau.
18. Cicerone KD: Evidence-based practice and the limits of rational rehabilitation, *Arch Phys Med Rehabil* 86:1073, 2005.
19. Cochrane Collaboration: *Cochrane brochure,* 2006. Retrieved from www.cochrane.org/resources/brochure.htm 8/6/06.
20. Cohen AM, Stavri PZ, Hersh WR: A categorization and analysis of the criticisms of evidence-based medicine, *Int J Med Inform* 73:35, 2004.
21. Coster W: International conference on evidence-based practice: a collaborative effort of the American Occupational Therapy Association, the American Occupational Therapy Foundation, and the Agency for Healthcare Research and Quality, *Am J Occup Ther* 59:356, 2005.
22. Culshaw HMS: Evidence-based practice for sale? *Br J Occup Ther* 58:233, 1995.
23. de Vet R, de Bie R: *Rehabilitation and Related Therapies Field,* 2006. Retrieved from www.fdg.unimaas.nl/epid/cochrane/field.htm.
24. Deighan M, Boyd K: Defining evidence-based health care: a health-care learning strategy, *NT Res* 1(5): 332, 1996.
25. Dowie J: *The research practice gap and the role of decision analysis in closing it,* Paper presented at European Medicine Decision Making conference, Lille, Norway, October 1994.
26. Dubouloz CJ, Egan M, Vallerand J et al: Occupational therapists' perceptions of evidence-based practice, *Am J Occup Ther* 53:445, 1999.
27. Edlund W, Gronseth G, So Y et al: *American Academy of Neurology clinical practice guideline process manual,* St. Paul, Minn, 2004, American Academy of Neurology.
28. Egan M, Dubouloz CJ, Rappolt S et al: Enhancing research use through online action research, *Can J Occup Ther* 71:230, 2004.
29. Egan M, Dubouloz CJ, von Zweck C et al: The client-centred evidence-based practice of occupational therapy, *Can J Occup Ther* 65:136, 1998.
30. Ely JW, Osheroff JA, Ebell MH et al: Obstacles to answering doctors' questions about patient care with evidence: qualitative study, *BMJ* 324:710, 2002.

31. Finnish Institute of Occupational Health: *Cochrane occupational health field,* 2006. Retrieved from www.cohf.fi.

32. Furlan AD, van Tulder M, Cherkin D et al: Acupuncture and dry-needling for low back pain: an updated systematic review within the framework of the Cochrane collaboration, *Spine* 30:944, 2005.

33. Gervais IS, Poirier A, Van Iterson L et al: Attempting to use a Cochrane review: experience of three occupational therapists, *Am J Occup Ther* 56:110, 2002.

34. Glanville J: Evidence-based practice: the role of NHS centres for reviews and dissemination, *Health Libr Rev* 11:243, 1994.

35. Glass GV, McGaw B, Smith ML: *Meta-analysis in social research,* Newbury Park, Calif, 1981, Sage.

36. Greengold NL, Weingarten SR: Developing evidence-based practice guidelines and pathways: the experience at the local hospital level, *Jt Comm J Qual Improv* 22:391, 1996.

37. Greenhalgh T: Is my practice evidence-based? (editorial), *BMJ* 313:957, 1996.

38. Greenhalgh T, Macfarlane F: Towards a competency grid for evidence-based practice, *J Eval Clin Pract* 3:161, 1997.

39. Grimshaw JM, Santesso N, Cumpston M et al: Knowledge for knowledge translation: the role of the Cochrane Collaboration, *J Contin Educ Health Prof* 26:55, 2006.

40. Gross AR, Aker PD, Goldsmith CH et al: *Conservative management of mechanical neck disorders. Part IV: Patient education, Abstract of Cochrane reviews, The Cochrane Library.* Oxford, United Kingdom, 1998, Cochrane Collaboration.

41. Hausman AJ: Implications of evidence-based practice for community health, *Am J Community Psychol* 30:453, 2002.

42. Hayes R, McGrath J: Evidence-based practice: the Cochrane Collaboration, and occupational therapy, *Can J Occup Ther* 65:144, 1998.

43. Hedges LV, Olkin I: *Statistical methods for meta-analysis,* New York, 1985, Academic Press.

44. Heymans MW, van Tulder MW, Esmail R et al: Back schools for nonspecific low back pain: a systematic review within the framework of the Cochrane Collaboration Back Review Group, *Spine* 30:2153, 2005.

45. Holm MB: Our mandate for the new millennium: evidence-based practice (2000 Eleanor Clarke Slagle Lecture), *Am J Occup Ther* 54:575, 2000.

46. Horn SD, DeJong G, Ryser DK et al: Another look at observational studies in rehabilitation research: going beyond the holy grail of the randomized controlled trial, *Arch Phys Med Rehabil* 86:8, 2005.

47. Hunt J: Towards evidence based practice, *Nurs Manage* 4:14, 1997.

48. Illot I: Challenges and strategic solutions for a research emergent profession, *Am J Occup Ther* 58:347, 2004.

49. Institute for Population Health of the University of Ottawa: *The Cochrane Musculoskeletal Group,* 2006. Retrieved from www.cochranemsk.org.

50. Institute for Work and Health: *The Cochrane Collaboration Back Review Group for spinal disorders,* 2006. Retrieved from www.cochrane.iwh.on.ca.

51. Johnston M, Sherer M, Whyte J: Applying evidence standards to rehabilitation research, *Am J Phys Med Rehabil* 85:292, 2006.

52. Karjalainen K, Malmivaara A, van Tulder M et al: Multidisciplinary bio-psychosocial rehabilitation for neck and shoulder pain among working age adults: a systematic review within the framework of the Cochrane Collaboration Back Review Group, *Spine* 26:174, 2001.

53. Kielhofner G: Scholarship and practice: bridging the divide, *Am J Occup Ther* 59:231, 2005.

54. Law M, Baum C: Evidence-based occupational therapy, *Can J Occup Ther* 65:131, 1998.

55. Lieberman D, Scheer J: AOTA's evidence-based literature review project, *Am J Occup Ther* 56:344, 2002.

56. London School of Hygiene & Tropical Medicine: *Cochrane Injuries Group,* 2006. Retrieved from www.cochrane-injuries.lshtm.ac.uk.

57. Malzahn DE, Fernandez JE, Kattel BP: Design-oriented functional capacity evaluation: the available motions inventory—a review, *Disabil Rehabil* 18:382, 1996.

58. Matias AC, Salvendy G, Kuczek T: Predictive models of carpal tunnel syndrome causation among VDT operators, *Ergonomics* 41:213, 1998.

59. McCluskey A: Occupational therapists report a low level of knowledge, skill and involvement in evidence-based practice, *Aust Occup Ther J* 50:3, 2003.

60. McKibbon KA, Wilczynski NL, Haynes RB: What do evidence-based secondary journals tell us about the publication of clinically important articles in primary healthcare journals? *BMC Med* 2:33, 2004.

61. Muir Gray JA: *Evidence-based healthcare: how to make health policy and management decisions,* London, 1997, Churchill Livingstone.

62. Partridge C: Evidence-based medicine—implications for physiotherapy? *Physiother Res Int* 1:69, 1996.

63. Raphael K, Marbach J: Evidence-based care of musculoskeletal facial pain: implications for the clinical science of dentistry, *J Am Dent Assoc* 128:73, 1997.

64. Rappolt S: The role of professional expertise in evidence-based occupational therapy, *Am J Occup Ther* 57:589, 2003.

65. Rosenberg W, Donald A: Evidence-based medicine: an approach to clinical problem solving, *BMJ* 310:1122, 1995.

66. Rosner B: *Fundamentals of biostatistics,* ed 6, Belmont, Calif, 2005, Duxbury Thomson.

67. Sackett DL, Rosenberg WM: The need for evidence based medicine, *J R Soc Med* 88:620, 1995.

68. Sackett DL, Rosenberg WM, Gray J et al: Evidence-based medicine: what it is and what it isn't, *BMJ* 312:71, 1996.

69. Sackett DL, Straus SE, Richardson WS et al: *Evidence-based medicine: how to practice and teach EBM,* Edinburgh, 2000, Churchill Livingstone.

70. Schiller MR: Linking outcomes research, education, and practice, *J Rehabil Outcomes Measure* 2:1, 1998.

71. Schonstein E, Kenny DT, Keating J et al: Work conditioning, work hardening and functional restoration for workers with back and neck pain, Cochrane Database Syst Rev (CD001822), The Cochrane Library, Oxford, UK, 2003, The Cochrane Collaboration.

72. Schuldt K, Ekholm J, Harms-Ringdahl K et al: Effects of changes in sitting work posture on static neck and shoulder muscle activity, *Ergonomics* 29:1525, 1986.

73. Shadish WR, Cook TD, Campbell DT: *Experimental and quasi-experimental designs for generalized causal inference,* Boston, 2002, Houghton Mifflin.

74. Sharpe M, Gill D, Strain J et al: Psychosomatic medicine and evidence-based treatment, *J Psychosomatic Res* 41:101, 1996.

75. Shaw L: *Cochrane Bone, Joint and Muscle Trauma Group,* 2006. Retrieved from http://cmsig.tees.ac.uk.

76. Siddle A: Pain assessment and management relating to an indwelling catheter, *Br J Nurs* 12:475, 2003.

77. Silagy C, editor: Registering a field. In *Cochrane collaboration handbook. Vol. III. Representing the interests of fields,* Oxford, United Kingdom, 1995, Cochrane Collaboration [updated 14 July 1995].

78. Stern P: A holistic approach to teaching evidence-based practice, *Am J Occup Ther* 59:157, 2005.

79. Sudsawad P: Concepts in clinical scholarship—a conceptual framework to increase usability of outcome research for evidence-based practice, *Am J Occup Ther* 59:351, 2005.

80. Taylor MC: What is evidence-based practice? *Br J Occup Ther* 60:470, 1997.

81. Tooth L, Bennett S, McCluskey A et al: Appraising the quality of randomized controlled trials: inter-rater reliability for the OTseeker evidence database, *J Eval Clin Pract* 11:547, 2005.

82. Tse S, Blackwood K, Penman M: From rhetoric to reality: use of randomized controlled trials in evidence-based occupational therapy, *Aust Occup Ther J* 47:181, 2000.

83. Tunis SR, Stryer DB, Clancy CM: Practical clinical trials: increasing the value of clinical research for decision making in clinical and health policy, *JAMA* 290:1624, 2003.

84. Turner P, Whitfield TWA: Physiotherapists' use of evidence based practice: a cross-national study, *Physiother Res Int* 2:17, 1997.

85. van Tulder MW, Assendelft WJ, Koes BW et al: Method guidelines for systematic reviews in the Cochrane Collaboration Back Review Group for Spinal Disorders, *Spine* 22:2323, 1997.

86. van Tulder MW, Koes BW, Bouter LM: Conservative treatment of acute and chronic nonspecific low back pain. A systematic review of randomized controlled trials of the most common intervention, *Spine* 22:2128, 1997.

87. Veiersted KB, Westgaard RH: Development of trapezius myalgia among female workers performing light manual work, *Scand J Work Environ Health* 19:277, 1993.

88. Veiersted KB, Westgaard RH, Andersen P: Electromyographic evaluation of muscular work pattern as a predictor of trapezius myalgia, *Scand J Work Environ Health* 19:284, 1993.

89. Verbeek J, Husman K, van Dijk F et al: Building an evidence base for occupational health interventions, *Scand J Work Environ Health* 30:164, 2004.

90. Verhagen AP, Bierma-Zeinstra SM, Feleus A et al: Ergonomic and physiotherapeutic interventions for treating upper extremity work related disorders in adults, Cochrane Database Syst Rev (CD003471), Cochrane Library, Oxford, United Kingdom, 2004, Cochrane Collaboration. Available at www.mrw.interscience.wiley.com/cochrane/clsysrev/articles/CD003471/frame.html.

91. von Zweck C: The promotion of evidence-based occupational therapy in Canada, *Can J Occup Ther* 66:208, 1999.

92. Wallace MC, Shorten A, Russell KG: Paving the way: stepping stones to evidence-based nursing, *Int J Nurs Pract* 3:147, 1997.

93. Watson-Landry D, Mathews M: Economic evaluation of occupational therapy: where are we at? *Can J Occup Ther* 65:160, 1998.

94. West S, King V, Carey TS et al: *Systems to rate the strength of scientific evidence. AHRQ Evidence report/technology assessment: Number 47,* AHRQ Publication No. 02-E016, Rockville, Md, 2002, Agency for Healthcare Research and Quality.

95. Westgaard RH, Aaras A: The effect of improved workplace design on the development of work-related musculo-skeletal illnesses, *Appl Ergon* 16:91, 1985.

SUGGESTED READING

Bannigan K: Clinical effectiveness: systematic reviews and evidence-based practice in occupational therapy, *Br J Occup Ther* 60:479, 1997.

Brown GT, Rodger S: Research utilization models: frameworks for implementing evidence-based occupational therapy practice, *Occup Ther Int* 6:1, 1999.

Cusick A, McCluskey A: Becoming an evidence-based practitioner through professional development, *Aust Occup Ther J* 47:159, 2000.

Illot I, Taylor MC, Bolanos C: Evidence-based occupational therapy: it's time to take a global approach, *Br J Occup Ther* 69:38, 2006.

Tickle-Degnen L: Using research evidence in planning treatment for the individual client, *Can J Occup Ther* 65:152, 1998.

Websites

Cochrane Collaboration: www.cochrane.org

Evidence-Based Occupational Therapy: www.otevidence.info

McMaster Occupational Therapy EBP Reviews: www.fhs.mcmaster.ca/rehab/ebp

Occupational Therapy Critically Appraised Topics: www.otcats.com

OT seeker: www.otseeker.com

PubMed: www.ncbi.nlm.nih.gov/entrez

Resource Center for Evidence-Based Practice: www.aotf.org/html/evidence.shtml

19

Certifications and Professional Associations in Ergonomics

Jill J. Page

Learning Objectives

After reading this chapter and completing the exercises, the reader should be able to do the following:
1. Identify options for pursuing ergonomic certification.
2. Articulate benefits from attaining ergonomic certification.
3. List opportunities for advanced ergonomic training.

Certified Professional Ergonomist (CPE) or Certified Human Factors Professional (CHFP). Professional ergonomic designations from the Board of Certification in Professional Ergonomics.

Associate Ergonomics Professional (AEP) or Associate Human Factors Professional (AHFP). Professional ergonomic designations from the Oxford Research Institute.

Certified Ergonomics Assessment Specialist (CEAS). Ergonomic designations from the Back School of Atlanta.

CASE STUDY

Jo Williams, an occupational therapist (OT), decided to expand her private practice and wanted to determine if ergonomic consulting to industry would be a viable avenue. After some basic market research that included interviewing the employers of some of her former clients and contacting the local chapter of the National Safety Council, she determined that there was a need in her area. Ergonomics had long been an interest area for Jo, and she had attended occasional continuing education seminars that addressed ergonomics but had never really pursued additional formal training in the field. Once Jo established that there was a need, she began to investigate training and certification options. Jo conducted Internet searches, reviewed the current literature, and contacted the American Occupational Therapy Association (AOTA) about ergonomic training and certification.

After reading through the chapter, think about each of the following questions:

1. What are some key areas to address before deciding to start an ergonomics practice?
2. Where would a therapist look for information about advanced training and certification in ergonomics?
3. List some of the benefits derived from achieving certification in ergonomics.

A s more health care dollars are spent on prevention and wellness, there is increased demand for therapists to demonstrate competency in these areas. Many therapists pursue ergonomics certification as a way to gain increased standing and visibility, as well as adding significant knowledge and training to their therapist designation.[5]

There are primarily two bodies extensively recognized for their ergonomic certifications: the Board of Certification in Professional Ergonomics (BCPE) and Oxford Research Institute, Inc. (ORI). Other certifications have been developed by companies that have traditionally offered industrial rehabilitation education programming to therapists: the Back School of Atlanta and Roy Matheson and Associates. This chapter discusses the certifications that are available to therapists and provides resources for readers to gain additional information about educational opportunities that are available in this area.

BOARD OF CERTIFICATION IN PROFESSIONAL ERGONOMICS

The BCPE, created in July 1990, is an independent, nonprofit organization that functions as a certifying body for professionals in the area of ergonomics. Before the formation of the BCPE, the only avenues available for professionals practicing in the fields of ergonomics and human factors to demonstrate competency were through other professional designations or state licensure.[2]

The BCPE offers three levels of certification:

- The Certified Professional Ergonomist (CPE) or Certified Human Factors Professional (CHFP)
- Associate Ergonomics Professional (AEP) or Associate Human Factors Professional (AHFP)
- Certified Ergonomics Associate (CEA)

It is important to note that the BCPE offers both a professional and an associate designation. This designation differentiates between the career problem solver involved with system design and methodology and the interventionist who deals more directly with evaluations, tools, and commonly approaches used in systems currently operating.[2] The requirements for attaining the CPE and CHFP credentials are more stringent and represent dedication and contribution to the field, whereas the AEP and the AHFP are temporary titles that permit individuals who have met the educational components, but not the experiential pieces, to work toward the attainment of CPE or CHFP over the course of 6 years. After the need for an additional level of certification was identified, the CEA was created for individuals with a background in engineering, health care or rehabilitation, industrial hygiene, and psychology that would allow practitioners to demonstrate entry-level awareness, understanding, and expertise. Currently, 915 individuals hold CPE or CHFP certificates, 104 AEP or AHFP, and 67 CEA. Of those, 31 are OTs and 30 are physical therapists (PTs) as of the writing of this chapter.[2]

| TABLE 19-1 | Criteria for Certification by the Board of Certification in Professional Ergonomics |

Level of Certification	Requirements
CPE or CHFP	1. A master's degree in human factors or ergonomics or an equivalent educational background in the life sciences, engineering sciences, and behavioral sciences to comprise a professional level of ergonomic education 2. Three years of full-time professional practice in human factors or ergonomics 3. A passing score on the CPE or CHFP written examination
AEP	1. Meets the education requirement for CPE or CHFP certification (MS in human factors or ergonomics or related field) 2. A passing score on Part I ("Basic Knowledge" of human factors or ergonomics) of the CPE or CHFP examination 3. Currently working toward fulfilling the requirement of 3 years of full-time experience as a human factors or ergonomics professional
CEA	1. A bachelor's degree from an accredited university 2. At least 200 contact hours of ergonomics training 3. Two years of full-time practice in ergonomics 4. A passing score on the CEA written examination

From Board of Certification in Professional Ergonomics, Copyright © 2006, www.bcpe.org.

The criteria for the certifications are listed in Table 19-1. The application kit for each designation can be obtained directly from the BCPE for a $10 USD fee, BCPE, PO Box 2811, Bellingham, WA 98227-2811 USA. The BCPE can also be contacted by telephone at 888-856-4685, fax at 866-266-8003 or e-mail at bcpehq@bcpe.org, and additional information is available at the BCPE homepage, http://bcpe.org. On receipt of the completed application package, the review board will determine if the applicant may sit for a written examination. The examination fee is $290 USD, and the annual maintenance fee is $125 USD. The application must be received no later than 4 months before the date of the examination that the applicant wishes to take. Examinations are offered at various sites throughout the United States and Canada. The BCPE does not sponsor coursework toward completion of the certification requirements but does make recommendations about courses, workshops, and written materials on its website. A handbook for candidates is available for free download on the website and includes more specific information about scope of practice and a Self-Screening for Eligibility to help the applicant determine the certification for which he or she is best qualified. In July 2005, the BCPE began a Continuance of Certification (CoC) process that requires certified professionals to complete a worksheet every 5 years, detailing active practice, continuing education, publications, service, and meetings in order to maintain certification. If an applicant lives in the European Economic Space (EES), it is recommended that he or she contact the Center for Registration of European Ergonomists (CREE) for information.[2]

Jo took the self-survey screening tool that she was able to download for free from the BCPE website (www.bcpe.org) and ascertained that her current experience was below the requirements for their certifications.

OXFORD RESEARCH INSTITUTE, INC.

ORI was founded in 1977 as a nonprofit corporation and provides certification for ergonomists, accreditation to university ergonomics programs and select commercial ergonomics training programs; independent product testing and certification; and international ergonomic training. ORI also offers its certificate holders free limited technical support, ergonomic technical materials, job placement support, and discounts on ergonomic training. ORI offers three levels of certification[3]:

- Certified Human Factors Engineering Professional (CHFEP)
- Certified Industrial Ergonomist (CIE)
- Certified Associate Ergonomist (CAE)

The criteria for the certifications are listed in Table 19-2. In both application procedures, the mailing address is Ergonomics Certification Program, Oxford Research Institute, 10153 Vantage Point Court, New Market, MD 21774 USA, telephone 301-865-4506 or 301-524-3895. ORI embraces a multidisciplinary team approach to ergonomics and believes that "no single individual or discipline can solve all of the ergonomic problems," without a coherent, multidisciplinary team.[3]

BACK SCHOOL OF ATLANTA

The Back School of Atlanta has developed curricula designed by therapists specifically to educate health and safety professionals, including OTs, occupational therapy assistants (OTAs), PTs, and physical therapy assistants (PTAs), in the area of ergonomics and musculoskeletal disorders. They offer basic training toward certification as a Certified Ergonomics Assessment Specialist (CEAS) on completion of coursework, written examination, and submission of completed job analysis reports. Advanced training focuses more on evaluation tools and solutions and results in certification as a Certified Ergonomics Assessment Specialist II (CEASII). The training is offered as a live, 2-day workshop in locations across the United States, a home-study course, or an online training program. More information can be obtained from Back School of Atlanta, 1962 Northside Drive, Atlanta, GA, 30318-2631 USA, telephone 800-783-7536, fax 404-355-3907, www.backschoolofatlanta.com, e-mail info@backschoolofatlanta.com.[1]

TABLE 19-2	Criteria for Certification by the Oxford Research Institute

Level of Certification	Requirements
CIE or CHFEP	1. Provide two copies of a detailed resume of professional education, ergonomics training, and experience that document 5 or more years of experience plus Masters or 3 or more years experience plus a PhD in a related field of employment or as a provider of human factors engineering, engineering psychology, or ergonomic technical services. 2. Offer evidence of specialized training or formal education in fields directly or closely related to ergonomics or human factors engineering or both. 3. Submit duplicate copies of transcripts and at least two, but not more than three, work samples or technical contributions to one or more of the above fields that reflect the experience and competence of the applicant. Such samples of the applicant's submittals may include books, published journal articles, technical reports, inventions, patents, awards, honors, technical evaluations, demonstrations, ergonomic training programs, video tapes, or other media in which the applicant was a major or primary contributor. At least one of the work samples should be "quantitative" and demonstrate an ability to use quantitative statistical methods in the context of ergonomics.

TABLE 19-2	Criteria for Certification by the Oxford Research Institute—cont'd

Level of Certification	Requirements
	4. Submit two letters of recommendation (and names and telephone numbers) from two professional ergonomist sponsors of the applicant who are familiar with his or her work in the specialty field to which the applicant is applying. It is desirable that the sponsor be a certified industrial ergonomist, certified human factors engineering professional, or a full member of the Human Factors Society or APA division 21, or have an equivalent of 8 years of combined education and work experience in the field of ergonomics or human factors engineering.
	5. Submit with the application a one-time fee of $375 USD, which will be refunded to unsuccessful applicants minus a $25 USD processing fee.
	6. A written examination is also required. Furthermore, all applications will be evaluated by a blind review panel of one or two judges who are highly qualified, experienced, and certified in the field selected by the applicant. If there is a concern about the applicant's qualifications, an additional reviewer will vote. On certification of the applicant he or she will be notified and issued a Certification designating a specialty, along with a registration number, which will be valid for the year in which the applicant was certified. An annual renewal fee of $95 USD will continue the certification in subsequent years on an annual basis. There is an additional requirement of 2 CEUs every 24 months to demonstrate continued education and training in either human factors engineering or ergonomics.
CAE	1. CAE applicant must provide two copies of a detailed resume that documents professional education, training, and experience.
	2. CAE applicant should have at least 1 year of experience in ergonomics.
	3. CAE applicant must have at least a BS/BA degree in an ergonomic-related or health and safety-related field.
	4. CAE applicant must submit one letter of recommendation from a sponsor who has known the applicant for at least three years. This sponsor does not have to be a CIE or CHFEP but may be an employer, professor, or work supervisor.
	5. Offer evidence (college transcripts) of specialized training or formal education in a field directly or closely related with ergonomics or human factors engineering. This may include attendance at seminars, workshops, or various lectures.
	6. Submit copies of one work sample if available. The CAE does not require a work sample, but it is desirable.
	7. A written CAE examination is required with a passing score of 60. The examination is about 2.5 hours in duration and contains an essay and multiple choice, true-false, and matching questions.
	8. Submit with the application a processing fee of $375 USD to cover the cost of the review process.

ROY MATHESON AND ASSOCIATES

A long-time leader in industrial rehabilitation products and education, Roy Matheson and Associates (RMA) developed their ergonomic certification in 1993. The Certified Ergonomic Evaluation Specialist (CEES) training is provided by Dr. John LaCourse, PhD, CPE, CEES and Louise Lynch, PT, CWCE, CEES, and is taught as a live, 4-day training that involves lectures and small group analysis of job tasks. On completion of the training, the individual can apply for the certification. The candidate must also submit a completed application package and 25 completed ergonomic assessments for successful review before being awarded the certification. More information can be attained from Roy Matheson and Associates, P.O. Box 492, Keene, NH 03431 USA, telephone 800-443-7690, fax 603-358-0116, www.roymatheson.com.[4]

After reviewing other offerings, Jo decided to sign up for the self-study course from the Atlanta Back School, which would allow her to progress at her own speed and balance the demands of advancing her education while running a business and preserving her family responsibilities. She chose to start her ergonomic training here, with an eye to the future for attaining certification to better serve her community, customers, and herself. Based on the information that she has collected, Jo believes that the eventual accomplishment of ergonomic certification will allow her greater access to employers, improved ability to plan, design, and execute ergonomic change, more opportunities for speaking and writing, and better outcomes for the persons under her care.

CONCLUSION

Therapists are encouraged to investigate the need for certification and advanced ergonomic training as they expand this area of practice. Certification can be a way for therapists to differentiate their practice from the competition and to ensure that they are providing a high-quality, consistent service to their customers. Box 19-1 contains a list of professional association Web links, and Box 19-2 contains a listing of universities and colleges that offer ergonomics and human factors educational programs.

Box 19-1   *Professional Association Resources*

American Occupational Therapy Association—
   www.aota.org
American Physical Therapy Association—
   www.apta.org
International Ergonomics Association—
   www.iea.cc
National Safety Council—www.nsc.org
Human Factors and Ergonomics Society—
   www.hfes.org
IIEE Applied Ergonomics Community—
   www.appliedergo.org
Foundation for Professional Ergonomics—
   www.ergofoundation.org
Canadian Centre for Occupational Health and
   Safety—www.ccohs.ca
Ergonomics Society of the United Kingdom—
   www.ergonomics.org.uk
International Society for Occupational
   Ergonomics and Safety—www.isoes.info

Human Factors and Ergonomics Society of
   Australia—www.ergonomics.org.au
Ergonomics Society of South Africa—
   www.ergonomicssa.com
Finnish Ergonomics Society—
   www.ergonomiayhdistys.fi/english.html
Federation of European Ergonomic Societies—
   www.fees-network.org
American National Standards Institute—
   www.ansi.org
Occupational Safety and Health
   Administration—www.osha.gov
Centers for Disease Control and Prevention—
   www.cdc.gov
National Institute of Occupational Safety and
   Health—www.cdc.gov/niosh/homepage.html

| **Box 19-2** | *Ergonomic Educational Programs: Universities Offering Ergonomic Programs* |

Ergonomics and human factors are now being taught in universities across the globe. In the United States and elsewhere, an increasing number of universities are offering graduate and postgraduate degrees in ergonomics and human factors:

Aston University—www.aston.ac.uk
Birkbeck College—www.bbk.ac.uk
Cardiff University of Wales (formerly UWIST)—www.cardiff.ac.uk
Carnegie Mellon University—www.cmu.
Center for Ergonomics, University of Michigan—www.engin.umich.edu
Cornell University—www.cornell.edu
Cranfield University—www.cranfield.ac.uk
Georgia Tech—www.gatech.edu
Harvard School of Public Health—www.hsph.harvard.edu
London Metropolitan University—www.londonmet.ac.uk
Loughborough University—www.lboro.ac.uk
Louisiana State University—www.lsu.edu
Napier University—www.napier.ac.uk
North Carolina State University—www.ncsu.edu/
Ohio State University—www.osu.edu
Penn State—www.pse.edu
San Jose State University—www.sjsu.edu
State University of New York at Buffalo—www.buffalo.edu
Texas A&M University—www.tamu.edu
Texas Tech University—www.ttu.edu
Tufts University—www.tufts.edu

University College London—www.ucl.ac.uk
University of Aberdeen—www.abdn.ac.uk
University of Birmingham—www.bham.ac.uk
University of California, Berkeley—www.berkeley.edu
University of California—www..ucla.edu
University of Cape Town—www.bme.uct.ac.za
University of Central Florida—www.ucf.edu/
University of Cincinnati—www.uc.edu/bert
University of Hull—www.hull.ac.uk
University of Iowa—www.uiowa.edu
University of Louisville—www.louisville.edu/
University of Lulea—www.itu.se
University of Maryland—www.umd.edu
University of Miami, Ohio—www.miami.muohio.edu
University of Minnesota—www.umn.edu
University of Nebraska, Lincoln—www.unl.edu
University of Nottingham—www.nottingham.ac.uk
University of Pennsylvania—www.upenn.edu
University of Surrey Robens Institute—www.eihms.surrey.ac.uk/robens/erg
University of Texas, Austin—www.utexas.edu
University of Twente—www.utwente.nl/en/
University of Virginia—www.Virginia.edu
University of Wales—www.swan.ac.uk
University of Washington—www.washington.edu
University of Wisconsin—www.wisc.edu
Virginia Polytechnic Institute and State University—www.vt.edu
Wright State University—www.wright.edu

Learning Exercise

Overview

This exercise is designed to help you determine your current level of ergonomic educational exposure and opportunity for increasing your knowledge base.

Purpose

The purpose of the exercise is to critically evaluate your current knowledge in ergonomics and identify areas for improvement and means to accomplish this end.

Exercise

Perform the Self-Survey Screening (Box 19-3). Determine if you are presently eligible for pursuing ergonomic certification. If not, identify areas for development and avenues in which to pursue additional training.

Box 19-3   *Self-Survey Screening Tool*

As an aide to deciding where any particular individual may fit into the overall ergonomics arena, this "self-screening" score sheet is offered for completion and guidance. More specific information is available in BCPE's *Candidate Handbook: Certification Policies, Practices and Procedures.*

Instructions

1. Read over the major categories (lettered), associated detailed topics (numbered) in the score sheet, plus the EFM subtopics list for further clarification.
2. Place your score on the line by each topic in accordance with the Point Assignments.
3. Compute the subtotal for each category, and enter it in the space provided for each category.
4. Compute the grand total and enter it in the space provided.

Self-Test

A. Ergonomics Principles
   1. Ergonomics Approach
   2. Systems Theory
B. Human Characteristics
   1. Anatomy, Demographics, and Physiology
   2. Human Psychology
   3. Social and Organization Aspects
   4. Physical Environment
C. Work Analysis and Measurement
   1. Statistics and Experimental Design
   2. Computation and Information Technology
   3. Instrumentation
   4. Methods of Measurement and Investigation
   5. Work Analysis
D. People and Technology
   1. Technology
   2. Human Reliability
   3. Health, Safety, and Well-Being
   4. Training and Instruction
   5. Occupational Hygiene
   6. Workplace Design
   7. Information Design (includes HCI)
   8. Work Organization Design
E. Application (projects pursued by the individual during education and training)
F. Professional Issues and Supporting Courses
   1. Ethics and Regulation
   2. Business and Economics
   3. Physics
   4. Quantitative and Qualitative Design and Analysis
   5. Engineering
   6. Architecture

Point Assignments

0 = Never exposed to this topic
1 = Learned from self-study or "on the job" experience
2 = Learned from seminars, short-courses, and workshops
3 = Part of my undergraduate program
4 = Part of my graduate program in another field

Box 19-3	*Self-Survey Screening Tool—cont'd*

5 = Part of my graduate program in human
    factors or ergonomics

Score Sheet

A.   (10 pts) Subtotal _____
1. 5 pts _____
2. 5 pts _____
B.   (30 pts) Subtotal _____
1. 15 pts _____
2. 5 pts _____
3. 5 pts _____
4. 5 pts _____
C.   (25 pts) Subtotal _____
1. 5 pts _____
2. 5 pts _____
3. 5 pts _____
4. 5 pts _____
5. 5 pts _____

D.   (50 pts) Subtotal _____
1. 5 pts _____
2. 5 pts _____
3. 10 pts _____
4. 5 pts _____
5. 5 pts _____
6. 5 pts _____
7. 10 pts _____
8. 5 pts _____
E.   (5 pts) Subtotal _____
1. 5 pts _____
F.   (30 pts) Subtotal _____
1. 5 pts _____
2. 5 pts _____
3. 5 pts _____
4. 5 pts _____
5. 5 pts _____
6. 5 pts _____
GRAND TOTAL _____

From the Board of Certification in Professional Ergonomics. Copyright © 2006, www.bcpe.org.

Multiple Choice Review Questions

1. The requirements for the BCPE certification of CEA include:
   A. a master's degree in engineering.
   B. 5 years of exclusive ergonomic work.
   C. a bachelor's degree from an accredited university.
   D. membership in the National Safety Council.

2. Therapists often pursue ergonomic certification because:
   A. it looks impressive on their resume.
   B. they wish to provide a higher standard of care to their customers.
   C. they want to meet continuing education requirements for their state licensure.
   D. there are lots of other therapists certified in their geographic area.

3. ORI offers the following certifications:
   A. Certified Industrial Ergonomist (CIE)
   B. Certified Ergonomist (CE)
   C. Certified Diplomat in Human Factors (CDHF)
   D. Certified Associate in Ergonomic Design (CAED)

4. Roy Matheson and Associates teaches ergonomic certification coursework in the form of:
   A. online training.
   B. self-study manual.
   C. live 4-day course, followed by the submission of 25 completed cases.
   D. no course work, certification test only.

5. ORI offers, in addition to ergonomic certification:
   A. independent product testing.
   B. online certification.
   C. training in functional capacity evaluation.
   D. training in impairment ratings.

6. To qualify for ongoing certification with the BCPE, the individual must:
   A. accrue 40 ergonomic continuing education contact hours annually.
   B. submit 10 work samples biannually.
   C. attend annual business meeting.
   D. pay annual maintenance fee of $125 USD.

7. The BCPE offers the following certifications:
   A. Certified Professional Ergonomist (CPE) or Certified Human Factors Professional (CHFP)
   B. Advanced Ergonomic Assistant (AEA)
   C. Certified Ergonomic Design Professional (CEDP)
   D. Designated Ergonomic Evaluator (DEE)

8. The BCPE Self-Survey Tool assesses an individual's exposure to:
   A. length of time in practice.
   B. chemistry education.
   C. design or number of patents filed.
   D. physics.

9. ORI embraces a philosophy of:
   A. a single discipline is best suited for solving ergonomic problems.
   B. a coherent multidisciplinary team is best suited for solving ergonomic problems.
   C. a partnership between an ergonomic professional and assistant is the only way to solve ergonomic problems.
   D. ergonomic problems usually solve themselves.

10. The Back School of Atlanta offers the following certifications:
    A. Certified Occupational Assessment Specialist (COAS)
    B. Certified Ergonomics Assessment Specialist I and II (CEAS I and II)
    C. Ergonomic Evaluator, Levels 1 and 2 (EE 1 and 2)
    D. Advanced Ergonomic Professional (AEP)

REFERENCES

1. The Back School of Atlanta: *The Back School of Atlanta Web page*, 2006, www.backschoolofatlanta.com.
2. Board of Certification in Professional Ergonomics: *Board of Certification in Professional Ergonomics Web page*, 2006, http://bcpe.org.
3. Oxford Research Institute: (2006) *Oxford Research Institute Web page*, 2006, www.oxfordresearch.org.
4. Roy Matheson and Associates: *Roy Matheson and Associates Web page*, 2006, www.roymatheson.com.
5. Snodgrass J: Getting comfortable: developing a clinical specialty in ergonomics has its own challenges and rewards, *Rehab Manag* July:24, 2004.

20

Economics and Marketing of Ergonomic Services

Denise M. Miller, Karen Jacobs

Learning Objectives

After reading this chapter and completing the exercises, the reader should be able to do the following:

1. Identify concepts for marketing in a new economy.
2. Describe components involved in marketing approaches.
3. Discuss the application of the marketing approaches in a case study analysis.

Consumer behavior. The study of how individuals, groups, and organizations select, buy, use, and dispose of goods, services, ideas, or experiences to satisfy their needs and desires.[13]

Exchange potential. Represents a core concept in marketing wherein five conditions must be satisfied in the process of obtaining a desired product from someone by offering something in return.[13]

Demographics. Data related to the size and growth rate of populations in different cities, regions, and nations; age distribution and ethnic mix; educational levels; household patterns; and regional characteristics and movements.[13]

Advertising. A specific communication task to be accomplished with a specific audience in mind in a specific target market during a specific period of time. The advertisement goals are based on achieving one of four aims: to inform, to persuade, to remind, and to reinforce.[13]

Understanding and implementing effective marketing strategies plays an important role in the delivery of ergonomics. This chapter provides an overview of marketing concepts in the new economy and discusses marketing approaches with a focus on ergonomic consultation.

Ergonomics consultation in occupational and physical therapy is a response to rising health care and workers' compensation costs that provides methods for preventing injuries in the workplace. Development of new product or service industries initiated in response to the changing needs of the consumer is part of a marketing approach. Since the early 1980s, marketing has become more common in health care. Drucker, a prominent management consultant, once said "that the aim in marketing is to know and understand the consumer so well that the product or service fits the consumer and sells itself."[4] Marketing is so enveloped in the business that it cannot be considered a separate function. The application of marketing techniques is necessary to survive in a competitive marketplace, and all therapists should therefore have an understanding of marketing approaches. Therapists must learn how to use marketing, just as they learned how to use the skills and techniques of their professions. Because little, if any, exposure to marketing is provided in the academic curriculum of occupational and physical therapy, therapists are encouraged to acquire additional knowledge about marketing concepts by attending workshops, taking continuing education courses, or pursuing degrees in business. In general, therapists need to become more business savvy.

MARKETING IN THE NEW ECONOMY

Marketing in the new economy, the so-called *digital age*, has ushered in a variety of opportunities for reaching and connecting with potential consumers 24/7, and marketing in the twenty-first century is different from marketing in previous years because of advances in technology. The Internet has allowed consumers the ability to do the following[13]:

- Find a significant amount of information about practically anything online. Advanced search engines provide consumers with the ability to search online for any information about goods and services or to search newspaper clippings, articles, and consumer reports at the click of the computer mouse.
- Find a greater variety of available goods and services. Almost anything a consumer thinks about and searches for can be ordered over the Internet, such as clothes, appliances, ergonomic office equipment, and even medical advice.
- Compare information about products and services. Customers can provide feedback about their purchases of goods and services, enter chat rooms to engage in dialogue with other consumers about their common interests, or post comments on their own specifically designed Web pages in order to exchange information, ideas, and opinions about any good or service.
- Increase buying power. Consumers can compare competitor prices and product features and even name the price they are willing to pay for the goods and services.
- Place and receive orders with ease. Consumers can place orders from home or the office, use wireless hookups, and even a mobile phone 24 hours a day, 7 days a week.

The Internet affords businesses new and innovative capabilities to reach consumers globally, about any subject and at any time of the day. Ergonomic consultants can create their own websites to market information about their services and products, describe the history and philosophy of their company, and list testimonials from satisfied customers about the services and/or products received. Ergonomic consultants can also use the Internet to perform market research about a potential customer or to review information about competitors. The amount of material freely available on the Internet has created vast opportunities for businesses large and small to market themselves in the new economy. However, understanding and knowing how best to market an ergonomic consultation business involves many more strategies beyond the click of a mouse.

DEFINITION OF MARKETING

According to the American Marketing Association, the term *marketing* is defined as "the process of planning and executing the conception, price, promotion and distribution of ideas, goods and services to create exchanges that satisfy individual and organizational objectives" (p. 21).[1] Central to this definition is a focus on the consumer. In the business of ergonomic services and consulting, this can emerge as satisfaction for the employee, employee's manager, occupational health nurse, safety officer, physician, or the organization contracting for the ergonomic service.

Marketing is a misunderstood term. It is often used synonymously with public relations, selling, fundraising, strategic planning, or development. According to Kotler, "Marketing is the analysis, planning, implementation and control of carefully formulated programs designed to bring about voluntary exchanges of values with target markets for the purpose of achieving organizational objectives. It relies heavily on designing the organization's offering in terms of the target market's needs and desires, and on using effective pricing, communication, and distribution to inform, motivate and service the markets" (p. 5).[13]

Paramount in this definition are needs and desires. Something that is identified as lacking in the market (an individual or group of individuals) reflects a *need;* a *desire* is a want or personal preference. The market is researched and analyzed to determine whether it reflects an absence of a good or service (need) or whether it prefers something in a different shape, format, time, or location (desire). According to Kiernan and colleagues, "Once the need or want is established, the potential buyer must view the good or service being offered as satisfying a need or want better than any other available good or service. It is the packaging and support of a good or service that assure an ongoing relationship with the customer both for purposes of repurchase and for influencing initial purchases by other potential buyers" (p. 50).[12]

According to Kotler, exchange is the process of obtaining a desired product from someone by offering something in return.[13] This exchange is

---

the core concept of marketing, and five conditions must be satisfied for the exchange potential to exist (Box 20-1). This activity is designed to be a value-creating process that leaves both parties better off because the exchange took place.

Marketing should be considered a dynamic activity that includes the successful analysis of a need, the design of a good or service to meet the need, the uniting of that good or service with a potential user, and the use of a good or service by the customer. In an ideal situation, marketing begins before a product or service is even developed. This has not always been the case. In particular, many industrial rehabilitation programs (e.g., work hardening) that may have begun with selling perspectives are now faced with the risk of becoming obsolete because they were developed as services for which no need currently exists at their cost, present locations, or format.[8]

MARKETING APPROACH

Four components are involved in a marketing approach (Figure 20-1): (1) analyzing market opportunities, (2) researching and selecting target markets and market segments, (3) developing marketing strategies, and (4) executing and evaluating a marketing plan.

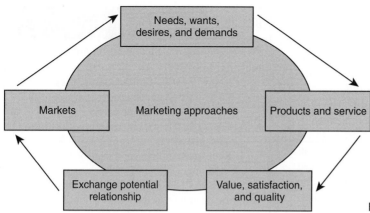

FIGURE **20-1** Core marketing concept.

Analyzing Market Opportunities

The first step in a marketing approach is the analysis of various elements of the marketplace. The market itself needs to be defined and may be selected simply on the basis of geography. The market includes all actual or potential buyers of a product, service, or idea. In the case of ergonomics consultation, example markets are businesses and industries, occupational health or rehabilitation nurses, insurance companies, safety officers, lawyers, workers with injuries, and other health professionals. Identifying attractive target markets includes analyzing the marketing opportunities, which necessitates a self-audit, consumer analysis, competition analysis, and environmental assessment.[11]

Self-Audit

A self-audit assesses *s*trengths and *w*eaknesses of, *o*pportunities for, and *t*hreats to the individual therapist, service, or business (SWOT analysis). Factors to assess include the following:

1. Reputation of the organization or therapist in the community.
2. Therapists' qualifications: What is the therapist's academic degree (e.g., BS, MS, OTD, DPT, EdD, PhD) or specialized training in ergonomics, human factors, or biomechanics? Are any of the therapists board-certified professional ergonomists (BCPE) or eligible for certification (see Chapter 19)?
3. Finances: Is advanced equipment available to perform work site analysis, or can it be

purchased if needed? Is the individual or company eligible to apply for grants or other means of funding (e.g., to develop "train the trainer" workshops at a designated work site)?

This self-audit assists in understanding how well or poorly prepared an individual or business is to meet the demands of the market. Ascertaining what an individual or business does well and maintaining that product or service at an optimal level is a critical aspect of marketing.

Consumer Analysis

Potential consumers must be identified for the provider to understand needs and desires for the product. Examples of consumers who might need or use ergonomic consultation are businesses and industries, occupational health or rehabilitation nurses, insurance companies, architects, attorneys, safety officers, workers with injuries, and health professionals. A potential consumer's behavior is influenced by cultural, social, personal, and psychologic factors (perceptions, beliefs, attitudes).[12] Many consumers play different roles in the decision process to implement a new program or service. It is important to analyze and understand how these factors can influence consumer's behaviors.

Competition Analysis

Identifying other providers of similar services can give an overview of the kinds of services being offered in particular locations. Analyzing these services reduces the potential for overlap and helps identify areas that are not being served. Opportunities for collaboration or joint ventures can be identified during a competition analysis. Knowing and understanding what the competition offers (e.g., location, hours of operation, services offered) further enhances an understanding of one's own strengths and weaknesses.

Environmental Assessment

An environmental assessment predicts the effect that demographics, political and regulatory systems, cultural and economic environments, psychographics, and technology may have on services. The following factors may have an impact on ergonomics.

Demographics

Because of economic necessity or preference, many older Americans continue to work after the traditional age of retirement. In the United States 35 million people have reached or passed the age of 65 years. This represents a 12% increase since 1990.[22] By 2034 this percentage is expected to increase to 18%, and by 2050 one fourth of the U.S. population will be over 65. To keep this working population active, occupational and physical therapists must become familiar with the aging process and learn to recognize the special needs of older workers (see Chapter 15). By becoming familiar with the physiologic effects of aging, therapists can develop intervention and prevention strategies that use ergonomics and thus assist in keeping this population actively engaged in the workforce.[3]

Political and Regulatory Agencies

The Occupational Safety and Health Administration (OSHA) published guidelines for the meatpacking industry that are still useful for developing an ergonomic program in most work sites today.[18] In addition, the Department of Labor released a document called "Ergonomics and the Americans with Disabilities Act (ADA)," which states that people with ergonomic disorders are covered by the ADA if the physical or mental impairment substantially limits their ability to perform essential functions of a job.[21] More than a decade ago, OSHA proposed an industry-wide ergonomics

standard called the "Ergonomics Protection Standard."[17] This standard, under review for many years, was finally approved in November 2000, only to be overturned by Congress in March 2001. The main objections to the now defunct rules were that federal law conflicted with state workers' compensation laws by specifically requiring predefined compensation, that the standards were too burdensome on small businesses, and that there was a lack of scientific support about musculoskeletal injuries related to work activities.

California, a state in crisis with mounting workers' compensation cases from 1997 to 2006, led the movement toward establishment of state guidelines by introducing ergonomic standards to protect workers from work-related repetitive strain injuries.[2] In the end, it does not seem to matter whether or not the federal standards were approved; it now appears that most states view work-related musculoskeletal disorders as one of the biggest health and safety problems facing the American worker. Therefore the need for qualified consultants to assist industry in compliance is an economic necessity in business and industry. Therapists interested in consulting in industry should develop an understanding of federal guidelines and be aware of any ergonomic standards within their own state of practice. Up-to-date information can be obtained from OSHA by phone (1-800-321-OSHA) and on the Internet (www. inquire@ergoweb.com).

Economic and Financial Factors

Thirty million Americans are presently dealing with a low back injury. Eighty percent of adults will experience low back pain sometime in their lives.[6] Low back pain accounts for millions of days of lost work and billions of dollars of lost productivity and workers' compensation claims. Clearly, injury prevention at the work site and health promotion are better alternatives to injury management.[9] The economic and financial benefits of injury prevention programs include decreased lost work time, increased safety and productivity, reduced errors, improved quality of service, and better employee relations.[20] As Hendrick stated in his 1996 presidential address at the Human Factors and Ergonomics Society (HFES) 40th Annual Meeting, "good ergonomics is good economics."[7]

Researching and Selecting Target Markets

After marketing opportunities have been analyzed, the needs of the market can be determined through research, which might include observation, surveys, or even experimentation. After research is completed, the market is divided into target markets (i.e., groups of consumers with similar needs, wants, or interests). The groups are further segmented into distinct groups of consumers who might require separate products and promotions. For example, industry can be segmented into types of businesses (e.g., service industries and manufacturing industries). Service industries can be further segmented into businesses within certain geographic areas and demographic groups (e.g., age, gender, or socioeconomic status). Targeting a market is the act of evaluating and selecting one or more markets to enter.

Developing Marketing Strategies

A marketing approach develops a marketing mix to meet the needs, desires, or interests of a well-defined target market. Marketing involves influencing the demand for a product or service. A marketing mix consists of the four Ps: product, place, price, and promotion.[16]

Product

The product is a marketing variable that needs to be designed for a specific target market. For example, for ergonomics consultation to a hospital, products can include work site analysis; audits for compliance with Titles II and III of the ADA; recommending intervention for workers with injury, such as splinting or redesigning a workstation; and implementing preventive programs, such as wellness and health promotion on the work site, including stress management or physical exercise.

Place

Where the product or service is provided is the place component of the marketing mix. Ergonomics consultation is usually provided at the work site; on occasion, therapists provide consultation in their own offices or provide expert testimony in court.

Price

The price, or fee schedule, for services should be based on cost, competitive factors, geography, and what the consumer is willing to pay. Four important methods for establishing a fee schedule are unit value system, cost-plus or overhead, local survey or usual and customary fee, and state code. Whatever method is selected, the price should be commensurate with perceived value.

Promotion

Promotion is the vehicle of communicating information to the consumer about the merits, place, and price of the product. According to Folts and co-workers, "[w]ork programs do not sell services; rather, they sell the benefits of those services. Clients do not want therapeutic modalities, exercises, or purposeful activities. Instead, clients desire the benefits treatment provides, such as pain reduction and the ability to return to work" (p. 13).[5]

The value of ergonomics must be promoted. Instruments of promotion are advertising, sales promotion, publicity, and personal selling.

Advertising

Advertising involves the use of a paid message presented in a recognized medium by an identified sponsor with the purpose of informing, persuading, and reminding. Some advertising vehicles include brochures, direct mail, and printed advertisements in the client company's monthly newsletter. Copy testing the brochure or direct mail piece invites potential target markets to provide feedback and direction about the concept of the material before an investment is made to print it. An ergonomic consultant could create a mock brochure, then copy test it with specific target markets, either individually or in a group format. The feedback is invaluable, and the time invested usually lends itself to producing materials about the product or service offered that are meaningful and useful to the consumer. Figure 20-2 is an example of a national awareness campaign developed by the American Occupational Therapy Association to promote occupational therapy in ergonomics. Figure 20-3 is an example of a copy

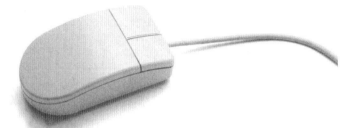

It seems like such a simple thing, but every time you move the mouse or your hand a certain way the pain is so sharp it forces you to stop being the productive, hardworking, get-it-done-now person you've always been, and that's the most painful thing of all.

This year, millions of Americans in all lines of work will get a painful reminder of just how much they depend upon their hands. They'll develop job-related injuries that will interfere with their work performance and their quality of life. Fortunately, these people will be in good hands if they receive occupational therapy as part of their treatment program. Studies show that O.T. shortens recovery time. And since it teaches people healthy, efficient ways to perform job and everyday life tasks, occupational therapy reduces the chance of re-injury. If O.T. can do all that for a hand injury, just think how it can help people who have had strokes and sports injuries and those with developmental disabilities and chronic illnesses. For more information, call 1-800-668-8255 for a free brochure. Or email us at: praota@aota.org.

OCCUPATIONAL THERAPY
Skills for the job of living.

ΛΟΤΛ *The American Occupational Therapy Association, Inc.• 4720 Montgomery Lane • Bethesda MD • 20814-3425*

FIGURE 20-2 Advertisement developed by the American Occupational Therapy Association to promote occupational therapy's role in ergonomics. (Reprinted with permission from the American Occupational Therapy Association, Bethesda, Md.)

Copy Test
Ergonomics Brochure

	Total #	Male #	Female #
1. Awareness top-of-mind			
2. What was said and shown?			
3. Main idea			
4. Interesting ad elements			
5. Confusing ad elements			
6. Hard-to-believe ad elements			
7. Objectionable ad elements			
8. Additional information			
9. Name of service advertised			
10. Other comments			

FIGURE 20-3 An example of sample copy testing questions used to survey target markets about their input regarding advertising materials.

testing format that could be used to survey the target audience about the advertised material.

Sales Promotion

Sales promotion is the use of a wide variety of short-term incentives to encourage purchase of the product. This approach is optimized when used in conjunction with advertising. For example, at an open house for an industrial rehabilitation program, a successful sales promotion to increase new referrals is a business card drawing for a free ergonomic work site analysis.[10] Other sales promotion strategies are giveaways with contact information, such as pens, pencils, visors, magnets, water bottles, sticky notes, and so on.

Publicity

An infrequently used marketing strategy, publicity is free promotion.[15] Despite this positive feature, one has little control over placement; thus, directing the message at target markets becomes difficult. Examples of publicity for promoting ergonomics consultation are newspaper articles and radio public service announcements on topics such as stress management in the workplace and preventing cumulative trauma disorders. Figure 20-4 is a press release promoting occupational therapy's role in ergonomics. Within 1 year of its release, the information had been broadcast on 744 radio stations in all 50 states and generated 436 newspaper articles in 26 different states. In 1 year alone, this publicity reached a total audience of 63,951,736 people.

Personal Selling

Personal selling, the most effective form of promotion, involves face-to-face communication between the therapist and the consumer. Word-of-mouth recommendations by recipients of ergonomics consultations are a powerful marketing tool, too. Some examples of personal selling are making presentations at meetings, providing continuing education workshops, and lecturing to professional organizations. Box 20-2 provides a creative example of personal selling.

Executing and Evaluating the Marketing Plan

After the target market has been selected and the marketing mix developed, the marketing plan should be initiated. Because marketing is a dynamic activity, a plan requires continual evaluation of its effectiveness. A time frame, such as a 12-month period, should be established to determine whether objectives and goals are being met. The marketing plan should be flexible to allow changes to be made as new opportunities and problems arise. The following case study demonstrates the use of marketing before the expansion of services.

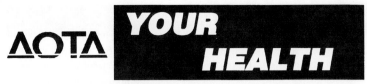

Facts From The American Occupational Therapy Association, Inc.

Preventing Carpal Tunnel Syndrome

by Karen Jacobs, EdD, OTR/L

(NAPS)—Here's some encouraging news: there are ways you may be able to help prevent repetitive motion injuries to your hands, wrists and fingers while on the job.

The American Occupational Therapy Association, Inc., offers the following advice:

Check your position

Keep shoulders erect, but relaxed, while sitting, place work close to you where it is easily accessible. Most work should be performed with elbows close to the body. Elbows should be bent to a 90 degree angle while working at your desk. Wrists should be only slightly bent, as they would look when you are holding a pencil.

If you use the telephone a lot, you may want to get a headset or speaker phone. Try not to cradle the telephone between your head and shoulder.

Check your equipment

The computer monitor should be placed about 26 inches from your eyes with the top of the screen at eye level.

You may be able to prevent shoulder, neck, and elbow problems by lowering the keyboard so its lowest point is positioned about an inch above your legs.

Give your body a break

Take a 10 minute break for every hour you spend at a computer terminal.

One of the better known workplace injuries is carpal tunnel syn-

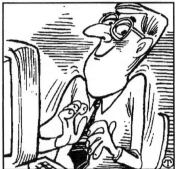

Some ways you may be able to help prevent repetitive motion injuries is by keeping shoulders erect, but relaxed, and taking 10 minute breaks every hour.

drome. It affects the hands, wrists and fingers. It is most often seen in keyboard operators and assembly line workers.

If you are experiencing any symptoms of carpal tunnel—such as numbness, weakness, pain and difficulty in moving your hands, wrists and fingers—you may want to see your doctor.

For more information about repetitive motion injuries, call The American Occupational Therapy Association, Inc., toll-free at 1-800-668-8255. Or you can visit www.aota.org on the Internet.

• *Dr. Jacobs is a faculty member at Boston University and currently president-elect of The American Occupational Therapy Association.*

FIGURE 20-4 Press release developed by the American Occupational Therapy Association to promote occupational therapy's role in ergonomics. (Reprinted with permission from the American Occupational Therapy Association, Bethesda, Md, 1998.)

Box 20-2	*Example of Creative Personal Selling*

Rachel Neuman, a doctoral student in physical therapy at Boston University, created "Ergonomics Day" at the Massachusetts State House, an event developed for legislators, their aides, and staff at the state house. An extensive literature review was conducted in order to find the most recent evidence on a variety of ergonomic topics. The evidence was summarized into 12 separate "ergonomic strategy" pages and/or pamphlets (examples of these are included in Appendix B). In addition, nine hands-on stations on various aspects of ergonomics were developed and set up around the grand staircase on the second floor of the Massachusetts State House. Members of the Boston University Sargent College Rotaract Club volunteered their time to help man the stations. Rachel Neuman and Karen Jacobs circulated and answered questions.

- Station 1 consisted of an adjustable notebook computer workstation, and safe and healthy computer ergonomics was addressed.
- Station 2 included appropriate seating for an office. Information was provided on what characteristics make a chair both safe and comfortable.
- Station 3 provided information on both stretching and rest breaks while at work. Various stretches were demonstrated.
- Station 4 was manned by a fellow doctoral physical therapy student, Theresa Conran, who created a website called "The Back Challenge" (www.thebackchallenge.com). She discussed a different tip each week for preventing chronic low back pain or helping to improve current episodes of low back pain. Her station provided information on these back pain prevention tips.

- Station 5 covered the topic of stress management. Specific techniques for managing stress, such as guided imagery, were discussed, and information was distributed on these techniques.
- Station 6 provided information on the proper method for shaking hands. This was obviously geared specifically toward the legislators, as hand shaking is an action they likely perform on a daily basis. Improper hand shaking can lead to overuse injuries, so a packet filled with helpful tips to prevent injury from excessive hand shaking was distributed.
- Station 7 was on backpack awareness. Although this is not a topic that specifically targets state officials, it is a topic that will likely hit "close to home," as it targets children. Handouts were provided with tips for backpack safety, as improper backpack use in childhood can lead to musculoskeletal problems in adulthood.
- Station 8 provided information on proper personal digital assistant (PDA) use, specifically on a condition termed "Blackberry thumb." A flier on helpful tips for PDA users, created by the American Physical Therapy Association, was available.
- Station 9 was a golf station. This topic, like the backpack station, was not specifically associated with workstation ergonomics. However, golf is a popular sport of legislators, and the Boston University Physical Therapy Clinic was recruited to promote their golf clinic and the use of proper ergonomics in golf.

CASE STUDY

A well-established, freestanding industrial rehabilitation center decided to start including ergonomics consultation as a service. The director of the center decided to perform a market analysis to determine the feasibility of such an expansion. In the first step, which involved identifying target markets, the director analyzed marketing opportu-

nities; the analysis included a self-audit, a consumer analysis, a competitive analysis, and an environmental assessment.

Self-Audit

A SWOT analysis was performed to determine the strengths and weaknesses of, opportunities for, and threats to the center.

Strengths
- Three occupational and physical therapists with master's degrees; two of these therapists are CPEs
- Excellent reputation in the community
- Located in an area with a high concentration of plastics and paper manufacturers

Weakness
- Limited financial resources for the purchase of equipment needed for work site analysis

Opportunities
- The medical director of the center had been appointed the medical director of a local plastics-manufacturing company.
- The center is eligible to apply for state funding provided by the Department of Industrial Accidents to develop a proposal for ergonomics training for companies with workers at risk for cumulative trauma disorders.

Threat
- Two local physical therapists in private practice are expanding services to include ergonomics consultation.

Consumer Analysis

The consumer analysis revealed the following markets as potential users of ergonomics consultation:
- Local industry, in particular manufacturers whose employees perform repetitive upper-extremity tasks and material handling (e.g., paper manufacturers)
- Employees who work extensively with computers, such as insurance agency personnel

Competitive Analysis

A competitive analysis revealed two competitors within a 30-mile radius of the center. These competitors were identified in the self-audit under the "threat" category.

Environmental Assessment

An environmental assessment indicated that the center was located in an industrial community with an aging workforce. One manufacturer of plastics noted that over the last 2 years an increasing number of workers sustained cumulative trauma disorders. Concurrently the number of lost work days per 100 workers increased steadily.

Market Segmentation

After the market analysis was completed in 2 weeks, a market segmentation was proposed. The potential consumers of ergonomics consultation were divided into distinct groups. For example, physicians were specified as orthopedic surgeons, occupational health practitioners, and neurologists. This market was further defined by the selection of only occupational health physicians as proposed primary referral sources for ergonomics consultation. Market segmentation was also performed for industrial sites.

The next step in the analysis involved developing marketing strategies specific to target markets by devising the optimal mix of product, place, price, and promotion. One of the target markets was a local plastics manufacturer. The center's product line for this manufacturer included baseline ergonomics screening surveys, work site analyses, customized education and training programs, work site modifications, and product design and evaluation (see Chapter 10 for more information on product design and evaluation). Ergonomics consultation would be provided at the work site, and the price of services would be based on cost-plus and consideration of what the competition was charging.

Promotion was aimed at the plastics industry. Personal selling was identified as the most effective sales mechanism. One of the center's therapists contacted the director of human resources of the plastics manufacturer to arrange for an appointment to promote ergonomics consultation. The development of a brochure was also suggested to delineate the center's expanded product line of ergonomics consultation. Copy testing of the new brochure was conducted with target markets, and valuable feedback from these consumers ensured an accurate understanding of the benefits of ergonomic consultation. A timeline was proposed to help determine whether these strategies resulted in contracts for ergonomics consultation.

When the market analysis was completed, expanding the center's product line to include ergonomics consultation on a trial basis (12 months) seemed feasible. The director evaluated the strategies after 6 months and again at the end of the year to determine whether the goals and objectives were being met.

CONCLUSION

Unlike the old economy, the new economy is based on the digital revolution and management of information about customers, products, prices,

Learning Exercises

1. Describe, design, and discuss content for a web page promoting your ergonomic consulting business.
2. Apply the definition of marketing and its importance to the development of an ergonomic consulting business.
3. Discuss the difference between needs and desires. Select three different target markets and discuss the needs and desires of those markets in relation to ergonomic consultation.
4. Discuss the exchange potential concept in an ergonomic consulting business, and identify how this process creates value for the consumers of this service.
5. Analyze the four components involved in a marketing approach, and apply components 1 and 2 in the development of new ergonomic business.
6. Develop marketing strategies for an ergonomic business.
7. Select an ergonomic product or service, and perform a SWOT analysis.
8. Perform a consumer analysis to analyze and discuss markets of potential users of ergonomic consultation.
9. Choose an ergonomic product or service and a location; analyze the competition.
10. Select an industry and complete an environmental assessment.
11. Collect data and demographics by performing market research on a selected target market.
12. Select one regulatory agency, and research that agency's contributions in the field of ergonomics.
13. Select a target market; select which ergonomic services to provide to that market, and develop marketing strategies to meet the needs, desires, or interests of that market. Incorporate the four Ps identified in the marketing mix.
14. Create one promotional piece about the occupational therapist's contribution to ergonomics.
15. Create an advertisement about your ergonomic consulting business. Copy test the advertisement with your target market.
16. Discuss ideas for promoting and publicizing the occupational therapist's role in ergonomic consulting.

competitors, and every other aspect of the marketing environment. Information can be infinitely differentiated, analyzed, personalized, and electronically dispatched to many people in a short period of time.[13] The understanding and implementation of marketing concepts allows therapists to take a proactive approach in the health care environment and be ready to meet the changing needs and wants of the marketplace. According to Schwartz, "[o]ccupational therapy is strategically placed to assume a leadership role in work place injury prevention. . . . Prevention services offered by occupational therapists both minimize the incidence and severity of disability, for a far lower cost than occupational health physicians and other primary care providers have traditionally charged" (p. 365).[19]

Multiple Choice Review Questions

1. Marketing on the Internet has provided consumers with the ability to do all but the following:
   A. Find a significant amount of information about practically anything online
   B. Find a greater variety of available goods and services
   C. Compare information about products and services
   D. Decrease buying power

2. Five conditions must be satisfied for an exchange potential to exist, and they include all but the following:

A. There must be at least two parties.
B. Each party has something that might be of value to the other party.
C. Each party is capable of communication and delivery.
D. Each party is obligated to accept or reject the exchange offer.

3. The four Ps of the marketing mix are:
   A. price, packaging, place, promotion.
   B. place, price, promotion, product.
   C. product, packaging, promotion, place.
   D. product, procedure, price, packaging.

4. What are the components of a marketing approach?
   A. Analyze market opportunities, research and select target markets and market segments, develop marketing strategies, and execute and evaluate the plan
   B. Develop a product or service, promote the product or service, and analyze the success of the product or service
   C. Market the product or service, research market segments, and evaluate the plan
   D. Analyze market opportunities, develop marketing strategies, and evaluate the plan

5. A SWOT analysis, or self-audit, evaluates:
   A. strengths, weaknesses, organization, and treatment.
   B. support, weaknesses, opportunities, and treatment.
   C. strengths, weaknesses, opportunities, and threats.
   D. segments, weaknesses, organizations, and threats.

6. Which is the most effective form of promotion?
   A. Advertising
   B. Publicity
   C. Personal selling
   D. Sales promotion

7. Eighty percent of repeat business for goods or services will come from what percent of your customer base?
   A. 10%
   B. 20%
   C. 30%
   D. 40%

8. Good ergonomics is good _____.
   A. economics
   B. entrepreneurship
   C. business planning
   D. efficiency

9. A refrigerator magnet with the logo, name, and contact information of the ergonomic consultant is an example of:
   A. publicity.
   B. personal selling.
   C. sales promotion.
   D. advertising.

10. Which type of promotion is typically free?
    A. Sales promotion
    B. Advertising
    C. Personal selling
    D. Publicity

REFERENCES

1. Bennett PD, editor: *Dictionary of marketing terms,* ed 2, Chicago, 1995, American Marketing Association.
2. California Code of Regulations: *The "Ergonomic" Regulation. Readopted,* Title 8, Section 5110, April 17, 1997; effective July 3, 1997.
3. Coy J, Davenport M: Age changes in the older adult worker: implications for injury prevention, *Work* 2:38, 1991.
4. Drucker PF: *Management challenges for the 21st century,* New York, 1999, HarperCollins.
5. Folts D, Jeremko J, Houk D: Marketing's role in work programs, *Work* 3:13, 1993.
6. Green J, Kelly L, Munn RD: Conquering the complex, *Rehab Manag* 17(7):22, 2004.
7. Hendrick H: Good ergonomics is good economics. Proceedings of the Human Factors and Ergonomics Society's 40th Annual Meeting, Philadelpha 1996.
8. Jacobs K: A marketing approach to work practice, *Work Programs Spec Interest Sect Newsl* 5:3, 1991.

9. Jacobs K: From the editor, *Work* 2:1, 1992.

10. Jacobs K: Marketing occupational therapy services. In Jacobs K, Logigian M, editors: *Functions of a manager in occupational therapy,* Thorofare, NJ, 1994, Slack.

11. Jacobs K: Work hardening in the health care system. In Ogden-Niemeyer L, Jacobs K, editors: *Work hardening: state of the art,* Thorofare, NJ, 1989, Slack.

12. Kiernan W, Carter A, Bronstein E: Marketing and marketing management in rehabilitation. In Kiernan W, Schalock R, editors: *Economics, industry, and disability,* Baltimore, 1989, Brookes.

13. Kotler P: *A framework for marketing management,* ed 2, Upper Saddle River, NJ, 2003, Prentice Hall.

14. Kotler P: *Marketing for non profit organizations,* Englewood Cliffs, NJ, 1975, Prentice-Hall.

15. Kotler P: *Principles of marketing: instructor's manual with cases,* Englewood Cliffs, NJ, 1983, Prentice-Hall.

16. McCarthy EJ: *Basic marketing: a managerial approach,* ed 13, Homewood, Ill, 1999, Irwin.

17. Occupational Safety and Health Administration (OSHA): Draft ergonomics protection standard, *Fed Regist* 57(149):34192, 1995.

18. Occupational Safety and Health Administration (OSHA): *Ergonomic program management guidelines for meatpacking plants,* Washington DC, 1991, U.S. Department of Labor.

19. Schwartz R: Prevention. In Jacobs K, editor: *Occupational therapy: work related programs and assessments,* Boston, 1991, Little, Brown.

20. Sehnal J, Christopher R: Developing and marketing an ergonomics program in a corporate office environment, *Work* 3:22, 1993.

21. Smith M: Ergonomic update: legislative, judicial, and other happenings, *Prev Inj* 2:8, 1993.

22. United States Census Bureau, U.S. Department of Commerce: *Economics and statistics administration. Census 2000 brief on the 65 years and over population 2000.* Retrieved January 1, 2007, from http://nationalatlas.gov/articles/people/a_age65pop.html.

SUGGESTED READING

Berkowitz EN: *Essentials of health care marketing,* New York, 1996, Aspen.

Hartley RF: *Marketing mistakes and successes,* ed 9, Hoboken, NJ, 2004, John Wiley & Sons.

Kotler, P: *A framework for marketing management,* ed 2, Saddle River, NJ, 2003, Prentice Hall.

Websites

American Marketing Association: www.marketingpower.com

American Occupational Therapy Association: www.aota.org

Board of Certification in Professional Ergonomics: www.bcpe.org

Centers for Disease Control and Prevention: www.cdc.gov/od/ohs/Ergonomics

Ergoweb: www.ergoweb.com

Guerilla Marketing: www.gmarketing.com

Occupational Safety and Health Administration: www.osha.gov

United States Department of Labor: www.dol.gov

Wikipedia: The Free Encyclopedia: www.en.wikipedia.org/wiki/marketing

21

Entrepreneurship

Charissa C. Shaw

Learning Objectives

After reading this chapter and completing the exercises, the reader should be able to do the following:

1. Define entrepreneurship and characteristics of entrepreneurs.
2. List the steps to take before starting your business.
3. Identify funding options for your entrepreneurial venture.
4. Describe the basics of writing a business plan.

Business. An occupation, profession or trade; the purchase and sale of goods in an attempt to make a profit.

Creative. Having the quality or power of creating; resulting from originality of thought or expression; imaginative.

Financing. The management of revenues; the conduct or transaction of money matters generally, especially those affecting the public, as in the fields of banking and investment.

At any one point, 7.2 million people are starting a business, making their dreams a reality.[20] Being an entrepreneur in the field of ergonomics means you are on what Malcolm Gladwell would call "the tipping point" of something big, an explosion of an industry that's just emerging.[8] The field of ergonomics is growing and getting more attention from corporations, schools, and product manufacturers that want to ensure consumer comfort, safety, and productivity. In the future we may see product manufacturers designing ergonomic products only because of fear of lawsuits and because of customer demand. This chapter discusses the various definitions of entrepreneurship, unravels the mystery of starting one's own business, covers what areas of practice are needed, and shares case studies of successful therapists turned entrepreneurs. This chapter should be read in conjunction with Chapter 20, Economics and Marketing of Ergonomic Services, as these are essential components of starting your entrepreneurial venture.

DEFINITIONS OF ENTREPRENEURSHIP

There are many definitions of entrepreneurs and entrepreneurship. According to Dollinger, entrepreneurship is "the creation of an innovative economic organization for the purpose of gain or growth under conditions of risk and uncertainty" (p. 4).[5] Sokolosky discusses the traits of successful entrepreneurs and says that "when change hits, entrepreneurs see the opportunity created by change and are able to capitalize on shifting markets and trends before others do."[20]

In her presentation on "Entrepreneurship for the Ergonomics Professional," Jacobs discussed the top 10 characteristics of an entrepreneur[11]:

1. Able to recognize and take advantage of opportunities
2. Resourceful
3. Creative
4. Independent thinker
5. Hard worker
6. Optimistic
7. Innovator
8. Risk taker
9. Visionary
10. Leader

Although this list itemizes critical characteristics for success, you do not need to have all of these qualities to be an entrepreneur. As an entrepreneur, I would say that I have seldom had more than two of these qualities at any one time. Sometimes we may feel lazy, not the strong leader we are perceived as, and may not take risks for fear of being embarrassed. At times we are extremely creative, coming up with ideas and solutions continuously. Yet we can also be blocked creatively, lacking optimism and realizing that we have limited resources to accomplish what we want. When motivation is low, it's important to reenergize by clarifying your vision and mission. Do not be too hard on yourself. If you can have most of the qualities 60% of the time, consider yourself an entrepreneur!

In *Starting from Scratch,* Moss identifies four common actions that the entrepreneurs he interviewed have mastered along the journey to success. These steps include the following: (1) harness what you have, (2) underestimate your obstacles, (3) notice your network, and (4) take the first step.[15] Moss reported one consistent factor among the entrepreneurs interviewed—they started their businesses on a part-time basis while working in another job. This point illustrates that anyone can start a business, even if he or she needs to keep a regular job for a while to make money. Taking the first step is the most important aspect that distinguishes entrepreneurs from employees.

Gerber, in his book *The E-Myth Revisited,* states that "the entrepreneur is the innovator, the grand strategist, the creator of new methods for penetrating and creating new markets" (p. 24).[7] Some examples he cites are Henry Ford, Tom Watson of IBM, and Ray Kroc of McDonalds. If you are considering starting your own venture, this last definition could be intimidating. But keep in mind that all giants started off small and built their companies over time. Even McDonalds started off with one small hamburger restaurant until one man saw an opportunity to franchise it, then in 20 years it grew into the giant you see today. In addition, being an entrepreneur does not mean you have to become a giant—only that you may, if you desire it. It all starts with a seed that grows when planted and watered with the right idea, plan, team, timing, and passion.

ERGONOMICS AND ENTREPRENEURSHIP

As an ergonomic consultant and product inventor, I believe that being an entrepreneur is about taking your desire and passion to create a service or product that will make this world a better place. Because of rising health care and workers' compensations costs, there has been a growing need for therapists to become involved with ergonomic consulting. In addition, product development in the field of ergonomics is an emerging niche with unlimited potential. Whether your business is consulting, offering seminars and certification, being an expert witness, developing video projects, selling, or evaluating or creating products, there are many opportunities for growth. As an expert witness in ergonomics, consultants are starting to see the need for a wide variety of testimony. For example, there have been cases in which an individual has sued a manufacturer, claiming that he or she developed a cumulative trauma disorder (CTD) as a result of poor ergonomic design. There are also many situations in which an expert witness will act as an authority in workplace ergonomics for either side. Such experts may use their knowledge of anatomy, physiology, biomechanics, and job task analysis to determine if the specific claim is valid. Another opportunity is as an expert witness consultant; these individuals can investigate whether a lawsuit is valid by evaluating the job tasks and work demands to determine if an injury could have been caused by a job.

In ergonomics consulting specifically, there are many opportunities to work with corporations and government organizations. One physical therapist turned ergonomist, Allison Heller-Ono of Worksite International, has become one of the most well-known ergonomics experts in the industry and has turned her *Developing an Ergonomic Process* guide into a training program for therapists interested in becoming entrepreneurs. Ms. Heller-Ono's approach is unique in the respect that she will go into a company and look toward changing the corporate culture to one that is more

aware of ergonomics by using a concept called *participatory ergonomics* (see chapter 3, Macroergonomics). This concept is applied to a small group of employees who are trained to work as a team to perform preventative evaluations and identify ergonomic problems or employees with discomfort early, before their symptoms become a CTD.

A growing trend for ergonomic consultants is integrating technology into the ergonomics process. A company called Atlas Ergonomics has implemented this concept extremely well with its clients. Drew Bossen, a physical therapist, has a web-based tool that inputs employee information into a database in which the company can easily track changes and the employee's progress. Another unique way Mr. Bossen runs his company is that he charges for his training program for physical therapists or other certified ergonomists to become subcontractors for Atlas. Drew has branded Atlas Ergonomics as the "truck driver" and "obesity in the office" specialist. This has included developing an extensive database of truck drivers and designing truck seats, as well as driver education.

Another avenue of ergonomic consulting is conducting physical demands analyses (PDA). These quantify the specific tasks, repetitions, vibration measures, time spent performing the tasks, weight lifted, and/or push and pull forces. When combined with the job description, this can be powerful documentation in implementing a postoffer preemployment screening program. It is critical that the therapist work with corporations' legal and human resources departments in order to make sure the work demands fall in line with their hiring procedures. Once the program is implemented, the therapist can work with a local rehabilitation clinic to provide consistent strength as well as range-of-motion testing. When a person's limits are defined, the therapist can clearly place him or her in a job that fits his or her physical capacity. This can offer substantial savings because most employees have minimized their risk of developing an ergonomic or other injury.

Another role therapists can play is providing "on-site return-to-work and therapy," which is much more cost-effective and returns an employee to work in as little as half the time of off-site therapy.[2] The therapist can provide ergonomics education and movement training along with the program. Wellness and stress management is another area of expertise that therapists can move into quite easily. Studies report that psychosocial issues such as stress contribute to CTDs, yet this aspect of injury management is often overlooked. Programs that a therapist can implement include site needs assessment, wellness surveys, postural retraining, massage/trigger point therapy, on-site fitness classes specifically for preventing ergonomic injuries, online wellness programs and information, employee newsletters, weight and nutrition management, and stretching and strengthening programs.

One example of a comprehensive wellness program can be found at the University of Southern California (USC) Department of Occupational Science and Therapy. The USC Occupational Therapy Faculty Practice specializes in wellness programs and services using the Lifestyle Redesign approach to help clients construct health-promoting habits and routines. The Lifestyle Redesign process enables clients to achieve a variety of health and wellness goals such as lowering cholesterol and blood pressure, increasing energy levels, and achieving satisfaction in their work-life balance.

Another example of this in practice is occupational therapist turned injury prevention specialist Michael Melnik. He works with numerous large corporations to develop strain and sprain prevention programs that use training and education, ergonomics, and stretching and warm-up activities to reduce injuries. In addition, he has just launched an online program, HealthEsite.com. Companies purchase access codes to the site and distribute them to employees. The site contains a variety of health, wellness, and injury prevention videos that employees can view at home.

CASE STUDY

Michael S. Melnik MS, OTR
President, Prevention Plus, Inc.
President, HealthEsite, LLC.

Type of Corporation: S Corporation

Funding Source: For consulting, no upfront funding was obtained. For videos, Mr. Melnik partnered with companies and paid them a percentage of the royalties.

Staff Profile: One full-time business development person, one part-time office manager, subcontractors as work warrants

Location: Minneapolis, Minnesota

My passion for entrepreneurship developed when I began my first job working in a clinic. Like most organizations, the clinic had its own idea of what I was supposed to do, when I was supposed to do it, and how much they would pay me to get it done. None of this sat well with me, and I learned something very important during my first work experience—I am basically unemployable. Not in the sense that no one would hire me, but unemployable in that I really, really don't want to work for anyone. So, despite the fact that I had a great boss, worked with wonderful people, and had numerous opportunities to develop my skills, I moved on. Although I worked closely with an entrepreneur for a few years after I left the clinic, I had no idea how to start a business. Things I had never considered before, such as office space, phone lines, copiers, fax machines, and paper clips, were all things I took for granted. Another thing I took for granted was clients. My previous employers had supplied me with all the work I needed. I now needed to start filling the pipeline myself. The good thing was that I knew I liked speaking. The trick was to find an audience. In the beginning I spoke at Rotary Clubs, the Chambers of Commerce in various communities, and any place that would let me speak. I didn't charge them, but I had one condition: the audiences had to critique my presentations. In short, I was perfecting my skills and marketing my services at the same time. Without fail, some of the audience members would want my card and would invite me to come speak at their companies. I had no clue 16 years ago that I would be doing what I am doing today. In fact, what I provide and how I provide it to clients has grown and changed continuously and dramatically over the years. It keeps me excited and motivated and has my clients asking "what's next." The latest project is an online health and wellness website that has led to the development of an entirely new company. My presentations, which have focused for years specifically on safety and injury prevention, are now expanding to the sales, marketing, and human resources departments of large companies. A year from now, who knows? What I do know is that if I continue to follow my passion and continue to try to get better at whatever I am doing, a year from now I will be in the right spot.

What are some of the traits Mr. Melnik has that make him a successful entrepreneur?

How does Prevention Plus differentiate itself in the market of ergonomic consulting?

Based on his story, how could a therapist transition to becoming an entrepreneur?

Petti Redding, OTR, of the Redding Group, has been successful with using wellness in her programs. Her approach is to use a method called the Human Structural Integrity Model, which uses trigger point deactivation, restoring neutral postural balance and behavior modifications. All methods are taught to the employee by an OT or PT, then the employee does his or her own treatment using these instructed methods. Depending where in the body the employee has pain, the employee works with an athletic trainer or other instructor to learn self-massage, stretches, and strengthening exercises that prevent the employee's discomfort from turning into a diagnosed injury. Ms. Redding's success speaks for itself; she has had as much as a 90% reduction in ergonomic injuries within a 1-year period.[18]

In addition, a therapist may decide to have his or her own clinic and include functional capacity evaluations in the product line and an ergonomics laboratory for training. Another option for the budding entrepreneur in ergonomics is to start a hand therapy clinic and include ergonomic consulting as part of the services offered.

Children and Youth

One relatively untapped niche market is ergonomics for children. There are many ways to break into working with kids, including providing presentations to children and youths, parents, teachers, and administrators on backpack safety, playground design, toy design, furniture design, ergonomic accessories design, computer use, and video game positioning and proper tools. You can write a book or create posters or workbooks and products for children. In addition, you may be able to get funding from local corporations that are looking to support their community in a positive way.

The Older Population

According to the National Institute for Occupational Safety and Health (NIOSH), in 2001 workers in the United States over age 55 represented 18.3 million or 13.6% of the total labor force.[9] This is important to ergonomists and therapists because as people get older, they may experience a loss of strength and a decrease in visual acuity, and we need to design the workspace around these parameters. According to Leeuwenburgh, after age 65 there is a measurable decrease in muscle strength that can affect a person's function.[14] As an ergonomist, when adjusting the environment to reflect the users' strengths, you may take into consideration special factors such as reach distances and use of assistive technology to assist with a person's sight.

In addition, there is some overlap between the elderly population and people with physical disabilities. For an entrepreneur in ergonomics, there are many avenues for consultation for both populations. These include ensuring Americans with Disabilities Act (ADA) compliance for the office and home, suggesting kitchen and bathroom modifications, and conducting presentations in community centers, group homes, and assisted-living centers.

Ergonomics and Telecommuting

Ergonomics for telecommuters and others working from home is also an emerging opportunity. A trend for corporations is to have employees telecommute either full-time or part-time to save company resources. Because every home is unique, these varied environments necessitate innovative product ideas. A therapist working with a corporation can develop a customized page on the company's website that is dedicated to the unique ergonomic needs of telecommuters including driving, workstation setup at home, and home activities that have ergonomic risk factors.

ROLES AS AN ERGONOMICS PROFESSIONAL

Sometimes, starting a new venture requires that the therapist play many roles—not only as the entrepreneur, but as the manager and the technician. When an entrepreneur is just starting out, it is easy to fall into the trap of doing marketing, attending sales meetings and making sales calls, handling operations, and performing the work. In order to work more efficiently, it is important to have a team in place so you do not end up in another job—your business! Think about systemizing your business and developing templates so that you can have subcontractors performing the work, trained with your expertise. Eker states that we need to spend more time "on the business rather than in the business. If you have to be physically present, it can only grow to the extent that you can handle" (p. 38).[6] Of course you need working income when you are just getting started, but the goal is to create ways to make passive income through your subcontractors, articles and books, and products.

As you gain expertise in ergonomic consulting, you may consider the following possibilities for avenues of passive income: workbooks, CDs and videos, books, software, newsletters (by subscription or offered free as a marketing tool), subcontractors, seminars (if someone else is running or conducting them), purchase of an already successful business, ergonomic products, and referral fees.

FROM THERAPIST TO ENTREPRENEUR

When considering transitioning to being an entrepreneur, Jacobs discusses the top five ways to transition into being an entrepreneur.[11] The first is to identify an area of practice within the field of ergonomics. In the previous section on ergonomics and entrepreneurship and throughout the book we have discussed many examples of ways to break into the field of ergonomics and develop a niche in the market. This can give you some ideas, but you really have to experiment and examine your feelings to figure out what is right for you. In his book, *Good to Great*, Collins dis-

cusses three things to make your entrepreneurial venture truly successful (and to identity your area of practice).[3] First, determine what you are deeply passionate about. What starts a "fire in your belly"? What does your intuition say the market is ready for? Second, look at what you can be the best in the world at. In the previous examples, the therapists turned ergonomists branded themselves and looked at a niche that they could fill and strive to be the best at. Third, what drives your "economic engine"? In other words, what will really make money for your new venture?

Jacobs' second step along the path to entrepreneurship is to summarize your idea.[11] In 50 words or less, describe where the idea originated (need), how you will bring it to market, and what makes your product unique (why people would buy it rather than another product), and list three qualifications that you have that will allow you to pursue this business. Also, it is helpful to come up with a "30-second elevator speech" to use when introducing yourself that includes your unique selling proposition (USP).

Here is an example of a USP:

Hello, my name is Charissa Shaw. I'm the President of Elysian Integrated Health Solutions, the only provider of ergonomics, wellness, and safety solutions for corporations. We keep people healthy, safe, and more productive at work. If you give me your card, I'll send you a free report on "Preventing Injuries at Work"!

The third step is to develop a business plan. It may be helpful to begin with a one-page business plan[10] to clarify your idea and just to get started. It is also important to collaborate with a professional mentor. Your mentor might even have a sample business plan you can look at and get ideas from. Some wonderful resources for this include the Service Corporation of Retired Executives (SCORE), which has retired business owners who mentor individuals through the process, and the Small Business Administration (SBA), which has sample business plans and other useful resources (see Resources at the end of this chapter).

Prebusiness Checklist

☐ What business am I interested in starting?

☐ What service or products will I market?

☐ Where is my optimal office location?

☐ Will I have a partner or employees?

☐ What skills and experience do I bring to the table?

☐ What will be my corporate identity? Logo? Brand? Colors?

☐ File my "Doing Business As" (DBA) with your local county clerk office

☐ Publish your DBA with your local paper and when published, bring both documents to the bank to set up your account.

☐ What financing will I need and how will I get it?

☐ Marketing materials: business cards, brochure, website(s)

☐ Business plan

☐ Network with local groups

☐ Determine corporate entities

☐ File a patent

☐ Contracts

FIGURE **21-1** A prebusiness check-list.

Prebusiness Checklist

A prebusiness checklist is shown in Figure 21-1. Each step is an important part of creating a successful business:

- What business am I interested in starting? Consider your passions, what you are good at, and what the marketplace needs at the time.
- What service or products will I market? Get specific about exactly what services and products you will offer—for example, in consulting you may decide to offer the following: ergonomic process implementation, train the trainer, ergonomics awareness training, and so on.
- Where is my optimal office location? Working from home might be a good option when you are just starting out. When clients are coming to you, you may want to consider sharing a space with a therapy clinic or other office setting. If products are your business, you may want to be in a visible part of the city where clients can easily find you.

- Will I have a partner or employees? If you decide you want a partner, make sure he or she complements what you do. Before deciding if you need a partner, identify what you need. This could include capital, business skills, or an area of expertise. The partner needs to add value to your business in order to really make a difference. When you take on a partner, you must consider the following: definition of responsibilities, due process, financial checks and balances, termination of the relationship, liquidation of the business, voting power, death, and profit sharing. As for employees, they are not really necessary until you have so many ongoing clients that you need full-time staff to manage the clients and deal with administrative concerns. Starting out, and maybe even for the life of your company, subcontractors work best because you do not have to pay employment taxes nor offer benefits.
- What skills and experience do I bring to the table? Writing your own experience or biosketch (Box 21-1) will clarify what skills

Box 21-1	*Sample of Professional Biography*

Profile

Charissa Shaw, President of Elysian Integrated Health Solutions, received her Master's degree from the number-one Occupational Therapy Graduate school in the nation, the University of Southern California (USC). After she received her Master's from USC, she began working as an Environmental Health and Safety Specialist for the University of California, Los Angeles (UCLA). While at UCLA, Ms. Shaw gained experience in Office and Industrial Ergonomics under the Department of Industrial Hygiene. In January 2001, Ms. Shaw began working as a Senior Ergonomic Consultant and Project Manager and has worked for AOL Time Warner, Bank of America, Union Bank of California, Brio Technology, Coldwell Banker, BART, Appgenesys and Transamerica Insurance and Investments Group. As an Environmental Health and Safety Consultant for AOL, Ms. Shaw worked under the department of Health and Wellness and facilitated the development of a crisis management team and an emergency response team.

As an ergonomic consultant, she has worked with AT&T (SBC), Google, Electronic Arts, Symantec, Trendmicro, Orange County Transportation Authority, AIG Sunamerica, City of Buena Park, City of San Gabriel, City of Upland, City of Downey, South Coast Air Quality Management District, YMCA, Sony Connect, Ameron International, Great American Custom Insurance, SES Insurance, Los Angeles County Department of Public Works, Colen & Lee, and Impact General. For Qualcomm, Ms. Shaw provided ergonomics and safety consulting for facilities in India and the United Kingdom. In addition, Ms. Shaw previously worked as an Adjunct Professor at USC, teaching Ergonomics to second-year graduate occupational therapy students. She has spoken at many national and international conferences regarding her ergonomics program success, including the Applied Ergonomics Conference, the Eastern Ergonomics Conference, the National Ergonomics Conference, and FIK International. Her international experience includes Malaysia and India, speaking on Office Ergonomics. She is a Certified Raytheon Six Sigma Specialist and has achieved as much as a 65% reduction in the ergonomic incident rate while managing various corporate ergonomic programs.

and experiences will serve you in your endeavor.

- What will be my corporate identity? An example of a corporate identity is Allison Heller-Ono, the President and CEO of Worksite International, where she provides ergonomics consulting, analysis, and training to global corporations and therapists around the world. Her logo is the shape of a globe with a red cross and a small stick figure, because of the desire to capture visually the international capabilities of her company to prevent and manage work injuries for a healthier workplace (Figure 21-2). You may want to consult a graphic designer to assist with your colors, logo, and branding.
- File your "Doing Business As" (DBA) with your local county clerk office.

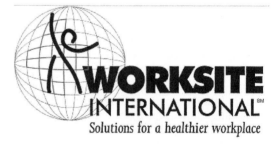

FIGURE 21-2 Example of a corporate logo. (Courtesy Worksite International.)

- Publish your DBA with your local newspaper, and when the announcement is published, take both documents to the bank to set up your account.

- What financing will I need, and how will I get it? Clarify the details in your business plan.
- Marketing materials: business cards, brochure, website(s). (See Chapter 20, Economics and Marketing of Ergonomic Services for detailed information.)
- Create a business plan (see the next section for more details).
- Network with local groups. Some suggestions include the local Rotary clubs, chambers of commerce, Toastmasters International, American Industrial Hygiene Association, Risk Management Association, International Facilities Management Association, Na-tional Human Resources Association, and so on. You can search on the Internet for contact information for these organizations, as websites and organizations change over time.
- Determine corporate entities. Box 21-2 gives a brief overview of the different types of business entities; it is recommended that

you do more research before making a decision.
- File a patent. Are you creating a unique product that is not on the market or modifying an existing product? You may need to do a patent search or hire a patent attorney to do one for you. Go to www.uspto.gov or call the U.S. Patent and Trademark office. They are extremely helpful with resources and assisting you with your search. The other option is filing the patent yourself. A great resource for this is the book *Patent It Yourself* by David Pressman.[17] Also, you may not need to have a patent and may be permitted to manufacture your product without it. Usually you will have approximately 6 months to develop your brand recognition before others start making it, and you can even come up with your own knock-offs! If you decide you are going to patent your idea, it's smart to get an industrial designer to draw a two-dimensional version of the

---

Box 21-2 | *Types of Business Entities*

Sole Proprietorship

You are the company, and the company is identified by your social security number. Typically, you do not have employees and you pay taxes only once. You are still able to make deductions for your business, but you do not need to have board members and hold regular meetings. This type of incorporation is acceptable when you are starting out because you do not have to pay the extra fees associated with incorporating.

Limited Liability Corporation (LLC)

You are a separate entity with your own tax identification number. However, there are fewer corporate formalities than those associated with a C or S corporation. Members and managers of an LLC need not hold regular meetings, reducing complications and paperwork. By default, LLCs are treated as a "pass-through" entity for tax purposes, much like a sole proprietorship or partnership. However, an LLC can also elect to be treated as a corporation for tax purposes, whether as a C

or an S corporation. An LLC can also deduct operational losses.

C Corporation

A corporation is a separate entity from you and has its own tax identification number. Corporations must hold regular meetings of the board of directors and shareholders and keep written corporate minutes. There are multiple deductions you can take, no ownership restrictions, and more credibility in the business community than with an LLC or sole proprietorship. Most corporations are C corporations.

S Corporation

Like a C corporation, an S corporation is a separate entity yet cannot have more than 100 stockholders, and each stockholder must be a resident or citizen of the United States. Also, it is difficult to place shares of an S corporation into a living trust, whereas a C corporation or LLC can do this easily.

product with all its features. Software is also available that will give a different, three-dimensional look to your product design. It is important to keep a bound notebook with dates and your signature. You may also want to mail yourself the documented idea so that there is proof of when you came up with the idea, if there is ever a question in court.[17] However, according to a Google search online, it appears this "poor-man's patent" does not hold up in a court of law and other methods should be considered (e.g., an inventor's journal signed by a witness).

- Contracts. There are many types of contracts you should consider obtaining before starting your business. You may also consider having an attorney review your clients' contracts before signing them, but usually your clients will not be willing to revise their contracts. The most important contracts to consider are "independent contractor" and "noncompete, nondisclosure" agreements that prevent you from working for another company or another person working for you as a subcontractor (Figure 21-3 is an example of an independent contractor agreement). For products, you need to be very careful that you do not share your idea indiscriminately. If you decide to share it, you should have the people with whom you share it sign a nondisclosure agreement (NDA). Once the product is patented or patent-pending, it is harder for people to steal an idea, but it does not stop them. Consult a specialist (patent attorney) for more information. You may also want to consider an NDA for your business plan and include this in the first two pages of your plan (Figure 21-4, p. 391).

Writing a Business Plan

In order to get motivated to write your first business plan, you should first understand why you need a business plan. The first reason is to bring together the necessary resources in one document: human, physical, technologic, and financial resources. According to Jacobs and Russo,[12] it can be used to raise money, but more important, it should be used and updated as a management

Box 21-3	*Sample Mission Statement*

The mission of Elysian Integrated Health Solutions is to implement the best team of ergonomics, safety, and health care professionals to provide optimal care to employees. At EiHS, our success depends on offering a complete range of customized injury prevention and wellness services including ergonomic consulting, postural retraining, and safety.

tool. A great business plan can assist with goal setting and your exit strategy.

When writing the plan, it is important to get organized and create a calendar of deadlines for yourself. Next, develop a list of names and contact information of people who could assist you in writing a good plan. Another task mentioned in the previous section is to look for free resources and mentors to assist you (e.g., SBA). As stated previously, a way to get started is simply to write a one-page business plan,[10] which can help to clarify what you really want to do. You can work out the rest of the details later.

Next, think about your vision for the company. What is your market, how many people can you serve, where will you be positioned 5 and 10 years from now? For your mission, ask what your purpose is and what services or specific products you will provide for your clients. A sample mission statement from Elysian Integrated Health Solutions is shown in Box 21-3.

According to Jacobs,[11] goals and objectives should clearly define what you are trying to accomplish in specific and measurable elements that you can track and that let you know when you have succeeded. As with your vision statement, it is important to think about what 5-year and 10-year goals you have for the company.

In your executive summary it may be helpful to include a SWOT analysis, which stands for strengths, weaknesses, opportunities, and threats. Also, a competitive analysis will clearly define what the existing competition or potential compe-

Text continued on p. 390.

INDEPENDENT CONTRACTOR AGREEMENT

This Agreement is made as of_____, between Charissa Shaw (hereinafter referred to as "Elysian Integrated Health Solutions") and _____ (Consultant) and the effective date of this Agreement shall be deemed for all purposes herein as _____ which is agreed upon as the date the Consultant was first approached by Charissa Shaw to consult with Elysian Integrated Health Solutions.

1. **Definitions.** The following definitions shall apply for purposes of this Agreement:

   (a) "Work Product" means all templates, programs, systems, data and materials, in whatever form, first produced or created by or for Consultant as a result of, or related to, performance of work or services under this Agreement.

   (b) "Background Technology" means all programs, systems, data and materials, in whatever form, that do not constitute Work Product and are: (1) included in, or necessary to, the Work Product; and (2) owned either solely by Consultant or licensed to Consultant with a right to sublicense.

Background Technology includes, but is not limited to, the following items:

   All platforms used to create Work Product; all evaluation forms, product forms, customer lists and contact information, and all Confidential Information of Client (as set forth in the Mutual Non-Disclosure Agreement between Client and Consultant, said terms being incorporated herein by this reference).

2. **Services Performed by Consultant:** Consultant agrees to perform the following services for Client:

The Consultant will perform workstation evaluations, develop and design products, perform expert witness testimony, present informational seminars and/or work on special projects (to be determined later) for Elysian Integrated Health Solutions and its clients. Elysian Integrated Health Solutions will fax or email client requests to the Consultant. For workstation evaluations, the Consultant will contact the client to schedule the work, provide necessary follow-up, and submit a written evaluation to Elysian Integrated Health Solutions within the specified timeframe.

The Consultant will report directly to Elysian Integrated Health Solutions and to any other party designated by Elysian Integrated Health Solutions in connection with the performance of the duties under this Agreement and shall fulfill any other duties reasonably requested by Elysian Integrated Health Solutions and agreed to by the Consultant.

3. **Consultant's Payment:** Consultant shall be compensated at the rate of $45.00 US per hour.

4. **Expenses:** The Consultant will be compensated at her hourly rate for any travel time over one hour. In addition, the Consultant will be compensated mileage expense calculated at the standard IRS rate. Also, the Consultant will be compensated for flights, hotel and $30 a day for meals while traveling over 200 miles outside Consultant's residence.

5. **Invoices:** Consultant shall submit invoices for all services rendered to Elysian Integrated Health Solutions. Elysian Integrated Health Solutions will then submit invoices to client for payment. Elysian Integrated Health Solutions will not be obligated to pay Consultant until Elysian Integrated Health Solutions has received payments from Client. Elysian Integrated Health Solutions shall make payments to Consultant within thirty days of receipt of payments from Client.

6. **Written Reports.** The Consultant shall prepare project plans, progress reports and evaluations (as specified by Elysian Integrated Health Solutions) provided to Elysian Integrated Health Solutions on a bi-monthly basis. A final evaluation report shall be due seven business days after the conclusion of the project and shall be submitted to Elysian Integrated Health Solutions in the form of a confidential written report at such time. The results report shall be in such form and setting and include employee discomfort, severity of discomfort, current work station set-up and equipment, ergonomic risk factors, pictures and recommendations (example should be provided) as is reasonably requested by Elysian Integrated Health Solutions.

FIGURE **21-3** Independent contractor agreement (subcontractor agreement).   *Continued*

7. **Independent Contractor:** Consultant is an independent contractor. Consultant and/or Consultant's staff are not employees of Client. In its capacity as an independent contractor, Consultant agrees and represents, and Client agrees, as follows:

(a) Consultant has the right to perform services for others during the term of this Agreement subject to non-competition provisions set forth in the Non-Competition Agreement executed concurrently herewith between Client and Consultant.

(b) Consultant has the sole right to control and direct the means, manner and method by which the services required by this Agreement will be performed.

(c) Consultant has the right to perform the services required by this Agreement at any place or location and at such times as Consultant may determine.

(d) Consultant will furnish all equipment and materials used to provide the services required by this Agreement, except to the extent that Consultant's work must be performed on or with Client's computer or existing software.

(e) The services required by this Agreement shall be performed by Consultant, or Consultant's staff, and Client shall not be required to hire, supervise or pay any assistants to help Consultant.

(f) Consultant is responsible for paying all ordinary and necessary expenses of its staff.

(g) Neither Consultant nor Consultant's staff shall receive any training from Client in the professional skills necessary to perform the services required by this Agreement.

(h) Neither Consultant nor Consultant's staff shall be required to devote full time to the performance of the services required by this Agreement.

(i) Client shall not provide any insurance coverage of any kind for Consultant or Consultant's staff.

(j) Client shall not withhold from Consultant's compensation any amount that would normally be withheld from an employee's pay.

8. **Business Development:** Elysian Integrated Health Solutions will pay Consultant a 20% commission on any new revenue or business generated or developed by Consultant. The commission shall be calculated after all taxes, expenses and costs including Consultant's fees, rates and expenses are deducted from any revenue received by Elysian Integrated Health Solutions. Consultant shall not be paid for their time or expenses to develop new business. Consultant shall pay a 10% commission on any lead resulting in new business or revenue that requires Elysian Integrated Health Solutions assistance in closing the deal. Consultant shall be paid the commission on a quarterly basis, but not until Elysian Integrated Health Solutions has been paid by Client.

9. **Ownership of Consultant's Work Product and Inventions:** Subject to full payment of the consulting fees due hereunder, Consultant hereby assigns to Client its entire right, title and interest in the Work Product including all patents, copyrights, trade secrets and other proprietary rights in or based on the Work Product. Consultant shall execute and aid in the preparation of any papers that Client may consider necessary or helpful to obtain or maintain any patents, copyrights, trademarks or other proprietary rights at no charge to Client, but at Client's expense. Contractor hereby certifies that for good and valuable consideration, the receipt and adequacy of which is hereby acknowledged by Contractor, Contractor's services rendered for and on behalf of the Client in connection with one or more projects, and that all Work Product rendered by Contractor hereunder were and/or will be created by Contractor as a "work-made-for-hire" specially ordered or commissioned by the Client for use as part of an print publication, as a contribution to a collective work or as a supplementary work; with Company being deemed the sole author of the Material and the sole and exclusive owner, throughout the universe in perpetuity, of all rights of every kind and nature, whether now known or hereafter devised (including, without limitation, copyrights and all renewals and extensions thereof) in and to the Material, including, without limitation, the right to make such changes and uses of the Material as it may

FIGURE **21-3,** cont'd

from time to time determine. To the extent, if at all, the Material may be determined not to be a "work-made-for-hire", all of the above-referenced rights in it shall be deemed transferred and assigned to Client by this agreement. Any and all inventions, discoveries, developments and innovations conceived by the Contractor during this engagement relative to the duties under this Agreement shall be the exclusive property of Elysian Integrated Health Solutions; and the Contractor hereby assigns all right, title, and interest in the same to Elysian Integrated Health Solutions. Any and all inventions, discoveries, developments and innovations conceived by the Contractor prior to the term of this Agreement and utilized by her in rendering duties to Elysian Integrated Health Solutions are hereby licensed to Elysian Integrated Health Solutions for use in its operations.

10. **Ownership of Background Technology:** Client agrees that Consultant shall retain any and all rights Consultant may have in the Background Technology. Subject to full payment of the consulting fees due hereunder, Consultant hereby grants Client an unrestricted, nonexclusive, perpetual, fully paid up worldwide license to use and sublicense the use of the Background Technology for the purpose of developing and marketing its products, but not for the purpose of marketing Background Technology separate from its products.

11. **Confidential Information:** During the term of this Agreement and two (2) years afterwards, Consultant will not use or disclose to others without Client's written consent Client's confidential information, except when reasonably necessary to perform the services under this Agreement, consistent with those terms and conditions set forth in the Mutual Non-Disclosure Agreement (hereinafter "NDA") executed concurrently herewith by Client and Consultant and that agreement is incorporated herein fully by reference.

(A) Client acknowledges and agrees that the confidentiality restrictions contained in this Agreement and the NDA shall not apply to the general knowledge, skills and experience gained by Consultant or Consultant's employees while engaged by Client.

(B) All information concerning the existence of this Agreement, the NDA and the existence of any business relationship between Consultant and Client shall be kept in confidence, unless Client grants written permission to Consultant to disclose same;

(C) Consultant will not disclose to Client information or material that is a trade secret of any third party.

(D) The provisions of this clause shall survive any termination of this Agreement and the NDA.

12. **Non-competition:** Consultant agrees that during performance of the services required by this Agreement and for two (2) years after completion, Consultant will not perform the same services for any competitor of Client in the specific field in which Consultant is performing services for Client subject to the terms and conditions set forth in the Non-Competition Agreement executed concurrently herewith by Client and Consultant and that agreement is incorporated herein fully by reference.

13. **Term of Agreement:** This Agreement will become effective on the date indicated in the introductory paragraph of this Agreement, and will remain in effect for 12 months from such date or until terminated as set forth in the section of this Agreement entitled "Termination of Agreement." Elysian Integrated Health Solutions may terminate this Agreement at any time by 10 business days' written notice to the Contractor.

14. **Termination of Agreement:**

(a) Each party has the right to terminate this Agreement if the other party has materially breached any obligation herein;

(b) If at any time after commencement of the services required by this Agreement, Client shall, in its sole reasonable judgment, determine that such services are inadequate, unsatisfactory, no longer needed or substantially not conforming to the descriptions, warranties or representations contained in this Agreement, Client may terminate this Agreement;

FIGURE **21-3, cont'd**

Continued

(c) If the Contractor is convicted of any crime or offense, fails or refuses to comply with the written policies or reasonable directive of Elysian Integrated Health Solutions, is guilty of serious misconduct in connection with the performance hereunder, or materially breaches provisions of this Agreement, Elysian Integrated Health Solutions at any time may terminate the engagement of the Contractor immediately and without prior written notice to the Contractor.

(d) Upon termination of this Agreement for any reason, each party shall be released from all obligations and liabilities to the other occurring or arising after the date of termination. However, any termination of this Agreement shall not relieve Client from the obligation to pay Consultant for services rendered prior to receipt of the notice of termination and for work performed or hours reserved for Client during the 30 day termination notice period.

15. **Return of Materials:** Upon termination of this Agreement, each party shall promptly return to the other all data, materials and other property of the other held by it.

16. **Warranties and Representations:** Consultant warrants and represents that:

(a) Consultant will not knowingly infringe upon any copyright, patent, trade secret or other property right of any former client, employer or third party in the performance of the services required by this Agreement.

(b) Consultant has the authority to enter into this Agreement and to perform all obligations hereunder, including, but not limited to, the grant of rights and licenses to the Work Product and Background Technology and all proprietary rights therein or based thereon.

(c) Consultant has not granted any rights or licenses to any intellectual property or technology that would conflict with Consultant's obligations under this Agreement.

17. **Indemnification:** To the maximum extent permitted by law, Consultant will indemnify, protect, defend and hold harmless Elysian Integrated Health Solutions from and against any and all claims, liabilities, liens, fines, demands, law suits, actions, losses, damages, injuries, judgments, settlements, costs or expenses whether asserted in law or in equity (hereinafter collectively, "Claims") made or asserted for any damages or injury of any kind or nature whatsoever to any person or property (including, without limitation, Claims for injury to or death of any employee of Consultant) including, without limitation, any such Claims resulting from, arising out of or caused in whole or in part by any activity in connection with (1) Subcontractor's performance or breach of its obligations pursuant to this Contract (2) the acts, omissions and execution of the Work provided by Consultant whether, its partners, officers, servants, representatives, affiliates, Subcontractors of Any Tier (3) Any other cause relating to or in connection with their work done pursuant to this contract whether or not such Claims are based upon actual or alleged active or passive negligence of Elysian Integrated Health Solutions except that Consultant will not be required to indemnify Elysian Integrated Health Solutions against Claims that are the result of the sole negligence or the willful misconduct of Company, its agents, servants or independent contractors who are directly responsible to Elysian Integrated Health Solutions. Consultant must provide a defense with counsel of Elysian Integrated Health Solutions' approval upon the first notice Elysian Integrated Health Solutions sends to Consultant and continue to provide such defense until the matter is fully resolved by either final judgment, settlement or other release executed by Elysian Integrated Health Solutions. Consultant will indemnify Elysian Integrated Health Solutions from and against all Claims including without limitation, all legal fees, legal costs (including, without limitation, paralegal costs, secretarial costs, copy costs, phone costs, facsimile costs and mail costs) and expert fees and costs that Elysian Integrated Health Solutions may directly or indirectly sustain, suffer or incur as a result thereof, and Consultant agrees to and does hereby assume on behalf of Elysian Integrated Health Solutions the defense of any Claims which may be brought against Elysian Integrated Health Solutions by reason of such Claims and will pay on behalf of Elysian Integrated Health Solutions, upon their demand, the amount of any costs allowed by law, any costs identified herein, any settlement reached or any judgment that may be entered against Elysian Integrated Health Solutions or any of them as a result of such Claims. Consultant will have the right to withhold from any payments due or that may become due to subcontractor, pursuant to the Contract Documents or otherwise, an amount sufficient to protect Elysian Integrated Health Solutions from such Claims including, without

FIGURE **21-3, cont'd**

limitation, all legal fees, legal costs (including without limitation, paralegal costs, secretarial costs, copy costs, phone costs, facsimile costs and mail costs) and expert fees and costs. Consultant's obligations pursuant to this Section will survive the expiration or termination of this Contract.

18. **Employment of Assistants:** Consultant may, at Consultant's own expense, employ such assistants or subcontractors as Consultant deems necessary to perform the services required by this Agreement. However, Client shall have the right to reject any of Consultant's assistants or subcontractors whose qualifications in Client's good faith and reasonable judgment are insufficient for the satisfactory performance of the services required by this Agreement.

19. **Mediation and Arbitration; Injunctive Relief Available:** Except for the right of Consultant to bring suit on an open account for simple monies due Consultant, in the event of any dispute arising under this Agreement the parties shall first attempt resolution of their disputes through mediation, excluding breaches of this Agreement that require injunctive relief. The parties agree to select a mutually agreeable, neutral third party to help them mediate any dispute that arises under the terms of this Agreement. If the mediation is unsuccessful, the parties agree that the dispute shall be decided by resorting to the Superior Court for the County of Los Angeles, Central District, State of California. The prevailing party in any proceedings shall be awarded reasonable attorney fees, expert witness costs and expenses, and all other costs and expenses incurred directly or indirectly in connection with the proceedings, unless the arbitrators shall for good cause determine otherwise.

The parties hereto acknowledge that the services to be rendered by the Contractor under this Agreement are of a special, unique, unusual, and extraordinary character which give them a peculiar value, the loss of which cannot be reasonably or adequately compensated by damages in any action at law, and the breach by the Contractor of any of the provisions of this Agreement will cause Elysian Integrated Health Solutions irreparable injury and damage. The Contractor expressly agrees that Elysian Integrated Health Solutions shall be entitled to injunctive and other equitable relief in the event of, or to prevent a breach of any provision of this Agreement by the Contractor. Resort to such equitable relief, however, shall not be construed to be a waiver of any other rights or remedies that Elysian Integrated Health Solutions may have for damages or otherwise. The various rights and remedies of Elysian Integrated Health Solutions under this Agreement or otherwise shall be construed to be cumulative, and no one of them shall be exclusive of any other or of any right or remedy allowed by law.

20. **General Provisions:**

(a) This Agreement is the sole and entire Agreement between the parties relating to the subject matter hereof, and supersedes all prior understandings, agreements and documentation relating to such subject matter. Any modifications to this Agreement must be in writing and signed by both parties.

(b) If any provision in this Agreement is held by a court of competent jurisdiction to be invalid, void or unenforceable, the remaining provisions will continue in full force without being impaired or invalidated in any way.

(c) This Agreement will be governed by the laws of the State of California.

(d) All notices and other communications required or permitted under this Agreement shall be in writing and shall be deemed given when delivered personally, or five days after being deposited in the United States mails, postage prepaid and addressed as follows, or to such other address as each party may designate in writing:

Elysian Integrated Health Solutions
Charissa Shaw
1806 Rockefeller Lane
Redondo Beach, CA 90278

Consultant: Insert address here

FIGURE **21-3, cont'd**   *Continued*

(e) This Agreement does not create any agency or partnership relationship.

(f) This Agreement is not assignable by either party without the prior written consent of the other.

(g) This Agreement may be executed in counterparts and facsimile signatures are deemed originals for purposes of this Agreement.

Elysian Integrated Health Solutions
Charissa Shaw, President

By: _____
(Signature)

_____
(Typed or Printed Name)

Title: _____

Consultant:
Insert name here

By: _____
(Signature)

_____
(Typed or Printed Name)

FIGURE **21-3, cont'd**

tition is and what differentiates you. Although the executive summary is listed first in the business plan, it is better to complete the entire plan first and finish this section last.

Some financial aspects you will want to include in your business plan are cash flow, profitability, and return on investment, especially if you are trying to attract investors.

To help you get started, a sample business plan outline from Palo Alto Software is shown in Box 21-4.

Obtaining Funding

The financial needs of the business will change as the business faces different challenges. As a new entrepreneur, you must be able to recognize where your firm is in the life cycle and be specific about the use of funding. If you decide to go into ergonomic consulting, you may need only enough money to pay your bills until you get clients. If you have a product, you might need seed capital for a prototype and market testing. This can tell

you whether or not the concept is viable. Startup capital is also known as *first-stage financing,* and it can be used for product development and marketing materials before there are any commercial sales.[5] Here is a short list of the pros and cons of various funding methods so that you know what your options are:

- Friends and family: Obtaining funding from people you know can be a delicate matter, because there may be other expectations from them. If you are not able to pay the money back, it can damage the relationship. The advantage of this funding source is that it can be easy to obtain.
- Presale of products: With this option, you must be very confident and be careful the deal goes through; otherwise you'll be stuck with the bill! You can pitch your idea to a distributor, get the order, and have them pay to make the product.
- Savings: This can be your best option for funding, if you have enough money saved.

CONFIDENTIAL INFORMATION AND NON-COMPETITION AGREEMENT

This Agreement is made with an effective date of _____, 2006, by Charissa Shaw on the one hand (hereinafter known as "TBE") and _____, (hereinafter known as "Consultant"). This agreement is included within and is part of the Independent Consultant Agreement between the Consultant and TBE.

RECITALS

Whereas, the parties acknowledge that TBE is engaged in a very narrow, unique facet of the ergonomic consulting and sales industry which is very limited in scope in that it is custom-tailored to a small group of clients who may potentially be interested in custom-tailored processes, designs and products, in addition to customer lists which have been compiled by the TBE through unique and proprietary processes; and

Whereas, the parties acknowledge that the existence and survival of the TBE depends on the protection of the processes, designs and products, client lists and related information, the customer lists and related information solicited to clients and/or potential clients, and information as to formulas and processes involved in compiling the business, customer and client lists and related information; and

TBE desires to appoint Consultant as advisor/consultant to TBE, whose duties are to service the needs of the clients, evaluate their ergonomic needs, design proper workspaces, sell appropriate products to facilitate same, and to help solicit sales to prospective and existing clients;

Whereas, to complete these duties, TBE must disclose to Consultant information related to TBE business operations, plans, manufacturing processes, including, without limitation, client lists, customer lists, techniques, methods, formulas, and products as well as other confidential information regarding the TBE, all of which is proprietary, confidential, and necessary for the existence and survival of the TBE (hereinafter referred to as "Confidential Information"), and TBE and Consultant wish to ensure that TBE interest in Confidential Information is protected and all information is retained in confidence by Consultant and remains proprietary information of the TBE;

Therefore, Consultant agrees to the following terms and undertakings in consideration of the TBE disclosure of such Confidential Information and for other good and valuable consideration. For purposes of this agreement, "TBE" shall also include all Consultants, subsidiaries and affiliates of TBE.

AGREEMENT

1. Use of Information Limited to Agreed Purpose

    1.01 The parties acknowledge that the TBE has or will make available to Consultant certain confidential information as defined below for the purpose of allowing Consultant to perform certain services with TBE, and such Confidential Information is to be used by Consultant on an as needed basis. The parties specifically acknowledge their understanding that the TBE would not make such disclosures of Confidential Information to the Consultant except for the sole purpose set forth in this section, and only with the protection provided in this Agreement.

2. Confidential Information

    2.01 Any written, printed, graphic, verbalized, electronically or magnetically recorded information furnished by TBE for Consultant's use, as stated above are the sole property of TBE. This proprietary information includes but is not limited to; (i) customer requirements, (ii) customer lists, (iii) marketing information, (iv) marketing strategies, (v) information concerning TBE Consultants, (vi) TBE products, (vii) TBE services, (viii) TBE prices, (ix) TBE operation, and (x) TBE related affiliates and subsidiaries.

    2.02 Consultant agrees to keep this Confidential Information in the strict confidence and will not disclose it by any means to any person(s) except with TBE approval, or as given by TBE president or other individual specifically empowered by TBE to approve use of Confidential Information and only to the extent

FIGURE **21-4** Nondisclosure agreement (NDA).   *Continued* necessary to perform the services under this Agreement. This prohibition also applies to Consultant, Consultant's agents, and sub-contractors. Upon termination of this Agreement, Consultant will return any Confidential Information in his/her possession to the TBE.

3. Proprietary Interest in TBE Competitors

3.01 The parties agree that while any contract for services between Consultant and TBE is in force, Consultant will not acquire any interest, either directly or deferred in any manner, including without limitation, stock, stock options, warrants, subscriptions, or other ownership vehicle, in any competitor's TBE who provides services within the ergonomic industry.

4. Non-Solicitation

4.01 For a period of two (2) years following either the termination of an executed contract for services between TBE and Consultant, or upon review of Confidential Information as set forth in the first paragraph of this Agreement, Consultant will not do either of the following: (i) call on, solicit, or take away any of TBE customers or potential customers Consultant became aware of as a result of performing services under any Agreement with TBE, or a result of reviewing TBE documents; or (ii) solicit or hire any of TBE Consultants or contractors Consultant became aware of as a result of performing services under any service Agreements with TBE or as a result of reviewing information as set forth in the first paragraph of this Agreement. TBE and Consultant agree that because TBE business is conducted nationwide there should not be a geographical limitation applied to this Agreement.

4.02 Consultant agrees not to seek or accept employment with any competitor of the TBE or any TBE which proprietary knowledge gained while under contract of the TBE could be used. Consultant will not work for contacts made during the terms of this contract, for a period of two (2) years after the termination of this Contract, unless such work would in no way involve the use of proprietary information obtained while under contract with the TBE.

5. No Warranties Provided As To Information Made Available

5.01 Consultant understands and agrees that TBE makes no warranties, whether expressed or implied concerning the validity, accuracy, or completeness of any information provided to Consultant and that such information is provided to Consultant with no warranties of merchantability or fitness whether expressed or implied.

6. Breach of Agreement

6.01 In the event of any violation of this Agreement by Consultant, TBE shall be entitled to: (i) immediately terminate any contract for services with Consultant, (ii) obtain injunctive and other equitable relief to reduce damages to TBE as a result of Consultant's breach, and to pursue all civil damages available against Consultant. The parties acknowledge and agree that time is of the essence and that immediate action by way of injunctive relief is appropriate in order to minimize any potential harm to the existence and survival of the TBE as a result of any breach of this Agreement by Consultant.

TBE
Charissa Shaw, President   Consultant:

By: _____   By: _____
(Signature)   (Signature)

_____   _____
(Typed or Printed Name)   (Typed or Printed Name)

Title: _____

FIGURE **21-4, cont'd**

Box 21-4	*Sample Business Plan Outline*

Courtesy Palo Alto Software: *Sample business plans.* Retrieved July 30, 2006, from www.paloalto.com/ps/bp/acmeconsulting_live.pdf.

As long as you believe in your business and stick with it, you will be sure to get a return on your own investment.

- Credit cards: This is another option to fund your business, especially if you can obtain a low teaser interest rate. You can even use your airline credit cards and get free tickets as you fund your business! With this option, it is important to work fast, get your cash flow positive, and be able to make monthly payments so your interest rate stays low.

- SBA or bank loans: Getting a loan is a great way to obtain financing for your business and still keep equity and control over your company. SBA loans can have lower interest rates than bank loans and, depending on your credit and interest rates, can be an amazing deal. Banks also require sources of collateral (personal assets like a house), down payment (that means you need to also invest your own money), credit record, management ability (resumes of the management team), and ability to repay the loan (cash flow projections). Make sure you make monthly payments; otherwise the bank will get your business!

- Grants: Believe it or not, there is free money set aside by the government to help you succeed in your business. For example, if you live in a U.S. Department of Housing and Urban Development (HUD) zone there are many government grants available to start a business in these underdeveloped areas. In addition, the National Institute of Health (NIH) has specific grants called the Small Business Innovation Research (SBIR) and Small Business Technology Transfer (STTR) programs (see Resources at the end of the chapter). However, these grants are not for product development and marketing, and it is important for you to contact NIH for details.[1] Also, certain cities may have special programs; for instance, the city in which I live offers $5000 for residents who are opening a store.

- Angel investing: This type of funding is applicable if you have been in your business less than 2 years and are asking for less than one million dollars. Angel investors will typically let you have more control of the company and more equity, as long as they receive a good return on their investment (ROI).

- Venture funding (also known as venture capital [VC] funding) is what you look for when you have had success on your own for 2 years or more, are looking for one million dollars or more, and are anticipating a viable ROI within a few years. For this option, your exit strategy needs to be clearly defined and your investors will want to know, "What's in it for me?" Venture capitalists will typically obtain equity and ownership in the company in addition to providing the management expertise to facilitate your success.
- Giving back: Developing a charitable trust for your organization is a great way to give back to your community. Once you achieve the point at which you have succeeded in your business, it is important to identify non-profit organizations that fall in line with your values and give time or money to these causes.

Exit Strategy

In Covey's classic, *The Seven Habits of Highly Effective People*, the seventh habit is to begin with the end in mind.[4] Think about your business exit strategy and your options, such as the following:

- Sell your business or merge
- Go public
- Stay private and grow

Give yourself a timeline, perhaps 10 years, and see yourself as a successful entrepreneur, then figure out what steps you need to take to achieve that level of success.[19] Who will want to buy your business? Identify potential "suitors" now and write them down. This is an important step in the business plan if you are looking for funding, so be very clear on this point.

CONCLUSION

Kiyosaki states that when owning a business, "growth and success are dependent on being strong and flexible."[13] Being an entrepreneur is a

---

Learning Exercise

Overview

This exercise is designed to apply the various examples of therapists-turned-entrepreneurs to your situation and learn the basics of starting a business.

Purpose

The purpose of the exercise is to evaluate your current status and what the next steps are in starting your business.

Exercise

Brainstorm all the areas of practice within ergonomics that you can see yourself doing. Write a one-page business plan using the outline provided. Do a competitive analysis of your practice area. Visualize yourself in the ideal business 5 years from now, then backtrack and list the steps required to get you there.

---

process, and you have to adapt to change, keeping your mind open to the ever-changing world. It is not an endpoint. There is a need to continuously learn, grow, and stay one step ahead of the competition.

The field of ergonomics is vast, and there are endless unexplored opportunities that are just beginning to emerge. Enjoy the journey, and may your new venture be successful and prosperous!

Multiple Choice Review Questions

1. What is an S Corporation?
   A. A sole proprietorship
   B. A sales corporation
   C. A service corporation
   D. A separate entity or company with no more than 100 stockholders

2. What does NDA stand for?
   A. Not doing anything
   B. Nondisclosure agreement
   C. Not disclosing anything
   D. Negotiating Deals Association

3. What is the value in developing products for your business?
   A. Passive income
   B. Brand recognition
   C. Expansion of the offering to your clients
   D. Opening up your mind to new possibilities

4. If you have a new product idea, do you need a patent?
   A. No
   B. Yes
   C. Sometimes; if you go to market fast and are the first to market you may not need a patent, but realize that other people make develop knockoffs within 6 months

5. Which one of the following statements is an exit strategy?
   A. Get out now
   B. Go public
   C. Move to Tahiti
   D. Put your money in a Swiss bank account

6. When receiving VC funding, it is understood that:
   A. the VC investors will have equity in the company.
   B. the funding is for one million dollars or less.
   C. there is low risk.
   D. you will get a low interest rate.

7. A vision statement is:
   A. necessary when starting your business.
   B. your company mission.
   C. your market and where you see your company 5 years from now.

8. When writing your business plan, the following component should be added under "Management Summary":
   A. Break-even analysis
   B. Organizational structure
   C. Sales strategy
   D. Company information

9. You should finish your executive summary of your business plan:
   A. first.
   B. last.
   C. halfway through the business plan.
   D. never.

10. One characteristic of entrepreneurs is that they are:
    A. frugal.
    B. creative.
    C. aggressive.
    D. organized.

REFERENCES

1. Abrams SL, editor: *The small business financial resource guide*, ed 7, Herndon, Va, 2003, Braddock Communications, Inc.
2. Argosy Health: Implementing an on-site return to work program, Presentation, El Segundo, Calif, 2004.
3. Collins J: *Good to great*, New York, 2001, Harper Collins.
4. Covey SR: *The seven habits of highly effective people*, New York, 1989, Fireside.
5. Dollinger MJ: *Entrepreneurship strategies and resources*, ed 2, Upper Saddle River, NJ, 1999, Prentice Hall.
6. Eker TH: *Speedwealth*, ed 2, 2001, Peak Potentials Publishing.
7. Gerber ME: *The E-myth revisited*, New York, 1995, Harper Collins.
8. Gladwell M: *The tipping point*, New York, 2002, Back Bay Books/Little Brown and Company.
9. Hamilton AC, Lunsford RA, Rosa RR et al, editors: *Worker health chartbook*, Washington DC, 2004, National Institute of Occupational Safety and Health.
10. Horan J: *The one page business plan*, Berkeley, 2004, The One Page Business Plan Company.
11. Jacobs K: *Entrepreneurship for ergonomics professionals*, Presentation at the Eastern Ergonomics Conference and Exposition, Boston, Mass, 2006.
12. Jacobs K, Russo P: *Entrepreneurship for the ergonomics professional*, Eastern Ergonomics Conference and Exposition, Boston, Mass, June 2006.
13. Kiyosaki R: Building the better biz, *Entrepreneur* June:172, 2006.

14. Leeuwenburgh C: *Preventing strength and muscle loss in the elderly, Florida, 2003.* Retrieved September 28, 2006, from http://www.napa.ufl.edu/2003news/oldmuscles.htm#contact.

15. Moss W: *Starting from scratch: secrets from 21 ordinary people who made the entrepreneurial leap,* Chicago, 2005, Dearborne Trade Publishing.

16. Petouhoff NL: *How to get your invention off the ground,* Marina Del Rey, Calif, 2004, Dr. Nat the Techno Cat Press.

17. Pressman D: *Patent it yourself,* 2003, Consolidated Printers.

18. Redding P: *Solving office ergonomic issues: where to focus and what to do,* Presentation at the Eastern Ergonomics Conference and Exposition, New York, 2005.

19. Robbins W: *Millionaire women's secrets of success* (CD), 1999. Available online at www.Millionaire-women.com.

20. Sokolosky V: *Do you have the right stuff to be an entrepreneur?* Retrieved August 2, 2006, from www.valerieandcompany.com.

RESOURCES

Alimed: www.alimed.com

Automate your ergonomics program: www.automateyourprogram.com

Business Incorporation, Forms, Attorney Search: www.nolo.com

Ergo Innovations (products): www.ergo-innovations.com

Ergonomics, Safety and Wellness Consulting: www.elysianhealth.com

Ergoboy: www.ergoboy.com

Ergolifestyle: www.ergolifestyle.com

Ergoweb: www.ergoweb.com

ErgoWorks: www.askergoworks.com

Humantech: www.humantech.com

National Venture Capital Association: www.nvca.org

Prevention Plus: www.preventionplusinc.com.

Questions about Ergonomics: www.asktheergonomist.com

Rotary International: www.rotary.org

Service Corporation of Retired Executives: www.score.org

Small Business Administration: www.sba.gov

Small Business Funding and Grants: http://grants.nih.gov/grants/funding/sbir.htm

U.S. Chamber of Commerce Small Business Institute www.uschamber.com

U.S. Department of Commerce: www.commerce.gov

U.S. Patent Office: www.uspto.gov

Writing Your Business Plan: www.planware.org

Sample Job Analysis and Design Considerations

Naomi Abrams

Learning Objectives

After reading this section and completing the exercises, the reader should be able to do the following:

1. Identify hazards assessed during an ergonomic job site analysis.
2. Identify engineering, administrative, and work practice controls.
3. Identify the differences in reporting recommendations from ergonomic job site assessments depending on referral source and client type.

Musician ergonomics. The study of the positions, methods, and factors influencing how musicians use their instruments.

Parenting. The daily routines, activities, and methods involved in caring for infants and young children.

Documentation. The method of reporting job site analysis findings and recommendations.

Methods of evaluating ergonomic concerns within the workplace have been discussed in detail in previous chapters. A therapist may be consulted regarding ergonomic issues in a variety of situations. Evaluations may take place in a therapy clinic, on a job site, in a simulated job site, or in a person's home. Therapists can approach the case with multiple frames of reference depending on their training, the type of job they are evaluating, and the location of the evaluation. Once the evaluation is completed, the therapist is responsible for presenting the recommendations to the referral source and the client in a method that encourages follow-through.

Recommendations may address engineering, administrative, or work practice controls. The cases described in this Appendix are examples of both consultation and the incorporation of ergonomic principles into the typical occupational or physical therapy treatment process.

Four case reports are presented and discussed. The first case is an evaluation completed in the client's home at the client's request. Recommendations were initiated using equipment immediately available in the client's home. A summary was provided for the client's reference as she attempts to follow through with the recommendations.

The second case is an evaluation that was completed as part of a comprehensive course of occupational therapy treatment. Recommendations were initiated over a period of 3 months and the client was given specifications for items to purchase that were later tested at home, at work, and in the clinic. The results of these changes were assessed, and the course of treatment was modified based on the level of integration and application by the client. Reports were generated for the referring physician, the client, and the insurance company.

The third case is an example of a worksite evaluation completed at the employee's request. Recommendations that addressed administrative controls and engineering controls were presented to the employer, and the employee was educated regarding work practice controls. The report provided a summary for both the employer and employee.

The final case example goes through the process of collecting data for a job database. Differences between collecting data for an individual worker versus for a population of workers and the values and limitations of this process are highlighted.

CASE STUDY 1: THE NEW MOTHER

Client Name: Trish
Occupation: Mother of 11-week-old son, Zeke
Date of Evaluation: May 3, 2006
Time Allotted for Evaluation: 1.5 hours
Evaluator: Naomi Abrams, MOT, OTR/L

History and Interview

An ergonomic evaluation was completed at the client's home on May 3, 2006. Trish reported that her current primary occupation is in the home, caring for her 11-week-old son. Before the birth of her son she was a practicing orthopedic physical therapist. At the time of evaluation, Zeke weighed 14 pounds, 7 ounces. Trish's primary complaints included low back pain, fatigue, and numbness and tingling in her left thenar eminence. She reported that pain typically occurred while carrying Zeke. She is right-hand dominant and tends to carry Zeke on her left side in order to use her right hand for home management tasks.

Past medical history is negative for any pregnancy-related carpal tunnel symptoms or significant low back pain. She noted that Zeke tends to hold his head to the right, and she recently had been trying to carry Zeke more in her right arm in order to promote a left gaze. She had tried wearing a prefabricated wrist cock-up splint on the left wrist while carrying Zeke in order to decrease pain. Also, she noted a decline in her own nutrition as a result of eating what she could with one hand while carrying Zeke.

Job Duties

1. *Feeding:* Trish breast-feeds using a Boppy pillow (a pillow shaped in a half-circle to fit around her body) while seated on the couch. The pillow provides support for most of Zeke's weight while he feeds and leaves both of her hands free for positioning his head.

2. *Diaper changing:* Trish uses the top of a clothing dresser as a changing table, with a baby pillow providing cushioning for Zeke.

3. *Car seat use:* Trish currently uses an infant car seat–carrier that weighs 9 pounds and is 28 inches long (head area to foot area), 16 inches at its widest including the handle, and 22 inches tall when the handle is in its most upright position. She uses this as a means of carrying Zeke when in the community. It fits into a holder in the car for transport. The coupling device is fixed to the center rear seat of her SUV. She feels that this is the most comfortable and safe position for her to keep watch over Zeke in the car.

4. *Carrying:* Trish reports that Zeke enjoys being held and walked. She reports that this is often the only way he calms down to sleep. It is also a method of interaction between the two of them, and they both enjoy dancing throughout the day as a form of play.

5. *Play time:* Trish has a play area for Zeke on the floor of the living area. It consists of a padded mat with a pillow to hold Zeke in a semi-reclined position to engage in play with overhead stimuli. Also, she often spends time interacting with him on the couch. During this time, he sits supported by the Boppy pillow and she sits on the couch.

Hazards Noted

1. *Feeding*

The couch used during feeding and play time provides poor postural support and is too deep for her to rest her feet on the floor (Figure A-1). This encourages a rounded kyphotic spine, which puts pressure on her back.

She uses feeding time to interact with Zeke, often spending longer than 10 minutes with a downward gaze. This further encourages a rounded posture.

2. *Diaper changing*

The changing dresser height is 46 inches (including the pillow). Trish is 63 inches tall; her elbow height from the floor is 41 inches. In order to place Zeke on the cushion, she has to lift him over her shoulder height. This places unnecessary

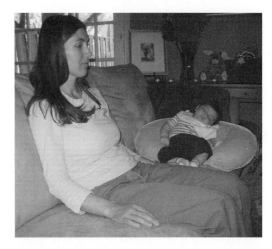

FIGURE **A-1** Seated posture on the couch without support.

strain on her back and upper extremities as well as placing her wrists at awkward angles.

The cushion on the changing dresser centers Zeke 12 inches away from the edge of the dresser. She tends to grasp Zeke under both axilla in order to place and lift him. This causes her to twist while lifting, placing strain on her back and shoulders.

To lift his legs while changing his diaper, she holds her shoulders in an elevated position because of the height of the changing surface.

3. *Car seat use*

While carrying Zeke in the baby carrier–car seat, Trish holds the carrier by the handle, in one hand off to her right or left, causing an awkward gait and compensatory lean (Figure A-2). This places strain on her low back and shoulder. Carrying Zeke in the carrier for an extended period using a two-handed grasp is not comfortable because the carrier has rough edges at the head and foot area. Also, the length of 28 inches causes her to abduct her shoulders, placing stress at her shoulders and neck.

She most often loads the carrier from the driver's side because of the location of the car in the driveway. In order to load and unload the carrier from the car, she lifts the carrier by the handle until it rests on the rear SUV seat, stabilizes herself

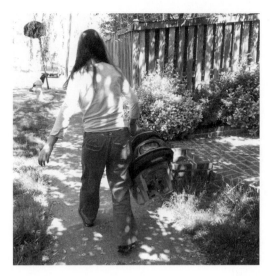

FIGURE **A-2** Mother carrying baby car seat–carrier with one arm.

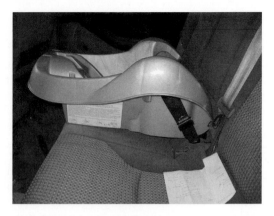

FIGURE **A-3** Car seat coupling device.

on the SUV seat, lifts the carrier with Zeke inside, and reaches more than 22 inches to place the carrier inside the coupler (Figure A-3). She also has to guide the carrier up and over the lip of the coupling component 12 inches above the car seat. She often bumps the ceiling of the car with the carrier handle during these maneuvers. With Zeke in the carrier, she is lifting approximately 23 pounds. This awkward movement places a large amount of strain on her spine and upper extremities.

4. *Carrying*

Trish tends to carry Zeke in her left arm with her left hand cupped under his buttocks and resting on her left hip. This places stress along her left wrist from the sustained wrist flexion and digital flexion force.

When carrying Zeke, she stands with an exaggerated lordotic curve in her lumbar spine, leaning back slightly to compensate for his weight. She reports this is the time she experiences the majority of her low back pain.

5. *Play time*

When placing Zeke in the Boppy pillow on the couch, she first sits with Zeke against her chest, then twists and bends in order to put him in the fold of the pillow. This places increased strain on her back and shoulders.

The play area on the floor is surrounded by the couch, wall, and coffee table in order to keep it out of reach of the family dog. Trish sits in a sustained full squat holding Zeke while she arranges the pillow in order to put Zeke inside the play area. She often uses a twisted position to get him in and out because of the location of the coffee table.

6. *General complaints*

Trish reports a decrease in overall nutrition because of time spent caring for Zeke.

Trish notes fatigue that limits tolerance for play and her own self-care. Fatigue could be caused by a general decrease in uninterrupted sleep, resulting from nighttime care of Zeke, common to mothers of infants.

Trish reports general musculoskeletal aches that have been persistent since Zeke's birth.

Recommendations

Engineering Controls

1. *Feeding:* Use a pillow behind her low back to increase postural support (Figure A-4). A pillow will also push her toward the edge of the couch, allowing her to rest her feet either on the floor or on the coffee table.

2. *Diaper changing:* Use a 10-inch stepstool to decrease the height of the lift when placing or lifting Zeke. This also addresses the elevated

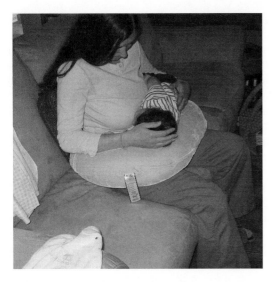

FIGURE **A-4** Seated posture while breast-feeding with back support and Boppy pillow.

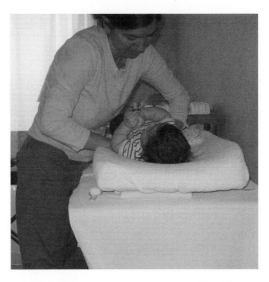

FIGURE **A-5** Reaching and twisting while lifting Zeke off changing table.

shoulder position when changing his diaper. The stool should be large enough for her to stand comfortably on both feet.

3. *Car seat use:* Limit carrying the baby carrier by using a stroller whenever possible.

4. *Play time:* Shift the coffee table away from the play area so that she is able to take Zeke in and out of the play area without twisting her spine.

Work Practice Controls

1. *Feeding*

Rest her foot on the coffee table (the same side Zeke is feeding on), in order to use her leg position to raise his head instead of using a sustained hold with that hand during feeding.

Use some of the time Zeke is feeding to complete neck and upper spine stretches. (Because of her professional training, it was not necessary to formally cover stretches during this evaluation.)

2. *Diaper changing*

Try using varying methods when lifting and lowering Zeke. Trish is able to use one hand to lift him into a seated position, then two hands to turn him to face her. Once in this position, she can more easily pull him to her shoulder without lifting his whole body weight or twisting her body (Figure A-5).

3. *Car seat use*

Various methods of loading and unloading the car seat were examined during the evaluation, including the following:

- Loading from the driver's side: Trish stands with her right foot on the runner and left foot inside the car. This increases the amount of reaching and leaning that she is required to use to load and unload the seat. Because of her hand dominance, she is not comfortable when she tries using the more stabilized version similar to the position she uses on the other side of the car. However, she reports less back discomfort using the stabilized method, and she should practice this method to see if it can become less awkward.

- Loading the seat from the passenger side of the car: In this position she is comfortable, stabilizing herself with her left knee on the seat and right foot firmly planted inside the car. This decreases her reach from over 22 inches to 12-15 inches. Decreasing her reach decreases the strain on her back and shoulders.

- Lowering the handle: She attempts to load the seat with the carrying handle raised to its highest carrying angle. When this handle is lowered, she has less of a tendency to hit the handle on the ceiling of the car and has more room for maneuvering. This decreases the amount of strain on her shoulders and arms and the amount of twisting of her spine.

4. *Carrying*

Trish reports using a wrist brace while carrying Zeke to decrease wrist pain. The splint provides a neuromuscular cue to keep her wrist and hand relaxed while carrying. However, she tends to compensate with her finger flexors while wearing the splint, placing her at risk for straining the muscles in her forearm. Instead of using the splint, she should continue to alternate arms, use both arms under his buttocks, and use a baby carrier. By using a front-mounted baby carrier, she has both hands free for home management tasks and her own self-care. Trish reports that Zeke does not particularly like the baby carrier; however, this could be a result of conditioning. She should primarily use the brace during the night to rest her wrist.

Two methods are suggested for addressing the lordotic lumbar curve. Both provide brief pain relief. As Zeke gets heavier, shorter periods of "dancing" should be used, perhaps replacing dancing with bouncing on her lap while Trish is seated. These include activating core musculature to straighten her spine for short periods of exercise (Figure A-6) and using a resting position against the wall.

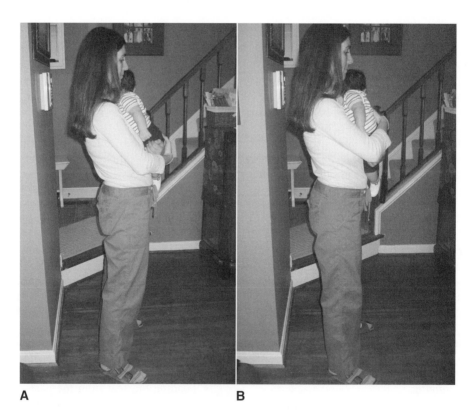

A   **B**

FIGURE **A-6 A,** Standing with baby without correcting for hyperlordotic posture. **B,** Standing with baby while correcting for hyperlordotic posture.

5. *Play time*

Trish should leave Zeke supported on the couch while she arranges the pillow in the play area, limiting the exposure time of the awkward squat and hold position.

6. *Generalized complaints*

Regarding Trish's nutritional needs, we determined that she could use his car seat in the house as a safe place for him to sit in the kitchen while she uses two hands to prepare and eat a meal. She understands that Zeke may become restless at first at not being held; however, she also understands that he will adjust. She verbalized awareness of how nutrition can affect her fatigue and believes that she can address this issue without added help.

Administrative Control

Trish should speak to her husband regarding providing care for Zeke for a few hours while she treats herself to a massage session at least a few times a month.

Summary

Trish noted multiple areas of concern during this evaluation including decreasing upper extremity pain, low back pain, and fatigue. During an evaluation of her current daily tasks around the home while caring for Zeke, areas for change were identified. These changes addressed her habits, techniques, and tools to initiate comprehensive change. Many of these changes will require practice and paying attention during what used to be rote tasks. She was reminded that these changes need to be gradual and was encouraged to ask her family for assistance.

Case Discussion

The evaluation of Trish and Zeke took place in their home, where Trish spends most of her time. Trish cares for Zeke 24 hours a day. An evaluation of her entire day needed to be compressed into an hour and a half. In one evaluation, we were able to examine many key aspects of Zeke's care and transportation. This allowed both the therapist and client to examine how the principles reviewed could be applied to other areas within Trish's day, including home management and self-care.

Engineering controls applied to the issues that arose concerning the care of Zeke include modifications to the couch she uses for feeding and the locations of play areas and care areas and the use of a step stool. These changes had to take into account that Zeke will continue to grow and that, although certain areas may not be causing direct strain now, the areas of potential stress need to be addressed.

Zeke's growth was an especially important factor in the consideration of the length of time that Trish spends carrying him around the house. As he gains weight and height, the stress of carrying him with one arm will become more hazardous. Trish's belief that it was important to always hold him had to be addressed as part of the work practice controls. Additional work practice controls included using Trish's background as a physical therapist to promote postural changes and stretches during her day and modifying how she carried Zeke. Many of the techniques recommended will require practice in order to apply them while also accounting for Zeke's needs.

Administrative controls took on a different meaning with this evaluation. While she did not have a supervisory structure to work within, she does have "co-workers": her husband and Zeke. Improved communication of needs between herself and her husband was necessary to establish a shorter work time and to add rest periods. She also needed to change her perception of Zeke's needs and remember to address her own needs. Protecting her own health will better assist her in dealing with Zeke's needs in the long term.

CASE STUDY 2: THE VIOLA PLAYER

Client Name: Pat
Medical Record Number: 12-34-45
Occupation: Professional viola player, music teacher (viola and violin)
Employer: Self-employed, contractor
Date of Evaluation: February 13, 2006
Referral Source: Dr. F.
Additional Services Prescribed: Occupational therapy

History and Interview

The client came to the clinic with diagnoses of left median nerve entrapment and right ulnar nerve entrapment. An ergonomic evaluation was ordered along with occupational therapy evaluation and treatment. The client is a 52-year-old woman who reported primary complaints of pain in bilateral upper extremities, left shoulder, and low back. Past medical history was significant for a bleeding disorder, which limits the client's ability to tolerate supine positions, thermal changes, and elevated heart rate (such as with exercise) and makes her prone to nosebleeds.

The client reported pain with driving, writing, hanging up clothes, and playing her viola and violin. At the time of the evaluation she was unable to play without symptoms. Her pain management techniques included gentle heat treatments and walking. Her paid occupations include performing by contract with various chamber orchestras and teaching the viola and violin. She reported that her chief concern was playing her viola (primary source of income), and therefore the evaluation and treatment focused on the viola playing. Her unpaid occupations included caring for three grandchildren under the age of 8.

Summary of Physical Findings

On evaluation it was noted that the client demonstrated poor postural stability with her core musculature. She tended to sit and stand with a posterior pelvic tilt. Sensation testing demonstrated minimal loss along the ulnar distribution on the right and median distribution on the left. Strength testing of her upper extremities found a decrease throughout (scored 4 of 5), including shoulder and scapular stabilizers. Tinel's test was negative for both upper extremities for the ulnar and median nerves.

Job Duties

Viola Performances

1. Dress appropriately for performances (black dress)
2. Attend rehearsals and performances with her instrument
3. Tune her instrument

4. Rehearse and perform for more than 1 hour pieces of varying difficulty and physical requirements chosen by the company

Music Teaching

1. Teach viola and violin to students with various levels of proficiency
2. Maintain schedule of classes and private students
3. Demonstrate viola and violin when appropriate
4. Contact students and their families as needed
5. Complete billing procedures
6. Organize end-of-semester performances by students

Summary of Ergonomic Evaluation

The client's viola playing was observed in the clinic using a chair without arms, similar to what the client reported she was required to use during performances.

Hazards Noted

1. *Viola playing*

She had the tendency to sit in a forward lean throughout her playing in order to see the conductor (Figure A-7). This position caused her to extend her cervical spine. She also played the viola with her shoulders elevated in a shrug. This placed strains on her low back, neck, and shoulders. These positions also increased her tendency toward nerve entrapment and forearm strain.

While playing, she had the tendency to keep her left wrist in a flexed position along the neck of the viola. This put pressure along her median nerve.

In order to stabilize her instrument while playing, she had a tendency to use forcible left lateral neck flexion at the chin rest. She also used this position during tuning to hold the instrument while making adjustments with her left hand (the right hand held the bow or plucked the strings). Additional force was used when she wore her performance dress because the fabric did not provide enough friction to secure the shoulder rest. These sustained forcible holds put stress

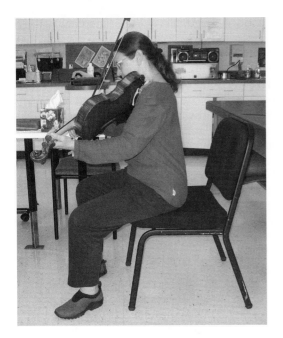

FIGURE **A-7** Pretreatment sitting posture while playing the viola.

along her cervical spine and shoulder musculature.

She reported additional back pain that occurred while playing the viola in a standing position. It was noted during the evaluation that she had a tendency to stand with a hyperlordotic posture, "slumping" her low spine while curving her upper spine forward into a C shape.

2. *Tuning*

The instrument required a forcible pinch with the left hand while ulnarly and radially deviating the wrist, putting strain on the wrist and fingers.

3. *Transporting*

Back pain was reported during carrying, lifting, and lowering the viola in the case and getting the viola out of the case. It was noted that the client often placed the viola on a chair or on the floor when getting it out of the case. This increased the compressive forces on her spine. She also had the tendency to twist and reach while lifting the case off the floor. These postures increased the risk of low back strain.

During her teaching, the client reported that she often carried her instrument for long periods of time.

Recommendations and Intervention

The following is a summary of interventions that took place over a series of 13 occupational therapy appointments in conjunction with treatment for the diagnosed conditions. Further discussion of OT treatment is included at the end of this summary.

Engineering Controls

1. *Viola playing*

Recommended the use of a back support pillow because of the straight-backed chairs typically provided for orchestra members. Also recommended the use of a seat cushion in the shape of a wedge (tilting down toward the front of the chair) to release client's hip muscles and encourage an upright posture while still allowing her to plant her feet on the floor to give her a stable base of support. The client was able to purchase a lightweight cushion and back pillow that she can comfortably transport to rehearsals and performances (Figure A-8).

The shoulder rest of the viola was built up using $^3/_4$-inch foam (Figure A-9). This was added to the sponges the client was already using for this same purpose. The added height decreased the amount of lateral neck flexion required as well as increasing the friction between the rest and her clothing.

2. *Tuning*

To address the pinch required for tuning and the hand pain noted, it was recommended that the client work with a viola maker to assess the potential for having larger tuning pegs installed.

Work Practice Controls

1. *Viola playing*

Educated the client regarding the effects of sustained forward postures on low back strain. Recommended using the music to guide weight shifts and pelvic tilts. The client was able to identify times when the music guided her to lean forward (intense and emotional measures) and "rest periods" (background or quiet measures)

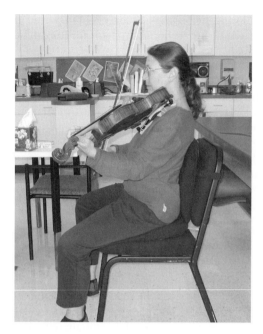

FIGURE **A-8** Modified viola playing posture with supportive cushions.

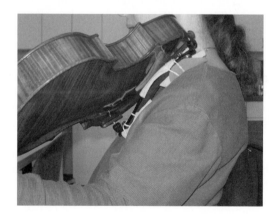

FIGURE **A-9** Modifications made to shoulder rest.

during which she could lean back and rest her low back.

Worked with the client in the clinic over several sessions to identify alternative wrist positions for both her right hand with the bow and left hand on the neck of the viola. The client was able to identify comfortable wrist positions available to various fingering techniques with the left hand. With her right hand, she was able to shift the movement from being primarily in the elbow and wrist with the shoulder held in a static shrug to being a combination of shoulder, elbow, and wrist movements. By varying her wrist position and arm use, she was able to decrease discomfort and muscle fatigue experienced during playing.

The client was coached to become aware of how much force was needed to stabilize the instrument versus what she was applying to the chin rest. She was able to determine that she was able to keep her head resting very lightly on the chin rest and was able to use certain measures in the music to straighten out her head for rest periods.

It was recommended that while standing to play (required only in classes, not performances) she alternate standing postures using a 2- to 4-inch step. Trying this in the clinic, she was able to alternate placing each foot on the step to release her lumbar spine. This improved her low back pain when she stands to play.

2. *Tuning*

It was recommended that she complete as much of the tuning as possible with the instrument resting on her lap, decreasing the duration and frequency of wrist flexion and neck lateral flexion required at a given time.

3. *Transporting*

Through practice, the client was taught how to decrease the amount of twisting while lifting from the floor as well as alternative lift positions to decrease lumbar strain. It was recommended that she practice placing her instrument on a higher surface, such as a table, during the loading and unloading.

With regard to carrying her instrument while teaching, she was able to identify an area in her teaching space where she felt safe resting her instrument and bow. She noted she was able to put the viola down more with practice and really carried it out of habit, not need.

Occupational Therapy Summary

Occupational therapy treatment focused on modulating pain, increasing strength and endurance, and modifying activities of daily living. Positions of comfort were identified so as to modulate pain. Gentle thermal modalities were also used to decrease pain. Exercises included shoulder stabilization, pelvic floor stabilization, and pelvic and back shifting to provide low back pain relief. Each exercise was completed seated or standing using gravity or small repeated pulses for resistance. Adaptive equipment and methods of joint protection were discussed, and the client was provided with time to try techniques in the clinic.

In addition, during the course of treatment it was noted that the client's pain was linked to her stress levels during her daily activities including caring for her family. Occupational therapy treatment included education regarding methods to decrease stress and decrease the body's response to stressful situations. This included deep breathing and assessment of priorities. The client was referred to a pain and stress management specialist for further training as needed.

Summary

The evaluation and recommendations summarized in this report were practiced during the course of occupational therapy treatment. During progressive treatments, the client noted decreased difficulty during performances and teaching. She also reported a decrease in general pain during her daily tasks. Further follow-up may be required as she reintegrates into her previous performance schedule.

Case Discussion

It is not typical to see clients for 13 visits for an ergonomic evaluation. In my clinic's setup, we combine occupational therapy treatment and ergonomic evaluations when needed per doctor's orders or client need. In this case it was determined that the client had underlying strength deficits and extenuating circumstances that required in-depth treatment. Ergonomic controls would not have addressed her primary complaints sufficiently to allow her to return to a demanding concert and rehearsal schedule. Therefore her treatment was based on a multilayer approach.

Engineering and work practice controls were recommended. Administrative controls were not applicable to this case because the client was self-employed and contracted into jobs that are not adaptable at the administrative level. The instrument itself limited the extent to which engineering controls could be applied.

Engineering controls were used to address contact stresses, postural stresses, and joint pain. These included changing the shoulder rest in order to raise the chin rest, adding portable cushions to her chair and changing the tuning knobs. Work practice controls were used to address postural stresses, nerve compression forces, and joint pain. These included using positional shifts during play, changing neck positions during play, using rest periods, and changing her movements while using the bow or strings.

A large portion of the occupational therapy treatment was used to address the client's body awareness. This included elevated muscular tension and body postures. During the initial ergonomic evaluation, it was noted that the client was not able to self-assess what type of posture she was in at each moment. When we discussed her "slumped" posture, she would self-correct into a hyperkyphotic posture. In essence, she would overcorrect into another harmful posture. Through practice in front of a mirror and with tactile cues provided by the therapist, she was able to become better aware of her body's position.

Pat reported that she had participated in prior courses of physical therapy in which her posture during playing was addressed. However, she was not able to sustain her ability to properly monitor and self-correct. She also stated that she remembered being taught how to protect her neck and arms while playing when she originally learned to play the viola. She found that, with practice in this clinic, she was able to use her previous learning as well as the new techniques addressed in this course of treatment. It was also recommended that she occasionally spend time with fellow viola players to problem-solve pains associated with playing in order to promote better follow-through after discharge from therapy.

Postural deficits and core strength deficits were addressed through both awareness exercises and strengthening exercises. Nerve compression also was treated in therapy through the use of splints, including a wrist cock-up splint for her left wrist and an elbow flexion block splint for her right arm. These splints were worn at night and provided rest for her nerves. Joint pain also was addressed through the use of modalities.

Stress was addressed during the extended occupational therapy treatment. It was found that the client could directly relate her pain levels to her stress level and that her stress levels were correlated to her unpaid occupations. These included caring for her elderly father, caring for her children and grandchildren who were living with her, taking care of the household activities, and managing her bleeding disorder. She was noticing decreased sleep patterns and increased overall muscular tension. Stress management techniques were addressed during the occupational therapy sessions including prioritizing activities, learning communication techniques, setting personal and family limits, and taking personal rest periods.

As a result of the holistic approach used by the therapist, the client has demonstrated a full return to her prior performance schedule. At the time of the last treatment, she was able to identify areas of physical and emotional stress and independently identify methods of self-correction.

CASE STUDY 3: THE CHEF INSTRUCTOR

Client Name: Kate
Date of Evaluation: June 10, 2006
Time Allotted: 4 hours (setup, class, and clean up)
Occupation: Chef instructor
Employer: XYZ Cooking School
Evaluator: Naomi Abrams, MOT, OTR/L

History and Interview

An ergonomic evaluation was completed at the XYZ Cooking School at the client's request. Kate reported that she had been teaching cooking for the XYZ Cooking School for the past 2 years. She reported that she has been a chef for the past 5 years, starting in a restaurant for $1\frac{1}{2}$ years and

then working as a caterer. Her current paid occupations include chef instructor and caterer, for both a catering company and a private client (cooking for one family in her own kitchen or in the client's kitchen).

Kate complained of right greater than left wrist pain and occasional numbness and tingling in her fingers. These symptoms have been fluctuating in intensity over the past few years but have recently gotten worse. She had not seen a doctor since the symptoms started. She had been using over-the-counter wrist braces at night as her primary form of symptom management. She reported that recently the symptoms had escalated to the point that a full day's work causes pain and wakes her up at night.

The ergonomic evaluation was completed during the preparation for, and teaching of, a demonstration-style soup-making class at the school. A demonstration class was chosen for observation because this style requires Kate to do most of the cooking. This school also offers a participation class; however, Kate often spends the bulk of that class watching and assisting students. A demonstration class provided the examiner with a better example of all of the tasks Kate was required to complete as a chef.

Job Duties

1. Plan and submit menus to the school, including ingredient lists.
2. Organize the classroom before classes, with the assistance of volunteers.
3. Assemble the items being prepared by the students during the participation classes or needed to cook the food for the demonstration class. This includes the following:
   - Carrying items purchased for the class from her car into the classroom
   - Carrying her uniform and personal cooking tools (usually in a few boxes or canvas bags) into the class from her car
   - Collecting and carrying items from different storage facilities around the building to the classroom
   - Planning the preparation and cooking schedule for herself and the assistants

- Precooking any items as needed; this could include parts of recipes, or entire recipes in cases in which cooking time exceeds class time
  - Directing volunteers in assisting with any of these tasks; the assistants have varying levels of proficiency in the kitchen, and she must adjust her plan based on their skill level
4. Teach the class. This includes preparing a variety of dishes while talking throughout each recipe and answering questions.
5. Participate in cleaning up after the class. This includes washing pots, pans, trays, utensils, and dishes. The amount of cleaning up she performs depends on the number of assistants and whether there is a staff dishwasher present. Often, she is not responsible for most of the cleaning in these classes.

Hazards Noted

1. *Carrying items*

Kate carries items from the car and from the storage areas using crates, sheet trays, or bowls of varying shapes, sizes, and weights, depending on content.

Often the crates, sheet trays, and bowls are awkward to carry or too heavy for her to keep core stability while carrying.

In order to decrease the number of trips to the refrigerators and storage areas, she gathers items in a large mixing bowl or on a sheet tray. She holds the tray or bowl in her right hand in a lateral pinch while loading with her left until the tray gets heavy, straining her wrist and thumb.

2. *Retrieving items from the cabinets and closets*

The large pans used most often are 14-inch sauté pans with 12-inch handles. The pans weigh 5 pounds. The cutting boards are stored vertically on the lowest shelf in the kitchen pantry area. Each cutting board weighs 10 pounds.

She holds large pots and pans from the end of the handles, putting strain on her wrist and hand.

She tends to pull the boards out and carry them with her right hand using a lateral grasp, putting strain on her wrist and thumb.

She twists while removing items from the cabinets, putting strain on her back.

3. *Cutting food*

Kate usually uses knives provided by the school, mostly a 9-inch chef's knife ($1/2$ pound). She may also bring her own knives. The classes require a sustained period of cutting and rapid cutting using various forces and angles depending on the item being cut (vegetables, meat, fish, fruit, etc.). During this class, she spends 1 to 10 minutes cutting at one time. Kate reports that the amount of cutting observed during this evaluation was light compared that in some classes. The school provides dense plastic cutting boards $1/2$ inch thick. The counter is 38 inches high and 29 inches deep. Her elbow height is 40 inches from the floor while wearing the shoes she finds most comfortable in the kitchen. She uses a damp paper towel under the cutting board to keep it from sliding.

The knives provided by the school are dull from frequent use.

She holds the knife tightly even when preparing other items for the cutting board with her left hand.

Because of the amount she is trying to accomplish, she often has multiple items on the cutting board, reducing the amount of space available for knife placement. This causes her to use the tip of the knife instead of the back of the knife (Figure A-10). The back of the knife is sharper and is where she has the most force during the cutting stroke.

Although the counter in this classroom is an appropriate comfortable height, she reports that counters in other classrooms have different heights. For example, the upstairs participation classroom counters are 36 inches high. At this height, she has to bend over while cutting.

4. *Stirring food*

Kate needs to stir items in pots on the stove, in a blender, or in the oven.

To stir items on the stove or in the blender, she reaches above or to her shoulder height (Figure A-11). She maintains this position for extended periods. She displays signs of shoulder girdle fatigue such as elevating her shoulder and decreased core stability such as leaning against the counter.

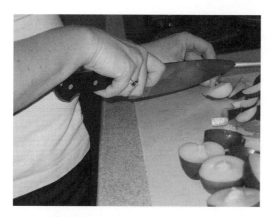

FIGURE **A-10** Using the tip of the knife to cut on a crowded board.

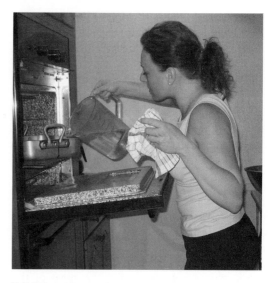

FIGURE **A-12** Working over shoulder height with extended reach in the oven.

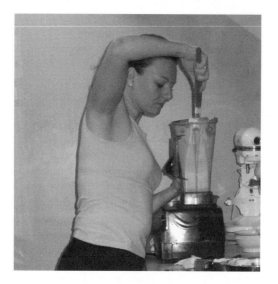

FIGURE **A-11** Stirring in a blender over shoulder height.

She uses a lateral grasp when stirring. This places strain on her thumb and wrist with repeated wrist deviation and circumduction.

She stirs in bowls on top of the cutting board or electric stove (rarely used to cook with). This further elevates the bowl and encourages additional shoulder strain.

5. *Working with ovens*

There are two stacked wall ovens in the demonstration kitchen. The top oven's highest shelf is

54 inches, and the bottom oven's lowest shelf is 24 inches from the floor. Kate has a 24-inch reach straight out from her shoulder. The doors extend 19 inches from the wall.

When loading and unloading from the ovens, Kate tends to reach from the front of the door, going up on her toes to reach the back of the oven. This puts strain on her shoulders, back, and legs. She is also at risk for losing her balance.

When stirring items in the oven, Kate pulls the pan from the oven with her left hand, holds it with one edge on the shelf, and stirs with her right (Figure A-12). This requires her to sustain a grasp on a hot and potentially heavy or unwieldy item.

6. *Static standing*

When Kate's posture is assessed, it is noted that she has the tendency to stand with a hyper-lordotic posture (with an anterior pelvic tilt) or with her left hip cocked. There is no room behind the counter for a stool.

7. *Teaching*

To make her demonstrations visible to the audience in the overhead mirrors (Figure A-13), Kate has to situate food items toward the far edge of the counter (29 inches deep). This amount of

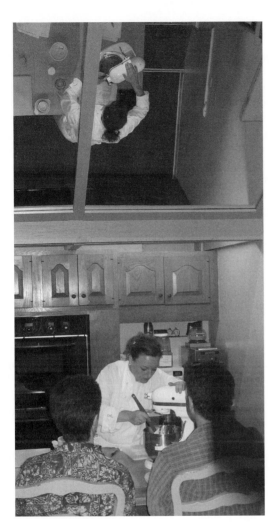

FIGURE **A-13** Using the overhead mirror to demonstrate a blender technique.

reaching puts strain on Kate's shoulders and puts her in an awkward position for tool use.

Recommendations

Engineering Controls

1. *Carrying items:* Use a rolling cart when transporting items from her car.
2. *Static standing:* The use of antifatigue, no-slip mats will help decrease strain on her back and feet and will also decrease the risk of slips caused by wet floors, common in a kitchen.

Work Practice Controls

1. *Carrying items*
   Enlist the help of the assistants
   Use team lifting for heavier items
2. *Retrieving items from cabinets and closets*
   When collecting items from around the school, she should put the tray or bowl down on the work surfaces before loading. Then, when the tray is loaded, she should adjust her grasp to distribute the weight to both hands and keep the tray close to her body. This will decrease the strain on her thumb and wrist.

   To decrease the amount of twisting, Kate should square herself to the cabinet before reaching or bending for items. This also allows her to use two hands for the heavier items such as the cutting boards or the items that are unevenly weighted, such as pots and pans.

   Slide items on trays to the edge of the counters instead of lifting.
3. *Cutting food*
   She should use only sharp knives in order to decrease the amount of force required for cutting. The school has a sharpening stone that she can use, or she can bring her own knives.

   She should keep her cutting board clear and allow adequate space for cutting items. When the crowding on her board was brought to her attention, she was able to identify methods to keep the board clear, methods that she often teaches to her students.

   If the counter is too low, she should use supplies available in the kitchen to raise the counter height. For example, in the upstairs classroom she can put two cutting boards together, one on top of the other, to raise the cutting surface by one inch. If she is at a private event with a very low counter she should use a packing crate, as long as it can be secured safely, with a cutting board on top.
4. *Stirring food*
   She should try to use a full-hand grasp on the spoons and spatulas instead of a lateral grasp to bring her elbow down near her body for the items that require sustained or forceful stirring. She reports this feels awkward, but she is willing to try this technique.

She should place the bowls on the counter rather than placing them on the cutting board or stove. This decreases the amount of shoulder elevation required. After trying this with multiple pots and bowls during the setup period, she was able to integrate this technique while teaching the class.

5. *Working with ovens*

Kate should first pull out the oven's shelf, then load the dish from the side of the oven. This decreases the distance she must reach. This also removes her need to stand on her toes.

She should use the same technique for stirring items in the oven. She does not have to hold up heavy trays if she pulls the whole shelf out of the oven instead of just the tray.

6. *Static standing*

Kate should use the postural corrections discussed during the evaluation. She was able to self-correct after different postures were demonstrated for her.

The cooking counter in the demonstration classroom has an open shelf running along its length 4 inches above the floor. She is able to prop one foot up on the shelf in order to relieve the pressure on her spine during static standing or cutting and stirring tasks, alternating her feet as needed.

She should use the classroom benches to elevate her feet between classes. This provides rest for her back and decreases the strain of prolonged standing and walking. Brief rest periods between classes will decrease the general fatigue Kate reports experiencing by the end of the day.

7. *Teaching*

She should stand along the side of the counter toward the far edge whenever possible in order to use tools within sight of the students.

Administrative Controls

1. *Carrying items*

The school should provide an adequate number of assistants to lift and carry items for the class. The number of assistants will need to be increased for classes requiring a large number of ingredients.

2. *Cutting food*

The school should provide professional sharpening services on a frequent basis to keep tools in good condition.

The school should provide an adequate number of volunteer assistants to allow more delegation of repetitive tasks and cutting. Classes that have a large amount of cutting, such as classes focused on fruits and vegetables, should have more assistants. Furthermore, the school should adjust for the experience of the volunteers. More assistants should be provided if one or more of the assistants are inexperienced, because assistants with less experience require more time to complete tasks and use tools. In cases in which she cannot rely on her assistants, Kate has to complete more of the preparation work in the same amount of time, increasing the risk for further injury.

3. *Static standing*

When planning out Kate's schedule, the class coordinator should budget time between classes for Kate to sit down and/or elevate her feet. Kate can be completing her paperwork during this time.

General Notes

1. During the evaluation process, Kate's resting wrist cock-up splints were evaluated.

   The splints were modified for wrist angle less than 20 degrees extension. This change decreases the pressure on her median nerve.

   The splints are stretched out from age. She should purchase replacement splints to improve their support.

   She should wear the splints during the day when she has rest periods, between classes, and at night.

2. Kate also was taught ways to modify her habit of holding onto tools, pots, and pans while lecturing or preparing items with her other hand. She was taught to put down her tools when not using them and to complete brief, unobtrusive stretches during the class. This helps to decrease any unnecessary prolonged strain on her hands.

3. She should resume the general cardiovascular and strengthening routine that she reports completing in the past. She was educated about choosing a routine that would strengthen core muscles and shoulder girdle muscles. If she feels she needs assistance developing this routine, it is recommended that she work with a personal trainer or occupational or physical therapist.

Summary

Kate reported that her primary concern was the pain in her arms and wrists. During an evaluation of the tasks required during the teaching of a demonstration class, areas for change were identified. Recommendations to address these changes include modifying her habits, tools, and techniques. Many of the recommendations made in this report were tested during the teaching phase of the class. During the follow-up after the class, Kate reported a decrease in the amount of upper extremity fatigue compared with what she normally felt after teaching. However, the habit changes recommended will require practice in order to be consistently used and adapted to other classrooms and situations.

Case Discussion

When completing an evaluation for an employee who performs many jobs within the same company, the evaluator must determine the best method to observe a representative set of job tasks. For this evaluation, the demonstration-style class was chosen in order to observe Kate completing the majority required of tasks within a condensed timeframe. The recommendations made then can be applied to multiple settings or tasks.

The ergonomic controls recommended include engineering, administrative, and work practice controls. The administrative controls include providing an adequate number of volunteer assistants, accounting for the number of assistants with limited cooking knowledge or experience, maintaining tools properly, and allotting time between classes for rest periods when organizing the class schedule.

In kitchens that are shared by many chefs, there is a limit to how many engineering changes can be implemented because changes will affect every instructor. The use of antifatigue mats, sharp knives, and a selection of tools can decrease the overall strain on Kate's body. One of the recommendations usually made to decrease strain in the kitchen includes large grip handles on tools. However, because this is a shared kitchen environment and because Kate moves from kitchen to kitchen, this recommendation was not made. In order to be implemented, the school would have to either supply all of their kitchens with these large-handled tools or supply Kate with a set of her own. She then would need to carry these tools with her from job to job. Also, large-grip tools often weigh more than standard kitchen equipment. This would increase the amount of carrying and lifting Kate needs to complete on a daily basis. To keep the amount of carrying to a minimum, it was recommended that she keep to a minimum the number of specialized tools she carries, such as her knives.

Although the doors on the ovens and the layout of the kitchen cannot be changed as part of a reasonable accommodation, Kate's use of each item or tool can be changed as part of work practice controls. The bulk of this report emphasizes Kate's responsibility for using tools properly and problem-solving postures in the kitchen. This includes decreasing the forces applied to tools with both the stabilizing hand and the hand using

---

Learning Exercises

1. As a student, what activities do you participate in on a daily basis that could be modified to decrease stress on your low back, neck, shoulders, and hands? Divide these modifications into the categories of engineering, administrative, and work practice controls. If you were trying to convince your teacher or school to modify the activities that present high risk, how would you write your report? What language would you use, and what topics would you highlight?

2. What hobbies do you engage in? How do these hobbies affect your body physically, your stress or emotional level, and your economic situation?

3. You are presented with a client in a therapy clinic who is a student and has the hobbies and habits you identified. The client is complaining of low back pain. Plan your course of treatment including evaluations, modalities, educational materials, exercises, and ergonomic adaptations.

the tool, using two hands to complete heavy tasks with a palmar grip instead of lateral pinch, positioning her body and her tools to decrease the amount of reaching or awkward grasp, and keeping her tools well maintained. A large portion of the evaluation and consultation process was spent assisting Kate in developing problem-solving skills related to ergonomic controls within the varied kitchens and tasks required. These techniques, combined with a general physical strengthening program, will decrease the strain of a physically and emotionally demanding job.

Multiple Choice Review Questions

1. A recommendation to use a stepstool is an example of:
   A. a work practice control.
   B. a method to increase productivity.
   C. an engineering control.
   D. an administrative control.

2. A recommendation to adjust type of grasp used with a tool is an example of:
   A. a purchase order.
   B. a neuromuscular cue for postural deficits.
   C. an engineering control.
   D. a work practice control.

3. It is important to address the height of a work surface because it:
   A. changes the amount of work that can be accomplished.
   B. affects the worker's posture, arm angle, and reach.
   C. is an engineering control.
   D. is the most common problem seen at a workstation.

4. When choosing the location of the evaluation, it is most important to determine:
   A. where the client is most comfortable.
   B. where the client is exposed to the most hazards.
   C. where the evaluator can spend the most time.
   D. where the evaluator can spend the least amount of time.

5. Administrative controls could not be applied in the case of the viola player because:
   A. the amount of time spent playing at performances was dictated by the music and was a requirement for employment.
   B. she was not employed by an administrator.
   C. the viola could not be adjusted.
   D. engineering changes provide better controls of workplace hazards.

6. Work practice changes are difficult to apply because they:
   A. require practice and worker acceptance and may initially decrease productivity.
   B. require a lot of money.
   C. require practice and may initially increase productivity.
   D. require a team approach.

7. In the case of the chef instructor, providing additional assistants during the cooking class is an example of:
   A. a workplace control.
   B. a method to keep the chef from not getting tired.
   C. an engineering control.
   D. an administrative control.

8. In the case of the mother, a pillow was placed behind her back while breast-feeding to:
   A. take into account that her child will be increasing in height and weight.
   B. correct her sitting posture and increase her back support.
   C. make the baby more comfortable.
   D. make her feet touch the floor.

9. It is important to convey to the client the rationale for each recommendation to:
   A. promote compliance.
   B. promote payment for services.
   C. improve the employee-employer relationship.
   D. decrease the likelihood of misunderstanding.

10. To decrease the amount of reaching for a job task, it is important to first change:
    A. the tool being using.
    B. the person's posture.
    C. the distance the item is from the body.
    D. the amount of time allowed for each task.

Sample Functional Job Analysis

Jenny Legge

CASE STUDY 4: THE DRAGLINE OPERATOR

Therapists are often the provider of choice for functional job analyses. Typically, referrals for a job analysis are made as part of a rehabilitation program to help a worker with an injury or disability return to the workforce. An alternative reason for referral is to build a job bank that would be applicable to a group of workers. These databases are often used to identify overall job demands for job-specific preplacement, postoffer screenings for new workers.

Background

The therapist was commissioned to build a job bank of all the job roles at a Queensland coal mine. The purpose of the database was to determine functional job demands for each role so that job-specific preemployment functional assessments that met Australian antidiscrimination legal requirements could be developed and implemented.

The job chosen for this case study is a dragline excavator operator. This job was chosen because it has a broad range of demands ranging from sedentary tasks to very heavy manual tasks. It illustrates the versatility required for an effective task database.

A dragline excavator (dragline) is a piece of heavy earth-moving equipment used in open-cut coal mines around the world to remove overburden and coal. The larger models that were used in this study weigh around 3500 tonnes (3858 tons) and are about 30 m (98 ft) wide. The boom extends approximately 80 m (262 ft) from the machine with buckets large enough to fit two four-wheel-drive vehicles. They can move 96,000 tonnes (106,000 tons) of dirt in 24 hours.

A dragline is operated by a team of two or three workers. Tasks vary from sedentary dragline operation using hand controls while seated in ergonomic chairs to manually handling cable weighing in excess of 35 kg (77 pounds) to climbing ladders and crawling around in cramped areas (Figure B-1). Three of these tasks will be presented.

Preparation

1. *Determine purpose of analysis and scope of work*

Meetings were held with management and experienced operators to develop a list of tasks to

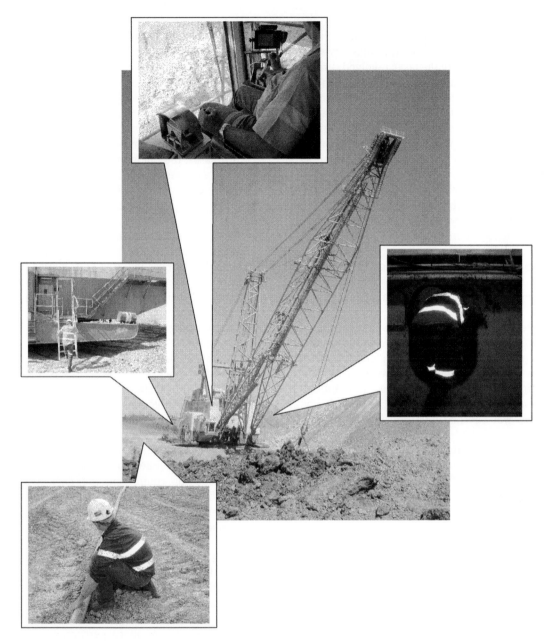

FIGURE **B-1** Anatomy of a dragline excavator.

be assessed. Several methods were used to identify tasks. The primary method was the workflow method, whereby the operator talks through a typical day to identify the tasks involved. Irregular tasks (those that are not performed on a daily basis) were then identified and added to the list. Time to complete the analysis was estimated to ensure adequate coverage so that disruption to production was kept to a minimum. The purpose of the analysis was clearly explained to the workers before the commencement of the analysis so that they understood what information was required and how it would be used as well as their role in the process. They were also given the opportunity not to participate in the analysis if they chose.

2. *Equipment preparation*

Standard equipment including a digital camera was used. The JobFit System software was the product chosen for the data collection and reporting.

3. *Site-specific preparation*

Site safety requirements specified that personal protective equipment (PPE), including hard hat, safety boots, and goggles, be worn at all times. Hearing protection was required intermittently. An escort was required at all times. The digital camera was checked by an onsite electrician before use.

4. *Other considerations*

The work environment of a dragline operator has a number of other requirements. These were an absence of susceptibility to motion sickness and an absence of fear of heights.

Job Analysis

Employer: Multinational Mining Company, Open Cut Coal Mine, Queensland, Australia
Worker: Typically male, average age 47 years
Roster: 12-hour rotating day-night shift, 4 days on, 4 days off

Step 1: Identification of Tasks

The following tasks were identified as part of the dragline operator role:

Dozer, operating
Dragline cable, coupling
Dragline cable, moving
Dragline cable, positioning

Dragline house, inspection
Dragline revolving frame, cleaning
Dragline revolving frame, inspection
Dragline, operation
Dragline boom, inspection
Light vehicle, operation

Step 2: Analysis of Tasks

Using the JobFit System software and standardized processes, the following information was collected for each task:

Overview: a step-by-step process of how the task is done and what equipment is used. It may include information such as heights, weights, and environmental factors

Duration and frequency

Postural tolerances requirements: scored based on the Department of Labor frequency classifications of Never, Occasional, Frequent, and Constant and described using nonmedical language to improve usability of the report

Material handling requirements: height, weight, and frequency

Additional information

Whenever possible, more than one worker was observed performing each task. This helped the therapist to differentiate between actual task demands and individual variations in methods. Workers were also questioned about other possible methods for completing the task. Weights were confirmed with engineering and purchasing departments. When working heights varied, this was noted and the worst case scenario was measured.

Task reports for (1) dragline, operation (Figure B-2), (2) dragline cable, moving (Figure B-3), and (3) dragline revolving frame, cleaning (Figure B-4) were recorded.

Once completed, the draft task reports were circulated to key workplace personnel including supervisors and experienced operators for feedback, primarily about the task overview and terminology used for naming tasks and equipment. Workers were not expected to comment on the measured postural tolerances and material handling requirements unless there was an obvious

Text continued on p. 422.

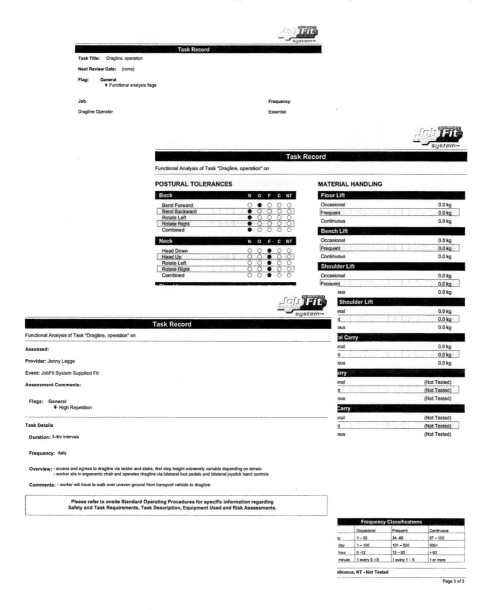

FIGURE **B-2** Task report for dragline, operation.

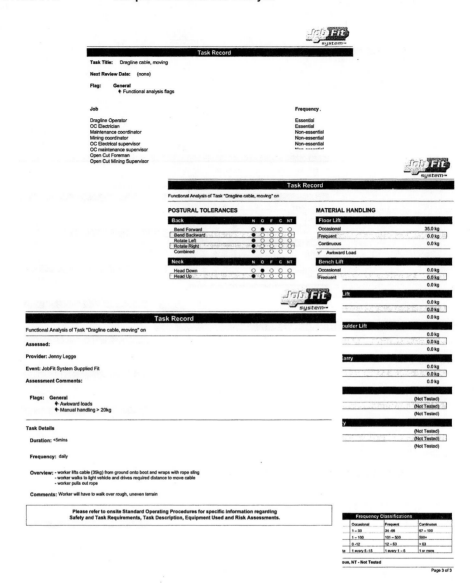

Task Record

Task Title: Dragline cable, moving

Next Review Date: (none)

Flag: **General**
          ✦ Functional analysis flags

Job	Frequency
Dragline Operator	Essential
OC Electrician	Essential
Maintenance coordinator	Non-essential
Mining coordinator	Non-essential
OC Electrical supervisor	Non-essential
OC maintenance supervisor	Non-essential
Open Cut Foreman	
Open Cut Mining Supervisor	

Task Record

Functional Analysis of Task "Dragline cable, moving" on

POSTURAL TOLERANCES

Back	N	O	F	C	NT
Bend Forward	○	●	○	○	○
Bend Backward	●	○	○	○	○
Rotate Left	●	○	○	○	○
Rotate Right	●	○	○	○	○
Combined	●	○	○	○	○

Neck	N	O	F	C	NT
Head Down	○	●	○	○	○
Head Up	●	○	○	○	○

MATERIAL HANDLING

Floor Lift	
Occasional	35.0 kg
Frequent	0.0 kg
Continuous	0.0 kg
✓ Awkward Load	

Bench Lift	
Occasional	0.0 kg
Frequent	0.0 kg
	0.0 kg

...Lift	
	0.0 kg
	0.0 kg
	0.0 kg

...oulder Lift	
	0.0 kg
	0.0 kg
	0.0 kg

...arry	
	0.0 kg
	0.0 kg
	0.0 kg

	(Not Tested)
	(Not Tested)
	(Not Tested)

...y	
	(Not Tested)
	(Not Tested)
	(Not Tested)

Task Record

Functional Analysis of Task "Dragline cable, moving" on

Assessed:

Provider: Jenny Legge

Event: JobFit System Supplied Fit

Assessment Comments:

Flags: **General**
          ✦ Awkward loads
          ✦ Manual handling > 20kg

Task Details

Duration: <5mins

Frequency: daily

Overview: - worker lifts cable (35kg) from ground onto boot and wraps with rope sling
             - worker walks to light vehicle and drives required distance to move cable
             - worker pulls out rope

Comments: Worker will have to walk over rough, uneven terrain

> **Please refer to onsite Standard Operating Procedures for specific information regarding
> Safety and Task Requirements, Task Description, Equipment Used and Risk Assessments.**

Frequency Classifications

	Occasional	Frequent	Continuous
	1 – 33	34 -66	67 – 100
	1 – 100	101 – 500	500+
	0 -12	12 – 63	> 63
te	1 every 5 -15	1 every 1 – 5	1 or more

...ous, NT - Not Tested

FIGURE B-3 Task report for dragline cable, moving.

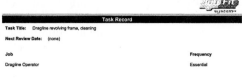

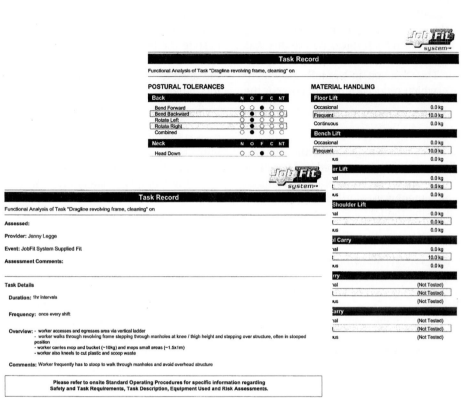

Task Record

Task Title: Dragline revolving frame, cleaning

Next Review Date: (none)

Job	Frequency
Dragline Operator	Essential

Task Record

Functional Analysis of Task "Dragline revolving frame, cleaning" on

POSTURAL TOLERANCES						**MATERIAL HANDLING**	
Back	N	O	F	C	NT	**Floor Lift**	
Bend Forward	○	○	●	○	○	Occasional	0.0 kg
Bend Backward	○	●	○	○	○	Frequent	10.0 kg
Rotate Left	○	●	○	○	○	Continuous	0.0 kg
Rotate Right	○	●	○	○	○	**Bench Lift**	
Combined	○	●	○	○	○	Occasional	0.0 kg
Neck	N	O	F	C	NT	Frequent	10.0 kg
						us	0.0 kg
Head Down	○	○	●	○	○	**er Lift**	

Task Record

Functional Analysis of Task "Dragline revolving frame, cleaning" on

Assessed:

Provider: Jenny Legge

Event: JobFit System Supplied Fit

Assessment Comments:

Task Details

Duration: 1hr intervals

Frequency: once every shift

Overview: - worker accesses and egresses area via vertical ladder
- worker walks through revolving frame stepping through manholes at knee / thigh height and stepping over structure, often in stooped position
- worker carries mop and bucket (~10kg) and mops small areas (~1.5x1m)
- worker also kneels to cut plastic and scoop waste

Comments: Worker frequently has to stoop to walk through manholes and avoid overhead structure

> **Please refer to onsite Standard Operating Procedures for specific information regarding Safety and Task Requirements, Task Description, Equipment Used and Risk Assessments.**

	al	0.0 kg
	t	0.0 kg
	us	0.0 kg
Shoulder Lift		
	al	0.0 kg
	t	0.0 kg
	us	0.0 kg
l Carry		
	al	0.0 kg
	t	10.0 kg
	us	0.0 kg
rry		
	al	(Not Tested)
	t	(Not Tested)
	us	(Not Tested)
arry		
	al	(Not Tested)
	t	(Not Tested)
	us	(Not Tested)

Frequency Classifications			
	Occasional	Frequent	Continuous
	1 – 33	34 -66	67 – 100
day	1 – 100	101 – 500	500+
our	0 -12	12 – 63	> 63
minute	1 every 5 -15	1 every 1 – 5	1 or more

inuous, NT - Not Tested

Page 3 of 3

Page 2 of 3

FIGURE B-4 Task report for dragline revolving frame, cleaning.

error. Errors were corrected and procedures were clarified as required.

Step 3: Classification of Tasks

Because of the isolated location of the work and the need to work in small teams, all tasks were considered essential.

Some tasks were also performed by workers employed in alternative job roles. Where this was the case, these job roles were also recorded on the task record. This resulted in organic growth of the job bank, which reduced time and cost for the client.

Step 4: Summation of Tasks

To identify the overall job demands, the requirements of all the tasks were compared and the most demanding measure for each postural and material handling requirement was recorded. This was done electronically using the JobFit System software.

Step 5: Report

The job report for the dragline operator is displayed in Figure B-5.

Case Discussion

Job banks are a valuable tool for therapists involved in the management and prevention of work-related musculoskeletal disorders. They are organic documents that continue to be reviewed and updated over time.

They have a number of advantages including, but not limited to, the following:

Providing a summary of the inherent requirements of a role to develop job-specific assessments

Facilitating the comparison of the physical demands of one job against those of another or against set criteria for risk management activities

Providing a quick reference to job demands for the development of workplace physical rehabilitation programs

They also have their limitations. Job banks are by nature, generic; they do not necessarily account for individual differences in body shape and habitual movement patterns. As a result, there is a risk of misinterpreting data and mismatching workers despite the best intentions. To fit the function for which a job database is designed, there is often the need to trade sensitivity with generic descriptors when populating job databases.

As with all work-related assessment tools, when conducting the task analyses used in this case study, the therapist addressed the five attributes of excellence recommended by NIOSH:

1. Safety: This was addressed by abiding by the workplace safety and emergency procedures at all times
2. Reliability: This was addressed by using consistent predetermined evaluation criteria, particularly with reference to working heights and frequencies and durations of movements and material handling
3. Validity: This was addressed through the descriptors used and the direct observation of the tasks being performed
4. Practicality: This was addressed by attempting to balance the need to collect detailed information in a timely cost-effective manner with minimal disruption to the workplace
5. Utility: This was addressed by communicating closely with the referrer to ensure that the final report met the referrer's needs and expectations.

Striving for excellence by addressing the safety, reliability, validity, utility, and practicality of the analysis method will assist therapists of all skill levels when developing a job database.

JobFit system

Job Record

Job Title: Dragline Operator

Description:

Departments

Open Cut -> Local site -> National division -> Global company

JobFit system

Job Record

Combined Functional Analysis of Job "Dragline Operator" at

POSTURAL TOLERANCES

Back	N	O	F	C	NT
Bend Forward	○	○	●	○	○
Bend Backward	○	○	●	○	○
Rotate Left	○	●	○	○	○
Rotate Right	○	●	○	○	○
Combined	○	○	●	○	○

Neck	N	O	F	C	NT
Head Down	○	○	●	○	○

MATERIAL HANDLING

Floor Lift	
Occasional	35.0 kg
Frequent	10.0 kg
Continuous	0.0 kg
✓ Awkward Load	

Bench Lift	
Occasional	35.0 kg
	10.0 kg
	0.0 kg
	0.0 kg
	0.0 kg
	0.0 kg
	0.0 kg
	0.0 kg
	0.0 kg
	0.0 kg
	10.0 kg
	0.0 kg
	(Not Tested)
	(Not Tested)
	(Not Tested)
	(Not Tested)
	(Not Tested)
	(Not Tested)

JobFit system

Job Record

Combined Functional Analysis of Job "Dragline Operator" at

The Combined Functional Analysis of this Job includes these tasks:

Task Name	Frequency
Dozer operation	Essential
Dragline boom, inspection	Essential
Dragline cable, coupling	Essential
Dragline cable, moving	Essential
Dragline cable, positioning	Essential
Dragline house, inspection	Essential
Dragline revolving frame, cleaning	Essential
Dragline revolving frame, inspection	Essential
Dragline, operation	Essential
Light vehicle operation	Essential

...ency Classifications		
...al	Frequent	Continuous
	34 -66	67 – 100
	101 – 500	500+
	12 – 53	> 53
-15	1 every 1 – 5	1 or more

Tested

Page 3 of 3

Page 2 of 3

FIGURE **B-5** Job report for the dragline operator.

Ergonomic Information Sheets for Consumers

ERGONOMIC STRATEGIES—*Computer Keyboards*

Problems Caused by Computer Keyboards

Computer keyboards can increase carpal tunnel pressure whenever the hands deviate sufficiently from a neutral position, which can prevent the free flow of fluids into the palm of the hand.

Research has shown that sustained increases in carpal tunnel pressure of >30 mm Hg disrupt blood flow and impair the nerves of the wrist and hand. Carpal tunnel pressure is typically ≥40 mm Hg when the wrists are flexed or extended during typing tasks.

Maintaining this position for an extended period of time can lead to injury of arm and hand musculature as well as the tendons and nerves within the wrist and hand.

In addition to increased carpal tunnel pressure, repetitiveness and exaggerated force application when using a keyboard are risk factors directly related to repetitive stress injury.

The standard, flat design of a typical keyboard requires users to make unhealthy postural adaptations to conform to the keyboard, and when a computer keyboard is used for longer than 5 hours, the likelihood of injury significantly increases.

Tips for Proper Keyboard Use

Using a downward-tilting keyboard tray (with no more than 15 degrees of tilt):

- Significantly reduces wrist extension while typing and at rest
- Considerably improves both low back pain and shoulder pain
- Allows wrists and hands to maintain a more neutral position for more than 60% of typing time

Open or fixed keyboards are ergonomically better than standard keyboards.

Open keyboards (with keys that slope up at an angle from the keyboard base) cause significantly less twisting of the wrist during typing.

Fixed keyboards (with keys split down the middle and angled) decrease the amount of wrist motion from left to right and maintain the wrist in a more neutral position.

Don't use a wrist rest! Research has shown that using a wrist rest doubles the pressure inside the carpal tunnel. This is because the floor of the carpal tunnel is a more flexible ligament that transmits external pressures directly into the carpal tunnel.

Keyboard keys should not stick or need excessive force to be operated.

Longer horizontal distances between the keyboard and the edge of the desk keep the wrist in a more neutral position and reduces chronic injury.

REFERENCES

Hedge A: *10 tips for using a computer mouse*, 2006. Retrieved December 1, 2006, from Cornell University Ergonomics Web,
http://ergo.human.cornell.edu/cumousetips.html.

Hedge A, Morimoto S, McCrobie D: Effects of keyboard tray geometry on upper body posture and comfort, *Ergonomics* 42(10):1333, 1999.

Kotani K, Barrero LH, Lee DL et al: Effect of horizontal position of the computer keyboard on upper extremity posture, *International Ergonomics Association*, 2006.

Pentikis J, Lopez MS, Thomas RE: Ergonomics evaluation of a government office building, *Work* 18(2):123, 2002.

Serina ER, Tal R, Rempel D: Wrist and forearm postures and motions during typing, *Ergonomics* 42(7):938, 1999.

Zecevic A, Miller DI, Harburn K: An evaluation of the ergonomics of three computer keyboards, *Ergonomics* 43(1):55, 2000.

QUESTIONS? Contact Rachel Neuman: raneuman@bu.edu or Karen Jacobs: kjacobs@bu.edu.

ERGONOMIC STRATEGIES—*Computer Mice*

How Does Mouse Use Lead to Discomfort?

When using a mouse, workers typically extend their arms, raise their shoulders, and/or position their elbows far away from the body for several minutes at a time without awareness of their position or breaks from mouse use.

Mouse use has been associated with an increased risk for upper extremity musculoskeletal disorders, such as carpal tunnel syndrome, because carpal tunnel pressures during mouse use are typically greater than pressures known to alter nerve function and structure.

Elevated carpal tunnel pressure during mouse use is an effect of both wrist extension and excessive fingertip force applied to depress the button and grip the sides of the mouse.

It has been estimated that workers use a mouse an average of 78 times per hour, accounting for approximately 23.7% of computer work time.

The highest levels of electromyographic (EMG) activity during computer work occur in the forearm during mouse activity compared with other computer tasks.

How Can I Prevent Symptoms?

Use an external mouse, and make sure the mouse is at elbow height.

Optimal positioning of the mouse is next to the keyboard on a sliding keyboard tray.

Minimize prolonged dragging tasks, and frequently perform other tasks with the hand used for the mouse.

Consider placing the mouse on the left side of the keyboard, as it reduces the postural constraints of the upper extremity using the mouse.

A quick-fix solution is using a "mouse bridge," which is a stand on which the mouse sits on top of the number keypad.

REFERENCES

Delisle A, Imbeau D, Santos B et al: Left-handed versus right-handed computer mouse use: effect on upper extremity posture, *Appl Ergon* 35:21, 2004.

Forsman M, Anteborn G, Thorn S: Variability in electromyographic measurements within and between individuals performing a computer work task, *International Ergonomics Association,* 2006.

Harvey R, Peper E: Surface electromyography and mouse use position, *Ergonomics* 40(8):781, 1997.

Keir PJ, Bach JM, Rempel D: Effects of computer mouse design and task on carpal tunnel pressure, *Ergonomics* 42(10):1350, 1999.

Luttmann A, Kylian H et al: Working conditions, musculoskeletal symptoms and muscular strain and fatigue at office work, *International Ergonomics Association,* 2006.

QUESTIONS? Contact Rachel Neuman: raneuman@bu.edu or Karen Jacobs: kjacobs@bu.edu.

ERGONOMIC STRATEGIES—*Computer Monitors*

How Can a Computer Monitor Become Problematic?

If a computer monitor is not positioned properly, it can lead to numerous types of chronic injury, especially of the neck, eyes, and back.

Computer monitors are often positioned too low for their users, which may bring about a downward eye glaze, an increased neck angle, and forward bending of the upper back.

With the neck and upper back in this position, stress on the spine significantly increases.

This position also causes fatigue to occur much earlier in the workday.

Vertical gaze direction, ocular surface area, and viewing angle are all affected as well.

Computer monitors positioned too high (i.e., above the horizontal of eye gaze) lead to shortening of the neck and upper back muscles beyond their optimum lengths and lengthening of the muscles in the front of the neck.

How Should I Properly Position My Computer Monitor, and Why Is This Important?

The monitor should be positioned directly in front of you at an arm's length away. Make sure it is perpendicular to the window, if you have one in your office, in order to avoid glare on the screen.

In order to minimize the load on the musculoskeletal system, the eye gaze inclination to a visual target, in this case the computer monitor, should be approximately 6° to 9° below the horizontal (about 10 cm [4 in] below eye height).

Large-sized monitors for convenient use of larger icons and symbols will likely necessitate a gaze at the proper angle and a more erect body posture.

Working within proper viewing angles will minimize the surface of the eyeball, which, in turn, will help the eye to retain its moisture and be better equipped to perform computer work.

REFERENCES

Delleman NJ, Berndsen MB: Touch-typing VDU operation: workstation adjustment, working posture and workers' perceptions, *Ergonomics* 45(7):514, 2002.

Pentikis J, Lopez MS, Thomas RE: Ergonomics evaluation of a government office building, *Work* 18(2):123, 2002.

Villanueva MBG, Sotoyama M, Jonai H et al: Adjustments of posture and viewing parameters of the eye to changes in the screen height of the visual display terminal, *Ergonomics* 39(7):933, 1996.

QUESTIONS? Contact Rachel Neuman: raneuman@bu.edu or Karen Jacobs: kjacobs@bu.edu.

ERGONOMIC STRATEGIES—*Golf*

The Swing

There is no "perfect" swing. Everyone has a different optimal swing position because of individual anatomic differences.

Think of the swing as a pathway, without emphasizing distinct positions.

Flexibility within a golf swing is important in order to allow for recovery from internal or external disturbances, such as when golfing on the side of a hill. Absolute invariance in a golf swing may actually be counterproductive.

Use sensory information in addition to visual information while swinging.

When practicing, use different types of clubs and different types of swings.

Facts About Golfing Injuries

Golfing injuries are often a result of poor swing mechanics, overzealous playing, or a traumatic event such as hitting the ground awkwardly.

The most common site of golfing injuries is the low back, followed by the elbow, then the wrist and hand, then the shoulder, especially the lead shoulder.

Pain and discomfort are usually experienced at extreme ranges of motion, such as at the top of backswing or the end of follow-through.

How to Prevent Golfing Injuries

Keep your hands and arms in front of your body as much as possible when taking a swing in order to limit the stresses applied to the shoulder.

Increase the flexibility of your hips and trunk in order to achieve appropriate shoulder turn during backswing.

Increase strength, flexibility, balance, and power in order to improve driving distance, carry distance, ball velocity, and clubhead speed.

Always stretch the muscles of the shoulder, lower back, and wrist (the major golf muscles) before playing, in order to prevent injury.

REFERENCES

Foster JB: Golfers swing to biomechanical research: research quantifies training's effect on performance, *Biomechanics* October:28, 2006.

Kim DH, Millett PJ, Warner JJ et al: Shoulder injuries in golf, *Am J Sports Med* 32(5):1324, 2004.

Knight CA: Neuromotor issues in the learning and control of golf skill, *Res Q Exerc Sport* 75(1):9, 2004.

QUESTIONS? Contact Rachel Neuman: raneuman@bu.edu or Karen Jacobs: kjacobs@bu.edu.

ERGONOMIC STRATEGIES—*Lighting*

What Are the Effects of Improper Office Lighting?

Inadequate office lighting may cause visual discomfort, which can lead to neck, shoulder, and/or forearm pain.

Severe headaches account for 48% of work-related aches and pains and are directly correlated with problematic office lighting.

Computer workers with improper office lighting may experience symptoms of visual discomfort such as red-eye, a gritty sensation within the eye, and sensitivity to light.

Visual discomfort has been proven to interfere with employees' job performance and overall productivity.

What Are the Causes and Effects of Glare?

Excessive office lighting via natural means (e.g., bright sun coming through the window) or artificial means (e.g., overhead lighting or one's own reflection when wearing light-colored clothes) can act as a major source of glare, which can become a significant problem.

Glare can significantly reduce visibility depending on the proximity of the source of glare to the viewer.

Glare has significant correlations to eye focusing problems and tired eyes and has been shown to lead to an increased number of typing errors.

Tips for Safe Office Lighting

The Human Factors and Ergonomics Society recommends that any luminous source within the computer user's field of view should not exceed three times the screen luminance.

There is considerable literature to support the fact that the room's surrounding light should be brighter than the central target, in this case, the computer display.

Why Is Proper Lighting Important?

Appropriate office lighting has been shown to increase creativity potential, especially if the office contains windows.

Higher visual acuity resulting from optimal office lighting conditions leads to better performance and/or lower levels of eyestrain.

REFERENCES

Aaras A, Horgen G et al: Does visual discomfort influence on muscle pain for visual display unit workers? *International Ergonomics Association*, 2006.

Brombach J, Schneider JV, Strasser H: Ergonomic impact of lighting scenarios on contrast and visual acuity, *International Ergonomics Association*, 2006.

Ceylan C, Dul J et al: Empirical evidence of the relationship between the physical work environment and creativity, *International Ergonomics Association*, 2006.

Pentikis J, Lopez MS, Thomas RE: Ergonomics evaluation of a government office building, *Work* 18(2):123, 2002.

Robertson MM, Larson NL et al: A cross-sectional survey of computer workers: examining the relationships of workstation design, tasks, psychosocial, work-related musculoskeletal and visual discomfort, *International Ergonomics Association*, 2006.

Sheedy JE, Smith R, Hayes J: Visual effects of the luminance surrounding a computer display, *Ergonomics* 48(9):1114, 2005.

QUESTIONS? Contact Rachel Neuman: raneuman@bu.edu or Karen Jacobs: kjacobs@bu.edu.

ERGONOMIC STRATEGIES—*Personal Digital Assistants (PDAs)*

What Is Blackberry Thumb?

Blackberry thumb is a repetitive stress injury caused by overuse of a handheld device with no one set of symptoms or one specific diagnosis.

Symptoms can include swelling, hand throbbing, muscle cramps, numbness, and pain that can become chronic if not addressed.

Because a PDA keyboard is so small, and the thumb, which is the least dexterous part of the hand, becomes overtaxed, the risk for injury skyrockets with overuse.

What Can I Do to Prevent Blackberry Thumb or Improve Current Symptoms?

Tips for preventing Blackberry thumb include the following:

1. Be selective in answering emails and text messages on hand-held devices.
2. Use abbreviations when text messaging and typing emails.
3. Type on handheld devices for no more than 10-minute sessions.
4. Try to avoid typing with your thumbs, and use other fingers to type.
5. Stretch the hands during typing sessions to enhance blood flow to the thumb muscles.

Some quick and easy exercises you can do include the following:

1. Tap each finger with the thumb of the same hand. (Repeat five times.)
2. Alternate tapping your palm and back of your hand against your thigh as quickly as you can. (Repeat 20 times.)
3. Open up your hands and spread the fingers as far apart as possible. Hold for 10 seconds. (Repeat eight times.)
4. Fold your hands together; turn your palms away from your body as you extend your arms forward. You should feel only a gentle stretch. Hold for 10 seconds. (Repeat eight times.)
5. Fold your hands together; turn your palms away from your body and extend your arms overhead. You should feel the stretch in your upper torso and shoulders to hand. Hold for 10 seconds. (Repeat eight times.)

Take personal responsibility; seek a physical therapist's care if symptoms persist.

REFERENCES

American Physical Therapy Association: *"Blackberry Thumb" causing digital distress in and out of the workplace,* 2006. Retrieved from www.apta.org.

American Physical Therapy Association: *Physical therapist tips for handheld users,* 2006. Retrieved from http://www.apta.org.

Amini D: Repetitive stress injuries and the age of communication, *OT Pract* 11(9):10, 2006.

QUESTIONS? Contact Rachel Neuman: raneuman@bu.edu or Karen Jacobs: kjacobs@bu.edu.

ERGONOMIC STRATEGIES—*Seating*

Facts About Prolonged Sitting Postures

Research suggests that joint forces in the lower back are significantly higher when in a prolonged seated position as opposed to a prolonged standing position.

Seated work increases the risk for low back pain because of sustained static loads imposed on the spine.

Sitting for prolonged periods of time also causes continuous compression on the intervertebral discs, which hampers the flow of fluid and decreases joint nutrition.

Why Is Office Seating Problematic?

When sitting, it is very easy to slump into a posture that significantly changes the shape of the spine and drastically increases the pressure on the intervertebral discs in the low back.

Slumping posture can result in low back pain and over a prolonged period of time can cause more serious back problems.

Many office chairs have traditional, padded, fixed-height lumbar (low back) supports that are unlikely to provide a comfortable or appropriate seat for people of various body types.

People do not always prefer chairs that correspond to their body's characteristics and therefore fail to adjust their chairs accordingly.

What Type of Office Chair Is Optimal?

Using a dynamic (adjustable) chair as opposed to a fixed chair is an easy way to help prevent low back pain associated with sitting.

Dynamic chairs allow opposite movements of the seat and back support, which accommodate a reclining posture, allowing for relaxation of the back muscles.

Office chairs should have a lumbar (low back) support positioned between the second and fifth lumbar vertebrae (lower four vertebrae of the spine).

A chair should allow for easily varied sitting postures in order to allow the spine to move rather than attempting to constrain people in an "ideal" sitting position.

REFERENCES

Callaghan JP, McGill SM: Low back joint loading and kinematics during standing and unsupported sitting, *Ergonomics* 44(3):280, 2001.

Coleman N, Hull BP, Ellitt G: An empirical study of preferred settings for lumbar support on adjustable office chairs, *Ergonomics* 41(4):401, 1998.

Van Dreën JH, de Looze MP, Hermans V: Effects of dynamic office chairs on trunk kinematics, trunk extensor EMG and spinal shrinkage, *Ergonomics* 44(7):739, 2001.

QUESTIONS? Contact Rachel Neuman: raneuman@bu.edu or Karen Jacobs: kjacobs@bu.edu.

ERGONOMIC STRATEGIES—*Stress Management*

What Can Stress Do to My Body?

Stress causes physical ailments such as headache, high blood pressure, insomnia, fatigue, and skin disorders as well as psychologic problems such as depression, anger, anxiety, resentment, and cynicism.

Stress can extend injury recovery time and interfere with pain management.

Chronic neuromuscular tension in conjunction with stress can lead to improper postural positions that easily become habitual.

How Can I Alleviate Stress?

Perform static stretches at your workstation in order to decrease muscular tension and allow for a brief period of relaxation.

After stretching, recline in your chair, close your eyes, and completely "let go" in order to allow for the natural reorganization of muscular tension, facilitating better posture.

Meditation is a mind and body strategy used to alleviate stress and can decrease blood pressure and increase the ability to sleep for longer periods of time.

Guided imagery is a healthy and effective method of coping with stress that involves imagining an image that is pleasing to the eye in order to decrease stress and anxiety and cause a sensation of peace and relaxation.

- Decreases blood pressure and heart and respiratory rate
- Increases a sense of self-control and reduces irritability

Other methods of alleviating stress include:

- Deep breathing exercises
- Prayer and spirituality
- Aromatherapy
- Massage
- Therapeutic touch
- Acupuncture

REFERENCES

Ackerman CJ, Turkoski B: Using guided imagery to reduce pain and anxiety, *Home Healthcare Nurse* 18(8):524, 2000.

Bixby N: *Yoga and posture.* Retrieved from www.posturepage.com/yoga.

Giese LA, Smith JJ: Stress management: the complementary alternative medicine approach, *Gastroenterol Nurs* 24(5):261, 2001.

QUESTIONS? Contact Rachel Neuman: raneuman@bu.edu or Karen Jacobs: kjacobs@bu.edu.

ERGONOMIC STRATEGIES—*Stretching and Rest Breaks*

Why Are Rest Breaks Beneficial?

Rest breaks reduce static loads on the musculoskeletal system and also reduce the incidence of repetitive strain injuries.

Breaks increase worker productivity and well-being, especially during continuous computer work.

Workers usually wait until they experience muscular discomfort before taking rest breaks; if rest breaks are taken before symptom onset, injuries can be prevented.

Research shows that breaks as short as 30 seconds are just as beneficial as longer breaks in allowing adequate time for overworked muscles to relax.

Tips for Stretching at the Workstation

Stretching at the workstation should target: fingers and wrists, hands and forearms, chest and upper back, shoulders and neck, both sides of the trunk, and the lower back.

Easy stretches that can be performed at work include the following:

1. Open up your hands, and spread fingers as far apart as possible. (Stretches hands, fingers, and wrist)
2. Cross your right arm straight across your body, and pull it closer with a bent left arm locked at the elbow. Repeat with the opposite arm. (Stretches shoulders)
3. Bring your right ear toward your right shoulder. Use your right hand to apply gentle overpressure to your head. Repeat to the left. (Stretches neck)
4. Stand up and cross your right leg over your left. Reach your arms above your head, and stretch all the way to the right, while pushing out your left hip. Repeat to the opposite direction. (Stretches trunk)
5. Bend trunk forward with knees slightly bent, and grab behind your knees. Slowly extend your knees and arch your back. (Stretches low back)

When stretching, make sure to maintain your position for at least 30 seconds per stretch, breathe calmly and regularly, avoid abrupt movements, and try to relax.

REFERENCES

Blangsted AK, Vedsted P, Sjøgaard G et al: Work-rest schedules and recovery in relation to computer work and low-force contractions, *International Ergonomics Association,* 2006.

Henning RA, Jacques P, Kissel GV et al: Frequent short rest breaks from computer work: effects on productivity and well-being at two field sites, *Ergonomics* 40(1):78, 1997.

Spring H, Illi U, Kunz HR et al: *Stretching and strengthening exercises,* New York, 1991, Thieme Medical Publishers.

QUESTIONS? Contact Rachel Neuman: raneuman@bu.edu or Karen Jacobs: kjacobs@bu.edu.

Answers to Review Questions

Chapter 1

1. C, D
   Note: This is because neither has been shown conclusively through outcome studies.
2. C
3. A
4. A
5. A
6. A, E
7. B
8. B, C
9. A, F
10. B

Chapter 2

1. B
2. D
3. D
4. D
5. B
6. C
7. B
8. D
9. B
10. A

Chapter 3

1. D
2. A, B, C, D
3. C
4. A
5. E
6. A
7. A
8. C
9. B, D
10. B, D

Chapter 4

1. C
2. D
3. A
4. B
5. D
6. D
7. C
8. B
9. A
10. C

Chapter 5

1. C
2. A
3. A
4. B
5. D
6. B
7. B
8. D
9. B
10. C

Chapter 6

1. A
2. C
3. D
4. A
5. D
6. A
7. A
8. B
9. B
10. D

Chapter 7

1. A
2. B
3. D
4. B
5. A
6. D
7. C
8. D
9. C
10. A

Chapter 8

1. E
2. C
3. C
4. C
5. B
6. A
7. B
8. A
9. A
10. B

Chapter 9

1. B
2. C
3. D
4. A
5. D
6. B
7. C
8. D
9. B
10. A

Chapter 10

1. F
2. D

   Note: Clients who can benefit from a particular type of equipment might not always be qualified to use the equipment (such as equipment that only qualified health care professionals are licensed to use), therefore B is not correct. Also, others such as flight attendants or other workers can also be called on to use certain types of medical equipment.

3. B, C
4. A
5. A, B
6. A
7. A
8. D
9. C, E
10. A

Chapter 11

1. B
2. A
3. A
4. B
5. B
6. A
7. B
8. A
9. C
10. D

Chapter 12

1. B
2. C
3. B
4. D
5. B
6. E
7. D
8. D
9. B
10. D

Chapter 13

1. E
2. A
3. E
4. E
5. A
6. B
7. D
8. E
9. D
10. E

Chapter 14

1. D
2. D
3. A
4. C
5. B
6. C
7. A
8. A
9. C
10. D

Chapter 15

1. B
2. D
3. B
4. D
5. B
6. B
7. C
8. A
9. D
10. D

Chapter 16

1. C
2. A
3. C
4. A
5. B
6. A
7. B
8. B
9. A
10. A

Chapter 17

1. C
2. A
3. C
4. B
5. D
6. D
7. A
8. B
9. C
10. A

Chapter 18

1. D
2. C
3. C
4. B
5. D
6. A
7. B
8. D
9. A
10. B

Chapter 19

1. C
2. B
3. A
4. C
5. A
6. D
7. A
8. D
9. B
10. B

Chapter 20

1. D
2. D
3. B
4. A
5. C
6. C
7. B
8. A
9. D
10. D

Chapter 21

1. D
2. B
3. A
4. C
5. B
6. A
7. C
8. B
9. B
10. B

Appendix A

1. C
2. D
3. B
4. B
5. A
6. A
7. D
8. B
9. A
10. C

Common Conversions

Common British to Metric Conversions

British Unit	×	=	SI Unit	×	=	British Unit
Length						
Inches (in.)	2.54		centimeters	0.3937		inches
Feet (ft.)	0.3048		meters	39.37		inches
Yard (yd.)	0.9144		meters			
Mile	1.609		kilometers			
Mass						
Pounds (lb.)	0.4536		kilograms	2.0205		pounds
Slug	14.594		kilograms			
Force						
Pound–feet (lb.–ft.)	4.4482		Newtons (N)	0.2248		pounds

From Roberts SL, Falkenburg SA: *Biomechanics: problem solving for functional activity,* St Louis, Mosby Year Book, 1992.

Temperature Conversion

$(^\circ C \times 1.8) + 32 = {^\circ}F$

$(^\circ F - 32) \div 1.8 = {^\circ}C$

Index

90-degree body links. *See* Ninety-degree body links

A

Page numbers followed by f indicated figures; b, boxes; t, tables.